Anti-Obesity Drug Discovery and Development

Editors

Prof. Dr. Atta-ur-Rahman, *FRS*

Prof. Dr. M. Iqbal Choudhary

Anti-Obesity Drug Discovery and Development

Bentham Science Publishers Ltd.
http://www.benthamscience.com/aoddd

Volume 1

Contents

Contd.....

PREFACE

Obesity is a disease which leads to a number of chronic illnesses and reduced life expectancy. It is a complex health problem, caused by a number of factors such as excessive food intake, lack of physical activity, genetic predisposition, endocrine disorders, medications and psychiatric illnesses. It has been identified as the leading preventable cause of mortality and morbidity, and substantial research work has been carried out to identify the strategies and molecular targets for pharmacological interventions. Onset of obesity in both developing and developed world has reached to epidemic proportions. In response to this, efforts to control and treat obesity have also been vigorously pursued, ranging from raising awareness about life style changes to the discovery and development of safe and effective anti-obesity drugs.

The book entitled of "***Anti-obesity Drug Discovery and Development***" is focused on this very important area of healthcare research. Fifteen well written reviews make this special volume an excellent compilation of state-of-the-art developments in the subject.

Hsu *et al.*, in the first chapter of the book set the stage for subsequent contributions by providing fundamental facts and statistics about obesity as well as the need of anti-obesity drugs. Constandi *et al.* review the current understanding about relationship between obesity and cardiovascular disorders (CVD). More specifically dyslipidemia in obesity is a major cause of CVD in obese patients, and strategies to increase HDL (good cholesterol) levels hold great promise. Barros-Mazon *et al.* in their chapter review studies conducted on inflammatory and metabolic aspects of obesity, and the positive changes that occur with sustained weight loss. The review contributed by Kusti *et al.* focuses on pharmacological interventions developed to treat obesity. It presents the diverse options currently available to shunt various points in the complex molecular cascade of obesity.

Modern technologies, such as proteomics and metabolomics, have been employed to study obesity and molecular markers associated with the disease. This important area is reviewed by Kim and Zakharkin in their article. Cynthia Arbeeny has contributed a review on the underlying mechanisms of cardiovascular risks, as well as targets which have been identified to develop pharmacological agents to reduce CVD related morbidity and mortality. Carpène and Iffiu-Soltesz have contributed a review focusing on discrepancies between the cultured adipocyte model and animal model in the discovery of anti-obesity drugs. The role of rimonabant as an anti-obesity drug and the associated adverse side-effects, along with its mechanism of action and results of clinical studies, have been reviewed by Curioni *et al.* This is an interesting account of the rise and fall of a "block-buster" drug and future prospects of its use. Secondary metabolites isolated from medicinal plants, have been used for a variety of therapeutic purposes. Park and Kim review the available information on various aspects of the potential uses of plant-based compounds against obesity and obesity-related co-morbidities. Some of the promising phytochemicals in the treatment of obesity have been discussed in this review. A greater understanding of obesity on molecular basis led to the discovery of opioid peptides and opiate receptors. These molecules are believed to mediate in the appetite towards palatable food. They are therefore regarded as an effective target in anti-obesity drug development. The role of opioid peptides and opiate receptors are reviewed by Reid and Davis. Rivera *et al.* present the studies conducted on the development of melanin concentrating hormone receptor 1 (MCH-R1) antagonists as a target for anti-obesity drug development. Structure-function of MCH-R1 and discovery of antagonists are the two main topics of this review. A review on the discovery of cannabinoid receptor 1 (CBR1) as a potential target for anti-obesity drug development is contributed by Hoareau *et al.* They emphasize the need for the development of safe and effective CBR1 antagonists after the failure of Torcetraqib. Recent studies confirm that food intake is regulated by certain receptors in brain. Similarly it has been discovered that specific endocrine cells, the X/A-like cells of gastric mucosa, play an important role in appetite. The role of endocrine cells, and acylated ghrelin released from these cells, in food intake is reviewed by Stengel *et al.* Flouris *et al.* have contributed a chapter focusing on the association between obesity and inflammation, along with efficacy of biochemical mimics in the control of obesity-related inflammation. Bariatric surgery is one of the most effective strategies to treat obesity disorder. Jacob *et al.* review the after effects of such surgeries such as vitamin deficiencies. They have also discussed various strategies developed to overcome post-operative problems.

We would like to express our deep gratitude to all the contributors for making this volume an excellent compilation of modern knowledge on the science of obesity and its treatment. We also wish to express our thanks to Ms. Taqdees Malik (Editorial Assistant), Ms. Sadaf Idrees Khan (Composer) and members of Bentham Science Publishers (The Netherlands) for their assistance in the timely completion of this assignment. We are also most grateful to Mr. Mahmood Alam (Managing Director) for efficiently leading the Bentham team in this project.

Prof. Dr. Atta-ur-Rahman, *FRS*
Prof. Dr. M. Iqbal Choudhary
Editors

Contributors

Ya-Wen Hsu	Department of Physical Medicine and Rehabilitation, Taipei Medical University-Shuang Ho Hospital, Taiwan Community Medicine Research Centre and Institute of Public Health, National Yang Ming University, Taipei, Taiwan
Po-Wen Ku	Graduate Institute of Sports and Health, National Changhua University of Education, Taiwan Community Medicine Research Centre and Institute of Public Health, National Yang Ming University, Taipei, Taiwan
Da-Chen Chu	Department of Neurosurgery, Taipei City Hospital, Taiwan Community Medicine Research Centre and Institute of Public Health, National Yang Ming University, Taipei, Taiwan
Tsan-Hon Liou	Department of Physical Medicine and Rehabilitation, Taipei Medical University-Shuang Ho Hospital, Taiwan Graduate Institute of Injury Prevention, Taipei Medical University, Taipei, Taiwan
Pesus Chou	Community Medicine Research Centre and Institute of Public Health, National Yang Ming University, Taipei, Taiwan
Justina Costandi	Department of Medicine, Henderson Research Centre, McMaster University, Hamilton, Ontario, Canada Graduate Department of Medical Sciences, McMaster University, Hamilton, Ontario, Canada
Michelle Melone	Department of Medicine, Henderson Research Centre, McMaster University, Hamilton, Ontario, Canada
Shirya Rashid	Department of Medicine, Henderson Research Centre, McMaster University, Hamilton, Ontario, Canada Graduate Department of Medical Sciences, McMaster University, Hamilton, Ontario, Canada
Silvia de Barros-Mazon	Department of Clinical Pathology, Faculty of Medical Sciences, University of Campinas (UNICAMP), Sao Paulo, Brazil
Daniela Miguel Marin	Department of Internal Medicine, Faculty of Medical Sciences, University of Campinas (UNICAMP), Sao Paulo, Brazil

Camila Puzzi de Carvalho	Department of Internal Medicine, Faculty of Medical Sciences, University of Campinas (UNICAMP), Sao Paulo, Brazil
Sarah Monte Alegre	Department of Internal Medicine, Faculty of Medical Sciences, University of Campinas (UNICAMP), Sao Paulo, Brazil
Mohannad Kusti	Department of Bariatric and Advanced Laparoscopic Surgery, Preston Memorial Hospital, Kingwood, West Virginia, USA
Forrest Olgers	Department of Bariatric and Advanced Laparoscopic Surgery, Preston Memorial Hospital, Kingwood, West Virginia, USA
Ehab Akkary	Department of Bariatric and Advanced Laparoscopic Surgery, Preston Memorial Hospital, Kingwood, West Virginia, USA
Kyoungmi Kim	Division of Biostatistics, University of California Davis School of Medicine and Technology and Innovation, Solae, St. Louis, MO, USA
Stanislav O. Zakharkin	Division of Biostatistics, University of California Davis School of Medicine and Technology and Innovation, Solae, St. Louis, MO, USA
Cynthia Arbeeny	Vice President Endocrine and Metabolic Diseases, Genzyme Corporation, 49 New York Ave., Framingham MA 01701-9322, USA
Christian Carpéné	INSERM, U858, Institut de Médecine Moléculaire de Rangueil, Toulouse, France Université de Toulouse III, UPS, IFR 150, Toulouse, France
Zsuzsa Iffiú-Soltész	Université de Toulouse III, UPS, IFR 150, Toulouse, France Department of Pharmacodynamics, Semmelweis University, Budapest, Hungary
Cintia Curioni	Departamento de Nutrição Social, Universidade do Estado do Rio de Janeiro, Rua S Francisco Xavier, 524 – Maracanã, Rio de Janeiro - RJ, 20550-900, Brazil
Cintia Azara	Faculdade Arthur Sá Earp Neto, Av. Barão do Rio Branco 1003, Centro Petrópolis/RJ, 25680-120, Brazil
Jane Capelli	Universidade Federal do Rio de Janeiro, Campus Macaé – Curso de Nutrição, Rua Aluísio da Silva Gomes, 50, Granja dos Cavaleiros – Macaé – RJ, CEP: 27930-560, Brazil

Taesun Park	Department of Food and Nutrition, Yonsei University, 262 Seongsanno, Seodaemun-gu, Seoul 120-749, Republic of Korea
Yunjung Kim	Department of Food and Nutrition, Yonsei University, 262 Seongsanno, Seodaemun-gu, Seoul 120-749, Republic of Korea
Caroline Reid	Department of Kinesiology and Health Science, York University 4700 Keele Street, Toronto, Ontario, Canada M3J 1P3, 503-10 Navy Wharf Court, Toronto, Ontario, M5V 3V2, Canada
Caroline Davis	Department of Kinesiology and Health Science, York University 4700 Keele Street, Toronto, Ontario, Canada M3J 1P3, 503-10 Navy Wharf Court, Toronto, Ontario, M5V 3V2, Canada
Gildardo Rivera	Departamento de Farmacia y Química Medicinal, Unidad Académica Multidisciplinaria Reynosa Aztlán, Universidad Autónoma de Tamaulipas, Calle 16 y Lago de Chápala, s/n, 88740, Reynosa, México
Antonio Monge	Unidad de Investigación y Desarrollo de Medicamentos, Centro de Investigación en Farmacobiología Aplicada (CIFA), Universidad de Navarra, Calle Irunlarrea, s/n, 31008, Pamplona, España
Virgilio Bocanegra-Garcia	Departamento de Farmacia y Química Medicinal, Unidad Académica Multidisciplinaria Reynosa Aztlán, Universidad Autónoma de Tamaulipas, Calle 16 y Lago de Chápala, s/n, 88740, Reynosa, México
Laurence Hoareau	Groupe d'Etude sur l'Inflammation Chronique et l'Obésité (GEICO), Plateforme CYROI - Université de La Réunion, 2 rue Maxime Rivière, 97490 Sainte Clotilde, France
Karima Bencharif	Groupe d'Etude sur l'Inflammation Chronique et l'Obésité (GEICO), Plateforme CYROI - Université de La Réunion, 2 rue Maxime Rivière, 97490 Sainte Clotilde, France
Régis Roche	Groupe d'Etude sur l'Inflammation Chronique et l'Obésité (GEICO), Plateforme CYROI - Université de La Réunion, 2 rue Maxime Rivière, 97490 Sainte Clotilde, France
Andreas Stengel	CURE: Digestive Diseases Research Center and Center for Neurovisceral Sciences and Women's Health, Digestive Diseases Division, David Geffen School of Medicine at UCLA and VA Greater Los Angeles Healthcare System, Los Angeles, California
Miriam Goebel	CURE: Digestive Diseases Research Center and Center for Neurovisceral Sciences and Women's Health, Digestive Diseases Division, David Geffen School of Medicine at UCLA and VA Greater Los Angeles Healthcare System, Los Angeles, California

Yvette Taché	CURE: Digestive Diseases Research Center and Center for Neurovisceral Sciences and Women's Health, Digestive Diseases Division, David Geffen School of Medicine at UCLA and VA Greater Los Angeles Healthcare System, Los Angeles, California
Andreas D. Flouris	FAME Laboratory, Institute of Human Performance and Rehabilitation, Centre for Research and Technology Thessaly, Karies, Trikala, 42100, Greece
Andres E. Carrillo	FAME Laboratory, Institute of Human Performance and Rehabilitation, Centre for Research and Technology Thessaly, Karies, Trikala, 42100, Greece
Giorgos S. Metsios	School of Sports, Performing Arts and Leisure, University of Wolverhampton, Walsall Campus, Gorway Road, Walsall, WS1 3BD, UK
Susan Jacob	Department of Veterans Affairs Loma Linda, Western University of Health Sciences, Pomona, CA, USA
Nhu Nguyen	Department of Veterans Affairs Loma Linda, Western University of Health Sciences, Pomona, CA, USA
Christian S. Jackson	Department of Veterans Affairs Loma Linda, Western University of Health Sciences, Pomona, CA, USA
Stewart Rendon	Department of Veterans Affairs Loma Linda, Western University of Health Sciences, Pomona, CA, USA

Prevalence of Obesity: The Global Epidemics

Ya-Wen Hsu[1,5], Po-Wen Ku[2,5], Da-Chen Chu[3,5], Tsan-Hon Liou[1,4] and Pesus Chou[*,5]

[1]*Department of Physical Medicine and Rehabilitation, Taipei Medical University-Shuang Ho Hospital, Taiwan*

[2]*Graduate Institute of Sports and Health, National Changhua University of Education, Taiwan*

[3]*Department of Neurosurgery, Taipei City Hospital, Taiwan*

[4]*Graduate Institute of Injury Prevention, Taipei Medical University, Taipei, Taiwan*

[5]*Community Medicine Research Centre and Institute of Public Health, National Yang Ming University, Taipei, Taiwan*

Abstract: Obesity, a widespread and growing problem in industrialized countries, engenders many medical, psychosocial and economic issues. In 1990s, the body mass index (BMI) became a universally accepted measure of the degree of overweight and now identical cutoff points are recommended. In the Western countries, cutoff points of 25 and 30 kg/m^2 are used for describing overweight and obesity. However, in Asian countries, the absolute health risk (particularly of type 2 diabetes mellitus) seems to be higher at the same level of BMI. The international obesity task force (IOTF) suggested the cutoff points to be 23 kg/m^2 for overweight and 25 kg/m^2 for obesity in Asian countries. Consensus for obesity treatment is that clinical therapy should begin with lifestyle changes focusing on behavioral modification, diet, and exercise. When lifestyle modification schemes are unsuccessful, drug therapy is an attractive option. The use of anti-obesity drug has become increasingly common in the last 30 years. In conclusion, the prevalence of obesity is increasing at an alarming rate in many parts of the world. Thus, increased attention should be paid to people who are at high risks. Anti-obesity drugs may be an option for weight control; however, they should be used under regulation and with caution.

Keywords: Obesity, overweight, orlistat, sibutramine.

INTRODUCTION

Obesity becomes more pervasive as individuals age. Whereas obesity was not a public health concern during the 19th century, all industrialized countries now pay increasing attention to this issue since it often leads to metabolic syndromes, cardiovascular diseases, diabetes, and many other diseases – all of which account for a substantial portion of health insurance expenditures [1].

The prevalence of obesity has increased rapidly in all industrialized countries in response to factors such as dietary and lifestyle changes. Diet with a relatively high amount of fat, protein and carbohydrates as well as low in fibers is much more common than previously. Modern technologies have brought conveniences and decreased physical activity simultaneously, which is increasingly focused in weight control studies. Since 1980, the prevalence of obesity has increased three-folds or higher in some areas of Australasia, China, Eastern Europe, the Middle East, North America, the Pacific Islands, and the United Kingdom. This trend appears to have accelerated in developing countries more than in industrialized ones. This chapter discusses the prevalence of obesity globally among adults and children. The pharmacotherapy for obesity is also briefly reviewed.

Definition of Obesity

As a chronic disease affecting adults and children, obesity poses a rapidly growing threat to the health of populations worldwide [2]. The recently coined term 'globesity' reflects the escalating prevalence of global obesity and overweight individuals [3]. Obesity refers to an excessive accumulation of body fat or

*Corresponding author: Tel: +886-2-22490088, Ext. 1600; Fax: +886-2-22480577; E-mail: chain_horn@yahoo.com.tw

Atta-ur-Rahman / M. Iqbal Choudhary (Eds.)

adipose tissue, possibly affecting individual health adversely [2]. However, overweight and obese individuals significantly differ in the quantity of excess fat, body weight distribution, and increased risk of health-related problems. Assessing fatness and classifying overweight and obese individuals precisely are of priority concern to identify individuals and groups at an increased risk of morbidity and mortality, as well as provide intervention programs for populations at risk. Comparisons have thus been made of weight status within and between populations [2].

Measurement of Fatness

Directly assessing the amount and distribution of an individual's body fat is complex and challenging for most body composition methods [4]. In practice, the conventional two-compartment model divides body weight into fat mass and fat-free mass. Approaches based on this model, e.g., under weighting (densitometry), have been adopted as a reference for evaluating body density. Subsequent approaches have been developed to assess body composition. For instance, body imaging is performed using dual energy X-ray absorptiometry (DEXA), magnetic resonance imaging (MRI) and computed tomography (CT). Although accurate and reproducible, such advanced methods are not extensively adopted given the demand for well-trained technicians, a lack of mobility, and high maintenance and service costs [4, 5]. Some simple assessments were commonly used, such as body mass index (BMI) or waist circumference [6]. The following paragraph briefly describes various methods for evaluating body fatness.

Anthropometry

Anthropometry includes measurements of weight, height, circumferences and length of various body regions, as well as skinfold thickness [4]. Individuals at risk for disease are identified based on anthropometry indices such as BMI and waist circumference [7]. Applicable to large samples, these approaches significantly contribute to national surveys that monitor obesity trends [5, 8].

Of the several weight-for-height indices, BMI is the most widely used one, which is calculated as weight in kilograms divided by the square of height in meters (kg/m^2) [9]. The validity of BMI in predicting body fatness based on a reference method is well-established in different age, gender, and racial groups [5]. BMI is simple, inexpensive, easily calculated, non-invasive and acceptable to subjects [10]. However, BMI does not distinguish between fat mass and lean body mass components, possibly yielding erroneous information. Moreover, BMI values indicating 'at risk of complication' vary among ethnic populations [5, 11, 12]. As an indirect measure of abdominal or central obesity, waist circumference is assessed at the natural waist (halfway between the lowest rib margin and the iliac crest), at the level of the umbilicus or the narrowest waist circumference by using an anthropometric tape [5, 10, 13]. Although waist circumference is a simple and conventional means of evaluating abdominal fat in order to predict the incidence rate of disease and mortality [5, 6], the different cut-off points make it difficult to define and clinically diagnose metabolic syndrome in diverse populations [5].

Skinfold is an indirect measurement of the thickness of two layers of skin and the underlying subcutaneous adipose tissue using skinfold callipers. Skinfold thickness is often adopted in deriving equations in order to estimate total body fat mass and percentage body fat. Skinfold is easily administered at a relative low cost, and appropriate for large-scale epidemiological surveys. However, the ability of skinfold thickness to estimate morbidity and mortality remains contentious [5, 7].

Body Volume Measurements

Densitometry, commonly referred to as underwater or hydrostatic weighing, involves estimating body composition by assessing total body density [7, 14]. It is based on the principle that fat is less dense than water and that an individual with more body fat will thus have a lower body density [5]. Widely considered as the 'gold standard' of assessing body composition, this approach has been adopted as the criterion in validation studies of other body composition methods [5, 14]. However, this time-consuming procedure requires active cooperation of the subjects [5]. The subject must be submerged under water completely, followed by exhaling of air in the subject's lungs to determine residual lung volume precisely, which often frightens subject lacking confidence in a water environment [4, 10].

Complete submersion in water might be difficult for young children, the elderly, and other unique populations [14]. An alternative approach, air displacement plethysmography (ADP), uses air displacement rather than water displacement, to estimate body volume and density. Deemed acceptable for children as young as four years old, this approach measures the raw body volume of subjects in minimal clothing as they sit in a chamber for approximately 5-10 minutes [5-7].

Body Water and Bioelectrical Impedance Methods

Hydrometry uses isotopes to calculate total body water, in which deuterium does the most widely utilized isotope owe to its safety and low cost. Hydrometry rests on the premise that the water content of fat-free mass is relatively stable (0.73 L/kg) [5]. Assay-based methods for total body water provide an indirect estimate of fat-free mass [4]. Total body water is determined using validated dilution equations based on the extent of the dilution of the isotopes by total body fluid [15]. Fat-free mass is then calculated as total body water/0.73, and total body fat is estimated as the discrepancy between body weight and fat-free mass [5].

Bioelectrical impedance analysis (BIA) assesses body impedance to a small electric current [6]. BIA is performed by attaching a pair of electrodes at the wrists and ankles [4]. The method rests on the premise that the electrical conductivities of lean and fat tissue differ from each other [10]. The current flows more easily throughout the body with a lean body mass or a large volume of total body water. Resistance to the current flow is greater for individuals with a large amount of body fat [7, 16]. This method is quick, easily used, non-invasive and relatively inexpensive for evaluating body composition [7, 10].

Imaging Methods

Developed to determine bone mineral mass, DEXA rests on the premise that transmitted X-rays at two energy levels passing through the body are attenuated differentially by bone mineral tissue and soft tissue. In addition to delivering low radiation exposure that subsequently makes it safe for use in a wide range of populations, including children [5, 17], the procedure is relatively simple, quick and capable of providing highly reproducible and accurate evaluations of body fat and lean body mass. Such advances facilitate the frequent assessment of body composition [5, 18]. However, the expensive equipment must be operated by experienced technicians [5, 10].

CT refers to a radiographic method that assesses the differences in the attenuation of X-ray beams as they pass through the subjects. A computer-generated image of the scanned area, created from the attenuated beams, allows for separate recognition of bone, adipose tissue, and lean tissue. In contrast to CT, MRI does not expose subjects to ionizing radiation, but forms a strong magnetic field to align the nuclear magnetization of hydrogen atoms in water in the body. MRI produces a computer-generated image from radio frequency signals released by hydrogen nuclei [7]. Capable of providing high-resolution images of selected tissues or organs, both approaches can be utilized to estimate the volume and distribution of subcutaneous versus visceral fat, muscle mass, and organ composition [5, 19].

In sum, of the several methods for evaluating body fatness, imaging methods are considered the most accurate means of assessing body composition [19]. However, limited availability, high costs and requirement of a technical skill prevent their regular use [7, 19]. Despite its use in research, densitometry is infeasible for clinical settings [20]. Simple methods, e.g., BMI, skinfold measurements and waist circumference, should not be rejected, especially in epidemiological studies [6]. Table **1** summarizes the merits and limitations of methods for assessing body composition.

Table 1. Merits and Limitations of Methods for Assessing Body Composition

Methods	Merits	Limitations
Anthropometry		
Body mass index (BMI)	Simple, inexpensive, easily calculated, non-invasive, acceptable to subjects, and available in nearly all epidemiological and clinical studies.	Incapable of distinguishing between fat mass and lean body mass components. Additionally, cut-off points indicating 'at risk of complications' vary across ethnic populations. Moreover, BMI values vary non-linearly with age in children.
Waist circumference	Easily assessed with simple and inexpensive equipment that is appropriate for large epidemiological studies and generally accepted for children and adults, as well as a major criteria for defining metabolic syndrome.	Varying cut-off points complicate efforts to define and clinically diagnose metabolic syndrome in different populations.

(Table 1) Contd…..

Methods	Merits	Limitations
Anthropometry		
Skinfold thickness	Easily obtained in large epidemiological studies and promising for use in determining total body fat and regional fat distribution.	Interobserver errors are relatively large. Raising a fold in extremely obese individuals could be problematic. Children may experience fear and discomfort during measurement. The accuracy of skinfold thickness in predicting morbidity and mortality remains contentious.
Body volume measurements		
Under weighting (Densitometry)	The 'gold standard' of assessing body composition.	Children and the elderly whom are unconfident in the water may find the experience frightening. The procedure is time consuming and requires active cooperation of the subjects. Cumbersome equipment is infeasible for general practice.
Air displacement plethysmography (ADP)	Efficient, comfortable, acceptable to children, as well as not requiring submersion of a subject in water	The equipment is moderately expensive for primary care. The subject must wear tightly fitted bathing costume and a tightly fitted bathing cap.
Body water and bioelectrical impedance methods		
Total body water	Simple and non-invasive Heavy water can be administered orally and distribu-tion estimated from saliva samples.	Infeasible for primary care. Total body water decreases with age during the first three years of life.
Bioelectrical impedance analysis (BIA)	Non-invasive, relatively inexpensive equipment, mobile and easily operated.	Operation of the equipment and use of prediction equations must be standardized. Analysis results depend on the instrument used, hydration and diet of subjects.
Imaging methods		
Dual energy X-ray absorptiometry (DEXA)	Extremely high reproducibility and accuracy in assessing body fat, as well as safe for children owing the low radiation exposure.	Expensive and immobile. It must be performed in a major medical facility and operated by well-trained technicians. Additionally, It cannot distinguish between visceral fat and subcutaneous fat. Moreover, subjects must remain still for approximately 20 minutes. DEXA is inappropriate for pregnant women.
Computed tomography (CT)	Capable of accurate quantifying intra-abdominal and subcutaneous fat.	The major limitation is the related radiation exposure. The equipment is expensive and skilled technicians are required for operations. Subjects must lie still in a supine position under a scanner for approximately 20 minutes.
Magnetic resonance imaging (MRI)	Capable of producing extremely detailed images with no radiation exposure. Capable of distinguishing the intra-abdominal area from subcutaneous fat.	The equipment is expensive, must be operated by highly-trained technicians and must be performed in a major medical facility. Subjects must lie still in a supine position under a scanner for approximately 20 minutes.

Sources: [4-6, 10, 17, 19].

PREVALENCE OF ADULT OBESITY

Obesity Classification for Adults

For practical concerns, the definitions are normally based on anthropometry, with BMI and waist circumference as the most conventionally adopted both clinically and in population studies [17]. Although less accurate than others, these methods can satisfactorily identify health risks [20]. As BMI classifies overweight and obesity in adults, the World Health Organization suggested a graded classification level for adults based on BMI, with a BMI of 25 kg/m^2 or above denoting overweight and a BMI of 30 kg/m^2 or above denoting obese. However, in Asian populations, morbidity and mortality occurs in individuals with low BMIs. In these populations, the cut-off points for overweight ($>$ 23 kg/m^2) and obese ($>$25 kg/m^2) are lower than the WHO criteria [2, 9]. WHO redefined the cutoff point for Asia-Pacific regions in 2000, and later modified that cutoff point again in 2004 after consulting with WHO experts [21], whom suggested setting 23 kg/m^2 as an increasing but acceptable risk and 27.5 kg/m^2 as an increased high risk. Table **2** displays the recommended classification of weight by BMI in adults.

Table 2. Classification of Weight by BMI in Adults

Classification	BMI (kg/m^2) (Caucasians)	BMI kg/m^2 (Asians)	Risk of Co-morbidities
Underweight	<18.5	<18.5	Low (but at increased risk of other clinical problems)
Normal range	18.5~24.9	18.5~22.9	Average
Overweight:	>25	>23	
Pre-obese/At risk	25~29.9	23~24.9	Increased
Obese I	30~34.9	25~29.9	Moderate
Obese II	35~39.9	≥ 30	Severe

Sources: [2, 9].

Although incapable of determining whether an individual is overweight or obese, waist measurement can accurately predict abdominal (central) obesity, which is related to cardiovascular risk factors of the Metabolic Syndrome. Recommended waist circumference cut offs are 102 cm for men and 88 cm for women. As with BMI, Asian populations appear to have a higher risk of diabetes and cardiovascular disease at a lower waist circumference than Caucasians. Therefore, using smaller waist circumference cut-off points has been recommended for Asian males with a circumference of 90 cm and women with a circumference of 80 cm [2, 5, 9].

Prevalence of Obesity Globally

According to WHO data, more than 1 billion adults are overweight, and at least 300 million among them are obese. The prevalence of obesity varies widely, ranging from below 5% in many regions of certain African nations, China and Japan to over 75% in urban Samoa. The prevalence also varies obviously even in a single country. For instance, obesity levels also increase to nearly 20% in some cities in China.

In recent years, a large-scale study called the International Day for Evaluation of Abdominal obesity (IDEA) was conducted for two and a half days between May 9 and July 6, 2005 in 63 countries with over 1,100 patients per country for ages ranging from 18 to 80 years old. The study evaluated abdominal adiposity (WC) and BMI with a cutoff point of 30 kg/m^2 for obesity as well as 25 kg/m^2 for overweight for 168, 000 patients who consulted with primary care physicians. According to those studies, the overall prevalence of overweight (BMI = 25-30 kg/m^2) and obesity (BMI > 30 kg/m^2) was 40 % and 20%, respectively, in men as well as 30% and 20%, respectively, in women, except for southern and eastern Asia (Fig. **1**).

Although the overweight percentage appears to be similar in different regions, the obesity percentage varied from just 7% in eastern Asia to 36% in Canada in men and women, and 38% to 40% in women in the Middle East and northern and southern Africa [22].

Prevalence of Obesity in America

The pervasiveness of obesity was nearly twice the level thirty years ago in the United States. In 2005–2006, 33.3% of men and 35.3% of women fit the criteria of obese [23]. The pervasiveness of obesity now is nearly twice the level thirty years ago in the United States (Fig. **2**).

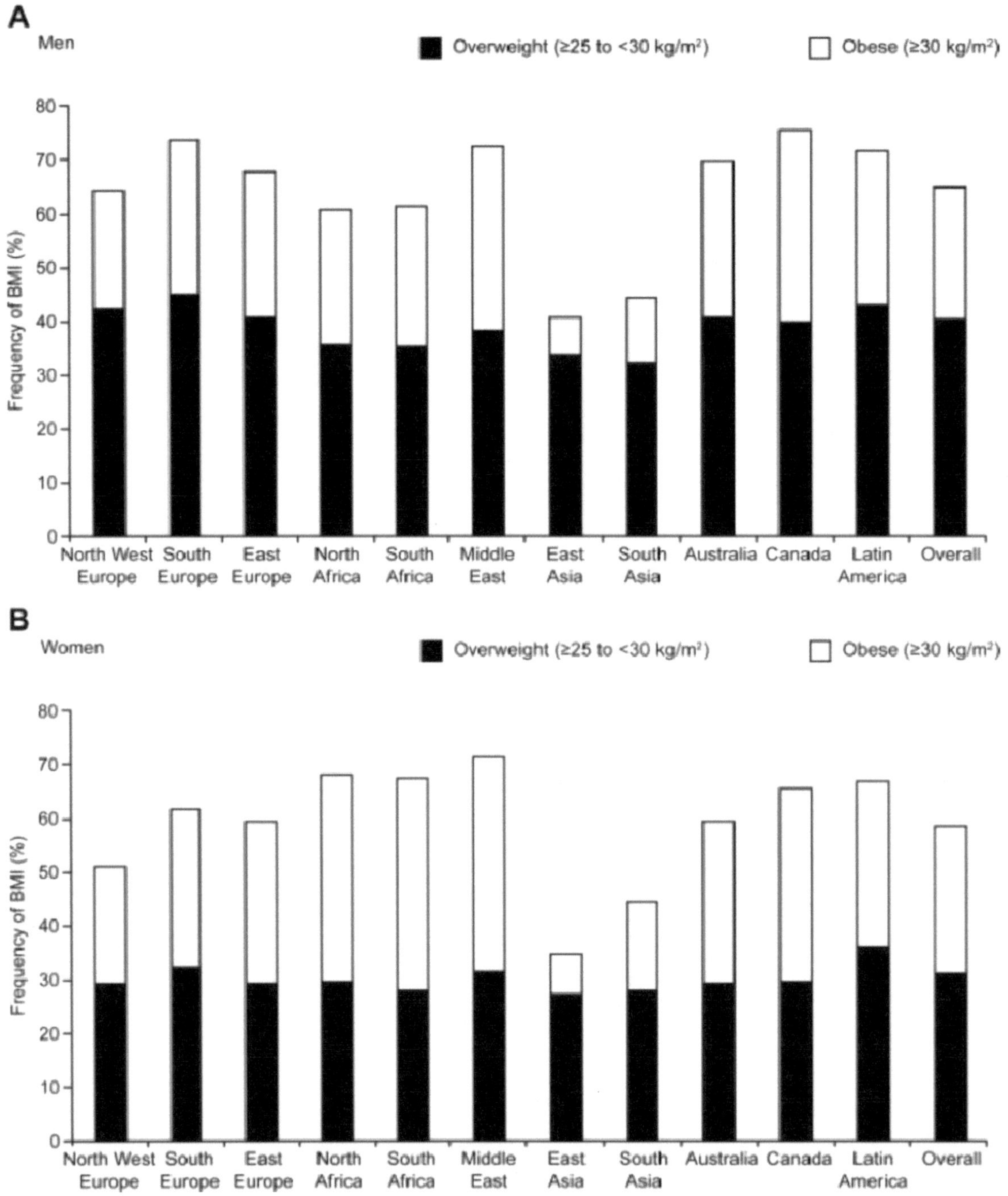

Fig. (1). (*From Circulation*. 2007; 116: 1942-1951) http://circ.ahajournals.org/cgi/content/full/116/17/1942?maxtoshow=&HITS=10&hits=10&RESULTFORMAT=&fulltext=International+Day+for+the+Evaluation+of+Abdominal+Obesity+%28IDEA%29&searchid=1&FIRSTINDEX=0&resourcetype=HWCIT.

Although the prevalence of obesity significantly increased between 1999 and 2006, the rate of increase did not change obviously between 2003-2004 and 2005-2006 for men and women. In 2007, all states failed to comply with the goals of the program Healthy People 2010, which strives to decrease the prevalence of obesity among adults by 15%. Many common deaths are related to obesity, including type 2 diabetes, hypertension and strokes, coronary heart disease, and certain cancers. Next, the prevalence of obesity in six states (i.e. Alabama, Mississippi, Oklahoma, South Carolina, Tennessee, and West Virginia) was found

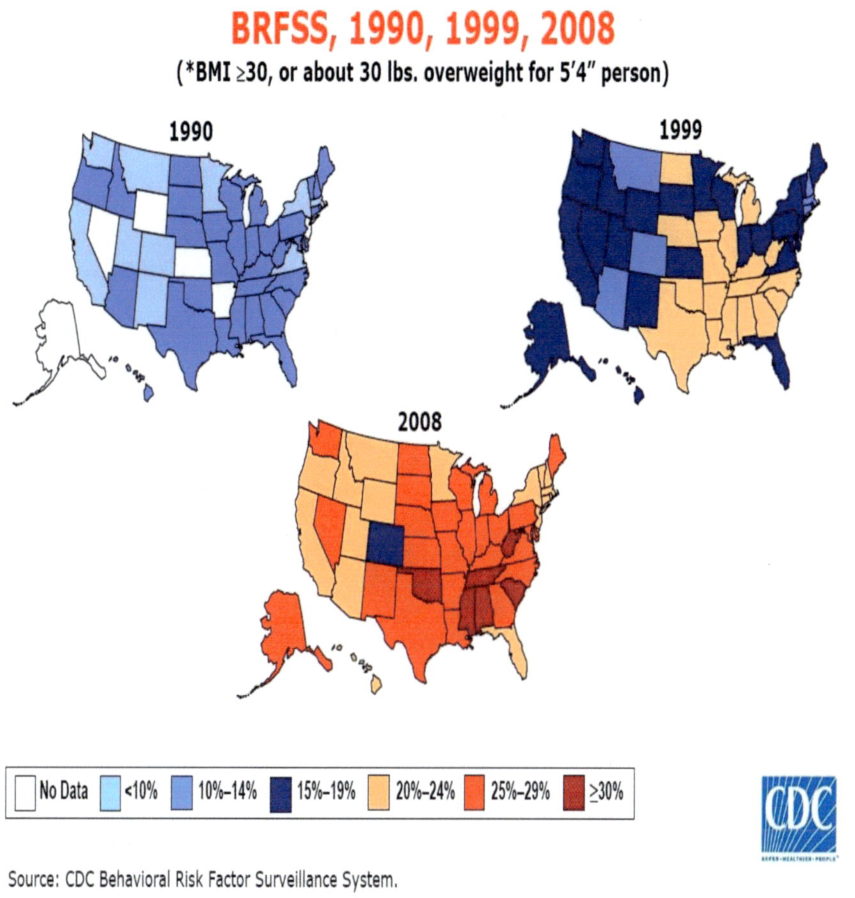

Fig. (2). http://www.cdc.gov/obesity/data/trends.html

with a BMI equal to or greater than 30% in 2008. Meanwhile, the other 32 states had a BMI equal to or greater than 25% [23]. Only Colorado was lower than 20%. According to a CDC analysis report based on data from the Behavioral Risk Factor Surveillance System (BRFSS) from 2006 to 2008 and the National Health and Nutrition Examination Survey (NHANES), the overall prevalence of obesity among non-Hispanic blacks, non-Hispanic whites, and Hispanics was 25.6%, 35.7% among non-Hispanic blacks, 28.7% among Hispanics and 23.7% among non-Hispanic whites (Fig. **3**).

Although the prevalence of obesity varies across states, this pattern seems to apply to all states, possibly owing to the different racial or ethnic groups with different behaviors to weight gain.

In Canada, the prevalence of obesity was 10% in 1970 (8 % in men and 13 % in women. In 2004, it had risen to 23% (23% in men and 22% in women) above age 20. That cost has significantly impacted the national health insurance system, as chronic diseases rank second to obesity [23, 24]. The rising trend of obesity appears more significant among rural adults, especially in young individuals. This phenomenon became apparent in Saskatchewan in 1977 (16.8%), 1983 (22.7%), 1993 (24.7%) and 2003 (34.5%) [25].

In Brazil, the prevalence of obesity increased from 17% to 24% (BMI > 30 kg/m^2) increased over the past decade with an increase of food consumption. The newest prevalence of obesity was 48.7% for BMI > 27 kg/m^2 and 25.3% for BMI > 30 kg/m^2. The factors associated with obesity were the female gender and age. BMI > 27 kg/m^2 was correlated with age and smoking while BMI > 30 kg/m^2 with a sedentary lifestyle [26]. Elevated food consumption of refined carbohydrates, including soft drinks and fast food, was a suspected predisposing factor of the pervasiveness of obesity among women in Brazil [27].

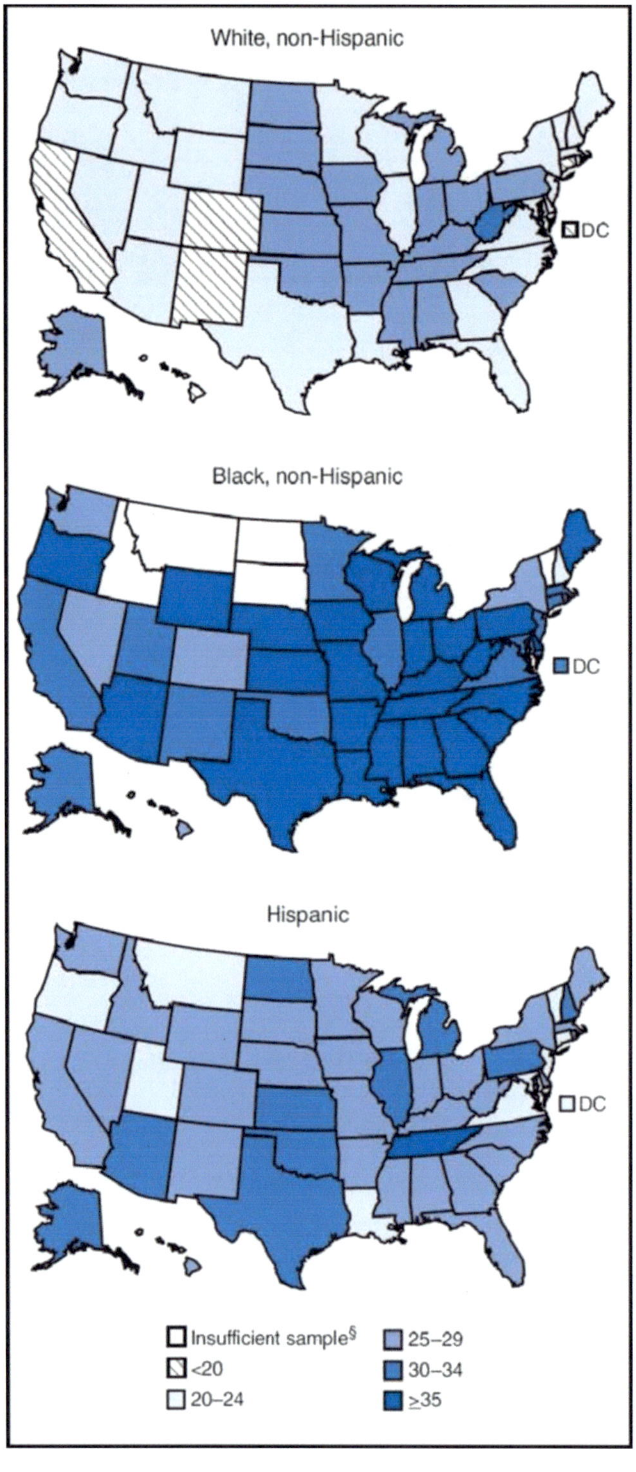

Fig. (3). http://www.cdc.gov/obesity/data/trends.html

Prevalence of obesity in Europe

In Germany, the prevalence of obesity increased with age according to data collected in Bavaria, 12-24 years old at three time intervals of 1995, 2000, 2005; data revealed an increasing prevalence of obesity from 1995 (2.1%) to 2000 (3.1%) and to 2005 (4%), revealing a rising trend of obesity among adolescents [28].

Even in France, the country with the lowest prevalence of obesity in Europe, its prevalence has grown over time. According to the French Social Security Health Examination Centers, 6.9% of men and 6.4% of women were obese in 1995 and 8.9% and 8.6% in 2005, respectively. Abdominal adiposity afflicted 5.6% of men and 8.5% of women in 1995 and 9.5% and 14.3% in 2005. Obesity prevalence regression slopes between 1995 and 2005 raise significantly [29].

In the United Kingdom, from 1993 to 2004, the pervasiveness of obesity significantly increased from 13.6% to 24.0% among men and from 16.9% to 24.4% among women. These figures are projected to reach 32.1% and 31.0% in men and women, respectively, by 2012 [30].

The latest data accumulated from eight Mediterranean islands in Greece and Cyprus from 2005-2007 revealed that the prevalence of obesity was 27% in males and 41% in females, and the prevalence of overweight individuals was 48% of males and 39% of females. The prevalence of obese elderly was positively correlated with the prevalence of diabetes, hypercholesterolemia and hypertension and negatively correlated with physical activity and the Mediterranean diet [31].

Crete, a traditional Greek island, is renowned for its agriculture, whose lifestyle was assumed for decades to be healthier than many other countries. However, according to the latest data accumulated from 502 farmers (18-79 years old) in Crete in 2005, the percentage of overweight individuals (BMI = 25.1-30 kg/m^2) and obese (BMI > 30 kg/m^2) was 42.9% while the percentage of body fat in men and women was 27.3% and 39.3%. Obesity is prevalent in both large cities and small villages [32].

In Croatia, weight-related data was accumulated most recently in 2003. The pervasive-ness of overweight, obesity and increased waist circumference was 38.11%, 20.34% and 43.52%, respectively, which was 43.2%, 20.1% and 34.98%, respectively, for men and 33.6%, 20.6% and 51.13%, respectively, for women. Regional differences became apparent following conflicting results. Individuals residing on the Adrian Sea coastal area of the country had a lower risk of cardiovascular disease for those living in the continental part of the country. Moreover, the prevalence of overweight individuals was the highest in northern region [33].

Prevalence of Obesity in the Asia-Pacific Region

The Department of Health in Taiwan defines the cutoff point of overweight and obesity, in which BMI > 24 is overweight and BMI > 27 is obese. Under such definition, the prevalence of obesity adjusted for the ages of the males and females was 10.5% and 13.2%, respectively, from 1993 to 1996 as well as 15.9% and 10.7%, respectively, from 2000 to 2001. The tendency of obesity appears to be more significant for children and men from 1980 to 2000 [34]. For data on Taiwanese aboriginals, according to the National Health Interview Survey (NHIS) in 2001, the prevalence of overweight (BMI = 25-30) and obese (BMI > 30) individuals was 45.1% and 10.5%, respectively, for men as well as 33.3% and 14.5%, respectively, for women, which implied that obesity is more prevalent among the Taiwan aboriginals [35].

Obesity trends in China accelerated from 1985 to 2000 [36, 37]. According to data of the China National Nutrition and Health Survey (NNAHS) database for the entire population in 2002, the prevalence of obesity was 17.6% and 5.6% for overweight individuals (BMI = 25-29.9 kg/m^2) and for obesity (BMI > 30 kg/m^2). The prevalence of overweight and obesity for adults age 18 and above was 22.8% and 7.1%. Meanwhile, for large city, middle-and-small city, class 1 rural, class 2 rural, class 3 rural and class 4 rural, it was 25.0% and 10.6%, 21.6% and 7.2%, 17.4% and 6.4%, 15.1% and 4.3%, 19.2% and 6.0%, as well as 12.8% and 2.7%, respectively. The government must closely monitor increasing obesity trends to sustain economic growth [38].

The pervasiveness of obesity in Japan appears to have not increased dramatically as in other industrial countries. The cutoff point for overweight individuals was a BMI of 23.0-24.9 kg/m^2, as suggested by the Western Pacific Region of the World Health Organization, with a high correlation of related metabolic disorders [39]. Although the percentage of overweight has risen in men from 15.2% to 29.7% over the past three decades, the equivalent has remained around 20% in women until now [40].

In Australia, the pervasiveness of overweight individuals was 48% in men and 30% in women while that of obesity was 19% in men and 22% in women. The prevalence rate resembled that of Europe and the United States, possibly owing to their their western-style diet and lifestyle [41].

The most recent data accumulated from Korean adults aged above 20 years old originated from Korean National Health Examination and Nutrition Survey data from 1998 to 2001. The pervasiveness of obesity

(BMI > 25 kg/m^2) in 2001 in men and women was 32.9% and 27.4%, respectively, which rose speedily from 1998. Interestingly, the prevalence of obesity in Korea has a significantly positive correlation with socioeconomic condition in men while having a significantly negative correlation with that in women [42].

The prevalence of obesity in Thailand has increased nearly 100 % over the past two decades. The BMI cutoff point was set at > 30 kg/m^2, leading to an underestimated pervasiveness of metabolic syndrome in Thailand [43]. Now, the cutoff point of obesity has been set at a body mass index > 25 kg/m^2 in adults. The pervasiveness elevated from 13.0% in men and 23.2% in women in 1991 to 18.6% and 29.5%, respectively, in 1997 and 22.4% and 34.3%, respectively, in 2004. The current trend of an increasing body weight has spread from urban to agricultural areas [44].

Prevalence of Obesity in the Middle East

Middle Eastern countries have witnessed a rapidly growing pervasiveness of obesity. Based on data from the Third National Surveillance of Risk Factors of Non-Communicable Diseases (SuRFNCD-2007), as accumulated in 2007, which included 5,287 Iranian citizens aged 15-64 years olds, obesity (body mass index > 30 kg/m^2) the pervasiveness and central obesity (waist circumference > 80 cm in females and > 94 cm in males) were 22.3% and 53.6%, respectively. The rates were the highest among females and urban residents [45].

The most recent nationwide cross-sectional study from Kuwait was collected in the adult Kuwaiti population of the Arabian Gulf region. The cutoff points of overweight and obesity were a body mass index > 25, and > 30. Pervasiveness of overweight and obesity was 80.4% and 47.5%, respectively, i.e. higher in women (81.9% and 53%) than in men (78% and 39.2%) [46].

Prevalence of Obesity in Africa

Pervasiveness of obesity of Tunisian women aged 20-59 years old at the national level was 22.6% (BMI > 30 kg/m^2), which obviously differed from environments, including major cities (30.2%), other cities (25.9%), rural clustered areas (19.4%) and rural dispersed areas (9.5%). The prevalence of obesity also rose with age and household wealth [47].

A favorable financial climate among the Beninese has led to increasing metabolic syndrome. A study from 541 Beninese healthy adults revealed that the pervasiveness of metabolic syndrome, as defined by the International Diabetes Federation, was 4.1%, 6.4%, and 11% in rural, semi-urban, and urban areas, respectively [48].

CHILDHOOD OBESITY

Similar to that of adults, the rate of overweight and obesity among children and adolescents is increasing rapidly. The prevalence of overweight and obesity among children and adolescents has reached unprecedented levels. Prevalence of overweight among the school-age populations overweight has increased in 25 countries, and in 42 countries for preschool age populations. The increase has been more dramatic in industrialized countries and in urbanized populations [49, 50]. One third of all children and adolescents in the United States are either obese or overweight. Global estimates identified 18,000,000 overweight children in 2002 [51]. Approximately 110 million children were classified as overweight or obese in 2005, defined as BMI above the 95th percentile for age and gender [52]. Over the past three decades, the prevalence of obesity has nearly tripled for children 2 to 5 years old and youth 12 to 19 years old, while quadrupling for children 6 to 11 years old [53]. Obesity poses an increasingly major threat to the health of children and adolescents [54].

Obesity Classification for Children and Adolescents

Using BMI to determine overweight and obesity in children is a contentious issue since the height and body composition of children is changing continuously. The correlation between adiposity and the ratio of weight to height may be weaker than that of adults [2, 55]. Classifications of overweight and obesity for children and adolescents are age- and gender-specific because the body composition of children varies as they age and varies between boys and girls [56]. Several countries have developed their own BMI-for-age gender-specific reference charts based on local data [17]. In the United Kingdom and the United States, a BMI exceeding the 85th percentile for a child's age and sex group is classified as overweight, and a BMI exceeding the 95th percentile is considered obese [56, 57].

Recently, the International Association for the Study of Obesity (IOTF) used an ethnically diverse database (Brazil, Great Britain, Hong Kong, the Netherlands, Singapore and the United States) to extend the adult cut-off values of BMI to childhood. Centile curves passing through the values of 25 kg/m^2 and 30 kg/m^2 at the age of 18 years old were derived [58]. These values provide age and gender specific BMI cut offs to define overweight and obesity in youth, corresponding to the adult cut-off points for overweight and obesity. These values also represent a reference for international comparisons [17].

Prevalence of Childhood Obesity

Obesity has increased among both genders and among all racial, ethnic, and socioeconomic groups [59]. According to the Centers for Disease Control and Prevention, in 2000, the prevalence of obesity among 12- to 19-yr-old non-Hispanic blacks was 23.6% and in Mexican-Americans, 23.4% compared with 12% of non-Hispanic white children. The prevalence of obesity, defined as the 95th percentile for age and gender, among 4-year-old US children (mean age, 52.3 months) was 18.4% (95% confidence interval [CI], 17.1%-19.8%) [60]. The prevalence of overweight and obese children in the United States increased from 15% in 1971 to more than 30% in 2000 [61]. Adolescent obesity has more than doubled in the United States over the past 25 years [62, 63]. According to National Health and Nutrition Examination Survey (NHANES) in the United States, from 1999–2002, an estimated 16% of children and adolescents aged 6-19 years old are overweight. This data represent an increase of 45% from previous studies among 1988-1994 from the National Center for Health Statistics, United States Department of Health and Human Services. The prevalence of obesity is disproportionately higher among African-Americans, Mexican-Americans, and Native Americans than other ethnic groups [62, 63], with an increase in more than 10% points between 1988 –1994 and 1999 –2000. The prevalence rates remained relatively stable in non-Hispanics during NHANES 1988 –1994 to 1999 –2000 [63].

However, as reported recently, the prevalence rates of childhood obesity may have reached a plateau recently in U.S. [64]. According to that report, 11.3% of children and adolescents were at or exceeded the 97th percentile of BMI for age; 16.3% had a BMI for age at or exceeded the 95th percentile and 31.9% were at or exceeded the 85th percentile from the 2000 Centers for Disease Control and Prevention growth charts [64] found no increase in prevalence between 2003 to 2006 data to the NHANES surveys.

The obesity rates in Mexico will exceed those in the United States in the near future, and is 1.5 times more common among Mexican American women, (http://www.4woman.gov/ minority/hispanicamerican). The values exceeded the 75th percentile for Mexican Americans [65]. In Brazil, an additional 0.5% of all children became overweight annually [17].

Approximately 10-30% of all European children between the ages of 7 and 11 years and 25% of adolescents are overweight or obese [66]. Hungary has reported that 20% of children between 11 and 14 years old are obese, with 6% of these children already diagnosed with hypertension [67]. In Poland, obesity rates increased from 8% to 18% from 1994 to 2000. Children from Mediterranean countries have a higher prevalence for overweight than in northern Europe, where rates tend to be within the 10-20% range.

Eighteen percent of all children in the Middle East are overweight, while 7% are obese [66]. In Israel, the rate of overweight is 13.9% and is still increasing, and ranks third after the United States and Greece for percentages of overweight children in general [68].

Of particular concern are those countries with traditionally low rates of childhood obesity [69]. Overweight and obesity are replacing the previous nutritional problem in developing countries, becoming significantly prevalent owing to easily available, inexpensive, high-caloric foods combined with sedentary lifestyles [70]. According to the World Health Organization, 14.9% of children under the age of 5 in Swaziland are overweight [67].

China is a developing country whose economy has expanded rapidly over the past two decades [71]. Economic growth during this period may have contributed to childhood obesity. The rise in childhood obesity has been restricted to urban areas with no or little increase in rural areas, as explained by differences in economic growth between cities. In Shanghai, where the household income is the highest nationwide, BMI increased dramatically between 1986 and 2000, and boys become more so than girls after 3 years old. This may reflect the additional attention that Chinese boys tend to receive more than girls, and that boys are expected to be strong while girls should be slender. The one-child family policy, which started in 1979 [49, 72], may have exacerbated this tendency. Chinese male adolescents are fatter than US male adolescents in early to mid-childhood but less so during adolescence and become thinner than US boys by age 18. Although Chinese boys have a year earlier of adiposity rebound than in the US/UK, BMI subsequently increases more gradually with age. Chinese girls have their rebound at nearly the same age as in the West, but they also slow afterwards and end up thinner [71]. Children in the more northern cities are fatter than those in southern China [73].

Australia's current rates of children obesity are among the highest in the industrialized world with 10% of all children obese and 20% overweight [74]. In New Zealand, 20% of all children between 5 and 14 years old are overweight with another 10% obese. Approximately 31% of Maori and Pacific Islander children are affected [75].

PHARMACOTHERAPY FOR OBESITY

Drug Treatment of Obesity

Even relatively modest decreases in body weight yield significant health benefits. Reducing body weight of only 5 to 10 % produces significant benefits for obese patients [76, 77]. Practitioners of obesity treatment generally concur that clinical therapy should begin with lifestyle modifications that address behavioral change, diet control, and regular exercise [78]. Pharmacotherapy provides a viable solution to obesity, but should be used in conjunction with non-pharmacological therapy. Only when lifestyle modifications are unsuccessful does drug therapy become a viable option. Obesity guidelines currently recommend that drug therapy be administered for patients with a BMI exceeding or equal to 30 kg/m^2 or a BMI of 27 to 30 kg/m^2 with one or more obesity related disorders [76, 79].

Anti-obesity drug use has become increasingly common over the past three decades. Based on 1998 BRFSS data, Khan estimated that 4.6 million American adults used prescription weight-loss pills from 1996 to 1998 [80]. According to U.S. Department of Health and Human Services estimates, from 1995 to 1997, 1.2–4.7 million residents in the United States were prescribed fenfluramine or dexfenfluramine for weight loss [81]. Stafford *et al.* [82] determined that 2.5 million Americans were prescribed anti-obesity medications in 1997, i.e. a 4-folds increase over the figure for the previous two years. Furthermore, Blanck *et al.* [83] identified that 7% of the BRFSS respondents consumed nonprescription weight-loss products, 2% reported using phenylpropanolamine (PPA), and 1% used ephedra between 1996 and 1998. However, drug treatment of obesity has not been entirely successful, as most anti-obesity drugs, e.g., fenfluramine-phentermine (fen-phen) [84, 85], PPA [86, 87], and ephedra [88], have been withdrawn from the market due to serious adverse effects. Only two drugs, i.e. orlistat (Xenical) and sibutramine (Meridia, Reductil), have been registered for long-term use and a third, i.e. rimonabant (Acomplia), was introduced to the global market in 2006. Furthermore, a few new drugs are undergoing clinical trials [89].

Currently Available Drugs for Treating Obesity

Only three medications have been approved for long-term use: orlistat, sibutramine and rimonabant. The following section discusses their pharmacological profiles in detail.

Orlistat (Xenical, Alli)

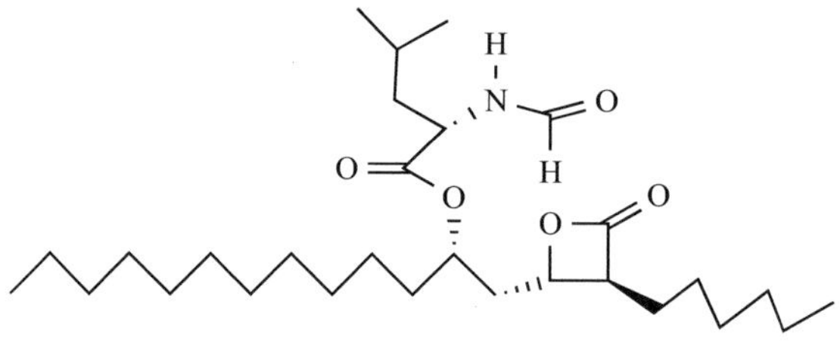

Xenical
$C_{29}H_{53}NO_5$

(S)-2-formylamino-4-methyl-pentanoic acid (S)-1-[[(2S, 3S)-3-hexyl-4-oxo-2-oxetanyl] methyl]-dodecyl ester

http://en.wikipedia.org/wiki/Xenical

Pharmacology and Mechanisms of Action

Orlistat is a hydrogenated derivative of a lipostatin isolated from soil bacteria (Streptomyces toxytincini). First approved in 1998, orlistat is a gastric and pancreatic lipase inhibitor that reduces dietary fat absorption by approximately 30% [81]. The drug acts in the lumen of the gut and inhibits the activity of gastrointestinal lipases. Only a minute fraction is absorbed after oral administration, which conveys considerable safety to this drug. Owing to low systemic absorption and first-pass metabolism, the bioavailability of orlistat is lower than 1%. Most of the drug is excreted unchanged in feces. The standard dose of orlistat is 120 mg three daily along with meals. The Food and Drug Administration (FDA) of the United States has approved half-strength orlistat (Alli) for over-the-counter use.

Efficacy

Sjostrom *et al.* [90] conducted a major trial to assess the efficacy of orlistat 120 mg in 743 obese patients. According to those results, orlistat treatment is an effective means of inducing weight loss and averting subsequent regain. XENical in the prevention of Diabetes in Obese Subjects (XENDOS), a 4-year double-blind placebo-controlled randomized study of 3,305 Swedish obese patients revealed that the mean weight loss in the orlistat group was 5.8 kg compared with 3.0 kg in the placebo and decreased the incidence of type 2 diabetes from 9.0% to 6.2% [91]. Orlistat has been under study in several double-blind, placebo-controlled trials for periods of up to two years. A meta-analysis of these trials revealed that body weight reduced by an average of 2.89 kg modified for weight changes in the placebo group after twelve months of treatment. Most of this loss of body weight occurred during the first six months of treatment. Body weight subsequently stabilized and remained reduced as long as treatment was continued [92]. A recent randomized controlled trial that specifically examined Orlistat administered 120 mg three times daily as a weight maintenance treatment after weight loss with very low energy diet (VLED) demonstrated a significantly reduced weight regain after 3 years (4.6 kg *vs.* 7 kg, $P < 0.02$) [93]. This moderate effect on body weight was sufficient to enhance several metabolic parameters. A retrospective analysis indicated reductions in triglyceride and cholesterol blood levels, enhanced oral glucose tolerance and a fall in systolic and diastolic blood pressure. The reduction in LDL cholesterol became more pronounced than would be expected from a reduction in body weight alone [94].

Some studies have assessed how orlistat affects adolescents. Chanoine *et al.* conducted a 54-week multi-center trial comparing Orlistat (N = 357) to placebo (N = 182) in obese 12 to 16 year olds. According to those results, BMI decreased by 0.55 kg/m^2 in those treated with orlistat and increased by 0.31 kg/m^2 in those in the placebo group ($P = 0.001$). Although decreasing in the orlistat group, waist circumference increased in the placebo group ($P < 0.05$) [95]. However, the findings were inconsistent in a 6-month randomized, double-blind, placebo-controlled trial involving forty adolescents ranging between 14 and 18 years old, in which orlistat did not significantly reduce BMI after 6 months [96]. Exactly how orlistat affects childhood obesity warrants further study.

Adverse Effects

Reported adverse effects of orlistat are gastrointestinal. Fatty and oily stool, fecal urgency, and oily spotting occurred in 15-30% of orlistat-treated patients. Fecal incontinence was observed in 7% of orlistat-treated patients compared with 1% of those on a placebo trial. Malabsorption of fat soluble vitamins, including vitamins A, D, E, and K, have also been reported; those taking orlistat are also advised to take vitamin supplements as well [97]. Systemic adverse effects are minimal owing to the lack of systemic absorption. These adverse effects are enhanced by a high dietary fat intake and may, therefore, serve as a component of behavioral feedback therapy. Most of these gastrointestinal side effects occur early during treatment and tend to disappear later on.

However, orlistat may be associated with an increased risk of colon cancer. Recent preliminary research on rats reveals a correlation with orlistat and increases in colonic preneoplastic markers [98]. Further research in humans is thus warranted. The increased presentation for free fatty acids to the lower gastrointestinal tract, as produced by combining a lipase inhibitor with a fatty diet, is assumed to increase oxalate absorption, thus heightening the risk of kidney stones and renal impairment [99].

Sibutramine (Meridia, Reductil)

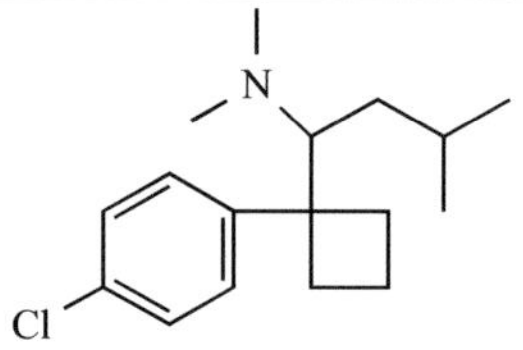

Reductil

$C_{17}H_{26}ClN$

1-[1-(4-chlorophenyl)cyclobutyl]-N,N,3-trimethyl-butan-1-amine

http://en.wikipedia.org/wiki/Reductil

Pharmacology and Mechanisms of Action

Sibutramine, originally developed as an antidepressant, is a centrally acting inhibitor of noradrenaline, serotonin and, to a lesser extent, dopamine reuptake. The drug was approved in the United States in 1997 and in the European Union in 1999. Sibutramine is the first centrally acting anti-obesity compound approved for use in most countries. Most of the drug and its active metabolites are renally excreted. Sibutramine acts mainly as an appetite suppressant, but may also increase energy expenditure by stimulating thermogenesis [100]. Sibutramine-induced hypophagia was accompanied by a reduction of pre-meal hunger and prospective consumption at the 30 mg dose.

Efficacy

The efficacy of sibutramine is significantly enhanced when used with a major lifestyle modification and regular frequent follow-up visits. Using sibutramine reduces body weight, most of which occurs during the first six months. Further treatment helps to maintain this body weight loss. In the sibutramine trial of obesity reduction and maintenance (STORM) randomized double blind trial; obese patients were prescribed sibutramine (10 mg) with a low caloric diet [101]. The patients lost 11.3 kg over six months. The group subsequently administered sibutramine (10 mg) appeared to show little weight-regain over the next 12 months. Conversely, the placebo group appeared to start to regain weight. Arterburn *et al.* systematically reviewed randomized controlled trials with sibutramine. According to that study, the average weight loss was 4.45 kg after one year and several metabolic parameters were improved during sibutramine therapy [102]. In three randomized double-blind, placebo-controlled weight-loss trials of one year, sibutramine reduced weight by 4.6% [103].

Two studies were conducted to determine whether Sibutramine is effective in obese adolescents [104, 105]. Berkowitz *et al.* demonstrated that sibutramine (10-15 mg/day) reduced body weight by a mean of 8.4 kg and BMI by a mean of 2.9 kg/m^2 more than the placebo trial group after 12 months in 498 obese adolescents [104].

Adverse Effects

Common adverse effects of sibutramine are related to increased adrenergic activity, including a dry mouth, headaches, insomnia, and constipation [106]. Other studies have demonstrated that sibutramine increases heart rate (3-7 beats per minute) and blood pressure (20% patients BP increase of 2-3 mmHg). These adrenergic adverse effects are of particular concern for patients with uncontrolled hypertension, pre-existing cardiovascular disease, or tachycardia. Concomitant treatment with monamine-oxidase inhibitors or serotoninergic drugs is also not recommended owing to the potential risk of serotonin syndrome.

Cardiovascular side effects include an increase in systolic and diastolic blood pressure, as well as an increase in heart rate, tachycardia and palpitations and vasodilatation. Such effects are probably related directly to its mechanism of action and can be explained as a consequence of its peripheral effects. A large trial, the Sibutramine Cardiovascular Outcome Trial (SCOUT), revealed that blood pressure decreased during 6-week treatment with sibutramine even when body weight remained unchanged in hypertensive patients. Small pulse rate increases were also observed regardless of blood pressure or weight change status [107, 108]. Recently, treatment with sibutramine was found to be associated with QT interval prolongation, possibly leading to ventricular fibrillation and cardiac arrest in rare cases. Therefore, monitoring of the electrocardiogram might be recommended for patients treated with sibutramine. Additionally, concomitant use of sibutramine with other drugs likely to prolong QT (e.g., certain antipsychotics, antidepressants, and antiarrhythmic agents) should be averted [109].

Rimonabant (Acomplias)

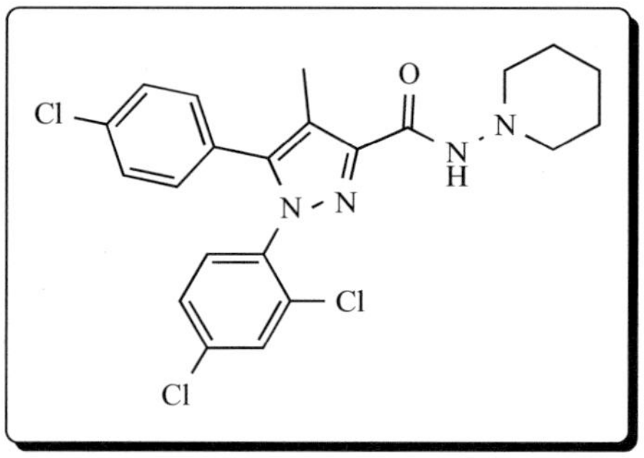

http://en.wikipedia.org/wiki/Rimonabant

Pharmacology and Mechanisms of Action

Having received approval in the European Union and other countries in 2006, rimonabant belongs to a novel class of antiobesity agents that block the cannabinoid-1 (CB-1) receptor subtype [110]. CB-1 receptor is a G-protein coupled receptor that is extensively expressed in the CNS, including in areas vital to the control of food intake. Endocannabinoids interact with several anorexic and orexigenic pathways within the CNS, including the central melanocortin and mesolimbic pathways, subsequently increasing the motivation to eat and stimulating food intake. Rimonabant is a potent CB-1-selective ligand, with 1000-fold greater affinity for the CB-1 receptor than the CB-2 receptor. Rimonabant acts by both central and peripheral mechanisms to decrease food intake and body weight [76].The drug is hepatically metabolized and excreted in bile.

Efficacy

Four double-blind trials, comprising the Rimonabant in Obesity (RIO) program, compared rimonabant 5 mg or 20 mg daily with a placebo in more than 6,600 individuals. The RIO Program enrolled patients with a BMI of 30 kg/m^2 or greater or BMI exceeding 27 kg/m^2 with co-morbidities. In contrast with the placebo group, rimonabant significantly reduced weight by 4.6 kg, reduced waist circumference, and enhanced triglyceride and HDL cholesterol profiles [111-115]. In RIO programs, rimonabant also significantly reduced the risk factors of metabolic syndrome [112].

The weight reduction observed during treatment with rimonabant is of the same order of magnitude as that found in the other available agents, orlistat and sibutramine. In the RIO-Europe study, patients with a BMI above 30 kg/m^2 or a BMI exceeding 27 kg/m^2 with co-morbidities received placebo or rimonabant treatment for one year. The final weight loss was 1.8 kg in the placebo group and 3.4 and 6.6 kg in the 5mg and 20mg rimonabant groups, respectively [115]. The maximum total drug induced reduction in body weight over placebo was around 4.8 kg. Waist circumference, HDL cholesterol, triglycerides and insulin resistance were also improved with 20mg of the drug. The most common adverse events were nausea and diarrhea. Mood disorders were more frequent in the rimonabant 20 mg group than in the other groups [115]. In the RIO-Lipids study [112], the drug was administered to overweight or obese patients with dyslipidemia in addition to a hypocaloric diet for 12 months. Rimonabant induced a significant weight loss and reduction in waist circumference with a dose of 20 mg daily. At the end of the study, weight loss was 2.3 kg in the placebo group, 4.2 and 8.6 kg in the groups receiving 5 or 20 mg rimonabant, respectively. Plasma triglycerides were reduced and HDL cholesterol increased. Glucose tolerance was enhanced and adioponectin plasma levels increased significantly after 20 mg of rimonabant daily. Systolic and diastolic blood pressure was lowered after 20 mg of rimonabant, particularly in patients with hypertension [112].

The improvement in HbAlc levels was more pronounced than estimated from body weight reduction. These additional actions are probably mediated directly via the blockade of peripheral CB-1 receptors or indirectly via the increased plasma concentrations of adiponectin, an adipokine that has been shown to enhance insulin sensitivity [112, 115]. Although a large clinical trial on how rimonabant affects the development of coronary atherosclerosis (STRADIVARIUS) has recently been initiated, the initial data failed to demonstrate that rimonabant affects the disease progression [116].

Adverse Effects

The most frequent adverse events are nausea, dizziness, diarrhea, and insomnia, each occurring 1-9% more frequently than in the placebo trial group. Adverse effects leading to drug discontinuation occurred in 13-16% of patients administered the 20 mg dose. In the 20mg rimonabant group, more patients discontinued treatment owing to adverse effects (i.e. depression, anxiety and nausea) than in the other groups [112]. An increased incidence of mood disorders is the major adverse effect. In RIO-Europe, RIO-North America, and RIO-Lipids, drug discontinuation due to psychiatric disorders (mainly depression) occurred in 6-7% of rimonabant-treated individuals, i.e. an absolute increase of 2-5% over that of placebo trial group. In Europe, rimonabant is contraindicated for patients with severe depression and/or patients treated with antidepressive medications; it is not advised for patients with other untreated psychiatric conditions.

Comparison and Clinical Applications of Available Drugs

Without head-to-head trials, no definitive data demonstrate the merits of one antiobesity drug over another [76]. Therefore, if drug treatment is to be initiated, the initial choice is largely based on patients' preferences, adverse effect profiles and clinical experience. Orlistat might benefit patients with high LDL cholesterol concentrations with cardiovascular disease, or those who are at high risk for developing type 2 diabetes. Patients with long-term use of orlistat should take vitamins for supplement. Sibutramine might be useful in patients lacking satiety or who snack frequently. Sibutramine should be not prescribed for patients with inadequately controlled hypertension, pre-existing cardiovascular disease, or tachycardia. Rimonabant might be used in patients with dyslipidemia related to the metabolic syndrome. However, rimonabant should be prescribed cautiously in patients with pre-existing psychiatric illness, especially depression or anxiety. Regardless of what drug is prescribed, treatment should be discontinued if no significant weight loss occurs within the first 3-6 months. Owing to the various mechanisms of action, although a combination treatment might be feasible, no strong evidence suggests substantial weight loss than with a single-drug treatment.

Drugs in Clinical Development

Following the development of rimonabant, Pfizer has begun to develop a new CB-1 receptor antagonist for appetite suppressants. This compound may result from a different balance between the central and peripheral effects of CB-1 antagonists. Despite a reduced adverse effect of central acting effect, including depression and anxiety, this agent may suffer from a reduced efficacy as appetite suppressants. A new appetite suppressing drug in clinical trials is APD 356, a 5-HT2c receptor agonist. Such compounds probably have anorexigenic effects comparable to those of 5HT-reuptake inhibitors. However, owing to their selectivity, a 5-HT receptor subtype should be less prone to induce adverse effects.

Since the identification of leptin as a circulating factor from adipose tissue that informs the brain of the status of the energy reserves, this pathway has been extensively studied [117]. However, no agonists or antagonists acting at these sites have so far entered clinical development. Conversely, numerous experimental and clinical findings strongly suggest a pivotal role of the melanocortin system in regulating food intake and energy expenditure. Ghrelin is the only gut hormone identified so far that stimulates the appetite. Antagonists of ghrelin receptors could therefore be novel anorexigenic agents that reduce the frequency of meals.

Uncoupling proteins 3(UCP3) are located in the skeletal muscle, and were assumed to be responsible for producing heat in this tissue and, therefore, represents an interesting pharmacological target [118]. Among the many compounds still under clinical development include those that reduce gastric emptying, pramlintide [119], an analogue of amylin that has been developed for type 2 diabetes. Inhibitors of gastrointestinal lipases (cetilistat), i.e. a possible alternative to orlistat, may offer a reduced frequency of adverse effects [120]. Compounds as above are still in preclinical or early clinical development stages. Whether these compounds can be prescribed as anti-obesity drug in the near future warrants further study.

CONCLUSION

Obesity has become a major public health concern with multiple high risks of chronic diseases. More than industrialized countries, developing countries should pay closer attention to the increasing prevalence of obesity and formulate appropriate policies and guidelines. Anti-obesity drugs maybe an option for weight control; however, they should be used under regulation and with caution.

REFERENCES

[1] Ryan JG. Cost and policy implications from the increasing prevalence of obesity and diabetes mellitus. Gend Med 2009; 6 (Suppl 1): 86-108.

[2] World Health Organization. Obesity: preventing and managing the global epidemic- Report of a WHO Consultation: World Health Organization. 2000; WHO Technical Report Series, No. 894.

[3] Eberwine D. Globesity: The Crisis of Growing Proportions. Perspectives in Health Magazine [serial on the Internet]. 2002; 7(3): Available from: http://www.paho.org/English/DPI/Number15_article2_2.htm

[4] Ellis KJ. Selected body composition methods can be used in field studies. J Nutr 2001; 131: 1589S-95S.

[5] Hu FB. Obesity epidemilogy. New York: Oxford University Press 2008.

[6] Well JCK, Fewtrell MS. Measuring body composition. Arch Dis Child 2006; 91: 612-7.

[7] Heyward VH, Wangner DR. Applied body composition assessment. Champaign: Human Kinetics; 2004.

[8] Bellisari A, Roche AF. Anthropometry and ultrasound. In: Heymsfield SB, Lohman TG, Wang ZM, Going SB, Eds. Human Body Composition. 2nd ed. Champaign: Human Kinetics 2005. pp. 109-28.

[9] World Health Organization Western Pacific Region, International Association for the Study of Obesity, International Obesity Task Force. The Asia-Pacific perspective: redefining obesity and its treatment. Sydney: Health Communications Australia Pty Limited 2000.

[10] Poskitt E, Edmunds L. Management of childhood obesity. New York: Cambridge University Press; 2008.

[11] Prentice AM, Jebb SA. Beyond body mass index. Obes Rev 2001; 2:141-7.

[12] World Health Organization. Appropriate body-mass index for Asian populations and its implications for policy and intervention strategies. Lancet 2004; 363: 157-63.

[13] World Health Organization Expert Committee on Physical Status. The use and interpretation of anthropometry. World Health Organization 1995; Technical Report Series, No. 854.

[14] Going SB. Hydrodensitometry and air displacement plethysmography. In: Heymsfield SB, Lohman TG, Wang ZM, Going SB, Eds. Human Body Composition. 2nd ed. Champaign: Human Kinetics; 2005; pp. 17-34.

[15] Schoeller D, A. Hydrometry. In: Heymsfield SB, Lohman TG, Wang ZM, Going SB, Eds. Human Body Composition. 2nd ed. Champaign: Human Kinetics 2005. pp. 35-50.

[16] Chumlea WC, Sun SS. Bioelectrical impedance analysis. In: Heymsfield SB, Lohman TG, Wang ZM, Going SB, Eds. Human Body Composition. 2nd ed. Champaign: Human Kinetics 2005. pp. 79-88.

[17] Lobstein T, Baur L, Uauy R. Obesity in children and young people: a crisis in public health. Obes Rev 2004; 5(Suppl 1): S4-104.

[18] Lohman TG, Chen Z. Dual-energy X-ray absorptiometry. In: Heymsfield SB, Lohman TG, Wang ZM, Going SB, Eds. Human Body Composition. 2nd ed. Champaign: Human Kinetics 2005. pp. 63-78.

[19] Ross R, Janssen I. Computed tomography and magnetic resonance imaging. In: Heymsfield SB, Lohman TG, Wang ZM, Going SB, Eds. Human Body Composition. 2nd ed. Champiagn: Human Kinetics 2005. pp. 89-108.

[20] Dehghan M, Akhtar-Danesh N, Merc AT. Childhood obesity, prevalence and prevention. Nutr J 2005; 4: 24.

[21] Appropriate body-mass index for Asian populations and its implications for policy and intervention strategies. Lancet 2004; 363:157-63.

[22] Balkau B, Deanfield JE, Despres JP, *et al.* International Day for the Evaluation of Abdominal Obesity (IDEA): a study of waist circumference, cardiovascular disease, and diabetes mellitus in 168,000 primary care patients in 63 countries. Circulation 2007; 116: 1942-51.

[23] Luo W, Morrison H, de GM, *et al.* The burden of adult obesity in Canada. Chronic Dis Can 2007; 27: 135-44.

[24] Belanger-Ducharme F, Tremblay A. Prevalence of obesity in Canada. Obes Rev 2005; 6: 183-6.

[25] Chen YR, D.C.; Dosman,J.A. Changing prevalence of obesity in a rural community between 1977 and 2003: a multiple cross-sectional study. Public Health Nutr 2009; 123: 15-9.

[26] Silveira EA, Kac G, Barbosa LS. Obesity prevalence and associated factors in the elderly in Pelotas, Rio Grande do Sul State, Brazil: obesity classification according to two cutoff points for body mass index. CadSaude Publica 2009; 25: 1569-77.

[27] Lobato JC, Costa AJ, Sichieri R. Food intake and prevalence of obesity in Brazil: an ecological analysis. Public Health Nutr 2009: 1-7.

[28] Schulz R, Guther B, Mutert S, Kuhn J. Obesity in bavarian adolescents: prevalence in trend, sociodemographic structural features and subjective health. Gesundheitswesen 2009.

[29] Czernichow S, Vergnaud AC, Maillard-Teyssier L, *et al.* Trends in the prevalence of obesity in employed adults in central-western France: a population-based study, 1995-2005. Prev Med 2009; 48: 262-6.

[30] Zaninotto P, Head J, Stamatakis E, Wardle H, Mindell J. Trends in obesity among adults in England from 1993 to 2004 by age and social class and projections of prevalence to 2012. J Epidemiol Commun Health 2009; 63: 140-6.

[31] Tyrovolas S, Bountziouka V, Papairakleous N, *et al.* Adherence to the Mediterranean diet is associated with lower prevalence of obesity among elderly people living in Mediterranean islands: the MEDIS study. Int J Food Sci Nutr 2009: 1-14.

[32] Vardavas CI, Linardakis MK, Hatzis CM, Saris WH, Kafatos AG. Prevalence of obesity and physical inactivity among farmers from Crete (Greece), four decades after the Seven Countries Study. Nutr Metab Cardiovasc Dis 2009; 19: 156-62.

[33] Fister K, Kolcic I, Milanovic SM, Kern J. The prevalence of overweight, obesity and central obesity in six regions of Croatia: results from the Croatian Adult Health Survey. Coll Antropol 2009; 33 (Suppl 1): 25-9.

[34] Chu NF. Prevalence of obesity in Taiwan. Obes Rev 2005; 6: 271-4.

[35] Ho CST. Prevalence of overweight and obesity and its associated factors in aboriginal Taiwanese: findings from the 2001 National Health Interview Survey in Taiwan. Asia Pac J Clin Nutr 2007; 16: 572-9.

[36] Tian H, Xie H, Song G, Zhang H, Hu G. Prevalence of overweight and obesity among 2.6 million rural Chinese adults. Prev Med 2009; 48: 59-63.

[37] Liu L, Ikeda K, Chen M, *et al.* Obesity, emerging risk in China: trend of increasing prevalence of obesity and its association with hypertension and hypercholesterolaemia among the Chinese. Clin Exp Pharmacol Physiol 2004; 31(Suppl 2): S8-10.
[38] Wu YF, Ma GS, Hu YH, *et al.* The current prevalence status of body overweight and obesity in China: data from the China National Nutrition and Health Survey. Zhonghua Yu Fang Yi Xue Za Zhi 2005; 39: 316-20.
[39] Sakuta HST. Overweight male personnel of the Japan Self-Defense Forces with body mass indices of 23.0-24.9 and obesity-related metabolic disorders. Environ Health Prev Med 2008; 13: 116-20.
[40] Murakami Y, Miura K, Ueshima H. Comparison of the trends and current status of obesity between Japan and other developed countries. Nippon Rinsho 2009; 67: 245-52.
[41] Thorburn AW. Prevalence of obesity in Australia. Obes Rev 2005; 6: 187-9.
[42] Park HS, Park CY, Oh SW, Yoo HJ. Prevalence of obesity and metabolic syndrome in Korean adults. Obes Rev 2008; 9: 104-7.
[43] Worachartcheewan A, Nantasenamat C, Isarankura-Na-Ayudhya C, Pidetcha P, Prachayasittikul V. Lower BMI cutoff for assessing the prevalence of metabolic syndrome in Thai population. Acta Diabetol 2009.
[44] Aekplakorn W, Mo-Suwan L. Prevalence of obesity in Thailand. Obes Rev 2009.
[45] Esteghamati A, Meysamie A, Khalilzadeh O, *et al.* Third national Surveillance of Risk Factors of Non-Communicable Diseases (SuRFNCD-2007) in Iran: methods and results on prevalence of diabetes, hypertension, obesity, central obesity, and dyslipidemia. BMC Public Health 2009; 9:167.
[46] Al Rashdan I, Al Nesef Y. Prevalence of Overweight, Obesity, and Metabolic Syndrome among Adult Kuwaitis: Results From Community-based National Survey. Angiology 2010; 61: 42-8
[47] Beltaifa L, Traissac P, El AJ, Lefevre P, Romdhane HB, Delpeuch F. Prevalence of obesity and associated socioeconomic factors among Tunisian women from different living environments. Obes Rev 2009; 10: 145-53.
[48] Ntandou G, Delisle H, Agueh V, Fayomi B. Abdominal obesity explains the positive rural-urban gradient in the prevalence of the metabolic syndrome in Benin, West Africa. Nutr Res 2009; 29: 130-39.
[49] Wang Y, Lobstein T. Worldwide trends in childhood overweight and obesity. [see comment]. Int J Pediat Obes 2006; 1: 11-25.
[50] Sturm R. Increases in clinically severe obesity in the United States, 1986-2000. [see comment]. Arch Intern Med 2003; 163: 2146-8.
[51] Ebbeling CB, Pawlak DB, Ludwig DS. Childhood obesity: public-health crisis, common sense cure. Lancet 2002; 360: 473-82.
[52] Haslam DW, James WPT. Obesity. Lancet 2005; 366:1197-209.
[53] Institute of Medicine Report Brief. Progress in Preventing Childhood Obesity: How Do We Measure Up?: Institute of Medicine Report Brief; Available from: http://www.iom.edu/Object.File/Master/36/984/ 11722_reportbrief.pdf
[54] Bradford NF. Overweight and obesity in children and adolescents. Primary Care; Clinics in Office Practice 2009; 36: 319-39.
[55] Anderson P, M., Butcher KF. Childhood obesity: Trends and potential causes. Future Child 2006; 16: 19-45.
[56] US Centers for Disease Control and Prevention. Defining childhood overweight and obesity. US Centers for Disease Control and Prevention; [cited 2009 0820]; Available from: http://www.cdc.gov/obesity/ childhood/defining.html
[57] UK Department of Health. Health Survey for England 2002. London: The Stationery Office; 2003.
[58] Cole TJ, Bellizzi MC, Flegal KM, Dietz WH. Establishing a standard definition for child overweight and obesity worldwide: international survey. BMJ 2000; 320: 1240-3.
[59] Whitlock EP, Williams SB, Gold R, Smith PR, Shipman SA. Screening and interventions for childhood overweight: a summary of evidence for the US Preventive Services Task Force. Pediatrics 2005; 116: 125-44.
[60] Anderson SE, Whitaker RC. Prevalence of obesity among US preschool children in different racial and ethnic groups. Arch Pediatr Adolesc Med 2009; 163: 344-8.
[61] Schwarzenberg SJ. Obesity in children: epidemic and opportunity. Minnesota Med 2005; 88: 62-6.
[62] Ogden CL, Flegal KM, Carroll MD, Johnson CL. Prevalence and trends in overweight among US children and adolescents, 1999-2000. JAMA 2002; 288(14): 1728-32.
[63] Ogden CL, Carroll MD, Curtin LR, *et al.* Prevalence of overweight and obesity in the US, 1999-2004. JAMA 2006; 295(13): 1549-55.
[64] Ogden CL, Carroll MD, Flegal KM. High body mass index for age among US children and adolescents, 2003-2006.[see comment]. JAMA 2008; 299(20): 2401-5.
[65] Martorell R, Khan LK, Hughes ML, Grummer-Strawn LM. Obesity in Latin American women and children. J Nutr 1998; 128: 1464-73.
[66] Lobstein T, Frelut ML. Prevalence of overweight among children in Europe. Obes Rev 2003; 4: 195-200.
[67] World Health Organization. The challenge of obesity in the WHO European Region: WHO Regional Office for Europe Fact sheet EURO/13/052005.
[68] Keinan-Boker L, Noyman N, Chinich A, Green MS, Nitzan-Kaluski D. Overweight and obesity prevalence in Israel: findings of the first national health and nutrition survey (MABAT). Israel Med Assoc J 2005; 7: 219-23.
[69] Lissau I, Overpeck MD, Ruan WJ, Due P, Holstein BE, Hediger ML. Health Behaviour in School-aged Children Obesity Working G. Body mass index and overweight in adolescents in 13 European countries, Israel, and the US. Arch Pediatr Adolesc Med 2004; 158: 27-33.
[70] Uauy R, Albala C, Kain J. Obesity trends in Latin America: transiting from under- to overweight. J Nutr 2001; 131: 893S-9S.
[71] Pan H, Jiang Y, Jing X, *et al.* Child body mass index in four cities of East China compared to Western references. Ann Hum Biol 2009; 36: 98-109.
[72] Potts M. China's one child policy.[see comment]. BMJ 2006; 333(7564): 361-2.
[73] Gu D, Reynolds K, Wu X, *et al.* Prevalence of the metabolic syndrome and overweight among adults in China. Lancet 2005; 365: 1398-405.
[74] Barnett AH. How well do rapid-acting insulins work in obese individuals? Diabetes Obes Metabol 2006; 8: 388-95.
[75] Baur L. The millennium disease. In: Barnett G, Ed. The Millenium Disease. Australian Parliament House, Launceston 2006; pp. 4-6.
[76] Padwal RS, Majumdar SR. Drug treatments for obesity: orlistat, sibutramine, and rimonabant. Lancet 2007; 369: 71-7.

[77] Poirier P, Giles TD, Bray GA, *et al.* Obesity and cardiovascular disease: pathophysiology, evaluation, and effect of weight loss: an update of the 1997 American Heart Association Scientific Statement on Obesity and Heart Disease from the Obesity Committee of the Council on Nutrition, Physical Activity, and Metabolism. Circulation 2006; 113(6): 898-918.
[78] Clinical guidelines on the identification, evaluation, and treatment of overweight and obesity in adults--The evidence report: National institutes of health. Obes Res 1998; 6: 51S-209S.
[79] Expert Panel on the Identification, Evaluation and Treatment of Overweight and Obesity in Adults. Executive summary of the clinical guidelines on the identification, evaluation, and treatment of overweight and obesity in adults. Arch Intern Med 1998; 158: 1855-67.
[80] Khan LK, Serdula MK, Bowman BA, Williamson DF. Use of prescription weight loss pills among U.S. adults in 1996-1998. Ann Intern Med 2001; 134: 282-6.
[81] Schwizer W, Asal K, Kreiss C, *et al.* Role of lipase in the regulation of upper gastrointestinal function in humans. Am J Physiol 1997; 273(3 Pt 1): G612-20.
[82] Stafford RS, Radley DC. National trends in antiobesity medication use. Arch Intern Med 2003; 163: 1046-50.
[83] Blanck HM, Khan LK, Serdula MK. Use of nonprescription weight loss products--result from a multistate survey. JAMA 2001; 286: 930-5.
[84] Connolly HM, Crary JL, McGoon MD, Hensrud DD, Edwards BS. Valvular heart disease associated with fenfluramine-phentermine. N Eng J Med 1997; 337: 581-8.
[85] Cardiac valvulopathy associated with exposure to fenfluramine or dexfenfluramine: U.S. Department of Heatlh and Human Services interim public health recommendations, November 1997. Morb Mortal Wkly Rep 1997; 46: 1061-6.
[86] Kernan WN, Viscoli CM, Brass LM, *et al.* Phenylpropanolamine and the risk of hemorrhagic stroke. N Eng J Med 2000; 343: 1826-32.
[87] Lake CR, Gallant S, Masson E, Miller P. Adverse drug effects attributed to phenylpropanolamine: a review of 142 case reports. Am J Med 1990; 89: 195-208.
[88] Morgenstern LB, Viscoli CM, Kernan WN, *et al.* Use of Ephedra-containing products and risk for hemorrhagic stroke. Neurology 2003; 60: 132-5.
[89] Gura T. Obesity drug pipeline not so fat. Science 2003; 299(5608): 849-52.
[90] Sjostrom L, Rissanen A, Andersen T, *et al.* Randomised placebo-controlled trial of orlistat for weight loss and prevention of weight regain in obese patients. European Multicentre Orlistat Study Group. Lancet 1998; 352: 167-72.
[91] Torgerson JS, Hauptman J, Boldrin MN, Sjostrom L. XENical in the prevention of diabetes in obese subjects (XENDOS) study: a randomized study of orlistat as an adjunct to lifestyle changes for the prevention of type 2 diabetes in obese patients. Diabetes Care 2004; 27: 155-61.
[92] Li Z, Maglione M, Tu W, *et al.* Meta-analysis: pharmacologic treatment of obesity. Ann Intern Med 2005; 142: 532-46.
[93] Richelsen B, Tonstad S, Rossner S, *et al.* Effect of orlistat on weight regain and cardiovascular risk factors following a very-low-energy diet in abdominally obese patients: a 3-year randomized, placebo-controlled study. Diabetes Care 2007; 30: 27-32.
[94] Davidson MH, Hauptman J, DiGirolamo M, *et al.* Weight control and risk factor reduction in obese subjects treated for 2 years with orlistat: a randomized controlled trial. JAMA 1999; 281: 235-42.
[95] Chanoine JP, Hampl S, Jensen C, Boldrin M, Hauptman J. Effect of orlistat on weight and body composition in obese adolescents: a randomized controlled trial. JAMA 2005; 293(23): 2873-83.
[96] Maahs D, de Serna DG, Kolotkin RL, *et al.* Randomized, double-blind, placebo-controlled trial of orlistat for weight loss in adolescents. Endocr Pract 2006; 12: 18-28.
[97] McNeely W, Benfield P. Orlistat. Drugs 1998; 56: 241-9.
[98] Garcia SB, Barros LT, Turatti A, *et al.* The anti-obesity agent Orlistat is associated to increase in colonic preneoplastic markers in rats treated with a chemical carcinogen. Cancer Lett 2006; 240: 221-4.
[99] Singh A, Sarkar SR, Gaber LW, Perazella MA. Acute oxalate nephropathy associated with orlistat, a gastrointestinal lipase inhibitor. Am J Kidney Dis 2007; 49: 153-7.
[100] Halford JC, Cooper GD, Dovey TM. The pharmacology of human appetite expression. Curr Drug Targets 2004; 5: 221-40.
[101] James WP, Astrup A, Finer N, *et al.* Effect of sibutramine on weight maintenance after weight loss: a randomised trial. STORM Study Group. Sibutramine Trial of Obesity Reduction and Maintenance. Lancet 2000; 356: 2119-25.
[102] Arterburn DE, Crane PK, Veenstra DL. The efficacy and safety of sibutramine for weight loss: a systematic review. Arch Intern Med 2004; 164: 994-1003.
[103] Padwal R, Li SK, Lau DC. Long-term pharmacotherapy for obesity and overweight. Cochrane Database Syst Rev 2004(3): CD004094.
[104] Berkowitz RI, Fujioka K, Daniels SR, *et al.* Effects of sibutramine treatment in obese adolescents: a randomized trial. Ann Intern Med 2006; 145(2): 81-90.
[105] Berkowitz RI, Wadden TA, Tershakovec AM, Cronquist JL. Behavior therapy and sibutramine for the treatment of adolescent obesity: a randomized controlled trial. JAMA 2003; 289: 1805-12.
[106] Luque CA, Rey JA. Sibutramine: a serotonin-norepinephrine reuptake-inhibitor for the treatment of obesity. Ann Pharmacother 1999; 33: 968-78.
[107] Torp-Pedersen C, Caterson I, Coutinho W, *et al.* Cardiovascular responses to weight management and sibutramine in high-risk subjects: an analysis from the SCOUT trial. Eur Heart J 2007; 28: 2915-23.
[108] Sharma AM, Caterson ID, Coutinho W, *et al.* Blood pressure changes associated with sibutramine and weight management - an analysis from the 6-week lead-in period of the sibutramine cardiovascular outcomes trial (SCOUT). Diabetes Obes Metab 2009; 11: 239-50.
[109] Ernest D, Gershenzon A, Corallo CE, Nagappan R. Sibutramine-associated QT interval prolongation and cardiac arrest. Ann Pharmacother 2008; 42: 1514-7.
[110] Pertwee RG. Cannabinoid pharmacology: the first 66 years. Br J Pharmacol 2006; 147 (Suppl 1): S163-71.
[111] Curioni C, Andre C. Rimonabant for overweight or obesity. Cochrane Database Syst Rev 2006(4): CD006162.
[112] Despres JP, Golay A, Sjostrom L. Effects of rimonabant on metabolic risk factors in overweight patients with dyslipidemia. N Engl J Med 2005; 353: 2121-34.

[113] Pi-Sunyer FX, Aronne LJ, Heshmati HM, Devin J, Rosenstock J. Effect of rimonabant, a cannabinoid-1 receptor blocker, on weight and cardiometabolic risk factors in overweight or obese patients: RIO-North America: a randomized controlled trial. JAMA 2006; 295: 761-75.

[114] Scheen AJ, Finer N, Hollander P, Jensen MD, Van Gaal LF. Efficacy and tolerability of rimonabant in overweight or obese patients with type 2 diabetes: a randomised controlled study. Lancet 2006; 368: 1660-72.

[115] Van Gaal LF, Rissanen AM, Scheen AJ, Ziegler O, Rossner S. Effects of the cannabinoid-1 receptor blocker rimonabant on weight reduction and cardiovascular risk factors in overweight patients: 1-year experience from the RIO-Europe study. Lancet 2005; 365: 1389-97.

[116] Nissen SE, Nicholls SJ, Wolski K, *et al.* Effect of rimonabant on progression of atherosclerosis in patients with abdominal obesity and coronary artery disease: the STRADIVARIUS randomized controlled trial. JAMA 2008; 299(13): 1547-60.

[117] Ahima RS, Osei SY. Leptin signaling. Physiol Behav 2004; 81(2): 223-41.

[118] Nagy TR, Blaylock ML, Garvey WT. Role of UCP2 and UCP3 in nutrition and obesity. Nutrition 2004; 20: 139-44.

[119] Ravussin E, Smith SR, Mitchell JA, *et al.* Enhanced weight loss with pramlintide/metreleptin: an integrated neurohormonal approach to obesity pharmacotherapy. Obesity (Silver Spring) 2009; 17: 1736-43.

[120] Kopelman P, de HGG, Kopelman P, *et al.* Weight loss, HbA(1c) reduction, and tolerability of cetilistat in a randomized, placebo-controlled phase 2 trial in obese diabetics: comparison with orlistat (Xenical). Obesity (Silver Spring) 2010; 18: 108-15.

HDL Levels in Obesity

Justina Costandi[1,2], Michelle Melone[1] and Shirya Rashid[*,1,2]

[1]*Department of Medicine, Henderson Research Centre, McMaster University, Hamilton, Ontario, Canada*

[2]*Graduate Department of Medical Sciences, McMaster University, Hamilton, Ontario, Canada*

Abstract: The incidence of obesity is increasing dramatically worldwide. In North America alone, approximately 60% of the population is either overweight or obese. Obese individuals are at high risk for the development of metabolic disorders, including insulin resistance, type II diabetes mellitus and cardiovascular diseases (CVD). In terms of CVD, in particular, obese individuals are at increased risk for heart diseases and stroke. Dyslipidemia in obesity is a major cause of obesity-related CVD. More specifically, the characteristic dyslipidemia of obesity is elevated plasma triglycerides and low plasma levels of high-density lipoprotein (HDL) particles. Since HDL particles carry the "good cholesterol" and are highly anti-atherogenic particles, the lowering of plasma HDL levels in obesity, is of particular concern. Moreover, with every 1% increase in plasma HDL levels, there is a 1-3% decline in CVD risk. Thus, HDL rising in obesity is an attractive therapeutic target. However, because of its complex metabolism, developing safe and potent HDL raising therapies has been a challege. In terms of nonpharmacological therapies, diet and exercise interventions only raise plasma HDL levels modestly at best (10-15%). Of the current anti-obesity therapies, orlistat and sibutramine do not raise plasma HDL levels, while rimonabant does directly increase HDL concentrations. There is concern, however, over the serious central nervous system side-effects of rimonabant. Furthermore, in terms of HDL raising pharmaceutical therapies, the most widely used are niacin and fibrates. Fibrates only achieve a modest rise (10-15%) in plasma HDL, while niacin produces a larger increase (25%); however, due to the induction of flushing with niacin, it's use is limited. More recently, non-flushing niacin has been developed which is a promising therapy. There is currently wide interest in developing new more potent HDL raising therapies that can induce greater reductions in CVD risk than current therapies. Foremost, the initially promising cholesteryl ester transfer protein (CETP) inhibitors proved to paradoxically increase CVD risk. In contrast, infusion of HDL or its protein apolipoprotein A-I has been more effective at reducing CVD risk. Overall, there are multiple points in the HDL metabolic pathway that may be targets for future HDL drug therapies and the future in HDL drug therapy holds great promise as we understand more about HDL's complex physiology.

Keywords: HDL, cholesterol, obesity, cardiovascular disease.

OBESITY AS A RISK FACTOR FOR CARDIOVASCULAR DISEASES

The incidence of obesity is increasing at an alarming rate in both developed and developing countries globally [1]. As socioeconomic conditions improve, there is a trend towards increased weight and sedentary lifestyle. Over 30% of US adults are obese [1]. In economically advanced urban regions in Africa and Asia, the incidence of obesity has reached levels comparable to those in industrialized countries [1].

The World Health Organization defines obesity as a chronic disease in which there is an excess accumulation of body fat to an extent that can compromise an individual's health [1]. It can be more specifically defined as having 25% or more total body fat in men; and 35% or more in women [2]. Obesity occurs when caloric intake exceeds energy expenditure, resulting in a positive caloric balance [3]. Total body fat can be measured by bioelectrical impedance, underwater weighing, and skin-fold thickness, all of which are impractical and costly methods for clinical use [2]. Some more anthropometric measures include body mass index (BMI) and waist circumference. BMI gives a measure of body fat content in terms of weight (kilograms) divided by height (meters) squared [2]. An overweight individual is classified as having a BMI of 25 – 29 kg/m^2, while an obese individual is classified by a BMI $\geq$ 30 kg/m^2 [4]. Waist circumference is an accurate way to measure abdominal obesity, where having a waist circumference of 102 cm or more in men and 88 cm or more in women is classified as obese [4]. It should be noted that there

*Corresponding author: Tel: 905-527-2299, Ext. 43780; Fax: 905-575-2646; E-mail: srashid@thrombosis.hhscr.org

are ethnic variations and these cut-offs are not applicable to children and adolescents, people aged 65 years and older, pregnant and breast-feeding women, and those with very muscular builds [1].

Obesity is a major risk factor for premature cardiovascular diseases (CVD) [5,6] as it is associated with a variety of CVD risk factors, such as type II diabetes mellitus, hypertension and dyslipidemia [7,8]. CVD, which include myocardial infarction and stroke, are among the leading causes of morbidity and mortality in the United States and worldwide [9]. Although the incidence of CVD has decreased in recent years, this trend is expected to reverse because of the global epidemic of obesity [1,5,9]. The landmark INTERHEART randomized, case-control trial investigated clinical parameters that can potentially increase the risk of heart attacks or myocardial infarction globally in 20,000 patients [6]. The trial findings showed that abdominal obesity accounted for a marked 24% of the global population burden of myocardial infarction [6]. Dyslipidemia, moreover, was the number one cause of myocardial infarction globally, accounting for 50% of myocardial infarction globally [6]. In fact, the effect of abdominal obesity, while large, was negated if dyslipidemia was incorporated in to the calculation [10]. Nonetheless, waist-to-hip ratio, which is a surrogate measure of visceral obesity, was highly correlated with the risk of CVD [10]. These findings further support and indicate that obesity increases the risk of CVD mainly because these individuals are dyslipidemic [11,12].

As the number of overweight and obese individuals increases worldwide, the incidence of CVD is predicted to reach epidemic proportions [6]. Consequently, this will contribute to a high social and economic cost in global health care systems. In order to address this growing concern, further research into the causes underlying the high risk of CVD in obesity is imperative to developing treatment and preventative strategies. Research aimed at expanding our understanding of the pathophysiology of dyslipidemia in obesity will greatly help in this regard.

THE CHARACTERISTIC DYSLIPIDEMIA OF OBESITY

Obese patients have a complex dyslipidemia characterized by elevated plasma levels of triglycerides (>1.7 mmol/L), increased plasma levels of low-density lipoprotein (LDL) particles (>0.9 g/L apolipoprotein (apo) B100, a marker of LDL numbers) and reduced levels of high-density lipoprotein (HDL) cholesterol (HDL-C) (<1.0 mmol/L) [13]. Each individual component of the characteristic dyslipidemia of obesity - increased triglycerides, which are incorporated in very-low density (VLDL) particles, elevated LDL plasma levels and decreased HDL plasma levels - is a major contributor to the high rates of CVD in obese individuals [14,15]. Since HDL particles are highly anti-atherogenic particles, the lowering of HDL plasma levels in obesity is of particular concern. HDL has in fact been described as the single most potent anti-atherosclerotic particle in human plasma [16]. In obese individuals, plasma HDL levels are consistently and markedly lower than HDL levels in normal individuals [17]. The remainder of this review will, therefore, focus on HDL metabolism and HDL treatment in obesity and dyslipidemia.

The Framingham Heart study reported that low HDL levels, independent of serum LDL or triglyceride levels, posed as much a risk to CVD as high LDL levels [18,19]. Thus, every 10% increase in HDL levels (normal levels are $\geq$ 1 mmol/L), correlates to a significant 30% decrease in the risk of CVD [20]. In fact, parallel with findings of the Israeli Ischemic Heart Disease Study, patients with the highest HDL-C were the least likely to develop CVD [19, 21]. Furthermore, the Prospective Cardiovascular Munster (PROCAM) subjects with a HDL-C concentration equal to or less than 0.9 mmol/L experienced a four-fold increase risk of CVD over 6 years compared with those having more than 0.9 mmol/L of HDL-C [22]. A ten year follow-up period of individuals with no baseline evidence of CVD in the Atherosclerosis Risk in Communities (ARIC) study further confirmed the inverse relationship between HDL and incidence of CVD [23]. The Physicians' Health Study demonstrated that even when total cholesterol serum levels were low, low HDL-C concentrations still increased the risk of developing CVD [24]. These clinical findings support and augment the importance of HDL as an atheroprotective particle.

HDL AS A PARTICLE

HDL are spherical particles consisting of a protein component and lipid component; although a distinct class of lipoproteins, HDL consists of many subfractions differing in lipid and protein composition, density, size and function [17,25]. The lipid components of HDL include a core of triglycerides and cholesteryl esters surrounded by free cholesterol and phospholipids [26] . The major protein components in HDL include apoAI, apoAII, apoAIII, apoCI, apoCI, apoCII, apoCIII, and apoE [26]. Both the cholesterol and apoAI components of HDL are lower in the plasma of obese individuals [17].

The most prominent ultracentrifugal HDL subfractions are HDL_2 and HDL_3 [27]. HDL_2 are larger, more cholesterol-ester rich and less dense compared to HDL_3 [17,26], with HDL_2 ranging 1.062 – 1.125 g/mL in density and 9 – 12 nm in diameter, and HDL_3 ranging 1.125 – 1.210 g/mL in density and 5 – 9 nm in diameter [28].

HDL can further be subdivided using two-dimensional gels, with the first dimension separating the particles by charge and the second dimension by size [29]. The subclasses that are seen include pre-β-HDL and α-1, α-2, α-3 and α-4 HDL particles, where the pre-β-HDL are disc-shaped and lipid poor while the α-HDLs are larger, spherical and lipid-rich [30-32]. Pre-β-HDL is the primary form of HDL secreted by the liver, while α-HDL is formed when pre-β-HDL is subsequently lipidated [31,33].

HDL can also be separated according to protein composition, using immunoaffinity chromatography [34]. Immunoaffinity chromatography is usually used to separate HDL particles into Lp(AI), containing apoAI only, and Lp(AI-AII), consisting of apoAI and apoAII [34]. Lp(AI) has similar properties to HDL_2 whereas Lp(AI-AII) matches HDL_3 [34].

HDL subclasses not only differ in physical properties but also in clinical relevance, with HDL_2 and pre-β-HDL, associated with cardioprotection [17]. Smaller HDL, representing HDL_3 are generally found in CVD patients [35], suggesting that the larger HDL, namely HDL_2, may be more cardioprotective [36]. Cross-sectional studies have indicated that both HDL_2 and HDL_3 levels are reduced in patients with atherosclerosis or myocardial infarction survivors compared to healthy patients [37]. Several similar studies investigating the relationship between HDL and coronary artery disease suggest that HDL_2 is inversely associated with CVD while HDL_3 subfractions are directly related to CVD severity [38-42]. As discussed below, pre-β-HDL is heavily involved in the removal of cholesterol from macrophages, such as those present in atherosclerotic plaques [43,44], thereby demonstrating its importance in preventing the development of atherosclerosis [17].

HDL METABOLISM

Plasma HDL levels are a balance between HDL synthesis and HDL clearance by the liver [43] and both the production and clearance rates of HDL are determinants of low HDL levels in obesity [45].

HDL particles are produced primarily by liver hepatocytes [46]. The most critical step in the cellular biosynthesis of HDL particles involves the activity of lipid transporters at the cell plasma membrane [44]. The first step in the synthesis of nascent or new HDL particles involves the ABCA1 transporter [43]. ABCA1 is a lipid transporter consisting of 12 transmembrane transporters at the hepatocyte plasma membrane [47]. ABCA1 lipid transporters act by mediating the efflux of phospholipids and cholesterol from inside the cell to the lipid-poor apoAI protein molecules which make up pre-β-HDL in the extracellular compartment [43,44]. Initially, HDL particles incorporate only small amounts of lipid into apoAI protein molecules, forming a disc shape, but they eventually become larger as they incorporate more and more lipid from cells [43,46]. As the HDL particles become larger, they accumulate more intracellular lipid *via* the ABCG1 lipid transporter and the SR-BI receptor [46,48]. Lecithin cholesterol acyltransferase (LCAT) esterifies the free cholesterol in nascent HDL, forming spherical HDL particles and further maturing the lipoprotein [49]. In addition, HDL-lipids are remodelled in the circulation by hepatic lipase, endothelial lipase, cholesteryl ester transfer protein (CETP) and phospholipid transfer protein (PLTP), all of which accelerate HDL catabolism [17].

The HDL particles in the circulation are eventually cleared from the circulation and taken up primarily by the liver [46,50]. A portion of the HDL particles that are cleared away from the circulation are taken up by receptor-mediated whole-particle uptake by liver hepatocytes [46]. However, the receptor carrying out this function has not yet been identified. The mechanism of action of cellular uptake of HDL-cholesterol (HDL-C) is better characterized. Both the ABCA1 and SR-BI hepatocyte receptors are involved in this HDL selective lipid uptake process, although the SR-BI-mediated process is better understood [51]. Both mediate the selective uptake of HDL cholesterol and cholesteryl esters. SR-BI appears to mediate internalization of whole particles of HDL, with subsequent removal of cholesterol and resecretion of smaller cholesterol-depleted HDL particles [29].

THE CARDIO PROTECTIVE ROLES OF HDL

Atherosclerosis is a widely prevalent chronic cardiovascular disease affecting the arterial wall, leading to ischemia and eventually infarction of the heart, brain or limbs [52]. HDL has long been known to have protective affects against the formation of atherosclerotic lesions.

HDL directly ameliorates the dysfunctional environment in atherosclerosis primarily by mediating a process called reverse cholesterol transport. Reverse cholesterol transport was first identified by Glomset in the late 1960's [53] and since then has been extensively studied. It is accepted as the main anti-atherogenic role of HDL [54] and is a critical target for HDL function enhancing therapy.

In reverse cholesterol transport, HDL directly removes cholesterol from foam cells, macrophages, and atherosclerotic plaques in the arterial wall, delivering them to the liver to be excreted as bile salts or biliary cholesterol [20]. This inhibits the formation of cholesterol-laden fatty streaks at the arterial wall, the first step in atherosclerosis development [20,55].

ApoAI, especially when deprived of lipids, such as when in the nascent or pre-β form of HDL, plays a key role in reverse cholesterol transport [36]. It is a key acceptor of free cholesterol effluxed from peripheral cells, such as macrophages, in a process mediated by ABCA1 [36]. Free cholesterol can also be transferred to mature HDL particles, including HDL_2 and HDL_3, *via* ABCG1 [56] and SR-B1 receptors [57], found in macrophages. Thus, excess cholesterol is transported from the arterial wall to the liver for excretion [36].

Atherosclerosis is defined as a chronic inflammatory disease [52] and interestingly, HDL particles have been found to mediate anti-inflammatory functions [58], adding to its anti-atherogenic repertoire. Monocyte adhesion to the activated arterial endothelium is one of the primary steps in inflammation [59]. HDL prevents the interaction between monocytes and endothelial cells through several mechanisms, such as the *in vitro* inhibition of the expression of endothelial cell adhesion molecules, including VCAM1, ICAM1, E-selectin, interleukin-1 and endotoxin [60-62]. In addition, HDL inhibits the formation of reactive oxygen species [63] and sphingosine kinase [64], resulting in the inhibition of NF-κB synthesis and subsequent expression of adhesion molecules on endothelial cells [65]. Monocyte transmigration across the endothelium with the help of the chemokine monocyte chemotactic protein-1 (MCP-1) has also been shown to be blocked by HDL [66,67].

Furthermore, platelet-activating factor (PAF) induction of leukocyte recruitment to the endothelium is inhibited by HDL [68]. Clinically, the inflammatory marker C-reactive protein (CRP) has been shown to negatively correlate with HDL levels in patients with the metabolic syndrome [69]. Thus, the adhesion and subsequent migration of monocytes into the subendothelial space of the arteries is inhibited by HDL, indicating its key role in anti-inflammation relating to atherosclerotic regression [58].

LDL oxidation is also crucial step in the pathogenesis of atherosclerosis, contributing to foam cell formation and the inflammatory response [70]. HDL serves as an antioxidant by inhibiting the oxidation of LDL at the arterial wall. HDL particles contain paraxonase-1 (PON1) and paraxonase-3 (PON3) and glutathione selenoperoxidase, and are associated with LCAT and PAF acetyl hydrolase (PAF-AH), all of which prevent the formation of and inactivate oxidized LDL [58,71]. PON1 may also stimulate HDL binding to ABCA1, thereby enhancing cholesterol efflux [72]. In addition, HDL inhibits the synthesis of the lipid hydroperoxides by blocking 12-lipoxygeniase, resulting in the prevention of LDL oxidation [73]. ApoAI mediates the removal and transport of LDL oxidizing agents [70] to the kidneys [65]. HDL has also been shown to inhibit the infiltration of LDL into the vessel wall [74]. Therefore, the anti-oxidant functions of HDL are crucial to the inhibition of atherosclerotic lesion progression and formation.

Nitric oxide (NO) is an endothelial vasodilator lacking in atherosclerosis [59]. This is attributed to the production of superoxides and endothelial dysfunction [59]. Consequently, smooth muscle cell proliferation, platelet aggregation and inflammation are promoted [75], thereby advancing atherosclerotic lesion and plaque rupture. HDL promotes the production of NO by upregulating endothelial nitric oxide synthase (eNOS) *via* multiple signalling pathways and mechanisms, including stimulation of eNOS activity [76,77] and prostacyclin (PGI_2) [78], resulting in increased NO production. The NO generated by eNOS improves the endothelium of the arterial wall, in addition to maintaining its integrity [79]. Specifically, NO dilates the blood vessel, prevents leukocyte adhesion and migration [80]. Along with PGI_2, NO attenuate platelet activation, adhesion and aggregation at the vessel wall, in addition to the decrease of vascular smooth muscle proliferation [80,81]. Conversely, HDL inhibits the synthesis of endothelin-1, a potent vasoconstrictor [82]. HDL also protects against endothelial apoptosis [83] and promotes survival and migration [84]. Thereby, the improvement of endothelial function and integrity by HDL serves to repair damaged caused by atherosclerosis.

HDL also has multiple antithrombotic functions, such as enhancing the protein C pathway [85], upregulating thrombomodulin [86], attenuating platelet activation and interfering with procoagulant interactions [79], thereby leading to the inhibition of thrombin generation and fibrin production. The interaction between fibrinogen and platelet glycoprotein IIb-IIIa is disrupted by HDL, which acts as an antagonist, thereby decreasing platelet aggregation [87]. In addition, tissue factor and adhesion molecule expression are downregulated [79], resulting in decreased thrombus formation [79]. Conversely, HDL enhances fibrinolysis by downregulating prothrombotic factors such as plasminogen activator inhibitor-1 and enhancing the antithrombitc factor, tissue plasminogen activator [88]. The inhibition of coagulation by HDL prevents plaque rupture and thrombus formation, which can obstruct the arterial lumen and lead to adverse myocardial events [59].

Hence, HDL reverses the processes leading to atherosclerosis by multiple processes, most notably by reverse cholesterol transport, and also by anti-inflammation, anti-oxidation, anticoagulation and endothelium amelioration. Thus, raising HDL in obesity is a highly attractive therapeutic drug target.

DETERMINANTS OF HDL LEVELS

HDL levels are highly heterogeneous in the general population as there are many factors that affect HDL metabolism and catabolism. Genetic heritability, environmental factors, and molecular mechanisms are among the main determinants of HDL levels in humans.

Genetic determinants account for 50% to 70% of HDL variability in humans [55]. Genome wide scans, in addition to specific gene association studies of key players in HDL metabolism and structure, have identified many polymorphisms with functional importance to the variations in HDL concentrations [89]. These genes include *ABCA1*, *APOA1*, *CETP*, *LIPC*, and *LCAT* [90]. Homozygous defects in *ABCA1* gene, results in Tangier disease, where there is an extreme decrease in HDL-C levels [91-93]. More than a dozen functional polymorphisms in the *APOA1* gene have been identified, and all result in a decrease in HDL-C [90]. Of note, there is also the apoA-I_{Milano} variant, which will be discussed in detail later. LCAT deficiency, associated with fish-eye disease, reduces HDL-C a marked 5-10%, compared to normal levels [90]. As previously discussed, CETP and hepatic lipase are regulators of HDL levels. Mutations in *CETP*, encoded by the *CETP* gene, have been associated with both increases and decreases in plasma HDL-C [90], while mutations in hepatic lipase, encoded by the *LIPC* gene, have been associated with increases in HDL-C [90].

Environmental factors which cannot be controlled - including gender, age and family history - also play a role in HDL concentration variability. In general, women have 10 mg/dL (0.26 mmol/L) higher plasma HDL-C levels than men [94]. 65% of their HDL is the larger, more atheroprotective HDL_2, while in men, only 47% of their HDL is HDL_2 [95]. This can be attributed to the presence of estrogen in women, which enhances hepatic formation of lipoproteins and apoplipoproteins [96-98]. Specifically, estrogen increases free fatty acid mobilization from lipid stores leading to heightened hepatic synthesis of VLDL and removal, LDLR upregulation [94], increased HDL lipids and enhanced liver synthesis of apoAI [99]. In addition, estrogen has been implicated in decreasing hepatic lipase activity and, thereby, reducing the rate of HDL_2 conversion to HDL_3 [99]. Thus men are associated with lower HDL concentrations [100] and therefore, greater CVD risk [101].

Age is another key factor leading to heterogeneous HDL levels. Throughout childhood, HDL levels steadily increase [102]. Due to hormonal changes, males experience progressive decreases in HDL during puberty, resulting in their lower HLD levels, as discussed above [103]. However, the decline in estrogen associated with menopause in females is implicated with up to a 10% decrease in HDL levels [101,104-106]. This is confirmed in prospective studies, which have shown that plasma HDL-C concentrations in male and female adults decrease with age [107,108]. In addition to hormonal changes, other mechanisms thought to be responsible for the decline in HDL with increasing age include the development of insulin resistance [109], inflammation [110] and lifestyle changes with age [102]. Insulin resistance is associated with decreased HDL formation, reduced HDL lipid efflux and HDL remodelling [109]. Similarly, inflammatory process in the aged population lead to increased HDL catabolism, decreased HDL formation, decreased apoAI-mediated lipid efflux, and HDL remodelling [110]. Furthermore, as an individual ages, changes in diet and physical activity may also affect HDL concentrations and function [102], as discussed below. Therefore, age is a major factor determining HDL levels.

Environmental factors which can be altered – including smoking, alcohol consumption, diet and exercise - also cause variability in HDL levels. Meta-analyses on smoking as an influential factor found that smoking decreases HDL-C by 5.7% [111]. Furthermore, multiple regression analysis of data collected from the Framingham Offspring study reported that smoking was associated with a 0.10-0.15 mmol/L decrease in HDL-C [112]. Autopsy studies of aortic segments revealed that the arteries of smokers had more fatty streaks and atherosclerotic lesions [113]. The mechanisms linking smoking, decreased HDL levels, and increased atherosclerotic progression is still unclear but is speculated to involved decreased LCAT activity [114]. On the other hand, cessation of smoking has been found to improve HDL-C concentrations [115]. These findings merit more attention and studies on the relationship between smoking and the development of CVD.

There is much evidence supporting a positive correlation between alcohol consumption and heart health. In particular, moderate alcohol consumption (30 g of alcohol per day) has been found to elevate HDL-C levels by 0.10 mmol/L and apoAI by 0.23 mmol/L [116]. While many mechanisms have been proposed, the most consistent finding is that alcohol consumption influences apoAI synthesis [117] and transportation [118], while reported changes in CETP activity and hepatic lipase are controversial. In some reports, alcohol consumption has been found to inhibit CETP activity, thereby stimulating early steps in reverse cholesterol transport [118]. On the other hand, many studies have reported that CETP activity is not affected [119-123]. Several studies reported subsequent decreases in hepatic lipase activity following alcohol consumption [124,125]. Conversely, others have reported no changes in hepatic lipase activity [126].

Diet and physical activity also influence HDL-C levels, as discussed in detail below. Briefly, diets low in saturated fat, in addition to those with increased unsaturated fatty acids and carbohydrates [127], are thought to adversely affect the HDL_2 subpopulation [128]. In addition, a sedentary lifestyle is associated with a lower HDL concentration when compared to a physically active lifestyle [129], discussed in further detail below.

HDL AS A THERAPEUTIC TARGET

The National Cholesterol Education Program (NCEP) Expert Panel published their third report classifying low serum HDL-C as <1.0 mmol/L and high levels as ≥ 1.5 mmol/L, for both men and woman [130]. The most widely used current lipid therapy, namely statins, are aimed at lowering LDL-C. Statins inhibit HMG CoA-reductase, a rate limiting enzyme in the cholesterol biosynthetic pathway [59]. By decreasing the production of endogenous cholesterol, statin therapy results in the upregulation of the LDL receptor in liver hepatocytes, which then leads to enhanced clearance of plasma LDL at the liver [59].

Nevertheless, statins are not a sufficient remedy in obese individuals, as they do not target the typical dyslipidemia of obesity, in which low plasma HDL levels are a significant factor. A low HDL level is a direct marker and direct inhibitor of atherogenic dyslipidemia, making it a highly attractive therapeutic target to reduce CVD development and risk [130]. However, because of HDL's complex metabolism, developing safe and potent HDL raising therapies has been a challenge.

Several nonpharmacological, lifestyle approaches to increasing HDL levels in patients with low HDL are weight reduction, diet and physical activity, the latter being the most effective [130]. In combination with these activities, a pharmacological approach of continually maintaining high levels of protective HDL may be achieved by such currently available therapies as: statins, nicotinic acid, fibric acids and their combinations.

LIFESTYLE INTERVENTIONS

While exercise and dietary changes are lifestyle interventions that are routinely prescribed for obese individuals, they only raise plasma HDL levels by modest amounts [17]. Decreasing caloric intake has in general been shown to have less of an impact on HDL levels than exercise [17]. Two prospective studies which measured HDL-C concentration after a period of reducing energy intake by 1000 kcal/day found HDL-C to increase in modest amounts [131,132]. Interestingly, a meta-analysis of 70 studies that looked at restricting caloric intake and lipoprotein profiles concluded that a temporary decrease in HDL by an average of 8% was observed when individuals were in the process of losing weight [133]. However, once a stable reduced weight was achieved, a 12% increase in HDL-C was observed [133]. An estimated 0.009 mmol/L increase in HDL-C occurs with every kilogram of weigh lost in individuals with stabilized body weights while a 0.007 mmol/L decrease in HDL-C per kilogram lost is associated with subjects actively losing weight [133,134].

Nevertheless, variations in diet composition often yield different affects on HDL-C levels. Recently, Volek *et al.* summarized the results of over 15 studies looking at the effects of very low carbohydrate diets [135]. In these studies, HDL increased by an absolute average of 11% [135]. Counter intuitively, diets lows in saturated fat generally decrease HDL-C concentrations [127,128,134,136-138]. This can be explained by the reduction in plasma cholesterol available for lipoprotein packaging associated with a reduction dietary intake of saturated fat [127,128,134,137,138]. The resulting relatively cholesterol-poor HDL particles are more susceptible to clearance, resulting in decreased levels [134].

Contradictory results have been published as to how exercise influences HDL-C. A major reason for this is accounted for by the differences in experimental design and heterogeneous baseline HDL-C levels in the different studies [17]. However, there is evidence suggesting that a certain threshold of exercise intensity or duration must be reached in order for HDL-C levels to be enhanced significantly. A dose response relationship was observed with increasing distances run, with significant improvements in HDL-C seen in individuals running 11 to 23 km/wk (7 to 14 miles/wk) [139]. This is equivalent to expending 700 to 1500 kcal/wk [140], which is easily attained by briskly walking or jogging for 30 minutes 3 to 5 times a week [139]. Other cross-sectional studies have reported that significant increases in HDL-C were seen after expending 1500 to 3000 kcal/wk, corresponding to 24 to 48 km/wk of moderate exercise [141,142]. This is further supported by the mean increases of HDL-C of 4 mg/dl seen in middle-aged men who expended over 2000 kcal/wk [143].

The mechanisms by which exercise enhances HDL-C are still not entirely clear. Changes in the activity level of lipases which affect HDL synthesis and catabolism seem to play a role [144]. Similar results were found in lipoprotein metabolism in endurance-trained men, who ran 16 km per day, compared to that in sedentary control subjects after an acute exercise session [129]. Lipoprotein lipase increased in activity by 80% in both groups of men [129]. This results in augmented lipid transfers to HDL, resulting in synthesis of new HDL particles [129]. In addition, a 38% reduction in hepatic lipase activity, seen after the exercise session, may have accounted for observed decrease in HDL clearance in both groups, which thereby increased the half-life of apoAI [129].

Altogether, the majority of the cross-sectional data indicates that a 3.5 to 6 mg/dL elevation in HDL-C can be expected in sedentary individuals who expend 1500 to 2200 kcal/wk in exercise [140]. Although this increase is modest, it can be translated to a 7-18% decrease in CVD risk, as every 1 mg/dL increase in HDL is associated with a 2-3% decreased risk in CVD [145].

ANTI-OBESITY DRUGS DECREASING CVD RISK: WHAT ARE THEIR EFFECTS ON PLASMA HDL LEVELS?

As discussed previously, obesity is considered a chronic disease, the prevalence of which will soon reach epidemic proportions globally. Its role as a major CVD risk factor has made it a prime target for therapy [146]. Much of the attention regarding CVD risk in obesity is currently focused on the relationship between obesity and plasma lipid levels and how they may be addressed in treatment. A remarkable 5-10% decrease in body weight may reduce the risk of various obesity related diseases such as hyperlipidemia, type II diabetes and hypertension [146-148]. Thus, patients with these diseases or a combination of them are the highest priority for anti-obesity drug prescriptions [148].

A change in lifestyle through augmented diet and exercise, although very useful, often requires supplementary assistance given through anti-obesity medications, especially in patients with a BMI greater than 30 kg/m^2, who are unable to lose weight from lifestyle modifications alone [149]. Over the past decade the development of such pharmacological agents has come forward, however, few are available in current practice [150].

ANTI-OBESITY DRUGS AIMED AT WEIGHT LOSS AND THEIR EFFECTS ON PLASMA HDL LEVELS

Orlistat

A key anti-obesity drug acting through its regulation of lipid metabolism is orlistat (xenical). Orlistat is a pancreatic and gastric lipase inhibitor that decreases ingested triglyceride hydrolysis [151,152]. The resulting dietary weight-loss is through the reduction of fat absorption, which was found to occur in a dose-dependent manner [151,152]. An approximate 30% reduction in fat absorption and subsequent excretion of fat in the faeces in patients treated with orlistat was observed as compared to placebo [151,152]. The largest placebo-controlled study of orlistat was XENical in the Prevention of Diabetes in Obese Subjects (XENDOS), which determined the effect of lifestyle modifications combined with orlistat therapy in the prevention of CVD in patients with type 2 diabetes and obesity [153]. This 4-year study reported a 37% CVD risk reduction in obese patients with combination therapy, increasing the evidence that changes in diet and exercise combined with drug therapy may decrease risk factors of the metabolic syndrome [153]. Orlistat is recommended for patients with high LDL levels, impaired glucose tolerance, and patients who lose weight and rapidly regain it [148]. Various clinical studies of orlistat and its effects on lipid metabolism have reported 5-8% reductions in LDL levels in the first 6 months [154]. The greatest decreases were shown to be after one year at 120 mg taken three times daily [154]. This was further validated in 2002 by Broom *et al.* which reported that orlistat decreased LDL-cholesterol levels in obese patients compared to placebo (-7.09% *versus* -0.55% $p < 0.0001$) [155]. Thus orlistat has been shown to decrease LDL levels, further decreasing the LDL/HDL ratio, a critical marker of cardiovascular risk [156].

The effect of lowering LDL may not always have the opposite effect on HDL levels. In a study by Hill *et al.*, a 2-4% increase in HDL levels was observed after 6 months of orlistat treatment [154]. However, at the one year mark of therapy, a slight decrease was reported, though not statistically significant [154]. Another study by Halpern *et al.* indicated that patients possessing normal HDL levels (1-1.2 mmol/L) maintained this level after treatment [157]. Only a small decrease in HDL levels of 1.8% was found with obese and non-insulin dependent diabetic patients [157]. HDL appears to be modestly affected by orlistat and its impact on increasing HDL may be linked to the patient's background, such as the baseline amount of HDL prior to treatment [130], the level of obesity and the progression of type 2 diabetes [156].

Overall, orlistat has been shown to be an effective therapy for decreasing long-term obesity-related CVD risk [154]. This in combination with a healthy and modest weight-loss over a long-term [148] may be a realistic therapy regime for obese patients.

Sibutramine

Another clinical anti-obesity drug also well accepted by patients is sibutramine (BTS54524), a norepinephrine and serotonin inhibitor [158,159]. Its weight loss mode of action is through the stimulation of satiety and subsequent reduction of food/caloric intake [160]. Sibutramine was found to increase weight loss in obese adolescents when combined with exercise and diet monitoring [161]. A meta-analysis of anti-obesity drugs reported a mean weight reduction of approximately 4.5 kg in 12 months with sibutramine, compared to orlistat, with a mean reduction of approximately 3.0 kg [162]. Its effects on HDL were to induce a significant increase by 15% compared to the placebo group [161]. The Sibutramine Trial of Obesity Reduction and Maintenance (STORM) reported in 2000, that HDL levels significantly rose in patients after 2 years of sibutramine (10-20 mg/day) treatment by 20.7%, compared to the placebo group, in which HDL increased by 11.7% ($p<0.001$), resulting from previous use of sibutramine in the placebo group [163]. Alongside the increase in HDL, a majority of patients lost 5-10% of their weight in 6 months [163]. In a 2005 study, sibutramine was found to increase HDL by 15% compared to the placebo group in adolescent obese patients complemented with a 15% reduction in weight [161]. The on-going Sibutramine Cardiovascular OUTcomes (SCOUT) trial, will further determine if the weight management in obese patients with high CVD risk will decrease CVD outcomes [164].

Rimonabant

Another appetite suppressing drug, rimonabant (acomplia), by Sanofi-Aventis$^{(R)}$, and released in 2006, produced interesting results in weight-loss [165,166]. The drug targets the endocannbinoid system, which is currently widely investigated due to its modulation of feeding behaviour [167] and maintenance of energy homeostasis in the body [168]. The Rimonabant in Obesity (RIO)-Europe Trial in 2005 sought to determine the efficiency of this cannbinoid receptor antagonist and found that with a weight loss of 5-10%, an increase in HDL by 22.3% ($p<0.001$), compared to the placebo group at 13.4%, was seen with a well tolerated 20 mg/day treatment [169]. Similar results were seen in the RIO Lipid trial [165] and the RIO-North America trial [170]. This increase in HDL with rimonabant may be mediated by its up-regulation of adiponectin, as seen by the increase in Acrp30 mRNA with rimonabant in animal and cell culture models [171]. Aside from rimonabant's promising results in the reduction of metabolic impairments in the metabolic syndrome in clinical trials [166], its success was short-lived as the beneficial results did not outweigh the adverse side effects of psychiatric disturbances, such as severe depression and suicide, forcing this drug to be suspended in 2008 [172,173].

PLE/Tannins

Alongside orlistat, sibutramine and rimonabant, increasing evidence is mounting for the potential of pomegranate leaf extract (PLE) to join the pancreatic lipase inhibitor family [174]. Lei *et al.* have shown that daily administering 400 mg/kg of PLE to high-fat fed mice for 5 weeks was able to restore total cholesterol to HDL-C ratio to the level found in normal diet fed mice [174]. Of interest, the effect of PLE treatment on increasing HDL levels was more efficient than sibutramine (4.6 mg/kg daily on high-fat diet) [174]. When the dose was increased to 800 mg/kg of PLE, fat absorption also decreased compared to the control group (determined by fecal fat) [174]. Furthermore, Lei *et al.* determined that PLE was a pancreatic lipase inhibitor by its ability to decrease the rate of free fatty acid release from triglycerides [174]. A 50% inhibition of enzymatic activity was noted using 1 g of PLE [174]. To break it down further, the team determined that the main bioactive component in PLE are tannins, compounds containing tannic acid and ellagic acid [174]. Remarkably, tannic acid alone had the most prominent effect by inhibiting pancreatic lipase activity by 99% *in vitro* and decreased intestinal fat absorption [174]. PLE was shown to be most effective in diet-induced obesity and the inhibition of obesity and hyperlipidemia, further meriting continued research in development of this anti-obesity medication to the clinical level [174].

Anti-obesity medication is an ever-evolving strategy that promotes synergy of pharmacological agents with a healthy lifestyle in terms of diet, exercise and accepting obesity as a disease rather than inappropriate eating habits. This has motivated researchers to take immediate action in this approach and prompt future studies to determine the efficacy of this approach towards decreasing metabolic impairments, including low HDL-C, in the metabolic syndrome.

LIPID ALTERING DRUGS AND THEIR EFFECTS ON HDL LEVELS AND ON REDUCING THE RISK OF CVD

The current focus on raising HDL levels in order to decrease CVD risk is expected to ameliorate the global burden of CVD. An obese individual may have an increased risk of CVD if their HDL levels are below 1 mmol/L, with a combination of two other factors that increase LDL levels above 4 mmol/L, such as hypertension or cigarette smoking [148]. Even a simple increase by 1 mg/dL (0.026 mmol/L) in HDL may decrease cardiovascular disease risk by 2-3% [145]. Therefore, exploring this avenue along with other chemotherapeutics to decrease plasma LDL-C and triglycerides creates a combination therapy to treat most non-obese and obese individuals with their associated risk of developing CVD.

Statins

As previously mentioned, statins are the most effective LDL-C lowering drugs. A meta-analysis of 14 randomized trials of statins reported that over a 5 year span there was a 12% reduction in all-cause mortality for every 1 mmol/L (39 mg/dl) reduction in LDL as well as a 21% reduction in CVD with statin treatment [175]. However, their effect on raising HDL is modest at approximately 5-15% [130,176]. Accordingly, in the post-hoc analysis of the Air Force/Texas Coronary Atherosclerosis Prevention Study (AFCAPS/TexCAPS), it was shown that with the use of lovastatin, HDL increased by 6% and reduced the risk of the first acute major coronary events (AMCE) by 37% ($p<0.001$) [177]. Interestingly, patients with no history of atherosclerotic CVD but with low initial HDL, and showing a greater than 7.5% increase in HDL and a decrease in LDL by greater than 25%, possessed the highest reduction in an AMCE [177]. This links the modest increase of HDL and substantial decrease in LDL to decreased risk of an AMCE [177]. With this in mind, decreasing LDL levels through the use of a statin in patients with low HDL has also proven to significantly reduce the progression of atherosclerosis [130,178]. This review will not discuss the various statins but it is important to note that although statins have minimal effect on HDL levels, their use in combination therapy with HDL raising compounds has contributed immensely to treatment regimens of CVD patients.

Niacin (Nicotinic Acid)

Reduction in the synthesis of larger VLDL particles by the liver results in increases in circulating HDL levels. This is because VLDL exchanges its core lipids with HDL in the circulation [179,180], resulting in the formation of more triglyceride-enriched HDL that are more easily catabolised by hepatic lipase at the liver [181]. Niacin is one key drug that inhibits hepatic synthesis of VLDL at the liver and prevents subsequent VLDL secretion [130]. Niacin mediates changes in plasma lipid concentrations to increase HDL-C levels and decrease both LDL-C and plasma triglyceride levels [182]. Grundy *et al.* found a 52% decrease in plasma triglyceride levels and a further reduction of VLDL by 36% in the first month of niacin treatment. His group further determined that triglyceride levels were decreased within each VLDL particles, resulting in a decrease in VLDL size rather than in VLDL numbers [182,183].

Alone, niacin has one of the highest impacts in the decrease of plasma triglycerides. Niacin has been reported to reduce plasma triglycerides by 20-50% [130]. At lower doses, niacin has been shown to increase HDL levels and does so markedly by up to 15-35% [130]. LDL levels have also been shown to decrease (5-25%), but a higher dose of niacin is required [130].

Niacin may be administered in three forms: immediate response (IR) taken three times daily, which has been shown to produce the most adverse side effects of skin redness or flushing and gastrointestinal symptoms. The second is long-acting (LA) taken once daily. This form has shown to reduce flushing but poses a higher risk of hepatotoxicity [184]. The preferred regime is with extended release (ER) niacin or Niaspan®, administered as a single dose at night. It produces a sustained release, resulting in a slower absorption rate of 8-12 hours in which it decreases the intolerable side effect of cutaneous flushing observed with regular niacin [130]. This is due to its delayed absorption [130].

Niacin has been shown to be the most favourable current therapy for altering plasma HDL levels [130]. It was more effective at raising HDL levels (30%) compared to lovastatin (6%) and gemfibrozil (fibrate) (10%). Interestingly, lovastatin was the preferred medication for lowering LDL levels, and in combination with niacin, could target dyslipidemia comprehensively [185]. The combination of niacin with a statin increased acceptance for patients who cannot tolerate the high doses of niacin required to lower LDL and at the same time need to raise beneficial HDL [185]. Monitoring for liver function is commonly performed for each patient to reduce any mild side effects and maximize the combinatory effect [186].

The first combination product of niacin with a statin was niacin/lovastatin (Advicor®, Kos Pharmaceuticals Inc.) [187]. This therapeutic approach was attempted to further decrease coronary artery disease risk factors than either agent alone as each medication acts on different mechanisms within the body and has different effects on blood lipid levels. The increase in its efficacy than each product alone has made it of interest for patients who would require combination therapies for complex dyslipidemias such as type 2 diabetes mellitus and metabolic syndrome [187].

Fibrates

A second approach to raising HDL levels and decreasing overall coronary heart disease risk is by fibrate therapy. The main effect of these hypolipidemic drugs is in lowering plasma triglyceride levels, shown to be in the range of 20-50% [184]. Fibrates also increase plasma HDL levels in the range of 5-15% [130]. The mechanism by which fibrates act is complex and interlinked with various protein signalling cascades. For example, fibrates are a well documented agonist for peroxisome proliferator-activated receptor-alpha (PPARα), which is mainly expressed in the liver [188-190] and which acts to increase liver HDL biosynthesis and decrease liver triglyceride biosynthesis [191]. In addition, fibrates mediate the down-regulation of the *apoCIII* gene (inhibitor of lipoprotein lipase) [192] and the up-regulation of *apoAI* (the main protein component of HDL particles) at the liver. Fibrates also increase fatty acid oxidation at the liver, which in turn reduces serum VLDL triglycerides [190].

Three fibrates are commonly administered in the US: gemifibrozil, fenofibrate, clofibrate, and internationally: bezafibrate and ciprofibrate [130]. The latter two will not be discussed as they do not present any changes in HDL-C.

Gemfibrozil

Gemfibrozil was found to have the largest effect within the fibrate class of drugs at reducing coronary heart disease and stroke in the 5 year Veterans Affairs High-Density Lipoprotein Cholesterol Intervention Trial (VA-HIT) study group [193]. Specifically, isolated low HDL and low-risk LDL cholesterol patients were targeted in the VA-HIT trial in which gemfibrozil therapy (1200 mg/day) produced a decrease in major coronary events attributed to the increase in HDL [193]. Robins *et al.* determined that the decrease in coronary heart disease of 11% was attributed to a 5 mg/dL increase in HDL [40]. The VA-HIT study demonstrated for the first time that lipid treatment in which there is no effect on LDL levels, but in which there is an increase in plasma HDL and a decrease in plasma triglycerides, has a tremendous impact on reduction of cardiac events [194].

Fenofibrate

Fenofibrate was administered at 300 mg/d for 8 weeks to 16 patients with coronary artery disease and produced an increase in HDL apoAII levels in plasma [190]. An increase in apoAII induces a protective effect against coronary artery disease [190]. To explain this result, the transcript levels (mRNA) of apoAII were examined *in vitro* within primary cultures of human hepatocytes, and in human heptablastomas (HepG2) cells, and were found to increase after 500 μmol/L of fenofibric acid treatment [190]. This further led Vu-Dac *et al.* to conclude that the secretion of apoAII particles in plasma, as a result of fibrate therapy, is enhanced through the transcription induction of apoAII by nuclear hepatic receptor PPARα [190]. PPARα-mediated transcriptional expression of lipoprotein lipase upon fenofibrate treatment also contributes to its cardioprotective effect [188,195]. In general, fenofibrate is well tolerated as a monotherapy [196] and it side effects are mild gastrointestinal upset, with a small risk in developing gallstones [197], which is much less in magnitude than with clofibrate therapy [198]. The Fenofibrate Intervention and Event Lowering in Diabetes (FIELD) study reported that over a 5 year trial of 200 mg/day, patients produced an initial 5% increase in HDL [199]; however, the HDL species changed from the larger athero-protective HDL_2 to smaller HDL_3 particles, perhaps due to the increase in lipoprotein lipase. Concomitantly, no change was noted in apoAI; however, apoAII protein levels increased [200]. The increase in apoAII, however, was not enough to show a reduced risk of primary coronary events [200]. However, the lack of risk benefit may also be the result of previous statin therapy in patients in the placebo group, which thus diminished the potential beneficial increase in cardioprotection by fenofibrate [200]. Perhaps fenofibrate should not be considered an HDL-raising therapy [200]; however, FIELD did reveal a decrease in total number of cardiovascular events, indicating that fenofibrate's benefits in metabolic syndrome patients still merit investigation [199].

Bezafibrate

Bezafibrate efficacy and safety was evaluated in the Bezafibrate Infarction Prevention (BIP) study. The study showed an increase in HDL by 18% and a decrease in triglycerides of 21% in patients with stable angina or a previous myocardial infarction [201]. Of note, in a post-hoc analysis, patients with baseline triglycerides of ≥ 200 mg/dL displayed a decreased risk of myocardial infarction or sudden death by 39.5 % with bezafibrate treatment [201]. This remarkable decrease in risk requires further analysis and validation by a controlled-randomized trial specifically examining a high triglyceride patient group [201]. In a 16 year follow up for long-term mortality and HDL levels in the BIP study, a 22% decrease in mortality was found in the patient group with a higher-tertile HDL-C level after benzafibrate therapy compared to those with a lower-tertile HDL-C response [202]. Patients with a smaller increase in HDL reported a risk similar to the placebo group [202]. Thus, the increase in HDL may be associated with the decrease in mortality seen in bezafibrate therapy [202].

Ciprofibrate

Ciprofibrate is yet another member of the fibrate family which has a beneficial effect on HDL serum levels. Ciprofibrate therapy in patients with hypertriglyceridemia and low HDL-C in the CIPROAMLAT study reported an increase in HDL by 10 % when 100 mg of ciprofibrate was administered daily for 4 months [203]. A smaller study determined the effect of 100 mg/d ciprofibrate therapy in patients with Frederickson's type IV dyslipidemia phenotype [204]. After 8 weeks of treatment, there was a 15% increase in HDL and an overall reduction in total cholesterol [204]. Ciprofibrate has also been associated with increasing paraoxonase PON1 activity in patients with metabolic syndrome. The antioxidant effect of HDL is attributed to the activity of PON1 within HDL particles. PON1 prevents LDL oxidation and subsequent atherosclerosis [205,206] and patients who experienced a myocardial infarction have been shown to have low PON1 activity [207]. A study by Paragh *et al.* demonstrated that administration of 100 mg/d of ciprofibrate in patients with metabolic syndrome resulted in a significant increase in their serum PON1 activity, alongside a marked 26% increase in HDL, and a decrease in oxidatively modified LDL [206]. Similar to the other fibrates, ciprofibrate cannot address comprehensively all of the metabolic impairments in the metabolic syndrome, but it does show a great deal of promise in improving both HDL concentrations and function and other lipid abnormalities in the metabolic syndrome when combined with other therapies, such as statins.

CHOLESTERYL ESTER TRANSFER PROTEIN (CETP) INHIBITORS

CETP is a hydrophobic plasma glycoprotein that is excreted by the liver and commonly circulates in the blood bound to HDL [208]. CETP stimulates the net transfer of cholesteryl esters from HDL to other apolipoprotein B containing particles, such as VLDL [209], as well as the subsequent transfer of triglycerides from VLDL to HDL [210]. HDL triglyceride enrichment by CETP enhances subsequent hydrolysis and catabolism of the HDL particles by hepatic lipase at the liver [210]. Thus, inhibition of CETP may increase plasma HDL levels as the circulating HDL particles then are not as susceptible to degradation by hepatic lipase [181]. The use of CETP inhibitors to treat hypercholesterolemia was discovered during an analysis of germ-line *CETP* mutations, such as a splicing defect found in the *CETP* gene of individuals of Japanese descent [211]. The resulting deficiency of CETP activity produced a marked increase in plasma HDL-C levels, potentially atheroprotective for the patient [211].

Several approaches to decreasing the activity of CETP to raise HDL levels have been studied, such as oligonucleotide antisense [212], small molecule inhibitors [213,214] and monoclonal antibodies [215]. Of these, small molecule inhibitors appear to have taken most of the attention; however, their long term effects on cardioprotection have been questioned as early trials have shown that some of these inhibitors can have adverse effects on cardiac health [208].

Torcetrapib

The small molecule inhibitor, torcetrapib ((CP-529,414) 4-[(3,5-Bistrifluoro-methylbenzyl)-methoxycarbonyl-amino]-2-ethyl-6-trifluoromethyl-3,4-dihydro-2H-quino-line-1-carboxylic acid ethyl ester), by Pfizer® [213], was originally found to be extremely beneficial in increasing HDL levels; more recently, however, there has been controversy regarding its long-term benefits and ability to decrease coronary atherosclerosis [216,217].

Clark *et al.* presented a 14 day study of torcetrapib administered in 10, 30, 60 and 120 mg per day quantities, and also 120 mg administered twice per day [218]. Torceptrapib alone was well tolerated in a patient group of 40 [218]. Their HDL-C concentrations increased in the range of 16-91% [218]. The highest responders in this range occurred with the double dose of 120 mg daily [218]. A subsequent increase in plasma apoAI levels of 27% was also noted [218]. A beneficial decrease of 9-42% was found in patient LDL-C concentrations, as well as a reduction in apoB concentrations of 26%, with 120 mg tor twice daily torcetrapib [218].

This spectrum was similar to that of partial CETP deficiency described in humans with mutations in the *CETP* gene [218]. Functional mutations include intron 14 G to A mutation in at the +1 position [211,219] and the exon 15 D442G mutation [220]. Complete CETP deficiency is seen in individuals with the homozygous G to A mutation, with HDL lipid levels increased by 3 to 4 fold and apoAI by 1.7 fold [211]. Individuals homozygous for the D442G mutation exhibit partial CETP deficiency and a 1 to 2 fold increase in HDL [220]. Overall, the double daily dose of 120 mg appeared to maintain a $\geq$ 80% inhibition of CETP activity over a two week period [218].

In a 2006 study, the mode of action of torcetrapib was further examined [213]; its main function was found to be to promote binding between CETP and HDL, thus rendering the CETP enzyme inactive, without affecting HDL function [213,218]. Further work in 2004 by Brousseau *et al.* demonstrated in patients with low levels of HDL-C (< 1mmol/L), when given 120 mg of torcetrapib daily, with and without a statin (atrovastatin), HDL levels increased remarkably by 61% and 46%, respectively [221]. Furthermore, HDL-C levels increased by 106% when 120 mg of torcetrapib was administered twice daily [221]. Similarly, McKenney *et al.* found in an 8 week trial that 20 mg/day of atrovastatin administered together with torcetrapib (10, 30, 60 and 90 mg/day or placebo) increased HDL-C levels by up to 40.2% and decreased LDL-C levels by 18.9%, at the highest dose or torcetrapib [222]. Although they did not report a difference in all-cause mortality versus the placebo group, they indicated that the drugs were well tolerated, with only a minor side effect of a small increase in systolic blood pressure [222].

In 2007, Barter *et al.* published the findings of the Investigation of Lipid Level Management to Understand its Impact in Atherosclerotic Events (ILLUMINATE) trial, a 12 month study that reported that with increasing doses of torcetrapib, an increase of 72.1% in HDL and decrease of 24.9% in LDL resulted [223]. The trial was, however, prematurely terminated due to a surprising increase in cardiovascular events and all-cause mortality [223]. This was attributed to the off-target pharmacologic effect of torcetrapib in increasing systolic blood pressure, which was much more severe in the analysis compared to that found in the McKenny *et al.* and Brousseau *et al.* investigations with torcetrapib [221,222]. This may be due to the longer duration of the Barter *et al.* trial, lasting 12 months [223], compared to 8 and 4 weeks during of the McKenny *et al.* and Brousseau *et al.* trials, respectively [221,222]. Barter *et al.* reported data to support a decrease in plasma potassium concentrations and increases in plasma sodium and bicarbonate concentrations in the torcetrapib groups compared to the group administered only the statin [223]. A post hoc analysis revealed an excess of mineralocorticoids, including aldosterone, in the torceptrapib group [223]. This could potentially lead to the increased blood pressure effect seen with this CETP inhibitor [223]. If the off-target effects could be avoided in future CETP inhibitors, their full benefits in increasing plasma HDL levels and cardioprotection could be achieved [216].

JTT-705

A second small molecule CETP inhibitor is JTT-705 (Roche R1658 or dalcetrapib) originally produced by Japan Tobacco Inc. [208]. JTT-705 is a thioester which inhibits CETP by binding to Cys-13, thereby providing structural inhibition of CETP [224]. This drug was examined by de Grooth *et al.* in subjects with normal plasma HDL levels in daily doses of 300, 600 or 900 mg [214]. HDL levels were reported to increase by 16, 25 and 34% in the subjects administered 300, 600 or 900 mg daily JTT-705, respectively [214]; however, LDL-C levels only decreased maximally by 7% at the highest dose [214]. Furthermore, changes in LDL-C levels affected patients more with initially high LDL-C [214]. Only mild gastrointestinal side effects were noted and subjects were highly compliant with the therapy (100% compliancy) [214].

Huang *et al.* further examined potential anti-atherosclerotic effects of JTT-705 [225]. They found that 100-300 mg per day of JTT-705 administered to rabbits that were severely hypercholesterolemic increased their HDL levels by up to 2 fold versus control, by inhibition of CETP activity [225]. However, these parameters, surprisingly, did not affect atherosclerotic lesion progression [225]. Instead, lesion progression was strongly correlated with a decrease in total non-HDL-C levels and an increase in triacylglycerol levels [225]. Although this was not found in the study described by de Grooth *et al.*, an important difference in the experiments conducted by de Grooth *et al.* was that the patients were not suffering from severe hypercholesterolaemia [214]. Nevertheless, these results do indicate that patients with familial hypercholesterolaemia may benefit from a combination therapy with a statin to maximize the effect of CETP inhibition in increasing plasma HDL levels without a pro-atherogenic outcome [225].

Anacetrapib

A current CETP inhibitor under investigation is anacetrapib [208]. In a phase I trial including 50 patients with dyslipidemia (specifically, mixed hypercholesterolemia), anacetrapib (MK-0859) was administered over a 28 day period at a maximum dose of 300 mg per day versus placebo after a 2 week diet run, where low fat meals were given (373 kcal and 20% fat) [226]. The anacetrapib group showed a 129% increase in plasma HDL-C levels, a 47% increase in plasma apoAI levels, a 38% decrease in plasma LDL-C levels and a 26% decrease in plasma apoB, at the maximum dose [226]. It is interesting to note that a lower dose of 150 mg per day of anacetrapib produced comparable increases in HDL-C of 104% and apoAI of 33%, without producing an increase in blood pressure, as was the case with the higher 300 mg per day dose of anacetrapib [226]. This study, however, did not report a significant change in total plasma cholesterol or triglyceride levels as a result of treatment [226]. Compared to JTT-705 and torcetrapib, anacetrapib treatment was well tolerated and produced a greater lipid altering effect in comparable trial sizes and study periods as the other CETP inhibitors [226]. A larger current trial underway is the Determining the EFficacy and Tolerability of CETP INhibition with AnacEtrapib (DEFINE), which is examining the safety and efficacy of anacetrapib treatment (100 mg per day versus placebo) in patients with coronary artery disease or risk equivalent over 18 months [227]. Findings from this trial on lipid and safety outcomes are expected to be released in 2010 [227]. It is with great hope and anticipation that the current investigations on anacetrapib and other CETP inhibitors are able to avoid the adverse effects seen with torcetrapib and allows this avenue of medication to become successful in treatment of low HDL-C and CVD.

THE BENEFITS OF COMBINATION LIPID ALTERING THERAPY

The overall goal of lipid treatment is to reduce atherosclerotic events [228]. Many of the therapies previously discussed were designed to do just that through their ability to raise HDL levels. In order maximize the remedial effect each therapy produces, often in separate pathways, combination drug therapies and regimes have been proposed. Here we highlight briefly some combination therapies and their heightened benefits on plasma lipids.

The conflict between the efficacy of niacin and fibrates and their combination has been extensively studied, in which each appears to have its own benefits, determined by the specific patient population under study. In a comparative study by Guyton *et al.*, patients administered 2g of Niaspan produced a 2-fold greater HDL-C increase (26 % increase) and improved the total- to HDL-cholesterol ratio better than gemfibrozil (1.2 g with a 13 % increase in HDL) [228]. Niaspan was also more effective with patients who began the trial with low HDL-C levels [228]. An increase in LDL-C by 9%, occurring with gemfibrozil, was found when treating patients with moderate to high triglyceride levels [228]. Conversely, gemfibrozil has a beneficial effect in lowering LDL levels, especially when the patients have high initial LDL, as in the Helsinki Heart Study [229]. Gemfibrozil did have a greater reduction in triglyceride levels (-40%) compared to Niaspan (-29.5%), indicating a different mode of action than Niaspan [228].

The amalgamation of a niacin and fibrate may be the most effective approach as each has its own benefits. For example, niacins decrease the catabolism of apoAI, while fibrates increase the production of apoAI; thus, together these therapies increase the stability of the HDL apoAI population in plasma to a greater extent compared to each therapy alone [230]. An example of such a combination therapy is clofibrate with niacin; this dual therapy raised plasma HDL levels, lowered triglycerides levels and reduced mortality in patients with hypertriglyceridaemia to a greater extent than either therapy alone [231].

Niacins have also been examined with statin therapy; this was tested by the combination of pravastatin and niacin [232]. The mixed drug therapy reduced LDL levels to a greater extent (-49%), compared to either niacin (-21%) and pravastatin (-33%) alone, and increased HDL more effectively when combined (16%), compared to niacin (12%) and pravastatin (13%) treatment alone [232]. The combination regime was also well tolerated in the patient population with type IIA or IIB primary hypercholesterolemia [232]. Furthermore, the combination of statins and fibrates produced beneficial effects for patients with type II diabetes and hyperlipdaemia [233]. The dual therapy of atorvastatin and fenofibrate created a 22% further increase in HDL compared to each monotherapy [233]. This combination decreased the risk of the 10-year probability of myocardial infarction by 17% [233].

Statin therapy has also been attempted with CETP inhibitors. Patients with high triglyceride levels treated with a CETP inhibitor may have more VLDL converted to LDL by lipoprotein lipase [222]. This is a counterproductive effect of CETP inhibitors. The combination of a CETP inhibitor with a statin to upregulate the LDL receptor and clear excess LDL from plasma would work in synergy with the CETP inhibitor [222]. This was done in a 4 week trial combining 600 mg of JTT-705 with 40 mg of pravastatin [234]. The two therapies were able to decrease CETP activity by 30%, increase HDL by 28% and decrease LDL by 5%, without any adverse effects previously seen with CETP inhibition [234]; however, an extended trial period is still needed to determine the long-term cardiovascular effects of the CETP-statin combination therapy, however promising [234].

THE FUTURE OF HDL RAISING DRUGS

While the prevalence of obesity is expected to reach epidemic proportions globally, the mounting concern of how to strategically treat obese patients to reduce their overall high CVD risk has been daunting for medical practitioners [235]. Traditionally, the lipid target has been to reduce plasma LDL levels in these individuals. However, reducing LDL levels is not enough when HDL levels are also low, as they frequently are in obese individuals, or are simultaneously being lowered, as indicated by the Treating to New Targets (TNT) trials [236]. When patients reduced their LDL-C to less than 70 mg/dL in the TNT trials with statin therapy, and also unfavourably decreased their HDL-C as a side effect of their therapy, there was a sharp increase in risk cardiovascular events immediately after [236]. This was seen in patients with a total cholesterol-to-HDL-C of greater than 5 [237]. This further proves that a total cholesterol-to-HDL-C ratio greater than 5 classifies is a main cardiovascular risk factor [237].

Given the long-standing association of low HDL-C with CVD, increasing HDL-C levels has been an established target of numerous current therapies. Although a number of HDL raising drugs and pharmacological interventions have been developed in the past, there are multiple points in the HDL metabolic pathway that may be novel targets for future HDL therapies. Given the complexity of HDL metabolism, two main strategies have evolved in HDL therapies - namely increasing HDL quantity and/or improving HLD function. From the discussion above, it is clear that increases in HDL levels does not necessarily correlate with increased quality and better CVD outcomes [238]. However, interrelations between the two are not only unavoidable, but possibly work synergistically. Both strategies will be discussed in light of future therapies and drug developments surrounding HDL.

LRH-1

Plasma apoAI levels are primarily controlled through transcriptional regulation of the *APOA1* gene at the liver [239]. Currently, fibrates, which work as PPARα agonists, upregulate apoAI transcription, as described above [239]. However, their net result on plasma apoAI levels is minimal [239]. Liver receptor homologue-1 (LRH-1), an orphan nuclear receptor in the liver, has been shown to directly enhance apoAI transcription by binding to the *APOAI* promoter region [240]. In addition, suppression of LRH-1 by small heterodimer partner (SHP) also inhibited *APOAI* gene expression [240]. These findings indicate that LRH-I is a potential target for augmenting apoAI transcription through an LRH-1 agonist [75].

ENDOTHELIAL LIPASE INHIBITION

As the name suggests, endothelial lipase is expressed by endothelial cells and is anchored to the extracellular surface by proteoglycans [238]. Its phospholipase activity and high affinity for circulating HDL renders it an important remodeler and modulator of HDL levels [241]. By hydrolyzing the phospholipids on apoAI containing particles, HDL size is reduced by endothelial lipase [242]. Overexpression of endothelial lipase in animal models led to reduced HDL-C and apoAI levels, while inhibition or loss of endothelial lipase function led to augmented HDL levels [241,243]. In addition, clinical studies indicate that endothelial lipase concentrations are inversely correlated with HDL-C and *in vivo* animal studies suggest that inflammation and other aspects of the metabolic syndrome are directly correlated with plasma endothelial lipase levels [244,245]. Loss of function mutations have been associated with increased plasma HDL-C levels [246] in addition to decreased incidence of CVD in certain populations [247]. These studies implicate the endothelial lipase is a negative regulator of HDL and apoAI levels. Therefore, these findings provide a good basis for the development of an endothelial lipase inhibitor, as inhibition could decrease apoAI catabolism leading to increased HDL levels while having no affect on normal reverse cholesterol transport [238]. Although potent and specific endothelial lipase inhibitors have been discovered [248], the clinically significant effects of these in mice and humans are yet to be determined.

HDL Infusions

ApoAI's close association with HDL and its role in mediating reverse cholesterol transport makes it a good therapeutic target. Methods to increase plasma apoAI levels, such as apoAI infusions and administration of apoAI mimetic peptides will be discussed below. Zhang *et al.* were the first to show that apoAI promotes reverse cholesterol transport *in vivo* in animal models [249]. Mice were intravenously administered apoAI adenovirus and subsequently injecting with macrophage foam cells containing radiolabeled cholesterol [249]. Plasma samples collected 24 and 48 hours later contained significantly higher plasma apoAI (26.8 versus 0.4 mg/L in control mice) and HDL-C (11.4 versus 5.5 mg/L) levels [249]. In addition, apoAI infusion resulted in significantly higher cholesterol in liver and feces, with tracer levels in the liver being 35% higher over 48 hr compared to controls [249]. Therefore, macrophage-specific reverse cholesterol was enhanced with the overexpression of apoAI [249].

Additional studies in mice and rabbits indicate that apoAI infusion can cause rapid regression of atherosclerosis [250,251]. Of interest, apoE-/- mice fed high cholesterol diets were administered 18 injections over 5 weeks of either 40 mg/kg of synthetic HDL (apoA-I_{Milano}/phospholipid complex (PC), which will be discussed in detail below) or PC alone [252]. With PC treatment, atherosclerotic lesion progression was prevented and plaque composition was altered [252]. Specifically, there was a reduction in macrophage content by 46% and lipid content by 40%, compared to control mice [252]. Mice treated with higher doses of the synthetic HDL complex (80 mg/kg) for the same time period resulted in atherosclerotic regression, as plaque surface area decreased by 3.6% versus control [252].

Rabbit injury models, which develop lipid-rich plaques at the site of injury [253], were infused with synthetic HDL for 90 minutes [251]. Significant plaque regression was observed using IVUS, where plaque size decreased by 30% [251]. These animal studies prompted HDL infusion compounds to be applied to human subjects [251]. Infusion compounds currently investigated and discussed below include: ETC-216, an apoA-I_{Milano} phospholipid complex compound, and CSL-111, an HDL construct with wild type apoAI.

APOA-I$_{MILANO}$ PHOSPHOLIPID COMPLEX

The involvement of a mutant apoAI associated with longevity in humans introduced a novel strategy in increasing HDL's beneficial effects. The initial discovery of an apoAI familial disorder in Italy in 1980 presented the first example of a variation in the primary sequence of a plasma apolipoprotein [254]. The Italian variant, classified as apoA-I$_{Milano}$, presented interesting features in their carriers [254]. Patients possessing this point mutation of cysteine to argenine (R173C) [255,256] had low HDL levels (0.25 – 0.78 mmol/L) and high triglyceride levels [254,257]. Counter-intuitively, these patients did not present clinical signs of clinical atherosclerosis or any adverse cardiovascular effects and enjoyed longevity [257]. The mutation was found to be autosomal dominant and heterozygous carriers were found to also enjoy the apparent longevity associated with the apoA-I$_{Milano}$ mutation [257].

The direct effect of this point mutation was further analysed in 2001 in the Limone sul Garda Study in which patients with apoA-I$_{Milano}$ where compared to patients with primary hypoalphalipoproteinemia (HA). The decrease in HDL seen in the patients with apoA-I$_{Milano}$ did not produce any adverse cardiovascular effects as would be expected. They also did not show any structural changes to the arteries of the heart compared to HA patients, who presented a higher prevalence of atherosclerotic plaque formation [258].

The point mutation of R173C described above causes the formation of a disulfide bond dimer [255]. By replacing the mutation to R173S and to the conserved R173K mutation, the disulphide bond was consequently disrupted [259]. It was found that R173K had the most effective lipid binding capacity [259]. Furthermore, R173S was intermediate to R173C, indicating that the loss of arginine and replacement of cysteine affected the lipid binding ability of apoA-I$_{Milano}$ [259] and allowed for the generation of HDL particles to potentially increase their stability [54].

ETC-216

The potential enhanced anti-atherogenic effects behind the variant apoA-I$_{Milano}$ is related to its increased stimulation of first steps of reverse cholesterol transport, in which free cholesterol is mobilized from tissue such as the arterial wall to nascent phospholipid rich cholesterol-poor apoA-I lipoproteins and subsequently transported to the liver [255,260]. Thus a phospholipid and apolipoprotein complex becomes the vehicle of cholesterol transport [255,260]. Esperion Therapeutics followed this logic in their ETC-216 compound [261]. To determine if the beneficial effects of apoA-I$_{Milano}$ could be used to mimic nascent HDL, the variant was complexed with dipalmitoylphosphatidylcholine (DPPC) known as ETC-216 (Esperion Therapeutics, Ann Arbour, Michigan) [261]. ApoE-/- knockout mice were given a single high dose of 400 mg/kg and reported rapid mobilization of tissue cholesterol by 1.6 fold in the first hour [261]. During the 48 hour treatment period, a decrease of 40-50% was seen in plaque lipid and a subsequent 29-36% decrease in inflammation by macrophage [261]. These findings increased the interest into this complex as the time frame of 48 hours versus weeks required for statin therapy to clear cholesterol was a highly attractive advantage [261]. With that, the first human trial began in 2003 [262].

Nissen *et al.* determined the effects of the complex ETC-216 in humans through intravenous administration of 15 or 45 mg/kg per week for 5 weeks in patients with coronary atheroma burden [262]. They monitored the percent change in atheroma volume through intravascular ultrasound (IVUS) [262]. Combined treatments resulted in an absolute reduction of coronary atherosclerosis of 4.2% compared to placebo (saline) at 0.8% reduction [262]. Interestingly, and in comparison, a combination treatment of niacin and simvastatin showed only a 0.4% decrease in angiographic percent stenosis (narrowing of blood vessels) after 3 years [263] while a decrease of 1% in atheroma volume was observed after a 5 week treatment period with ETC-216 [262].

Although the above results showed a promising decrease in coronary atherosclerosis with ETC-216, larger clinical trials are needed to validate these finding and determine any potential side effects along with morbidity and mortality of this treatment [262].

CSL-111

The concept of using reconstituted HDL as a chemotherapeutic to treat atheroma burden was undertaken in 2007 by the Effects of Reconstituted High-Density Lipoprotein Infusions on Coronary Atherosclerosis (ERASE) trial [264]. The trial used infused reconstituted HDL (rHDL) consisting of apolipoprotein A-1 from human plasma combined with phosphatidylcholine from soybean (CSL-111) [264]. 183 patients were assigned to receive 40 or 80 mg/kg of CSL-111 versus placebo (saline) per week for 4 weeks [264]. Overall, the trial indicated that the effects of intravenous administration of HDL do not reduce the percentage change in atheroma volume as the absolute change in plaque volume was not significantly different between treatment and control [264]. However, significant plaque improvement was seen when measuring the change in plaque characterization indexes by IVUS and by change in coronary score when atherosclerosis progression and regression was measured by quantitative coronary angiography [264]. It should be noted that complications arose in the higher 80 mg/kg group as the treatment was discontinued due to liver function abnormalities [264].

In another study, individuals were given either a single infusion of placebo or 20 mg/kg·h of CSL-111 for 4 h [265]. Treatment with CSL-11 resulted in an approximate 1.3-fold increase in plasma HDL cholesterol and a greater than 2-fold increase in plasma apoAI above baseline [265]. These values were maintained after 72 hours of treatment, increasing HDL-C by approximately 1.4-fold and apoAI by 1.7-fold, above baseline [265]. *Ex vivo* studies of patient plasma after treatment revealed a greater than 50% decrease in platelet aggregation [265]. Similarly, *in vitro* experiments with platelets from healthy individuals demonstrated a 50% reduction in thrombus formation and a reduction of platelet function with CSL-111 treatment [265]. Of interest, the apoAI component of HDL or its receptor, scavenger receptor-B1 (SR-B1), had little effect in the above mentioned assays to reduce platelet aggregation [265]. However, incubation of platelets with soybean phosphocholine, representing the phospholipid component of HDL, attenuated aggregation and enhanced cholesterol efflux from platelet membranes, similarly to CSL-111 [265], which contributed to the loss of platelet hyper-reactivity [266]. Together, this data indicates that CSL-111 has the potential to be extremely useful in the treatment of atherosclerotic burden *via* multiple HDL anti-atherogenic functions – that is by mediating reverse cholesterol transport and also by anti-thrombotic effects.

The ability for CSL-111 to maintain its safety and efficacy in humans is yet to be determined. Furthermore, differences in individual benefits and combinatorial effects are yet to be investigated with HDL CSL-111 and the mutant apoAI complex, ETC-216, described in the previous section, meriting larger and long-term trials. In addition, intravenous administration for these infusion treatments is not usually tolerated well or practical. A less invasive method of drug delivery should be developed.

HDL MIMETIC PEPTIDES

Since the benefits of raising HDL through infusions potentially extended to reducing atherosclerotic progression and increasing longevity, other methods of directly raising HDL were pursued. This led to the development of HDL mimetic peptides, which hold many advantages over HDL infusions. Similar to the rationale of using apoAI for the HDL infusions, apoAI mimetic peptides are currently being studied. These mimetic peptides are a fraction of the size of the original apoAI protein, allowing for more convenient modes of administration – that is oral adiministration [267]. In addition, because of its small size, the peptides are not as difficult and expensive to manufacture as the HDL infusion constructs [267]. ApoAI mimetic peptides comprise only 18 amino acids (~2 kDa) versus 243 amino acid (~27 kDa) for normal apoAI [267]. However, their secondary structures are similar to apoAI, consisting of the lipid-binding class A amphipathic helices [268,269]. After screening and modifying many peptides, the most successful in terms of mimicking HDL functions at the arterial wall, and having optimal chemical and physical properties, was 4F, so named because of the 4 hydrophobic phenylalanines in the short amino acid sequence (Ac-D-W-F-K-A-F-Y-D-K-V-A-E-K-F-K-E-A-F-NH_2) [267]. Other peptides, including 2F and 5F were also screened, but they did not have the favourable chemical and physical properties of 4F, thereby inhibiting their biological function, or they had to be administered parenterally [270].

D-4F and L-4F

The stability of peptides once administered is extremely important in the drug's efficacy [271]. Some peptides may be rapidly degraded by various gut peptidases before reaching their target, reducing their efficacy. To overcome this, researchers have been generating peptide therapeutics with L or D-amino acids to improve their stability *in vivo* [270].

To examine this, LDL receptor null mice on a Western diet were orally administered twice daily both L and D-amino acid forms of 4F, named L-4F and D-4F respectively [270]. The investigators found that L-amino acid peptides were degraded and excreted while D-amino acids were not recognized by the peptidases and were found to remain intact in the circulation [270]. In addition, D-4F was able to decrease lesion formation remarkably by 79% [270]. Interestingly, there was no reported significant change in total plasma cholesterol or HDL-cholesterol levels [270]. Similarly, when D-4F was administered to apoE null mice, there was a 75% reduction in lesions shown with the lowest dose of 0.5 mg/mL peptide [272]. Recently, administration of multiple doses of D-4F to apoE null mice resulted in increased LCAT activity, apoAI and HDL levels after 24 hrs [273].

In addition to these findings, it was shown that D-4F may have an interesting anti-inflammatory functions. D-4F was reported to reduce inflammation in mice with influenza A by preventing the trafficking of macrophages within arteries after infection [274]. Subsequently, this function of D-4F was attributed to its ability to inhibit human type II pneumocytes (A549) from activating caspases and secreting pro-inflammatory molecules [275]. Researchers have also noted that HDL levels decrease as a result of infection, but with D-4F treatment, HDL levels rise past the pre-infection values [274]. Thus, D-4F as an apoAI mimic might have anti-inflammatory functions, which is significant considering patients with heart disease are at risk of complications such as myocardial infarction due to infection [276,277]. Moreover, the effects of inflammation and cytotoxicity of enlarged adipocytes in obesity may be alleviated by this treatment [278,279].

Recently, progress has also been made in L-4F treatments. When administered intravenously to cholesterol fed rabbits, L-4F was found to inhibit atherosclerotic lesions and improve the HDL and LDL inflammatory indices by the same degree as D-4F [280]. The obstacle, therefore, remained in its susceptibility to degradation in the digestive tract [281]. In 2009, Navab *et al.* found that orally co-administering L-4F with niclosamide, a drug traditionally used for treating tapeworm and other parasitic infections [282], in apoE null mice, rendered the peptide resistant to degradation by trypsin [281]. The successful absorption of L-4F subsequently led to atherosclerotic lesion regression and reduced inflammation [281]. The advantage of L-4F over D-4F is that, similar to apoAI, L-4F is rapidly degraded once taken up by peripheral tissues [283], while D-4F remains undegraded in tissues for extended periods of time, potentially leading to long-term toxicity and other unwanted side effects [281]. More studies investigating the association of niclosamide with L-4F, in addition to alternative agents, are needed to properly characterize this treatment.

The evolution of the D-4F treatment and safety in human trials was performed in 2008 in which patients with coronary artery disease were administered a single dose between 30-500 mg of D-4F under fasting conditions or 500 mg with a low-fat meal [284]. A single dose of orally administered D-4F was considered to be safe [284]. Moreover, absorption was greater under fasting conditions and increased in a dose dependent manner [284]. Although the authors made it clear that the study was not powered to study clinical effects on CVD or HDL function, plasma was taken from the subjects at various time points after treatment and was used to measure lipid parameters and the HDL inflammatory index in human aortic cells [284]. HDL inflammatory index is a measure of the inflammatory response induced by oxidized LDL in human aortic cells after the addition of the subject's HDL [284]. No marked changes were seen in HDL-C or apoAI levels in plasma after treatment, however, patients' HDL inflammatory indexes did significantly increased after 4 h of 300 mg and 2 h of 500 mg, compared to placebo [284]. Similarly, the addition of L-4F (10 ng/mL) to cultured human aortic endothelial cells significantly reduced the LDL inflammatory index, or the ability of LDL to induce an inflammatory response [284]. These findings indicated that the functions of HDL mimetics could substitute for the full-length HDL molecule.

DRUG THERAPIES IN DEVELOPMENT THAT TARGET IMPROVED HDL FUNCTION

As previously described, the most important anti-atherogenic function of HDL is its stimulation of reverse cholesterol transport. Strategies targeting reverse cholesterol transport are expected to reduce CVD incidence and are described below. However, HDL therapeutic targets should not be limited to enhancing only this anti-atherogenic aspect of HDL particles, as HDL is implicated in many other athero-protective effects, including anti-inflammatory effects, anti-oxidation actions, anti-coagulation and improvement of endothelial function. Hence, enhancing these properties in future HDL therapies are anticipated to augment the beneficial effects of HDL on atherosclerotic inhibition.

LXR Agonists

A novel therapeutic target still in its infancy stage is the liver X receptor (LXR) agonist. LXR is a transcription factor belonging to the superfamily of ligand-activated nuclear receptors [285]. LXRs are important modulators of cholesterol homeostasis and inflammation [286]. LXRs reside in the nucleus and complex with retinoid X receptor (RXR) upon LXR ligand stimulation; this complex then acts on LXR response elements (LXRE) in the promoters of target genes [287]. In the absence of an activating ligand, the LXR-RXR complex is bound to co-repressors of LXR action, including silencing mediator of retinoic acid and thyroid hormone receptor (SMRT) [288] and nuclear receptor co-repressor (N-Cor) [289]. Upon ligand binding, the co-repressors are replaced with co-activators and transcription of LXR/RXR target genes is initiated [290]. Both LXRα and LXRβ are activated by oxysterol ligands, which are oxidized cholesterol metabolites [285].

As previously described, ABCA1 and ABCG1 transporters play important roles in reverse cholesterol transport. LXRs directly upregulate ABCA1 [291-293] and ABCG1 [294-296] transcription, thereby enhancing reverse cholesterol transport [287].

In atherosclerotic mouse models, including apoE-/- and LDLR-/- knockout mice, the administration of the LXR agonist, GW3965, resulted in enhanced reverse cholesterol transport and regression of atherosclerotic lesions [54]. However, these benefits were offset by the increase in plasma triglycerides also induced by the LXR agonists, which can lead to increased risk for hepatic steatosis [297,298]. This is due in large part to LXRs also upregulating sterol regulatory element-binding protein-1c (SREBP1c) [299,300]. This leads to the activation of transcription of lipogenic genes, such as fatty acid synthase (FAS) [301], acetyl-CoA carboxylase (ACC), and stearoyl-CoA desaturase 1 (SCD1), as reviewed by Tontonoz *et al.* [302].

Recently however, Naik *et al.* were successful in showing that administering the LXR agonist, GW3965, to LDLR/apobec double knockout mice, resulted in enhanced reverse cholesterol transport devoid of increased triglyceride levels [303]. This was shown by injecting the mice with radiolabeled cholesterol-loaded macrophages and monitoring tracer levels in plasma and feces [303]. GW3965 treated mice excreted 64% more radiolabeled cholesterol compared to control [303]. In addition, GW3965 increased HDL concentrations by 54% in all treated mouse models [303]. These findings imply that reverse cholesterol transport is enhanced upon LXR agonist treatment [303]. Of interest, LXR-623, a synthetic LXR ligand, has been shown to decreases atherosclerotic progression and upregulate ABCA1 and ABCG1 upon oral administration in several animal models [304]. These findings suggest a novel means of managing and preventing atherosclerosis.

The development of LXR agonists appropriate for human therapeutics is still in its infancy. To date, there has only been one such trial. Katz *et al.* recently published their findings on the safety of administering a single oral dose of LXR-623 to healthy individuals [304]. In this randomized, double-blind study, the subjects were either given a placebo, or a single LXR-623 dose between 12.5-300 mg [304]. ABCA1 and ABCG1 mRNA was found to be significantly upregulated by 2 to 5 fold at 75 mg and higher, although further studies are merited in order to characterize the full impact of the LXR agonist [304]. LXR-623 was found to be relatively safe at lower doses, however, participants who received 150 mg or more suffered mild to moderate adverse affects relating to the central nervous system [304]. Blood parameters, such as HDL-C, apoAI and triglyceride levels were not measured in the study [304]. The full potential of LXR agonists is yet to be determined as further studies in humans are required in order to elucidate the mechanisms by which they enhance reverse cholesterol transport, and how they alter blood parameters such as HDL and triglyceride levels, in addition to the atheroma burden in humans. In the meantime, the findings to date suggest that enhanced ABCA1 and ABCG1 function and expression *via* LXR agonist ligands are good therapeutic targets for raising HDL concentrations.

HDL DELIPIDATION AND INFUSION

As discussed above, pre-β-HDL is more atheroprotective than mature, α-HDL subclasses, as it activates ABCA1 [305] and is an excellent acceptor for free cholesterol [36]. Consequently, pre-β-HDL is a key player in reverse cholesterol transport [17], and a continual supply of lipid-poor HDL is required in order to maintain effective levels of this anti-atherogenic function [306]. The notion of delipidating lipid-rich α-HDL led to the production of a delipidating agent called LSI-S955 (Lipid Sciences) [307]. In 2009, Sacks *et al.* determined whether such an agent could be used to enhance reverse cholesterol transport in human and nonhuman primate plasma [306]. They mixed plasma with sevoflourane and n-butanol, creating a delipidating environment which selectively removed cholesterol from HDL without affecting the other lipoprotein components in plasma [306]. After treating the human plasma with the delipidating reagents, HDL-C decreased by approximately 75% ($p<0.0001$) and VLDL slightly increased, however, LDL-C did not change [306]. The apoB concentration or proportion of VLDL and LDL was not affected [306]. In addition, ABCA1 mediated cholesterol efflux increased 7 fold compared to control treated plasma, whereas, SR-B1 mediated efflux slightly decreased [306]. After selectively delipidating pooled African Green monkey plasma, α-HDL decreased by approximately 20 – 30%, while pre-β-HDL levels increased by 30% compared to baseline [306]. Furthermore, weekly treatment of selectively delipidated monkey plasma to 12 monkeys with diet-induced atherosclerosis resulted in a significant reduction atheroma volume per mm lesion length, however, the atheroma volume percent decrease was not significant [306]. Importantly, no control monkeys were used in this portion of the study [306]. Of interest, no adverse side effects were observed when delipidated plasma was administered to animal models, including mice, pigs and monkeys [307]. These findings implicate that with more studies, HDL delipidation has potential therapeutic application to CVD patients [306].

CONCLUSION

The growing concern about the high and expanding prevalence of obesity globally, and its associated high CVD risk, is focusing attention on comprehensive evaluation of current therapies aimed at ameliorating the multiple metabolic impairments in obesity. Reduced plasma HDL levels is amongst the most frequent and deleterious metabolic impairment in obese individuals. With its multiple potent direct anti-atherogenic functions, including stimulating reverse cholesterol transport, evaluation of the HDL lowering effects of current anti-obesity therapies, lipid-altering drugs, and combination therapies is of intense current interest and focus. These current therapies include statins, fibrates, nicotinic acids and CETP inhibitors. Currently niacin is the best available pharmaceutical HDL raising therapy but has associated unpleasant, intolerable side effects. Future therapies aimed at raising plasma HDL levels and improving HDL anti-atherogenic functions are currently in development and hold high hopes in improving the HDL profile in obese humans. Some of the key drug therapies in development include apoAI mimmetics and LXR agonists, both of which can enhance HDL mediated reverse cholesterol transport. As with many multivariant disorders, obesity is considered a heterogenous disorder requiring multiple levels of treatment and, thus, both pharmacological and lifestyle interventions should be included in any therapies to ameliorate obesity-related metabolic impairments, including low plasma HDL[148]. The greatest concern lies in reducing the high CVD risk in obese individuals [235] which not only inflicts suffering in the patient but produces a great social and economic burden on health care systems globally [148]. Fortunately, with the intense focus on development of new more effective anti-obesity therapies which reduce CVD, the future in anti-obesity therapies is bright.

REFERENCES

[1] WHO. Obesity: Preventing and Managing the Global Epidemic,WHO, Geneva 2000.

[2] Grundy SM. Obesity, metabolic syndrome, and cardiovascular disease. J Clin Endocrinol Metab 2004; 89: 2595-600.

[3] Bays HE. "Sick fat," metabolic disease, and atherosclerosis. Am J Med 2009; 122: S26-S37.

[4] 1998 Clinical Guidelines on the Identification, Evaluation, and Treatment of Overweight and Obesity in Adults-the Evidence Report. National Institutes of Health. Obes Res 1998; 6: 51S-209S.

[5] The growing burden of heart disease and stroke in Canada, 2003, Heart and Stroke Foundation Canada, Ottawa 2003.

[6] Yusuf S, Hawken S, Ounpuu S, *et al.* Effect of potentially modifiable risk factors associated with myocardial infarction in 52 countries (the INTERHEART study): case-control study. Lancet 2004; 364: 937-52.

[7] Bays H, Ballantyne C. Adiposopathy: why do adiposity and obesity cause metabolic disease? Future Lipidol 2006; 1: 389-420.

[8] Bays HE, Gonzalez-Campoy JM, Bray GA, *et al.* Pathogenic potential of adipose tissue and metabolic consequences of adipocyte hypertrophy and increased visceral adiposity. Exper Rev Cardiovasc Ther 2008; 6: 343-68.

[9] Murray CJ, Lopez AD. Mortality by cause for eight regions of the world: Global Burden of Disease Study. Lancet 1997; 349: 1269-76.

[10] Yusuf S, Hawken S, Ounpuu S, *et al.* Obesity and the risk of myocardial infarction in 27,000 participants from 52 countries: a case-control study. Lancet 2005; 366: 1640-9.

[11] Lee JW, Im JA, Lee HR, *et al.* Visceral adiposity is associated with serum retinol binding protein-4 levels in healthy women. Obesity (Silver Spring) 2007; 15: 2225-32.

[12] Miller WM, Nori-Janosz KE, Lillystone M, Yanez J, McCullough PA. Obesity and lipids. Curr Cardiol Rep 2005; 7: 465-70.

[13] Despres JP. Cardiovascular disease under the influence of excess visceral fat. Crit Pathw Cardiol 2007; 6: 51-9.

[14] Adeli K, Taghibiglou C, Van Iderstine SC, Lewis GF. Mechanisms of hepatic very low-density lipoprotein overproduction in insulin resistance. Trends Cardiovasc Med 2001; 11: 170-6.

[15] Chan DC, Barrett HP, Watts GF. Dyslipidemia in visceral obesity: mechanisms, implications, and therapy. Am J Cardiovasc Drugs 2004; 4: 227-46.

[16] Nofer JR, Assmann G. Atheroprotective effects of high-density lipoprotein-associated lysosphingolipids. Trends Cardiovasc Med 2005; 15: 265-71.

[17] Rashid S, Genest J. Effect of obesity on high-density lipoprotein metabolism. Obesity (Silver Spring) 2007; 15: 2875-88.

[18] Castelli WP, Garrison RJ, Wilson PW, *et al.* Incidence of coronary heart disease and lipoprotein cholesterol levels. The Framingham Study. JAMA 1986; 256: 2835-8.

[19] Castelli WP. Cholesterol and lipids in the risk of coronary artery disease--the Framingham Heart Study. Can J Cardiol 1988; 4 (Suppl A): 5A-10A.
[20] Toth PP. High-density lipoprotein as a therapeutic target: clinical evidence and treatment strategies. Am J Cardiol 2005; 96: 50K-8K.
[21] Goldbourt U, Yaari S, Medalie JH. Isolated low HDL cholesterol as a risk factor for coronary heart disease mortality. A 21-year follow-up of 8000 men. Arterioscler Thromb Vasc Biol 1997; 17: 107-13.
[22] Assmann G, Schulte H, von EA, Huang Y. High-density lipoprotein cholesterol as a predictor of coronary heart disease risk. The PROCAM experience and pathophysiological implications for reverse cholesterol transport. Atherosclerosis 1996; 124 (Suppl): S11-S20.
[23] Sharrett AR, Ballantyne CM, Coady SA, *et al.* Coronary heart disease prediction from lipoprotein cholesterol levels, triglycerides, lipoprotein(a), apolipoproteins A-I and B, and HDL density subfractions: The Atherosclerosis Risk in Communities (ARIC) Study. Circulation 2001; 104: 1108-13.
[24] Stampfer MJ, Sacks FM, Salvini S, Willett WC, Hennekens CH. A prospective study of cholesterol, apolipoproteins, and the risk of myocardial infarction. N Engl J Med 1991; 325: 373-81.
[25] Schmitz G, Lackner K. High-density lipoproteins and atherosclerosis. Curr Opin Lipidol 1993; 4: 392-400.
[26] Kwiterovich PO, Jr. Lipoprotein heterogeneity: diagnostic and therapeutic implications. Am J Cardiol 2002; 90: 1i-10i.
[27] Anderson DW, Nichols AV, Pan SS, Lindgren FT. High density lipoprotein distribution. Resolution and determination of three major components in a normal population sample. Atherosclerosis 1978; 29: 161-79.
[28] Kane JP, Havel RJ. Introduction: Structure and Metabolism of Plasma Lipoproteins. In: Scriver CR, Beaudet WS, Sly WS, Valle D, Eds. The metabolic and molecular bases of inherited disease. New York: McGraw Hill; 2001, pp. 2705-16.
[29] Rashid S, Marcil M, Ruel I, Genest J. Identification of a novel human cellular HDL biosynthesis defect. Eur Heart J 2009; 30(18): 2204-12.
[30] Asztalos BF, Llera-Moya M, Dallal GE, *et al.* Differential effects of HDL subpopulations on cellular A. J Lipid Res 2005; 46: 2246-53.
[31] Kunitake ST, La Sala KJ, Kane JP. Apolipoprotein A-I-containing lipoproteins with pre-beta electrophoretic mobility. J Lipid Res 1985; 26: 549-55.
[32] Rye KA, Barter PJ. Formation and metabolism of prebeta-migrating, lipid-poor apolipoprotein A-I. Arterioscler Thromb Vasc Biol 2004; 24: 421-8.
[33] Yokoyama S. Assembly of high-density lipoprotein. Arterioscler Thromb Vasc Biol 2006; 26: 20-7.
[34] von EA, Huang Y, Assmann G. Physiological role and clinical relevance of high-density lipoprotein subclasses. Curr Opin Lipidol 1994; 5: 404-16.
[35] Vega GL, Grundy SM. Hypoalphalipoproteinemia (low high density lipoprotein) as a risk factor for coronary heart disease. Curr Opin Lipidol 1996; 7: 209-16.
[36] Rader DJ. High-density lipoproteins and atherosclerosis. Am J Cardiol 2002; 90: 62i-70i.
[37] Miller NE. Associations of high-density lipoprotein subclasses and apolipoproteins with ischemic heart disease and coronary atherosclerosis. Am Heart J 1987; 113: 589-97.
[38] Drexel H, Amann FW, Rentsch K, *et al.* Relation of the level of high-density lipoprotein subfractions to the presence and extent of coronary artery disease. Am J Cardiol 1992; 70: 436-40.
[39] Freedman DS, Otvos JD, Jeyarajah EJ, *et al.* Relation of lipoprotein subclasses as measured by proton nuclear magnetic resonance spectroscopy to coronary artery disease. Arterioscler Thromb Vasc Biol 1998; 18: 1046-53.
[40] Robins SJ, Collins D, Wittes JT, *et al.* Relation of gemfibrozil treatment and lipid levels with major coronary events: VA-HIT: a randomized controlled trial. JAMA 2001; 285: 1585-91.
[41] Rosenson RS, Otvos JD, Freedman DS. Relations of lipoprotein subclass levels and low-density lipoprotein size to progression of coronary artery disease in the Pravastatin Limitation of Atherosclerosis in the Coronary Arteries (PLAC-I) trial. Am J Cardiol 2002; 90: 89-94.
[42] Salonen JT, Salonen R, Seppanen K, Rauramaa R, Tuomilehto J. HDL, HDL2, and HDL3 subfractions, and the risk of acute myocardial infarction. A prospective population study in eastern Finnish men. Circulation 1991; 84: 129-39.
[43] Yokoyama S. Assembly of high-density lipoprotein. Arterioscler Thromb Vasc Biol 2006; 26: 20-7.
[44] Matsuura F, Oku H, Koseki M, *et al.* Adiponectin accelerates reverse cholesterol transport by increasing high density lipoprotein assembly in the liver. Biochem Biophys Res Commun 2007; 358: 1091-5.
[45] Ooi EM, Watts GF, Farvid MS, *et al.* High-density lipoprotein apolipoprotein A-I kinetics in obesity. Obes Res 2005; 13: 1008-16.
[46] Lewis GF, Rader DJ. New insights into the regulation of HDL metabolism and reverse cholesterol transport. Circ Res 2005; 96: 1221-32.
[47] Fitzgerald ML, Mendez AJ, Moore KJ, *et al.* ATP-binding cassette transporter A1 contains an NH2-terminal signal anchor sequence that translocates the protein's first hydrophilic domain to the exoplasmic space. J Biol Chem 2001; 276: 15137-45.
[48] Zannis VI, Chroni A, Krieger M. Role of apoA-I, ABCA1, LCAT, and SR-BI in the biogenesis of HDL. J Mol Med 2006; 84: 276-94.
[49] Dobiasova M, Frohlich J. Understanding the mechanism of LCAT reaction may help to explain the high predictive value of LDL/HDL cholesterol ratio. Physiol Res 1998; 47: 387-97.
[50] Rashid S, Uffelman KD, Lewis GF. The mechanism of HDL lowering in hypertriglyceridemic, insulin-resistant states. J Diabetes Complications 2002; 16: 24-8.
[51] Trigatti BL, Krieger M, Rigotti A. Influence of the HDL receptor SR-BI on lipoprotein metabolism and atherosclerosis. Arterioscler Thromb Vasc Biol 2003; 23: 1732-8.
[52] Ross R. Atherosclerosis--an inflammatory disease. N Engl J Med 1999; 340: 115-26.
[53] Glomset JA. The plasma lecithins:cholesterol acyltransferase reaction. J Lipid Res 1968; 9: 155-67.
[54] Toth PP. Novel therapies for increasing serum levels of HDL. Endocrinol Metab Clin North Am 2009; 38: 151-70.
[55] Rader DJ. Molecular regulation of HDL metabolism and function: implications for novel therapies. J Clin Invest 2006; 116: 3090-100.
[56] Wang N, Lan D, Chen W, Matsuura F, Tall AR. ATP-binding cassette transporters G1 and G4 mediate cellular cholesterol efflux to high-density lipoproteins. Proc Natl Acad Sci USA 2004; 101: 9774-9.

[57] Yancey PG, Bortnick AE, Kellner-Weibel G, *et al*. Importance of different pathways of cellular cholesterol efflux. Arterioscler Thromb Vasc Biol 2003; 23: 712-9.
[58] Barter PJ, Nicholls S, Rye KA, *et al*. Antiinflammatory properties of HDL. Circ Res 2004; 95: 764-72.
[59] Glass CK, Witztum JL. Atherosclerosis. the road ahead. Cell 2001; 104: 503-16.
[60] Baker PW, Rye KA, Gamble JR, Vadas MA, Barter PJ. Ability of reconstituted high density lipoproteins to inhibit cytokine-induced expression of vascular cell adhesion molecule-1 in human umbilical vein endothelial cells. J Lipid Res 1999; 40: 345-53.
[61] Calabresi L, Franceschini G, Sirtori CR, *et al*. Inhibition of VCAM-1 expression in endothelial cells by reconstituted high density lipoproteins. Biochem Biophys Res Commun 1997; 238: 61-5.
[62] Cockerill GW, Rye KA, Gamble JR, Vadas MA, Barter PJ. High-density lipoproteins inhibit cytokine-induced expression of endothelial cell adhesion molecules. Arterioscler Thromb Vasc Biol 1995; 15: 1987-94.
[63] Robbesyn F, Garcia V, Auge N, *et al*. HDL counterbalance the proinflammatory effect of oxidized LDL by inhibiting intracellular reactive oxygen species rise, proteasome activation, and subsequent NF-kappaB activation in smooth muscle cells. FASEB J 2003; 17: 743-5.
[64] Xia P, Vadas MA, Rye KA, Barter PJ, Gamble JR. High density lipoproteins (HDL) interrupt the sphingosine kinase signaling pathway. A possible mechanism for protection against atherosclerosis by HDL. J Biol Chem 1999; 274: 33143-7.
[65] Florentin M, Liberopoulos EN, Wierzbicki AS, Mikhailidis DP. Multiple actions of high-density lipoprotein. Curr Opin Cardiol 2008; 23: 370-8.
[66] Barter PJ, Baker PW, Rye KA. Effect of high-density lipoproteins on the expression of adhesion molecules in endothelial cells. Curr Opin Lipidol 2002; 13: 285-8.
[67] Mackness B, Hine D, Liu Y, Mastorikou M, Mackness M. Paraoxonase-1 inhibits oxidised LDL-induced MCP-1 production by endothelial cells. Biochem Biophys Res Commun 2004; 318: 680-3.
[68] Sugatani J, Miwa M, Komiyama Y, Ito S. High-density lipoprotein inhibits the synthesis of platelet-activating factor in human vascular endothelial cells. J Lipid Mediat Cell Signal 1996; 13: 73-88.
[69] Patel DA, Srinivasan SR, Xu JH, *et al*. Distribution and metabolic syndrome correlates of plasma C-reactive protein in biracial (black-white) younger adults: the Bogalusa Heart Study. Metabolism 2006; 55: 699-705.
[70] Navab M, Ananthramaiah GM, Reddy ST, *et al*. The oxidation hypothesis of atherogenesis: the role of oxidized phospholipids and HDL. J Lipid Res 2004; 45: 993-1007.
[71] Navab M, Berliner JA, Subbanagounder G, *et al*. HDL and the inflammatory response induced by LDL-derived oxidized phospholipids. Arterioscler Thromb Vasc Biol 2001; 21: 481-8.
[72] Rosenblat M, Vaya J, Shih D, Aviram M. Paraoxonase 1 (PON1) enhances HDL-mediated macrophage cholesterol efflux *via* the ABCA1 transporter in association with increased HDL binding to the cells: a possible role for lysophosphatidylcholine. Atherosclerosis 2005; 179: 69-77.
[73] Navab M, Hama SY, Cooke CJ, *et al*. Normal high density lipoprotein inhibits three steps in the formation of mildly oxidized low density lipoprotein: step 1. J Lipid Res 2000; 41: 1481-94.
[74] Galle J, Ochslen M, Schollmeyer P, Wanner C. Oxidized lipoproteins inhibit endothelium-dependent vasodilation. Effects of pressure and high-density lipoprotein. Hypertension 1994; 23: 556-64.
[75] Hausenloy DJ, Yellon DM. Targeting residual cardiovascular risk: raising high-density lipoprotein cholesterol levels. Heart 2008; 94: 706-14.
[76] Mineo C, Yuhanna IS, Quon MJ, Shaul PW. High density lipoprotein-induced endothelial nitric-oxide synthase activation is mediated by Akt and MAP kinases. J Biol Chem 2003; 278: 9142-9.
[77] Nofer JR, van der Giet M, Tolle M, *et al*. HDL induces NO-dependent vasorelaxation *via* the lysophospholipid receptor S1P3. J Clin Invest 2004; 113: 569-81.
[78] Fleisher LN, Tall AR, Witte LD, Miller RW, Cannon PJ. Stimulation of arterial endothelial cell prostacyclin synthesis by high density lipoproteins. J Biol Chem 1982; 257: 6653-5.
[79] Mineo C, Deguchi H, Griffin JH, Shaul PW. Endothelial and antithrombotic actions of HDL. Circ Res 2006; 98: 1352-64.
[80] Davignon J, Ganz P. Role of endothelial dysfunction in atherosclerosis. Circulation 2004; 109: III27-III32.
[81] Vane JR, Botting RM. Pharmacodynamic profile of prostacyclin. Am J Cardiol 1995; 75: 3A-10A.
[82] Ong AC, Jowett TP, Moorhead JF, Owen JS. Human high density lipoproteins stimulate endothelin-1 release by cultured human renal proximal tubular cells. Kidney Int 1994; 46: 1315-21.
[83] Kimura T, Sato K, Kuwabara A, *et al*. Sphingosine 1-phosphate may be a major component of plasma lipoproteins responsible for the cytoprotective actions in human umbilical vein endothelial cells. J Biol Chem 2001; 276: 31780-5.
[84] Okajima F. Plasma lipoproteins behave as carriers of extracellular sphingosine 1-phosphate: is this an atherogenic mediator or an anti-atherogenic mediator? Biochim Biophys Acta 2002; 1582: 132-7.
[85] Griffin JH, Kojima K, Banka CL, Curtiss LK, Fernandez JA. High-density lipoprotein enhancement of anticoagulant activities of plasma protein S and activated protein C. J Clin Invest 1999; 103: 219-27.
[86] Nicholls SJ, Cutri B, Worthley SG, *et al*. Impact of short-term administration of high-density lipoproteins and atorvastatin on atherosclerosis in rabbits. Arterioscler Thromb Vasc Biol 2005; 25: 2416-21.
[87] Nofer JR, Walter M, Kehrel B, *et al*. HDL3-mediated inhibition of thrombin-induced platelet aggregation and fibrinogen binding occurs *via* decreased production of phosphoinositide-derived second messengers 1,2-diacylglycerol and inositol 1,4,5-tris-phosphate. Arterioscler Thromb Vasc Biol 1998; 18: 861-9.
[88] O'Connell BJ, Genest J, Jr. High-density lipoproteins and endothelial function. Circulation 2001; 104: 1978-83.
[89] Dastani Z, Engert JC, Genest J, Marcil M. Genetics of high-density lipoproteins. Curr Opin Cardiol 2006; 21: 329-35.
[90] Klos KL, Kullo IJ. Genetic determinants of HDL: monogenic disorders and contributions to variation. Curr Opin Cardiol 2007; 22: 344-51.
[91] Bodzioch M, Orso E, Klucken J, *et al*. The gene encoding ATP-binding cassette transporter 1 is mutated in Tangier disease. Nat Genet 1999; 22: 347-51.
[92] Brooks-Wilson A, Marcil M, Clee SM, *et al*. Mutations in ABC1 in Tangier disease and familial high-density lipoprotein deficiency. Nat Genet 1999; 22: 336-45.
[93] Rust S, Rosier M, Funke H, *et al*. Tangier disease is caused by mutations in the gene encoding ATP-binding cassette transporter 1. Nat Genet 1999; 22: 352-5.

[94] Knopp RH, Paramsothy P, Retzlaff BM, *et al.* Sex differences in lipoprotein metabolism and dietary response: basis in hormonal differences and implications for cardiovascular disease. Curr Cardiol Rep 2006; 8: 452-9.

[95] Johnson JL, Slentz CA, Duscha BD, *et al.* Gender and racial differences in lipoprotein subclass distributions: the STRRIDE study. Atherosclerosis 2004; 176: 371-7.

[96] Knopp R, Zhu XD, Lau J, Walden C. Sex hormones and lipid interactions: implications for cardiovascular disease in women. Endocrinologist 1994; 4: 286-301.

[97] Mendelsohn ME, Karas RH. Molecular and cellular basis of cardiovascular gender differences. Science 2005; 308: 1583-7.

[98] Seed M, Knopp RH. Estrogens, lipoproteins, and cardiovascular risk factors: an update following the randomized placebo-controlled trials of hormone-replacement therapy. Curr Opin Lipidol 2004; 15: 459-67.

[99] Tilly-Kiesi M, Lichtenstein AH, Joven J, *et al.* Impact of gender on the metabolism of apolipoprotein A-I in HDL subclasses LpAI and LpAI:AII in older subjects. Arterioscler Thromb Vasc Biol 1997; 17: 3513-8.

[100] Applebaum-Bowden D, McLean P, Steinmetz A, *et al.* Lipoprotein, apolipoprotein, and lipolytic enzyme changes following estrogen administration in postmenopausal women. J Lipid Res 1989; 30: 1895-906.

[101] Collins P. HDL-C in post-menopausal women: An important therapeutic target. Int J Cardiol 2008; 124: 275-82.

[102] Walter M. Interrelationships among HDL metabolism, aging, and atherosclerosis. Arterioscler Thromb Vasc Biol 2009; 29: 1244-50.

[103] Kreisberg RA, Kasim S. Cholesterol metabolism and aging. Am J Med 1987; 82: 54-60.

[104] Hall G, Collins A, Csemiczky G, Landgren BM. Lipoproteins and BMI: a comparison between women during transition to menopause and regularly menstruating healthy women. Maturitas 2002; 41: 177-85.

[105] Kannel WB, Wilson PW. Risk factors that attenuate the female coronary disease advantage. Arch Intern Med 1995; 155: 57-61.

[106] Matthews KA, Meilahn E, Kuller LH, *et al.* Menopause and risk factors for coronary heart disease. N Engl J Med 1989; 321: 641-6.

[107] Ferrara A, Barrett-Connor E, Shan J. Total, LDL, and HDL cholesterol decrease with age in older men and women. The Rancho Bernardo Study 1984-1994. Circulation 1997; 96: 37-43.

[108] Wilson PW, Anderson KM, Harris T, Kannel WB, Castelli WP. Determinants of change in total cholesterol and HDL-C with age: the Framingham Study. J Gerontol 1994; 49: M252-M257.

[109] Rohrer L, Hersberger M, von EA. High density lipoproteins in the intersection of diabetes mellitus, inflammation and cardiovascular disease. Curr Opin Lipidol 2004; 15: 269-78.

[110] van der Westhuyzen DR, de Beer FC, Webb NR. HDL cholesterol transport during inflammation. Curr Opin Lipidol 2007; 18: 147-51.

[111] Craig WY, Palomaki GE, Haddow JE. Cigarette smoking and serum lipid and lipoprotein concentrations: an analysis of published data. BMJ 1989; 298: 784-8.

[112] Garrison RJ, Kannel WB, Feinleib M, *et al.* Cigarette smoking and HDL cholesterol: the Framingham offspring study. Atherosclerosis 1978; 30: 17-25.

[113] Ginsberg HN. Nonpharmacologic management of low levels of high-density lipoprotein cholesterol. Am J Cardiol 2000; 86: 41L-5L.

[114] Imamura H, Teshima K, Miyamoto N, Shirota T. Cigarette smoking, high-density lipoprotein cholesterol subfractions, and lecithin: cholesterol acyltransferase in young women. Metabolism 2002; 51: 1313-6.

[115] Maeda K, Noguchi Y, Fukui T. The effects of cessation from cigarette smoking on the lipid and lipoprotein profiles: a meta-analysis. Prev Med 2003; 37: 283-90.

[116] Rimm EB, Williams P, Fosher K, Criqui M, Stampfer MJ. Moderate alcohol intake and lower risk of coronary heart disease: meta-analysis of effects on lipids and haemostatic factors. BMJ 1999; 319: 1523-8.

[117] Okamoto Y, Fujimori Y, Nakano H, Tsujii T. Role of the liver in alcohol-induced alteration of high-density lipoprotein metabolism. J Lab Clin Med 1988; 111: 482-5.

[118] van der Gaag MS, van TA, Vermunt SH, *et al.* Alcohol consumption stimulates early steps in reverse cholesterol transport. J Lipid Res 2001; 42: 2077-83.

[119] Hendriks HF, Veenstra J, van TA, Groener JE, Schaafsma G. Moderate doses of alcoholic beverages with dinner and postprandial high density lipoprotein composition. Alcohol Alcohol 1998; 33: 403-10.

[120] Ito T, Nishiwaki M, Ishikawa T, Nakamura H. CETP and LCAT activities are unrelated to smoking and moderate alcohol consumption in healthy normolipidemic men. Jpn Circ J 1995; 59: 541-6.

[121] Nishiwaki M, Ishikawa T, Ito T, *et al.* Effects of alcohol on lipoprotein lipase, hepatic lipase, cholesteryl ester transfer protein, and lecithin:cholesterol acyltransferase in high-density lipoprotein cholesterol elevation. Atherosclerosis 1994; 111: 99-109.

[122] Riemens SC, van TA, Hoogenberg K, *et al.* Higher high density lipoprotein cholesterol associated with moderate alcohol consumption is not related to altered plasma lecithin:cholesterol acyltransferase and lipid transfer protein activity levels. Clin Chim Acta 1997; 258: 105-15.

[123] van TA, Groener JE, Scheek LM, *et al.* Induction of net mass lipid transfer reactions in plasma by wine consumption with dinner. Eur J Clin Invest 1995; 25: 390-5.

[124] Goldberg CS, Tall AR, Krumholz S. Acute inhibition of hepatic lipase and increase in plasma lipoproteins after alcohol intake. J Lipid Res 1984; 25: 714-20.

[125] Taskinen MR, Valimaki M, Nikkila EA, Kuusi T, Ylikahri R. Sequence of alcohol-induced initial changes in plasma lipoproteins (VLDL and HDL) and lipolytic enzymes in humans. Metabolism 1985; 34: 112-9.

[126] Valimaki M, Taskinen MR, Ylikahri R, *et al.* Comparison of the effects of two different doses of alcohol on serum lipoproteins, HDL-subfractions and apolipoproteins A-I and A-II: a controlled study. Eur J Clin Invest 1988; 18: 472-80.

[127] Mensink RP, Zock PL, Kester AD, Katan MB. Effects of dietary fatty acids and carbohydrates on the ratio of serum total to HDL cholesterol and on serum lipids and apolipoproteins: a meta-analysis of 60 controlled trials. Am J Clin Nutr 2003; 77: 1146-55.

[128] Berglund L, Oliver EH, Fontanez N, *et al.* HDL-subpopulation patterns in response to reductions in dietary total and saturated fat intakes in healthy subjects. Am J Clin Nutr 1999; 70: 992-1000.

[129] Herbert PN, Bernier DN, Cullinane EM, *et al.* High-density lipoprotein metabolism in runners and sedentary men. JAMA 1984; 252: 1034-7.

[130] Third Report of the National Cholesterol Education Program (NCEP) Expert Panel on Detection, Evaluation, and Treatment of High Blood Cholesterol in Adults (Adult Treatment Panel III) final report. Circulation 2002; 106: 3143-421.

[131] Rossner S, Bjorvell H. Early and late effects of weight loss on lipoprotein metabolism in severe obesity. Atherosclerosis 1987; 64: 125-30.

[132] Wolf RN, Grundy SM. Influence of weight reduction on plasma lipoproteins in obese patients. Arteriosclerosis 1983; 3: 160-9.

[133] Dattilo AM, Kris-Etherton PM. Effects of weight reduction on blood lipids and lipoproteins: a meta-analysis. Am J Clin Nutr 1992; 56: 320-8.

[134] Mooradian AD, Haas MJ, Wehmeier KR, Wong NC. Obesity-related changes in high-density lipoprotein metabolism. Obesity (Silver Spring) 2008; 16: 1152-60.

[135] Volek JS, Sharman MJ, Forsythe CE. Modification of lipoproteins by very low-carbohydrate diets. J Nutr 2005; 135: 1339-42.

[136] Meksawan K, Pendergast DR, Leddy JJ, *et al.* Effect of low and high fat diets on nutrient intakes and selected cardiovascular risk factors in sedentary men and women. J Am Coll Nutr 2004; 23: 131-40.

[137] Pelkman CL, Fishell VK, Maddox DH, *et al.* Effects of moderate-fat (from monounsaturated fat) and low-fat weight-loss diets on the serum lipid profile in overweight and obese men and women. Am J Clin Nutr 2004; 79: 204-12.

[138] Slyper A, Jurva J, Pleuss J, Hoffmann R, Gutterman D. Influence of glycemic load on HDL cholesterol in youth. Am J Clin Nutr 2005; 81: 376-9.

[139] Kokkinos PF, Holland JC, Narayan P, *et al.* Miles run per week and high-density lipoprotein cholesterol levels in healthy, middle-aged men. A dose-response relationship. Arch Intern Med 1995; 155: 415-20.

[140] Durstine JL, Grandjean PW, Davis PG, *et al.* Blood lipid and lipoprotein adaptations to exercise: a quantitative analysis. Sports Med 2001; 31: 1033-62.

[141] Drygas W, Jegler A, Kunski H. Study on threshold dose of physical activity in coronary heart disease prevention. Part I. Relationship between leisure time physical activity and coronary risk factors. Int J Sports Med 1988; 9: 275-8.

[142] Lakka TA, Salonen JT. Physical activity and serum lipids: a cross-sectional population study in eastern Finnish men. Am J Epidemiol 1992; 136: 806-18.

[143] Drygas W, Kostka T, Jegier A, Kunski H. Long-term effects of different physical activity levels on coronary heart disease risk factors in middle-aged men. Int J Sports Med 2000; 21: 235-41.

[144] Thompson PD, Yurgalevitch SM, Flynn MM, *et al.* Effect of prolonged exercise training without weight loss on high-density lipoprotein metabolism in overweight men. Metabolism 1997; 46: 217-23.

[145] Gordon DJ, Probstfield JL, Garrison RJ, *et al.* High-density lipoprotein cholesterol and cardiovascular disease. Four prospective American studies. Circulation 1989; 79: 8-15.

[146] Eckel RH, Krauss RM. American Heart Association call to action: obesity as a major risk factor for coronary heart disease. AHA Nutrition Committee. Circulation 1998; 97: 2099-100.

[147] Goldstein DJ. Beneficial health effects of modest weight loss. Int J Obes Relat Metab Disord 1992; 16: 397-415.

[148] Royal College of Physicians of London, Anti-obesity drugs: Guidance on appropriate prescribing and management.Sarum ColourView group, Salisbury, Wiltshire 2003.

[149] Fujioka K. Management of obesity as a chronic disease: nonpharmacologic, pharmacologic, and surgical options. Obes Res 2002; 10 (Suppl 2): 116S-23S.

[150] Coutinho W. The first decade of sibutramine and orlistat: a reappraisal of their expanding roles in the treatment of obesity and associated conditions. Arq Bras Endocrinol Metabol 2009; 53: 262-70.

[151] Zhi J, Melia AT, Guerciolini R, *et al.* Retrospective population-based analysis of the dose-response (fecal fat excretion) relationship of orlistat in normal and obese volunteers. Clin Pharmacol Ther 1994; 56: 82-5.

[152] Guerciolini R. Mode of action of orlistat. Int J Obes Relat Metab Disord 1997; 21 (Suppl 3): S12-S23.

[153] Torgerson JS, Hauptman J, Boldrin MN, Sjostrom L. XENical in the prevention of diabetes in obese subjects (XENDOS) study: a randomized study of orlistat as an adjunct to lifestyle changes for the prevention of type 2 diabetes in obese patients. Diabetes Care 2004; 27: 155-61.

[154] Hill JO, Hauptman J, Anderson JW, *et al.* Orlistat, a lipase inhibitor, for weight maintenance after conventional dieting: a 1-y study. Am J Clin Nutr 1999; 69: 1108-16.

[155] Broom I, Wilding J, Stott P, Myers N. Randomised trial of the effect of orlistat on body weight and cardiovascular disease risk profile in obese patients: UK Multimorbidity Study. Int J Clin Pract 2002; 56: 494-9.

[156] Kiortsis DN, Filippatos TD, Elisaf MS. The effects of orlistat on metabolic parameters and other cardiovascular risk factors. Diabetes Metab 2005; 31: 15-22.

[157] Halpern A, Mancini MC, Suplicy H, *et al.* Latin-American trial of orlistat for weight loss and improvement in glycaemic profile in obese diabetic patients. Diabetes Obes Metab 2003; 5: 180-8.

[158] Buckett WR, Thomas PC, Luscombe GP. The pharmacology of sibutramine hydrochloride (BTS 54 524), a new antidepressant which induces rapid noradrenergic down-regulation. Prog Neuropsychopharmacol Biol Psychiatry 1988; 12: 575-84.

[159] Luque CA, Rey JA. The discovery and status of sibutramine as an anti-obesity drug. Eur J Pharmacol 2002; 440: 119-28.

[160] Correa LL, Platt MW, Carraro L, *et al.* [Evaluation of the sibutramine effect on satiety with a visual analogue scale in obese adolescents]. Arq Bras Endocrinol Metabol 2005; 49: 286-90.

[161] Godoy-Matos A, Carraro L, Vieira A, *et al.* Treatment of obese adolescents with sibutramine: a randomized, double-blind, controlled study. J Clin Endocrinol Metab 2005; 90: 1460-5.

[162] Li Z, Oben JA, Yang S, *et al.* Norepinephrine regulates hepatic innate immune system in leptin-deficient mice with nonalcoholic steatohepatitis. Hepatology 2004; 40: 434-41.

[163] James WP, Astrup A, Finer N, *et al.* Effect of sibutramine on weight maintenance after weight loss: a randomised trial. STORM Study Group. Sibutramine Trial of Obesity Reduction and Maintenance. Lancet 2000; 356: 2119-25.

[164] James WP. The SCOUT study: risk-benefit profile of sibutramine in overweight high-risk cardiovascular patients. Eur Heart J 2005; 7 Supplement L: L44-L48.

[165] Despres JP, Golay A, Sjostrom L. Effects of rimonabant on metabolic risk factors in overweight patients with dyslipidemia. N Engl J Med 2005; 353: 2121-34.

[166] Kyrou I, Valsamakis G, Tsigos C. The endocannabinoid system as a target for the treatment of visceral obesity and metabolic syndrome. Ann N Y Acad Sci 2006; 1083: 270-305.

[167] Mechoulam R, Fride E. Physiology. A hunger for cannabinoids. Nature 2001; 410: 763, 765.
[168] Cota D, Marsicano G, Tschop M, *et al*. The endogenous cannabinoid system affects energy balance *via* central orexigenic drive and peripheral lipogenesis. J Clin Invest 2003; 112: 423-31.
[169] Van Gaal LF, Rissanen AM, Scheen AJ, Ziegler O, Rossner S. Effects of the cannabinoid-1 receptor blocker rimonabant on weight reduction and cardiovascular risk factors in overweight patients: 1-year experience from the RIO-Europe study. Lancet 2005; 365: 1389-97.
[170] Pi-Sunyer FX, Aronne LJ, Heshmati HM, Devin J, Rosenstock J. Effect of rimonabant, a cannabinoid-1 receptor blocker, on weight and cardiometabolic risk factors in overweight or obese patients: RIO-North America: a randomized controlled trial. JAMA 2006; 295: 761-75.
[171] Bensaid M, Gary-Bobo M, Esclangon A, *et al*. The cannabinoid CB1 receptor antagonist SR141716 increases Acrp30 mRNA expression in adipose tissue of obese fa/fa rats and in cultured adipocyte cells. Mol Pharmacol 2003; 63: 908-14.
[172] Hill MN, Gorzalka BB. Impairments in endocannabinoid signaling and depressive illness. JAMA 2009; 301: 1165-6.
[173] Janero DR, Makriyannis A. Cannabinoid receptor antagonists: pharmacological opportunities, clinical experience, and translational prognosis. Exper Opin Emerg Drugs 2009; 14: 43-65.
[174] Lei F, Zhang XN, Wang W, *et al*. Evidence of anti-obesity effects of the pomegranate leaf extract in high-fat diet induced obese mice. Int J Obes (Lond) 2007; 31: 1023-9.
[175] Baigent C, Keech A, Kearney PM, *et al*. Efficacy and safety of cholesterol-lowering treatment: prospective meta-analysis of data from 90,056 participants in 14 randomised trials of statins. Lancet 2005; 366: 1267-78.
[176] LaRosa JC, He J, Vupputuri S. Effect of statins on risk of coronary disease: a meta-analysis of randomized controlled trials. JAMA 1999; 282: 2340-6.
[177] Cui Y, Watson DJ, Girman CJ, *et al*. Effects of increasing high-density lipoprotein cholesterol and decreasing low-density lipoprotein cholesterol on the incidence of first acute coronary events (from the Air Force/Texas Coronary Atherosclerosis Prevention Study). Am J Cardiol 2009; 104: 829-34.
[178] Herd JA, Ballantyne CM, Farmer JA, *et al*. Effects of fluvastatin on coronary atherosclerosis in patients with mild to moderate cholesterol elevations (Lipoprotein and Coronary Atherosclerosis Study [LCAS]). Am J Cardiol 1997; 80: 278-86.
[179] Foger B, Ritsch A, Doblinger A, Wessels H, Patsch JR. Relationship of plasma cholesteryl ester transfer protein to HDL cholesterol. Studies in normotriglyceridemia and moderate hypertriglyceridemia. Arterioscler Thromb Vasc Biol 1996; 16: 1430-6.
[180] Mann CJ, Yen FT, Grant AM, Bihain BE. Mechanism of plasma cholesteryl ester transfer in hypertriglyceridemia. J Clin Invest 1991; 88: 2059-66.
[181] Rashid S, Watanabe T, Sakaue T, Lewis GF. Mechanisms of HDL lowering in insulin resistant, hypertriglyceridemic states: the combined effect of HDL triglyceride enrichment and elevated hepatic lipase activity. Clin Biochem 2003; 36: 421-9.
[182] Bays H. Safety of niacin and simvastatin combination therapy. Am J Cardiol 2008; 101: 3B-8B.
[183] Grundy SM, Mok HY, Zech L, Berman M. Influence of nicotinic acid on metabolism of cholesterol and triglycerides in man. J Lipid Res 1981; 22: 24-36.
[184] McKenney J. New perspectives on the use of niacin in the treatment of lipid disorders. Arch Intern Med 2004; 164: 697-705.
[185] Vega GL, Grundy SM. Lipoprotein responses to treatment with lovastatin, gemfibrozil, and nicotinic acid in normolipidemic patients with hypoalphalipoproteinemia. Arch Intern Med 1994; 154: 73-82.
[186] Guyton JR, Capuzzi DM. Treatment of hyperlipidemia with combined niacin-statin regimens. Am J Cardiol 1998; 82: 82U-4U.
[187] Bays HE. Extended-release niacin/lovastatin: the first combination product for dyslipidemia. Expert Rev Cardiovasc Ther 2004; 2: 485-501.
[188] Fruchart JC, Brewer HB, Jr., Leitersdorf E. Consensus for the use of fibrates in the treatment of dyslipoproteinemia and coronary heart disease. Fibrate Consensus Group. Am J Cardiol 1998; 81: 912-7.
[189] Staels B, Dallongeville J, Auwerx J, *et al*. Mechanism of action of fibrates on lipid and lipoprotein metabolism. Circulation 1998; 98: 2088-93.
[190] Vu-Dac N, Schoonjans K, Kosykh V, *et al*. Fibrates increase human apolipoprotein A-II expression through activation of the peroxisome proliferator-activated receptor. J Clin Invest 1995; 96: 741-50.
[191] Duez H, Chao YS, Hernandez M, *et al*. Reduction of atherosclerosis by the peroxisome proliferator-activated receptor alpha agonist fenofibrate in mice. J Biol Chem 2002; 277: 48051-7.
[192] Staels B, Vu-Dac N, Kosykh VA, *et al*. Fibrates downregulate apolipoprotein C-III expression independent of induction of peroxisomal acyl coenzyme A oxidase. A potential mechanism for the hypolipidemic action of fibrates. J Clin Invest 1995; 95: 705-12.
[193] Rubins HB, Robins SJ, Collins D, *et al*. Gemfibrozil for the secondary prevention of coronary heart disease in men with low levels of high-density lipoprotein cholesterol. Veterans Affairs High-Density Lipoprotein Cholesterol Intervention Trial Study Group. N Engl J Med 1999; 341: 410-8.
[194] Rubins HB, Robins SJ. Conclusions from the VA-HIT study. Am J Cardiol 2000; 86: 543-4.
[195] Schoonjans K, Peinado-Onsurbe J, Lefebvre AM, *et al*. PPARalpha and PPARgamma activators direct a distinct tissue-specific transcriptional response *via* a PPRE in the lipoprotein lipase gene. EMBO J 1996; 15: 5336-48.
[196] Keating GM, Croom KF. Fenofibrate: a review of its use in primary dyslipidaemia, the metabolic syndrome and type 2 diabetes mellitus. Drugs 2007; 67: 121-53.
[197] Palmer RH. Effects of fibric acid derivatives on biliary lipid composition. Am J Med 1987; 83: 37-43.
[198] Havel RJ, Kane JP. Drugs and lipid metabolism. Annu Rev Pharmacol 1973; 13: 287-308.
[199] Keech A, Simes RJ, Barter P, *et al*. Effects of long-term fenofibrate therapy on cardiovascular events in 9795 people with type 2 diabetes mellitus (the FIELD study): randomised controlled trial. Lancet 2005; 366: 1849-61.
[200] Hiukka A, Leinonen E, Jauhiainen M, *et al*. Long-term effects of fenofibrate on VLDL and HDL subspecies in participants with type 2 diabetes mellitus. Diabetologia 2007; 50: 2067-75.
[201] Secondary prevention by raising HDL cholesterol and reducing triglycerides in patients with coronary artery disease: the Bezafibrate Infarction Prevention (BIP) study. Circulation 2000; 102: 21-7.
[202] Goldenberg I, Boyko V, Tennenbaum A, *et al*. Long-term benefit of high-density lipoprotein cholesterol-raising therapy with bezafibrate: 16-year mortality follow-up of the bezafibrate infarction prevention trial. Arch Intern Med 2009; 169: 508-14.

[203] Aguilar-Salinas CA, Assis-Luores-Vale A, Stockins B, *et al.* Ciprofibrate therapy in patients with hypertriglyceridemia and low high density lipoprotein (HDL)-cholesterol: greater reduction of non-HDL cholesterol in subjects with excess body weight (The CIPROAMLAT study). Cardiovasc Diabetol 2004; 3: 8.
[204] Bermudez-Pirela V, Souki A, Cano-Ponce C, *et al.* Ciprofibrate treatment decreases non-high density lipoprotein cholesterol and triglycerides and increases high density lipoprotein cholesterol in patients with Frederickson type IV dyslipidemia phenotype. Am J Ther 2007; 14: 213-20.
[205] Mackness MI, Durrington PN. HDL, its enzymes and its potential to influence lipid peroxidation. Atherosclerosis 1995; 115: 243-53.
[206] Paragh G, Seres I, Harangi M, *et al.* Ciprofibrate increases paraoxonase activity in patients with metabolic syndrome. Br J Clin Pharmacol 2006; 61: 694-701.
[207] McElveen J, Mackness MI, Colley CM, *et al.* Distribution of paraoxon hydrolytic activity in the serum of patients after myocardial infarction. Clin Chem 1986; 32: 671-3.
[208] Joy T, Hegele RA. The end of the road for CETP inhibitors after torcetrapib? Curr Opin Cardiol 2009; 24: 364-71.
[209] Tall AR. Plasma cholesteryl ester transfer protein. J Lipid Res 1993; 34: 1255-74.
[210] Barter PJ, Brewer HB, Jr., Chapman MJ, *et al.* Cholesteryl ester transfer protein: a novel target for raising HDL and inhibiting atherosclerosis. Arterioscler Thromb Vasc Biol 2003; 23: 160-7.
[211] Inazu A, Brown ML, Hesler CB, *et al.* Increased high-density lipoprotein levels caused by a common cholesteryl-ester transfer protein gene mutation. N Engl J Med 1990; 323: 1234-8.
[212] Sugano M, Makino N, Sawada S, *et al.* Effect of antisense oligonucleotides against cholesteryl ester transfer protein on the development of atherosclerosis in cholesterol-fed rabbits. J Biol Chem 1998; 273: 5033-6.
[213] Clark RW, Ruggeri RB, Cunningham D, Bamberger MJ. Description of the torcetrapib series of cholesteryl ester transfer protein inhibitors, including mechanism of action. J Lipid Res 2006; 47: 537-52.
[214] de Grooth GJ, Kuivenhoven JA, Stalenhoef AF, *et al.* Efficacy and safety of a novel cholesteryl ester transfer protein inhibitor, JTT-705, in humans: a randomized phase II dose-response study. Circulation 2002; 105: 2159-65.
[215] Swenson TL, Hesler CB, Brown ML, *et al.* Mechanism of cholesteryl ester transfer protein inhibition by a neutralizing monoclonal antibody and mapping of the monoclonal antibody epitope. J Biol Chem 1989; 264: 14318-26.
[216] Nicholls SJ, Tuzcu EM, Brennan DM, Tardif JC, Nissen SE. Cholesteryl ester transfer protein inhibition, high-density lipoprotein raising, and progression of coronary atherosclerosis: insights from ILLUSTRATE (Investigation of Lipid Level Management Using Coronary Ultrasound to Assess Reduction of Atherosclerosis by CETP Inhibition and HDL Elevation). Circulation 2008; 118: 2506-14.
[217] Nissen SE, Tardif JC, Nicholls SJ, *et al.* Effect of torcetrapib on the progression of coronary atherosclerosis. N Engl J Med 2007; 356: 1304-16.
[218] Clark RW, Sutfin TA, Ruggeri RB, *et al.* Raising high-density lipoprotein in humans through inhibition of cholesteryl ester transfer protein: an initial multidose study of torcetrapib. Arterioscler Thromb Vasc Biol 2004; 24: 490-7.
[219] Brown ML, Inazu A, Hesler CB, *et al.* Molecular basis of lipid transfer protein deficiency in a family with increased high-density lipoproteins. Nature 1989; 342: 448-51.
[220] Inazu A, Jiang XC, Haraki T, *et al.* Genetic cholesteryl ester transfer protein deficiency caused by two prevalent mutations as a major determinant of increased levels of high density lipoprotein cholesterol. J Clin Invest 1994; 94: 1872-82.
[221] Brousseau ME, Schaefer EJ, Wolfe ML, *et al.* Effects of an inhibitor of cholesteryl ester transfer protein on HDL cholesterol. N Engl J Med 2004; 350: 1505-15.
[222] McKenney JM, Davidson MH, Shear CL, Revkin JH. Efficacy and safety of torcetrapib, a novel cholesteryl ester transfer protein inhibitor, in individuals with below-average high-density lipoprotein cholesterol levels on a background of atorvastatin. J Am Coll Cardiol 2006; 48: 1782-90.
[223] Barter PJ, Caulfield M, Eriksson M, *et al.* Effects of torcetrapib in patients at high risk for coronary events. N Engl J Med 2007; 357: 2109-22.
[224] Okamoto H, Yonemori F, Wakitani K, *et al.* A cholesteryl ester transfer protein inhibitor attenuates atherosclerosis in rabbits. Nature 2000; 406: 203-7.
[225] Huang Z, Inazu A, Nohara A, Higashikata T, Mabuchi H. Cholesteryl ester transfer protein inhibitor (JTT-705) and the development of atherosclerosis in rabbits with severe hypercholesterolaemia. Clin Sci (Lond) 2002; 103: 587-94.
[226] Krishna R, Anderson MS, Bergman AJ, *et al.* Effect of the cholesteryl ester transfer protein inhibitor, anacetrapib, on lipoproteins in patients with dyslipidaemia and on 24-h ambulatory blood pressure in healthy individuals: two double-blind, randomised placebo-controlled phase I studies. Lancet 2007; 370: 1907-14.
[227] Cannon CP, Dansky HM, Davidson M, *et al.* Design of the DEFINE trial: determining the EFficacy and tolerability of CETP INhibition with AnacEtrapib. Am Heart J 2009; 158: 513-9.
[228] Guyton JR, Blazing MA, Hagar J, *et al.* Extended-release niacin vs gemfibrozil for the treatment of low levels of high-density lipoprotein cholesterol. Niaspan-Gemfibrozil Study Group. Arch Intern Med 2000; 160: 1177-84.
[229] Frick MH, Elo O, Haapa K, *et al.* Helsinki Heart Study: primary-prevention trial with gemfibrozil in middle-aged men with dyslipidemia. Safety of treatment, changes in risk factors, and incidence of coronary heart disease. N Engl J Med 1987; 317: 1237-45.
[230] Kashyap ML. Mechanistic studies of high-density lipoproteins. Am J Cardiol 1998; 82: 42U-8U.
[231] Carlson LA, Rosenhamer G. Reduction of mortality in the Stockholm Ischaemic Heart Disease Secondary Prevention Study by combined treatment with clofibrate and nicotinic acid. Acta Med Scand 1988; 223: 405-18.
[232] Davignon J, Roederer G, Montigny M, *et al.* Comparative efficacy and safety of pravastatin, nicotinic acid and the two combined in patients with hypercholesterolemia. Am J Cardiol 1994; 73: 339-45.
[233] Athyros VG, Papageorgiou AA, Athyrou VV, Demitriadis DS, Kontopoulos AG. Atorvastatin and micronized fenofibrate alone and in combination in type 2 diabetes with combined hyperlipidemia. Diabetes Care 2002; 25: 1198-202.
[234] Kuivenhoven JA, de Grooth GJ, Kawamura H, *et al.* Effectiveness of inhibition of cholesteryl ester transfer protein by JTT-705 in combination with pravastatin in type II dyslipidemia. Am J Cardiol 2005; 95: 1085-8.
[235] Adan RA, Vanderschuren LJ, la Fleur SE. Anti-obesity drugs and neural circuits of feeding. Trends Pharmacol Sci 2008; 29: 208-17.
[236] Barter P, Gotto AM, LaRosa JC, *et al.* HDL cholesterol, very low levels of LDL cholesterol, and cardiovascular events. N Engl J Med 2007; 357: 1301-10.

[237] Paccaud F, Schluter-Fasmeyer V, Wietlisbach V, Bovet P. Dyslipidemia and abdominal obesity: an assessment in three general populations. J Clin Epidemiol 2000; 53: 393-400.
[238] Duffy D, Rader DJ. Update on strategies to increase HDL quantity and function. Nat Rev Cardiol 2009; 6: 455-63.
[239] Mooradian AD, Haas MJ, Wong NC. Transcriptional control of apolipoprotein A-I gene expression in diabetes. Diabetes 2004; 53: 513-20.
[240] Delerive P, Galardi CM, Bisi JE, Nicodeme E, Goodwin B. Identification of liver receptor homolog-1 as a novel regulator of apolipoprotein AI gene transcription. Mol Endocrinol 2004; 18: 2378-87.
[241] Jaye M, Lynch KJ, Krawiec J, *et al.* A novel endothelial-derived lipase that modulates HDL metabolism. Nat Genet 1999; 21: 424-8.
[242] Jahangiri A, Rader DJ, Marchadier D, *et al.* Evidence that endothelial lipase remodels high density lipoproteins without mediating the dissociation of apolipoprotein A-I. J Lipid Res 2005; 46: 896-903.
[243] Jin W, Millar JS, Broedl U, Glick JM, Rader DJ. Inhibition of endothelial lipase causes increased HDL cholesterol levels *in vivo*. J Clin Invest 2003; 111: 357-62.
[244] Badellino KO, Wolfe ML, Reilly MP, Rader DJ. Endothelial lipase concentrations are increased in metabolic syndrome and associated with coronary atherosclerosis. PLoS Med 2006; 3: e22.
[245] Badellino KO, Wolfe ML, Reilly MP, Rader DJ. Endothelial lipase is increased *in vivo* by inflammation in humans. Circulation 2008; 117: 678-85.
[246] deLemos AS, Wolfe ML, Long CJ, Sivapackianathan R, Rader DJ. Identification of genetic variants in endothelial lipase in persons with elevated high-density lipoprotein cholesterol. Circulation 2002; 106: 1321-6.
[247] Tang NP, Wang LS, Yang L, *et al.* Protective effect of an endothelial lipase gene variant on coronary artery disease in a Chinese population. J Lipid Res 2008; 49: 369-75.
[248] Goodman KB, Bury MJ, Cheung M, *et al.* Discovery of potent, selective sulfonylfuran urea endothelial lipase inhibitors. Bioorg Med Chem Lett 2009; 19: 27-30.
[249] Zhang Y, Zanotti I, Reilly MP, *et al.* Overexpression of apolipoprotein A-I promotes reverse transport of cholesterol from macrophages to feces *in vivo*. Circulation 2003; 108: 661-3.
[250] Chiesa G, Sirtori CR. Use of recombinant apolipoproteins in vascular diseases: the case of apoA-I. Curr Opin Investig Drugs 2002; 3: 420-6.
[251] Chiesa G, Sirtori CR. Recombinant apolipoprotein A-I(Milano): a novel agent for the induction of regression of atherosclerotic plaques. Ann Med 2003; 35: 267-73.
[252] Shah PK, Nilsson J, Kaul S, *et al.* Effects of recombinant apolipoprotein A-I(Milano) on aortic atherosclerosis in apolipoprotein E-deficient mice. Circulation 1998; 97: 780-5.
[253] Chiesa G, Monteggia E, Marchesi M, *et al.* Recombinant apolipoprotein A-I(Milano) infusion into rabbit carotid artery rapidly removes lipid from fatty streaks. Circ Res 2002; 90: 974-80.
[254] Weisgraber KH, Bersot TP, Mahley RW, Franceschini G, Sirtori CR. A-Imilano apoprotein. Isolation and characterization of a cysteine-containing variant of the A-I apoprotein from human high density lipoproteins. J Clin Invest 1980; 66: 901-7.
[255] Franceschini G, Maderna P, Sirtori CR. Reverse cholesterol transport: physiology and pharmacology. Atherosclerosis 1991; 88: 99-107.
[256] Weisgraber KH, Rall SC, Jr., Bersot TP, *et al.* Apolipoprotein A-IMilano. Detection of normal A-I in affected subjects and evidence for a cysteine for arginine substitution in the variant A-I. J Biol Chem 1983; 258: 2508-13.
[257] Gualandri V, Franceschini G, Sirtori CR, *et al.* AIMilano apoprotein identification of the complete kindred and evidence of a dominant genetic transmission. Am J Hum Genet 1985; 37: 1083-97.
[258] Sirtori CR, Calabresi L, Franceschini G, *et al.* Cardiovascular status of carriers of the apolipoprotein A-I(Milano) mutant: the Limone sul Garda study. Circulation 2001; 103: 1949-54.
[259] Alexander ET, Tanaka M, Kono M, *et al.* Structural and functional consequences of the Milano mutation (R173C) in human apolipoprotein A-I. J Lipid Res 2009; 50: 1409-19.
[260] Tall AR, Small DM. Body cholesterol removal: role of plasma high-density lipoproteins. Adv Lipid Res 1980; 17: 1-51.
[261] Shah PK, Yano J, Reyes O, *et al.* High-dose recombinant apolipoprotein A-I(milano) mobilizes tissue cholesterol and rapidly reduces plaque lipid and macrophage content in apolipoprotein e-deficient mice. Potential implications for acute plaque stabilization. Circulation 2001; 103: 3047-50.
[262] Nissen SE, Tsunoda T, Tuzcu EM, *et al.* Effect of recombinant ApoA-I Milano on coronary atherosclerosis in patients with acute coronary syndromes: a randomized controlled trial. JAMA 2003; 290: 2292-300.
[263] Brown BG, Zhao XQ, Chait A, *et al.* Simvastatin and niacin, antioxidant vitamins, or the combination for the prevention of coronary disease. N Engl J Med 2001; 345: 1583-92.
[264] Tardif JC, Gregoire J, L'allier PL, *et al.* Effects of reconstituted high-density lipoprotein infusions on coronary atherosclerosis: a randomized controlled trial. JAMA 2007; 297: 1675-82.
[265] Calkin AC, Drew BG, Ono A, *et al.* Reconstituted High-Density Lipoprotein Attenuates Platelet Function in Individuals With Type 2 Diabetes Mellitus by Promoting Cholesterol Efflux. Circulation 2009; 120(21): 2095-104.
[266] Shattil SJ, Anaya-Galindo R, Bennett J, Colman RW, Cooper RA. Platelet hypersensitivity induced by cholesterol incorporation. J Clin Invest 1975; 55: 636-43.
[267] Navab M, Anantharamaiah GM, Reddy ST, Fogelman AM. Apolipoprotein A-I mimetic peptides and their role in atherosclerosis prevention. Nat Clin Pract Cardiovasc Med 2006; 3: 540-7.
[268] Anantharamaiah GM, Jones JL, Brouillette CG, *et al.* Studies of synthetic peptide analogs of the amphipathic helix. Structure of complexes with dimyristoyl phosphatidylcholine. J Biol Chem 1985; 260: 10248-55.
[269] Anantharamaiah GM. Synthetic peptide analogs of apolipoproteins. Methods Enzymol 1986; 128: 627-47.
[270] Navab M, Anantharamaiah GM, Reddy ST, *et al.* Apolipoprotein A-I mimetic peptides. Arterioscler Thromb Vasc Biol 2005; 25: 1325-31.
[271] Frokjaer S, Otzen DE. Protein drug stability: a formulation challenge. Nat Rev Drug Discov 2005; 4: 298-306.
[272] Navab M, Anantharamaiah GM, Hama S, *et al.* Oral administration of an Apo A-I mimetic Peptide synthesized from D-amino acids dramatically reduces atherosclerosis in mice independent of plasma cholesterol. Circulation 2002; 105: 290-2.
[273] Chen X, Burton C, Song X, *et al.* An apoA-I mimetic peptide increases LCAT activity in mice through increasing HDL concentration. Int J Biol Sci 2009; 5: 489-99.

[274] Van Lenten BJ, Wagner AC, Anantharamaiah GM, *et al.* Influenza infection promotes macrophage traffic into arteries of mice that is prevented by D-4F, an apolipoprotein A-I mimetic peptide. Circulation 2002; 106: 1127-32.
[275] Van Lenten BJ, Wagner AC, Navab M, *et al.* D-4F, an apolipoprotein A-I mimetic peptide, inhibits the inflammatory response induced by influenza A infection of human type II pneumocytes. Circulation 2004; 110: 3252-8.
[276] Pesonen E, Siitonen O. Acute myocardial infarction precipitated by infectious disease. Am Heart J 1981; 101: 512-3.
[277] Spodick DH, Flessas AP, Johnson MM. Association of acute respiratory symptoms with onset of acute myocardial infarction: prospective investigation of 150 consecutive patients and matched control patients. Am J Cardiol 1984; 53: 481-2.
[278] Heilbronn LK, Campbell LV. Adipose tissue macrophages, low grade inflammation and insulin resistance in human obesity. Curr Pharm Des 2008; 14: 1225-30.
[279] Sommer G, Kralisch S, Stangl V, *et al.* Secretory products from human adipocytes stimulate proinflammatory cytokine secretion from human endothelial cells. J Cell Biochem 2009; 106: 729-37.
[280] Van Lenten BJ, Wagner AC, Navab M, *et al.* Lipoprotein inflammatory properties and serum amyloid A levels but not cholesterol levels predict lesion area in cholesterol-fed rabbits. J Lipid Res 2007; 48: 2344-53.
[281] Navab M, Ruchala P, Waring AJ, *et al.* A novel method for oral delivery of apolipoprotein mimetic peptides synthesized from all L-amino acids. J Lipid Res 2009; 50: 1538-47.
[282] Perera DR, Western KA, Schultz MG. Niclosamide treatment of cestodiasis. Clinicial trials in the United States. Am J Trop Med Hyg 1970; 19: 610-2.
[283] Glass CK, Pittman RC, Keller GA, Steinberg D. Tissue sites of degradation of apoprotein A-I in the rat. J Biol Chem 1983; 258: 7161-7.
[284] Bloedon LT, Dunbar R, Duffy D, *et al.* Safety, pharmacokinetics, and pharmacodynamics of oral apoA-I mimetic peptide D-4F in high-risk cardiovascular patients. J Lipid Res 2008; 49: 1344-52.
[285] Peet DJ, Janowski BA, Mangelsdorf DJ. The LXRs: a new class of oxysterol receptors. Curr Opin Genet Dev 1998; 8: 571-5.
[286] Castrillo A, Tontonoz P. Nuclear receptors in macrophage biology: at the crossroads of lipid metabolism and inflammation. Annu Rev Cell Dev Biol 2004; 20: 455-80.
[287] Zelcer N, Tontonoz P. Liver X receptors as integrators of metabolic and inflammatory signaling. J Clin Invest 2006; 116: 607-14.
[288] Chen JD, Evans RM. A transcriptional co-repressor that interacts with nuclear hormone receptors. Nature 1995; 377: 454-7.
[289] Horlein AJ, Naar AM, Heinzel T, *et al.* Ligand-independent repression by the thyroid hormone receptor mediated by a nuclear receptor co-repressor. Nature 1995; 377: 397-404.
[290] Glass CK, Rosenfeld MG. The coregulator exchange in transcriptional functions of nuclear receptors. Genes Dev 2000; 14: 121-41.
[291] Borst P, Elferink RO. Mammalian ABC transporters in health and disease. Annu Rev Biochem 2002; 71: 537-92.
[292] Costet P, Luo Y, Wang N, Tall AR. Sterol-dependent transactivation of the ABC1 promoter by the liver X receptor/retinoid X receptor. J Biol Chem 2000; 275: 28240-5.
[293] Repa JJ, Turley SD, Lobaccaro JA, *et al.* Regulation of absorption and ABC1-mediated efflux of cholesterol by RXR heterodimers. Science 2000; 289: 1524-9.
[294] Kennedy MA, Venkateswaran A, Tarr PT, *et al.* Characterization of the human ABCG1 gene: liver X receptor activates an internal promoter that produces a novel transcript encoding an alternative form of the protein. J Biol Chem 2001; 276: 39438-47.
[295] Sabol SL, Brewer HB, Jr., Santamarina-Fojo S. The human ABCG1 gene: identification of LXR response elements that modulate expression in macrophages and liver. J Lipid Res 2005; 46: 2151-67.
[296] Venkateswaran A, Repa JJ, Lobaccaro JM, *et al.* Human white/murine ABC8 mRNA levels are highly induced in lipid-loaded macrophages. A transcriptional role for specific oxysterols. J Biol Chem 2000; 275: 14700-7.
[297] Li AC, Glass CK. PPAR- and LXR-dependent pathways controlling lipid metabolism and the development of atherosclerosis. J Lipid Res 2004; 45: 2161-73.
[298] Pal M, Pillarisetti S. HDL elevators and mimetics--emerging therapies for atherosclerosis. Cardiovasc Hematol Agents Med Chem 2007; 5: 55-66.
[299] Horton JD, Goldstein JL, Brown MS. SREBPs: activators of the complete program of cholesterol and fatty acid synthesis in the liver. J Clin Invest 2002; 109: 1125-31.
[300] Repa JJ, Liang G, Ou J, *et al.* Regulation of mouse sterol regulatory element-binding protein-1c gene (SREBP-1c) by oxysterol receptors, LXRalpha and LXRbeta. Genes Dev 2000; 14: 2819-30.
[301] Joseph SB, Laffitte BA, Patel PH, *et al.* Direct and indirect mechanisms for regulation of fatty acid synthase gene expression by liver X receptors. J Biol Chem 2002; 277: 11019-25.
[302] Tontonoz P, Mangelsdorf DJ. Liver X receptor signaling pathways in cardiovascular disease. Mol Endocrinol 2003; 17: 985-93.
[303] Naik SU, Wang X, Da Silva JS, *et al.* Pharmacological activation of liver X receptors promotes reverse cholesterol transport *in vivo*. Circulation 2006; 113: 90-7.
[304] Katz A, Udata C, Ott E, *et al.* Safety, pharmacokinetics, and pharmacodynamics of single doses of LXR-623, a novel liver X-receptor agonist, in healthy participants. J Clin Pharmacol 2009; 49: 643-9.
[305] Asztalos BF, Schaefer EJ, Horvath KV, *et al.* Role of LCAT in HDL remodeling: investigation of LCAT deficiency states. J Lipid Res 2007; 48: 592-9.
[306] Sacks FM, Rudel LL, Conner A, *et al.* Selective delipidation of plasma HDL enhances reverse cholesterol transport *in vivo*. J Lipid Res 2009; 50: 894-907.
[307] Brousseau ME. Emerging role of high-density lipoprotein in the prevention of cardiovascular disease. Drug Discov Today 2005; 10: 1095-101.

Inflammatory and Metabolic Markers in Pre- and Post-Treatment of Obesity

Silvia de Barros-Mazon[1], Daniela Miguel Marin[2], Camila Puzzi de Carvalho[2] and Sarah Monte Alegre[*,2]

[1]*Department of Clinical Pathology,* [2]*Department of Internal Medicine, Faculty of Medical Sciences, University of Campinas (UNICAMP), Sao Paulo, Brazil*

Abstract: Obesity is a challenging health problem in the industrialized world and in recent population studies the prevalence of overweight, obesity and abdominal obesity is constantly increasing, reaching to an epidemic proportions. The excess of body weight is associated with a low-grade systemic inflammation and a cluster of metabolic alterations such as insulin resistance, hypertension and dyslipidemia, which is presumed to play a role in the development of cardiovascular disease and type 2 diabetes mellitus. It is now well-established that adipocytes secrete proteins (adipokines) that actively control energy homeostasis, glucose and lipid metabolism, neuroendocrine and cardiovascular function and inflammatory response. Excessive levels of some adipokines such as TNF-α and IL-6 can disturb the metabolism suggesting the adipose tissue as a link between obesity, low grade inflammation and insulin resistance. In obesity, sustained weight loss has several beneficial effects on lipid metabolism, glucose tolerance and arterial blood pressure. There have been an increasing number of obese patients requiring treatment (bariatric surgery and/or diet) for weight loss. The weight loss induced by bariatric surgery causes a reduction in the inflammatory state, increasing levels of adiponectin and GLP-1, which are all related to beneficial metabolic changes described above. GLP-1 is especially related to insulinotropic properties through induced expansion of insulin secreting B-cell mass and enhanced insulin secretion. GLP-1 acts also in insulin action enhancing B-cell glucose sensitivity contributing to glycemic control after surgical procedure. So our focus in this chapter is to emphasize metabolic and inflammatory profile in obesity and its metabolic changes after weight loss.

Keywords: Obesity, adipokines, inflammatory cytokines, insulin resistence, GLP-1, weight loss.

1. INTRODUCTION

During evolution, humans have faced various periods of famine and scarcity which have been a substantial threat to survival. As a result, this necessity became the basis for a greater capacity for storing energy whenever food was available and replacing the consumed stores as soon as supplies became available again. People who survived in those conditions developed strategies and complex rituals that revolved around shared meals. Social status was assessed by the acquisition of resources and to be well-endowed with a layer of fat was a clear sign of success, wealth and social dominance [1]. However, these same properties that constituted an evolutionary advantage can make individuals more susceptible to obesity during times of abundance [2].

In more recent times, in industrialized societies, people face a different challenge: overnutrition, an excessive intake of energized foods high in fat and sugar, which when combined with a sedentary lifestyle or low physical activity can lead to the development of obesity [3]. Current more prevalent negative health consequences of obesity in association with the modern idealism of slimness represents the new prototype of the species, glamorized by fashion and art.

While prevalence of obesity increases worldwide, the understanding of its pathogenesis and metabolic consequences have markedly advanced.

Adipose tissue has been classified into two major forms on the basis of gross appearance, cell type-specific gene expression, and a predominant type of adipocytes: brown and white adipose tissue [4].

* Corresponding author: Tel: +55 19 35217044, +55 19 35217098; Fax: +55 19 32894107; E-mail: salegre@fcm.unicamp.br

Atta-ur-Rahman / M. Iqbal Choudhary (Eds.)

Recent data have demonstrated the plasticity conditions in which fully differentiated white adipocytes can transdifferentiate into brown adipocytes, and vice versa [5]. Brown adipose tissue is derived from a rich blood supply with an extensive capillary network and an enormous number of mitochondria per cell. Its primary function is heat generation and is considered to be at most a minor component of human adipose tissue [4, 6, 7].

Brown adipose tissue is capable of responding to various environmental stimuli to generate heat from stored metabolic energy. This thermogenic mechanism in brown fat mitochondria is recognized as being due to a brown-specific mitochondrial uncoupling protein (UCP) which provides an alternative flow of protons through the inner mitochondrial membrane to re-enter the mitochondrial matrix, thereby uncoupling the oxidation of fuel from ATP production [8, 9].

The abundance of brown adipose tissue peaks at about the time of birth and is less pro-eminent after the postnatal period. In humans, the importance of brown adipose tissue is not known [10].

White adipose tissue (WAT) is a specialized loose connective tissue that is extensively laden with adipocytes, which are differentiated cells specialized in the storage of fat. These adipocytes have a single large lipid inclusion resulting in displacement of the cytoplasm and a flattening of the nucleus to the cytoplasmatic membrane [11]. WAT contains various other cell types in addition to adipocytes. Heavier connective tissue septa separate white adipose tissue depots into lobules of various sizes. The connective tissue surrounding white adipocytes contains precursor cells, fibroblasts, immune cells, reticular fibers and nerves and in obesity is often infiltrated by macrophages [12-14]. It is endowed with a well-organized vasculature [11, 15]. However, capillaries are often observed at the junctions where adipocytes meet. Blood vessels and nerves link adipose tissue to the whole body for metabolic regulation. Anatomic and histological observations have shown direct sympathetic innervations of white adipocytes originating from the central nervous system [16].

The morphology of WAT is affected by nutritional status and is the predominant form in adult humans. It accounts for 15% to 20% of body weight in healthy men and 20% to 25% in healthy women. In healthy adults, it remains constant over prolonged periods and can increase volume with obesity or decrease with anorexia, cancer and other diseases or during periods of food shortage and calorie deficit or threat of starvation [17]. It is comprised of 70% to 90% lipid, 3% to 5% water and 2% to 3% protein.

WAT is the main lipid storage depot in the body and is of crucial importance in buffering the daily influx of dietary fat entering the circulation. Its primary functions are storage and release of metabolic fuel that occur through very well orchestrated mechanisms. Adipocytes accumulate and release fatty acids which is the basis of their function. They store energy as triglycerides during calorie abundance and facilitate retrieval during periods of food shortage and calorie deficit, such as fasting, starvation, and long-term exercise [18].

The amount of triglycerides stored within adipocytes must be an accurate reflection of the imbalance between energy intake and energy expenditure, integrated over a long period.

Under normal conditions, adipocytes are highly capable of fine-tuning the balance between synthesis (lipogenesis) and breakdown (lipolysis) of triglycerides in response to physiological needs. The adipose triglyceride-storage capacity provides the means to keep energy homeostasis and to prevent an abnormal increase in plasma of the non-esterified fatty acids (NEFAs), a product from triglycerides breakdown that is lipotoxic to the body.

In humans, triglycerides are mainly taken up from the circulation and the contribution of *de novo* lipogenesis in adipose tissue to overall metabolism generally appears to be insignificant compared to the liver [19].

Dietary triglycerides and *de novo* synthesized triglycerides from the liver are transported to adipose tissue as lipoprotein particles, respectively as quilomicrons and very low density lipoprotein (VLDL). Triglycerides are not taken up directly but are first hydrolyzed by an extracellular lipoprotein lipase (LPL), which is stimulated by insulin [20] and then enter the cell as fatty acids. In adipocytes these fatty acids are then rapidly activated and the resulting CoA derivatives are transferred to glycerol in the form of glycerol 3-phosphate. This essential intermediate in lipid biosynthesis comes mainly from glycolysis, which renders glucose an important substrate in the formation of triglycerides by adipocytes. In adipocytes, glucose is stored primarily as lipid. This is the result of increased uptake of glucose and activation of lipid synthetic enzymes, including pyruvate dehydrogenase, fatty acid synthase and acetyl CoA carboxilase [21].

Adipocytes are one of the most highly insulin-responsive cell types and this hormone is a regulator of important aspects of adipocyte biology [20]. Insulin's actions on lipid metabolism is analogous to its role in glucose metabolism. Insulin upregulates LPL and stimulates gene expression of intracellular lipogenic enzymes, such as acetyl-CoA carboxilase and fatty acid synthase. On the other hand, insulin also profoundly inhibits lipolysis in adipocytes, primarily through inhibition of hormone-sensitive lipase (HSL) phosphorylation. Insulin inhibits the activity of this lipase primarily via reductions in cAMP levels due to the activation of a cAMP-specific phosphodiesterase in fat cells [22, 23] (Fig. **1**).

Normal – Functional Adipose Tissue

Under normal conditions, in postprandial moments, the increase in glucose and lipid stimulates insulin release and increases fatty acid transport and lipogenesis in adipocytes. On the other hand, reductions in glucose and insulin during fasting and sympathetic nervous system action lead to lipolysis and the release of fatty acid for use by other tissues.

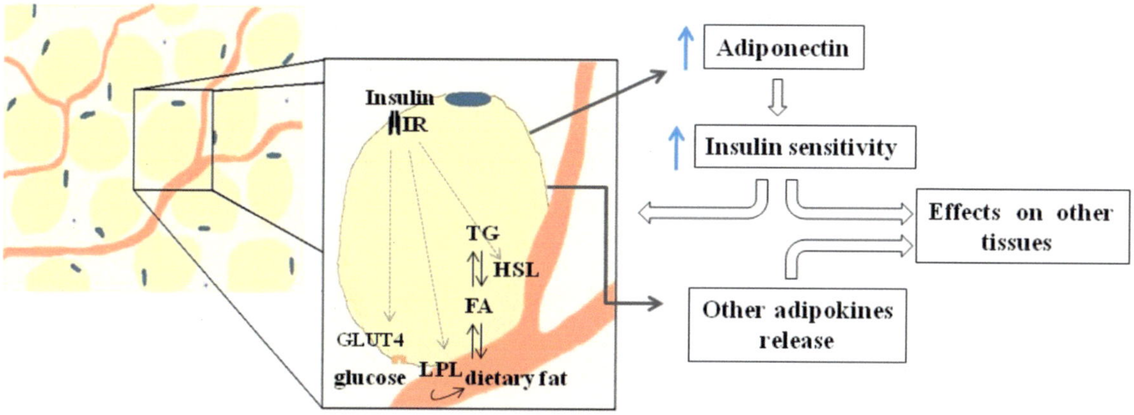

Fig. (1). Adipose tissue is the main lipid storage depot in the body and is of crucial importance in buffering the daily influx of dietary fat entering the circulation. Adipocytes accumulate and release fatty acids which is the basis of their function. The amount of triglycerides stored within adipocytes must be an accurate reflection of the imbalance between energy intake and energy expenditure, integrated over a long period. Under normal conditions, adipocytes are highly capable of fine-tuning the balance between synthesis (lipogenesis) and breakdown (lipolysis) of triglycerides in response to physiological needs. The adipose triglyceride-storage capacity provides the means to keep energy homeostasis and to prevent an abnormal increase in plasma of the non-esterified fatty acids (NEFAs), a product from triglycerides breakdown that is lipotoxic to the body. Adipocytes are one of the most highly insulin-responsive cell types and this hormone is a regulator of important aspects of adipocyte biology. Insulin upregulates LPL and stimulates gene expression of intracellular lipogenic enzymes and inhibits lipolysis in adipocytes, primarily through inhibition of HSL phosphorylation. Adipose tissue is also considered an endocrine organ. Among numerous factors which have physiologic effects on other tissues, it releases adiponectin, an important adipokine related to insulin sensitivity. Illustration by Natalia Mazon.

When the body needs lipids, lipolysis occurs in adipocytes and triglycerides are hydrolyzed to glycerol and non-esterified fatty acids (NEFAs). In this step, the major rate-limiting factor in stimulated lipolysis is HSL, but additional lipases, such as adipose tissue triglyceride lipase, may play an essential role in basal lipolysis [24]. NEFAs, as energy substrates, are released into the circulation and are transported to the different tissues bound to albumin. There they are oxidized to provide energy, in particular in muscle [24, 25] and to provide signaling molecules and substrates for lipoprotein production by the liver [25].

Until the 1990's, adipose tissue had largely been considered an inert storage depot for excess metabolic fuel. With the discovery of leptin [26] as an adipose-derived hormone, and thereafter the discovery of the many other secreted proteins involved in health and disease, adipose tissue is now considered not only an energy reservoir but also has reached the status of a true endocrine organ [27-29].

Nowadays, adipose tissue is characterized as a complex and highly metabolic and endocrine organ that actively produces various hormones, cytokines and chemokines, collectively called adipokines, and is involved in many functions through local and/or systemic action, exerting interaction between efferent (from adipocytes) and afferent signals and constituting a feedback system, a cross-talk of adipose tissue with other organs as well as within the adipose, capable of adapting to the numerous challenges of energy metabolism [30]. They play important roles in cell differentiation, and growth, in homeostasis of glucose, energy balance, metabolism of lipids, fibrinolytic system/vascular homeostasis, inflammation and insulin resistance [28, 30-32].

These adipokines are made up of adipocytes, stromal vascular cells, connective tissue matrix and nerve tissue [27-29]. Adipocytes express and secrete several endocrine hormones such as leptin and adiponectin, while many secreted proteins, such as cytokines, are preponderantly derived from the nonadipocyte fraction of adipose tissue [11].

Among the secreted factors having endocrine function, the following should be mentioned: estrogens, resulting from aromatization of androgens by adipose tissue, stimulated by insulin and cortisol [33] leptin, reflecting fat hypertrophy, being regulated by factors other than the size of adipose tissue, such as energy balance and hormones (glucocorticoids and insulin) and tumor necrosis factor-α (TNF-α) modulating positively leptin secretion [34-36]; angiotensinogen, which via angiotensin II, produced locally, induces differentiation of preadipocytes into adipocytes [37]; and adiponectin, which is inversely correlated with body weight [38]. On the other hand, TNF-α and interleukin-6 (IL-6) are examples of factors which have an autocrine/ paracrine activity on adipose tissue. Adipose tissue are a source and target tissue of TNF-α, which is expressed equally in the different fat depots and is a regulator of fat cell size and adipose tissue cellularity and also induces insulin resistance. IL-6 is released more by visceral than subcutaneous abdominal adipocytes [39], is induced by TNF-α and participates in insulin resistance [40]. IGF-1 is also produced by adipocytes and is a potent factor in the proliferation of preadipocytes [41].

As will be detailed in the next section, some of these adipokines appear to play an important role in obesity associated with insulin resistance, cardiovascular complications and other co-morbidities. In fact, since it was shown that adipose tissue acts as a true secretory organ [42, 43] high plasma levels of inflammatory cytokines in obese people have been reported [44, 45]. As a result, a growing number of researchers started to investigate the relationship between obesity and inflammation, the basic mechanisms in which cytokines are expressed in adipose tissue, their circulating levels and inflammatory process, as well as the stimulus for the production of acute phase proteins produced by the liver [43, 45]. Moreover, studies in human obesity and insulin resistance have revealed a clear association between the chronic activation of pro-inflammatory signaling pathways and decreased insulin sensitivity. To date, elevated levels of inflammatory cytokines have been reported in various diabetic and insulin resistant states [46-51].

One of the adipose tissue dysfunctions in obesity is primarily characterized by its increased mass. Expansion of adipose tissue mass is caused by a combination of size increase of pre-existing adipocytes (hypertrophy) and *de novo* adipocyte differentiation (hyperplasia) [11].

During continued positive caloric balance, energy must be store. This chronic storage of positive caloric balance is usually first accomplished through enlargement of fat cells (lipogenesis) and adipocyte hypertrophy. The accumulation of fat may result in pathological fat dysfunction manifested by an increased net release fatty acids and an increased pro-inflammatory response.

2. OBESITY, INSULIN RESISTANCE AND INFLAMMATION

Obesity is currently an epidemic disease, treated as a complex problem, and several factors may be involved in its etiology, including genetic factors, environmental and evolutionary. Population studies have explored the issue of obesity as a public health problem. Developed countries such as the USA, UK, Netherlands and Germany have shown prevalence estimated between 5-15% of the obese population [52].

The prevalence of obesity has reached epidemic proportions globally. In 2005, the World Health Organization estimated that approximately 1.6 billion adults were overweight (body mass index –BMI – over 25kg/m^2) and at least 400 miliion of them clinically obese (BMI over 30) [53-55].

This poses a major public health issue, since obesity is a large contributor to the global burden of chronic diseases. In addition, the prevalence of obesity-related disorders is also increasing at an alarming rate [56].

Even more alarming than adult obesity is the marked increasing rate of obese children. The association between the ascending epidemiological curves of obesity, particularly in children, and the metabolic burden, brought about an estimation of decreased life expectancy at birth in the United States for the first half of this century [57, 58].

Obesity is characterized by chronic excessive accumulation of fat which leads to an undermining of health. This excessive accumulation can represent a substantial risk of developing serious diseases such as type 2 diabetes mellitus, cardiovascular disease, hypertension, dyslipidemia, respiratory problems, sleep apnea, gastrointestinal diseases, arthritis, venous circulatory disease, strokes and certain types of cancers. The health consequences range from increased risk of premature death to serious chronic diseases that affect the quality of life of the individual [59, 60].

Metabolically, obesity is characterized by hyperinsulinemia and peripheral insulin resistance [61] and is the major risk factor for developing type 2 Diabetes Mellitus. In obesity and also in Type 2 Diabetes Mellitus, insulin resistance occurs in skeletal muscle, liver, fat, and pancreas. Although it was found that muscle was the main site of insulin resistance [62], today, the adipose tissue has been identified as having this role [63].

Obesity has been associated with a low-grade inflammation process in adipose tissue, observed in rodents and humans, and is characterized by the activation of some pro-inflammatory signalling pathways, such as c-jun N-terminal kinase (JNK) and nuclear factor κB (NFκB), leading to increased expression of downstream cytokines such as tumor necrosis factor-α (TNF-α), interleukin-6 (IL-6) and monocyte chemoattractant protein-1 (MCP-1) among others [39, 40, 49, 64]. Furthermore, some of those cytokines can lead to stimulation of several circulating factors such as C-reactive protein (CRP) and serum amyloid A (SAA) [65-72] amplifying the existing inflammatory process (Fig. **2**).

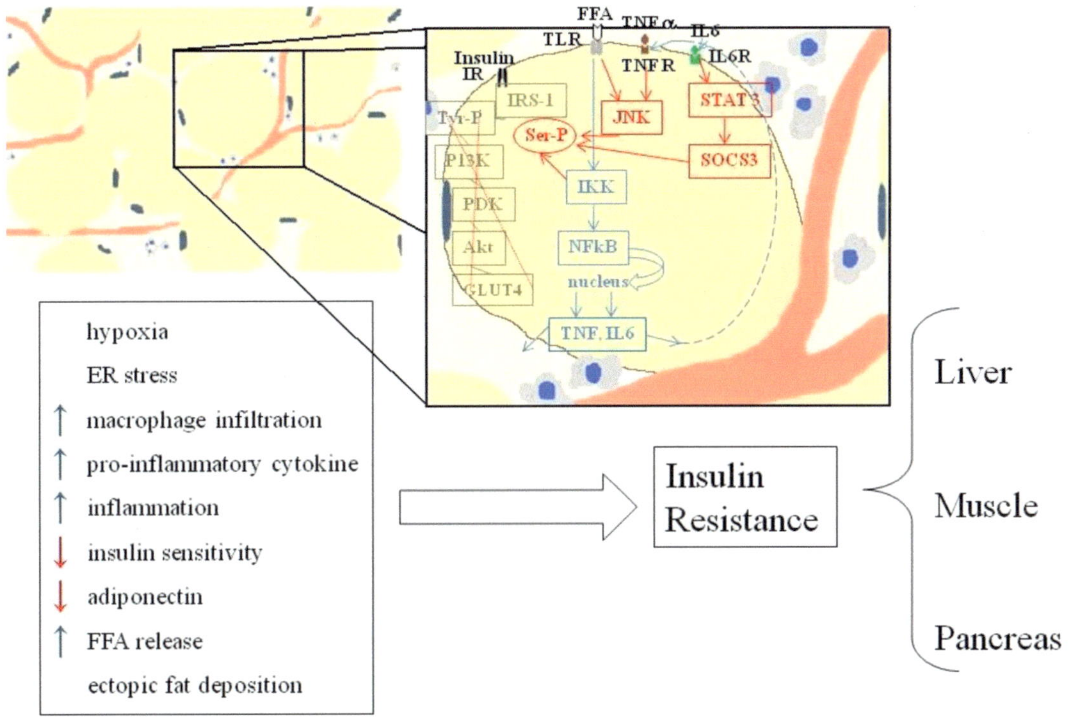

Fig. (2). Expansion of the adipose tissue leads to an increase in lipid storage in the TG droplet. Hypoxia and endoplasmic-reticulum (ER) stress are proposed mechanisms to explain the macrophage infiltration and the development of chronic, low-grade inflammation. The pro-inflammatory cytokines and free fatty acids (FFAs) have been demonstrated to activate inflammation and to inhibit insulin signaling pathways. FFAs bind to TLR4 (toll-like receptor 4) to activate IkB-kinase (IKK) which stimulates nuclear translocation and expression of NF-κB associated genes such as interleukin (IL)-6 and tumor necrosis factor (TNF)-α. Activated IKK, c-Jun amino-terminal kinase (JNK) increase serine phosphorylation of insulin receptor substrate (IRS-1) that downregulates insulin signaling associated with IRS tyrosine phosphorylation, PI3-kinase (P13K), PDK and Akt, resulting in reduced glucose transport into cells. IL-6 has been demonstrated to activate directly, as well as FFA indirectly, the suppressor of cytokine signaling 3 (SOCS3) pathways, which also inhibits the insulin signaling pathways. The ultimate effect is insulin resistance in adipose tissue and on peripheral organs which may each independently exacerbate the other, culminating in severe adipocyte dysfunction. *Illustration by Natalia Mazon.*

Enlarged – Dysfunctional Adipose Tissue

Many of these pro-inflammatory mediators have been shown to be detrimental to insulin signaling, linking the obesity and the inflammation with numerous diseases, including insulin resistance, type 2 diabetes and cardiovascular disease. The elevation of pro-inflammatory cytokines such as tumor necrosis factor (TNF-α) and interleukin-6 (IL-6), can cause insulin resistance by interfering with its signaling [73, 74]. In addition, CRP has been considered a predictor of cardiovascular risk, related to the degree of sensitivity to insulin and endothelial dysfunction [75-77] and, more recently, it has been recognized as having a role in the pathogenesis of cardiovascular diseases, diabetes and cancer [78].

It seems likely that the adipocytes initiate the inflammatory response because they are the first cells affected by the development of obesity. Adipocytes appear to share some properties with immune cells such as pro-inflammatory cytokine production, complement activation [79] and toll-like receptor expression [80]. Likewise, preadipocytes share some characteristics with macrophages such as phagocytosis in response to several stimuli [81,82]. However, studies on the source of cytokine secretion from adipose tissue have demonstrated that although adipocytes are able to secrete cytokines, macrophages are probably the major producer [83, 84]. To reinforce this, some studies have demonstrated the increased presence of macrophages in adipose tissue in obesity [12, 14] and others have shown macrophage expression of functional genes that code for transcription factors, cytokines, inflammatory signalling molecules and fatty acid transporters, all of them considered essential for adipocyte biology [85-87].

One of the hypotheses proposed for the origin of the low-grade inflammation process comes from the fact that the expansion of adipose tissue leads to local hypoxia and thus to the recruitment and the infiltration of macrophages around dead adipocytes [88]. Macrophages would be recruited into adipose tissue to scavenge the adipocyte debris, in particular the residual lipid droplets, from dead adipocytes. In fact, the necrosis of adipocytes is approximately 3-times higher in obese than in lean human subjects, and is also increased with adipocyte hypertrophy [14].

Another hypothesis considers that the excess of lipid in adipocytes may initiate a state of cellular stress and activation of inflammatory signaling pathways, which leads to increased adipocyte production of pro-inflammatory cytokines, including TNF–α, IL6, and chemoattractant molecules such as MCP-1. This last one, with the help from endothelial cells via interaction of adhesion molecules with integrins and chemokine receptors on the monocyte surface, recruits them to adipose tissue, where they differentiate into macrophages [89].

The activation of inflammatory pathways by endoplasmic reticulum (ER) stress appears to be of central importance in the low-grade inflammation process. According to recent data, obesity generates conditions that increase the demand on the ER [90-92]. This is particularly the case for adipose tissue which undergoes severe changes in tissue architecture, increases in protein and lipid synthesis and perturbations in intracellular nutrient and energy fluxes. In fact, adipose tissue ER stress was found to be a common feature of obesity, insulin resistance and diabetes [90]. In both, cultured cells and whole animals, ER stress leads to activation of JNK and thus contributes to insulin resistance [90]. Oxidative stress is a major source of ER stress and is associated with dysregulation of various adipocytokines [93]. ER stress may provide additional reactive oxygen species (ROS) and may induce inflammation through activation of the JNK and NF-κB pathways [94, 95]. In the cytoplasm, JNK acts to inhibit insulin signaling through the phosphorylation of the insulin receptor substrate 1 (IRS-1) on serine 307 [96]. JNK mediated serine phosphorylation of IRS-1 inhibits insulin receptor signaling through several mechanisms, including the loss of its ability to serve as a substrate, disruption of insulin receptor-IRS-1 interaction, and, when the stress is severe and prolonged, IRS-1 degradation. Indeed, mice with a genetic deficiency of JNK1 display marked protection from diet-induced obesity and insulin resistance [97].

So, the accumulation of macrophages and the communication between adipocytes and macrophages may aggravate the state of inflammation, resulting in increased secretion of inflammatory cytokines, adipokines and angiogenic factors [88] that will act on different sites aggravating part of the insulin resistance [98]. To date, there is a large body of evidence suggesting that inflammation is the "link" between obesity, insulin resistance and endothelial dysfunction [99].

Nowadays, it is clearly established that a strong interaction occurs between cytokine and insulin signalling pathways, resulting in an impaired biological effect of insulin. Although the exact mechanisms have not yet been clearly elucidated it has been clearly demonstrated that cytokines such as TNF-α and IL-6 are able to decrease insulin action [100-105] (Fig. **2**).

TNF-α, which is cytokine expressed by adipose tissue, monocytes and macrophages, has been studied longer and has many pro-inflammatory and immunoregulatory actions. Its expression by adipose tissue is increased in obese people compared to lean [42, 106]. Recombinant TNF-α decreases insulin sensitivity, while TNF-α- or TNF-α receptor-null mice have an increased sensitivity in response to this hormone suggesting that the overproduction of TNF-α by adipose tissue from obese animal models contributes to insulin resistance [64, 107]. TNF-α is thought to play a major role in the pathophysiology of insulin resistance in rodents [64] and is able to inhibit the signaling of insulin in human adipocytes *in vitro* [108]. The proposed mechanisms involved in the serine phosphorylation of IRS-1 prevent its association with PI-3 kinase (fosfatilinositol 3-kinase) [109] or the reduction of the tyrosine kinase of the insulin receptor [48, 104].

In addition, some studies have demonstrated that TNF-α induces the decrease of important functional genes in 3T3-L1 adipocyte, including GLUT4 [110], HSL, long-chain fatty acyl CoA synthetase, adiponectin (ADIPOQ), the transcription factor CCAAT/ enhancer binding protein-alpha (C/EBP), and the nuclear receptors PPARγ and retinoic acid X receptor (RXR). Because all of these genes are both directly and indirectly critical for glucose homeostasis, changes in their expression probably contribute to insulin resistance in obesity induced-chronic inflammation [111].

IL-6, the other very important pro-inflammatory cytokine present in obesity, appears to play a central role in the connection between obesity, inflammation and coronary heart diseases [112]. Moreover, one of the main effects of IL-6 is the induction of hepatic C-reactive protein (CRP) production, which is known to be the main mediator of acute inflammatory response [113] and an independent, major risk marker of cardiovascular complications [114]. It has been demonstrated that visceral adipose tissue produces higher IL-6 amounts than subcutaneous adipose tissue [39, 83], which could explain the relationship between central fat deposits and enhanced cardiovascular risk complications in humans, because visceral adipose tissue is in close contact with the liver through the venous portal system. In addition, IL-6 production by adipose tissue has been suggested to affect liver metabolism by inducing VLDL secretion and hypertriglyceridaemia [115]. Further, IL-6 appears to be involved in insulin resistance and its complications [40, 42]. The IL-6 receptor belongs to the cytokine class I receptor family involving the JAK/STATs (Janus kinases/signal transducers and activators of transcription) signal transduction pathway. Janus kinase activation induces STAT phosphorylation, dimerisation and translocation to the nucleus to regulate target gene transcription [116]. And, as it was demonstrated in study in human skeletal myotubes, IL-6 inhibited insulin signaling and induced expression of suppressor of cytokine signaling 3 (SOCS-3), a negative regulator of insulin cascade [117]. In addition, adiponectin production in adipocytes is inhibited by IL-6 what contribute to IL-6-induced hepatic insulin resistance [118].

It has been suggested that not only the pro-inflammatory effects of cytokines, but also of reactive oxygen species and FFAs in obesity, are mediated through specific intracellular signalling pathways, involving NF-κB, IκB kinase, (IKK), Activating Protein-1 (AP-1) and c-Jun NH2-terminal kinase (JNK) signalling molecules. All these pathways could interact with insulin signalling *via* serine/threonine inhibitory phosphorylation of IRS.

Overnutrition and obesity are often accompanied by elevations in tissue and circulating FFA concentrations, and saturated FFAs can directly activate pro-inflammatory responses in vascular endothelial cells, adipocytes and myeloid-derived cells [119]. More recently the role of TLR4 has been demonstrated as a key component in fatty acid-induced inflammation in cultured macrophages [120]. TLR4 stimulation results in the activation of both IKK/NFκB and JNK/AP-1 signaling, culminating in the expression and secretion of pro-inflammatory cytokines/chemokines, including, IL1b, IL-6, TNF, MCP-1, among others [121].

Recently, Shi *et al.* [80] demonstrated the link between TLR4 and fatty acid and obesity-induced insulin resistance. They showed that FFAs activate the NFκB signaling pathway in primary macrophages from wildtype mice but not in macrophages derived from TLR4 deficient ($Tlr4^{-/-}$) mice. In addition, they demonstrated that saturated fatty acids are the most potent inducers of this inflammatory response and that obese mice have increased TLR4 expression in adipose tissue compared to lean controls. On the other hand, they found that male $Tlr4^{-/-}$ mice are protected from FFA infusion-induced insulin resistance, which is probably due to decreased FFA-induced NFκB transcriptional activity, resulting in reduced adipose tissue TNF-α, IL6 and MCP-1 expression. So the authors concluded that TLR4 seems to have a role in the development of FFA- and obesity-induced insulin resistance since it acts as a sensor of elevated tissue and/or serum FFA concentrations that are commonly associated with obesity [80].

In contrast to an overall highly enhanced inflammatory environment, in obesity, the secretion of peptide hormones such as leptin and adiponectin, is disturbed, which in turn is associated with diseases such as metabolic syndrome, insulin resistance [122, 123] and cardiovascular disease [124].

In normal condition, adiponectin has anti-inflammatory effects by inhibiting the phagocytic activity and production of TNF-α by macrophages [125] and have been related to insulin sensitivity.

Unlike leptin, adiponectin is decreased in obese subjects and in patients with type 2 diabetes,as demonstrated by Weyer *et al.* [126]. These low concentrations of adiponectin are associated with reduced ability of insulin to phosphorylate their receptors, the initial step of insulin action [127, 128]. Reduced levels of adiponectin were observed in obesity and type 2 diabetes and appear to be more related to the degree of insulin resistance than to obesity and glucose, suggesting that the low levels found in obesity and type 2 diabetes would be explained as representing states of insulin resistance [126]. Moreover, the decrease of adiponectin has also been associated with increased risk of developing coronary heart disease [129-132]. In mice, deletion of the adiponectin gene resulted in insulin resistance, dyslipidemia and increased neointimal proliferation and its overexpression or pharmacological administration improved insulin sensitivity and protected against atherosclerosis [133-136]. Additionally some reports link low concentrations of adiponectin to myocardial infarction [137] and to the progression of subclinical coronary heart disease [138]. To date, adiponectin is the only protein secreted by adipose tissue that has its expression decreased in states of obesity and T2DM. The relative contribution of the deficiency in this cytokine versus the overabundance of the proinflammatory cytokines remains unclear.

Insulin is important to both antilipolysis and the stimulation of LPL. In insulin-resistant states the responses of both LPL and HSL to insulin are blunted. An inefficient trapping of dietary energy occurs because of both decreased LPL-mediated lipolysis of chylomicron-TG and ineffective inhibition of HSL-mediated lipolysis in adipose tissue [139].

The inhibition of lipolysis in adipose tissue has been considered the most sensitive pathway of insulin action [140]. As a consequence, when insulin resistance develops, the increased amount of lipolysis of stored triacylglycerol molecules in adipose tissue produces more fatty acids, which could further inhibit the antilipolytic effect of insulin, creating additional lipolysis.

In obesity, the most consistent lipid disorder is hypertriglyceridemia which is attributable to increased plasma concentrations of VLDL apolipoprotein(apo) B-100 and chylomicron apoB-48 [141, 142]. Over secretion, reduced hydrolysis, and/or impaired clearance of triglyceride-rich lipoproteins have been proposed as mechanism for this lipid abnormality [141, 143].

On the other hand, hyperlipidemia is responsible, in part, for inducing peripheral tissue insulin resistance, and dyslipidemia contributes to the development of atherosclerosis. Beside this, metabolic changes characteristic of the acute-phase response, are also proatherogenic. Nevertheless, the precise relationships between dyslipidemia, adiposity and insulin resistance are complex and still poorly defined [141, 144, 145].

Some reports have been highlighted the role of certain adipocytokines such as adiponectin, leptin, resistin, interleukin-6 (IL-6) and TNF-α on glucose and lipid metabolism [146-148].

As mentioned before, unlike other adipocytokines, plasma adiponectin concentrations are decreased in obese and insulin-resistant individuals, including those with type 2 diabetes [38, 149]. Furthermore, diminished plasma adiponectin concentrations were correlated with hypertriglyceridemia, low high density lipoprotein (HDL)-cholesterol concentrations and decreased low density lipoprotein (LDL) particle size independent of the amount of intra abdominal fat and degree of insulin resistance [150, 151].

Some effects of adiponectin on lipid metabolism have been proposed such as decreasing accumulation of triglycerides in skeletal muscle by enhancing fatty acid oxidation through activation of acetyl-CoA oxidase, carnitine palmitoyltransferase- 1, and AMP kinase [152], and stimulanting LPL on VLDL hydrolyzes [153] and, decreasing the supply of NEFAs to the liver for gluconeogenesis, thus decreasing triglyceride synthesis.

3. WEIGHT LOSS

The increased levels of inflammatory markers and acute phase proteins have been demonstrated in morbidly obese individuals [154].

The goals towards treating patients with obesity is improve adipose tissue functional capacity, improve adipose tissue-mediated nutrient metabolism, reduce systemic inflammation and corrected the production of clinically relevant adipocyte factors which may all in association or contribute to type 2 diabetes, hypertension, cardiovascular disease and dyslipidemia.

Follow-up studies demonstrated that a massive weight loss associated with lifestyle interventions is related to improvement in insulin sensitivity and in glycemic control [155-157], blood pressure, lipid profile [158] and delayed progression from impaired glucose tolerance to diabetes mellitus [159].

Furthermore, weight loss reverts the metabolic complications of obesity [160,161] and this effect may be due to a higher decrease in visceral than in subcutaneous fat [162,163] or may be due to a reduction in the lipid content within muscles [163].

Improvements in insulin resistance, glycemic control and decrease of hyperinsulinemia were also observed in subjects submitted to gastric bypass [164-166] but the strategies used to bring on weight loss can exert different impacts on metabolic parameters.

Madsen *et al.* [167] observed that a 10 % weight loss after diet, exercise counseling and drug or placebo use are necessary for long-term improvement of adiponectin and insulin sensitivity and reduction in CRP and fibrinogen levels. Further, Jazet *et al.* [168] found that 50% of weight loss after a very low calorie diet reduced basal endogenous glucose production and improved hepatic, adipose tissue and skeletal muscle insulin sensitivity in obese, insulin-treated type 2 diabetic patients and also improved insulin-stimulated glucose disposal by approximately 100% in those patients. This improvement is comparable with the improvements seen in obese nondiabetic patients in whom restrictive bariatric surgery was used to induce weight loss [164].

Seven days of aerobic exercise were related to improvements in β-cell function and in insulin sensitivity in older people with impaired glucose tolerance despite no change in body weight, fasting glucose or circulating levels of lipid, catecholamine, leptin or adiponectin levels [169].

A meta-analysis carried out by Wu *et al.* [170] showed that diet and exercise in a weight loss program are more effective interventions to produce greater long-term weight loss than interventions that only included a diet program. Furthermore, the degree of weight loss is an important issue concerning metabolic improvements and a 5-10% weight loss is associated with reduction in diastolic blood pressure [171], lipid profile [172] insulin sensitivity [128] improvement in quality of life [173] and in symptoms such as shortness of breath, sweating and osteoarthritic abnormalities [174]. In fact, smaller rates of weight loss of about 2.5-5% are also related to improvements in insulin sensitivity [175].

Reducing body weight by 10% or more was also effective in reducing circulating levels of inflammatory markers [128, 176], as well as a smaller decline in body weight (~7%) due to lifestyle change was related to a 30% reduction in CRP levels. However, it still remains to be known what the magnitude of weight loss should be reached in order to obtain long-term improvements in metabolic and inflammatory markers.

Recent epidemiological studies and clinical interventions have reported contradictory findings related to dietary or exercise interventions and the resulting alterations in plasma cytokines. Moderate diet-induced weight loss accompanied by aerobic or resistive exercise training was not associated with changes in adiponectin levels despite decreased total fat mass, fasting plasma glucose, insulin, and leptin [177]. Xydakis *et al.* [178] observed that after a 7% weight loss through caloric restriction there was a significant decrease in plasma levels of insulin, HOMA-IR, leptin, and CRP but not adiponectin, NEFA and TNF-α levels changes. Kopp 2003 [179] showed a reduction of circulating levels of CRP, IL-6 after weight loss by gastric surgery in morbidly obese individuals associated with a reduction in inflammation and inflammatory markers along with an improvement in IR, weight and blood glucose.

Lifestyle modification associated to anti-obesity drugs has been applied as a part of obesity management. Controversial results are found about additional effects of drug therapy on improving weight loss and metabolic parameters.

In a trial, the use of sibutramine with a lifestyle management program was associated with maintaining weight loss over a period of 18 months. Those subjects who maintained lifestyle interventions over a period of 18 months but stopped sibutramine after 6 months of treatment, regained weight at the end of 18 months [180]. Malone *et al.*, 2005 [181] also observed that patients who received sibutramine had greater weight loss and decrease in body mass index than subjects that enrolled in a weight management program without sibutramine use.

On the other hand, Madsen *et al.* 2008 [167] found no additional effects of orlistat treatment on plasma levels of adiponectin, CRP, and fibrinogen in a program of diet/exercise induced weight loss.

Other drugs from separate classes of treatment like insulin-sensitizers [182,183], statins [184,185], fibric acids [186,187], angiotensin-converting enzyme (ACE) inhibitors [188] seems to promote reductions in inflammatory markers as TNF-α, CRP, IL-6, IL-7, IL-18. However, no drugs are currently approved for the indication of metabolic syndrome or for treatment of inflammation in a isolate manner [189,190].

More recently, a meta-analysis of the use of insulin sensitizing drugs for weight loss, compared with diet or a lifestyle modification program, shows that treatment with metformin resulted in a statistically significant decrease in BMI compared with placebo. Nevertheless, the main conclusion is that a structured lifestyle modification program to achieve weight loss should still be the first line treatment in obese women [191].

However, surgical treatment in severe obesity has been considered an effective method for reducing weight. The general measures to control weight, such as caloric restriction, use of medications, behavioral changes, among others, have been insufficient to cause weight loss in these patients [192,193]. As shown by Tuomilehto 2001 [194], weight loss has increasingly been linked to decreased incidence of type 2 Diabetes in the very obese. It is known that weight loss after surgery is usually quick and most occurs in the first 6 to 12 months of follow up continuing for up to 2 years, with maintenance for several years [195,196], and is accompanied by the improvement of several comorbidities.

Linscheid *et al.* 2008 [197], observed steady increases in total and high molecular weight (HMW) adiponectin during a 24 month period after surgery. After gastroplasty, adiponectin concentrations increased significantly [198] and pro-inflammatory cytokines such as tumor necrosis factor-alpha receptors and CRP were decreased [199]. We observed similar results with previous studies [200,201].

Other studies demonstrated that reduced circulating levels of adiponectin could be partially reversed after weight loss in obese individuals and in situations of insulin resistance [149,202].

Fruebis *et al.* 2001 [203], demonstrated that administration of adiponectin in mice induced weight loss despite the maintenance of food intake. The mechanisms involved seem to be related to the reduction of circulating fatty acids and increased lipid oxidation in muscle, thus improving insulin sensitivity. The same author showed improvement in glucose levels linked to decrease hepatic glucose release and increased glucose uptake in muscle.

Bariatric surgery-induced weight loss has been related to changes in inflammatory markers and adiponectin. We have recently demonstrated that weight loss after diet (~10%), compared to gastric bypass (~39%) produces a small improvement in insulin resistance, insulin secretion and incretin levels. However, surgical weight loss improved the carbohydrate metabolism through the improvement of insulin sensitivity, reducing type 2 diabetes at the same time that it enhanced the adiponectin and GLP-1 levels [204]. Our results are in agreement with previous studies.

Incretins, which are hormones secreted by the digestive system, improve metabolic action, or have an anti-diabetic action. One of these incretins is the glucagon-like peptide-1 (7-36) amide (GLP-1) which is a peptide secreted by L cells in the region of the distal ileum, after cleavage of proglucagon. This peptide, in response to ingestion of food, stimulates or enhances the secretion of insulin, inhibits the action of glucagon, and delays gastric emptying [205, 206]. GLP-1 is responsible for increased secretion of insulin as a result of ingestion of food [205].

In the pancreas, GLP-1 is a powerful secretagogue in beta cells. The insulinotropic action in the beta cells occurs at three levels: secretion, production of insulin by the action of insulin gene expression and proliferation of beta cells and neogenisis [207-209]. In the human pancreas, receptors for GLP-1were found in alpha and delta cells, in which the action causes the secretion of somatostatin and inhibition of secretion of glucagon [210, 211]. In the stomach, GLP-1 slows gastric emptying and is responsible for the decrease of nutrients available for intestinal absorption and a lower demand for insulin to maintain the post-euglycemic prandial state [212, 213]. In the central nervous system, GLP-1 suppresses the intake of food by the induction of satiety during the meal [214, 215]. In hepatic cells and skeletal muscle in humans, the GLP-1 reduces glycogenesis and in adipocytes, leading to increased lipolysis [216-219].

Several studies have proposed mechanisms by which weight loss surgery improves the metabolism of glucose, insulin resistance and DM2. The role of the digestive system in the modulation of insulin secretion was proposed by Unger and Eisentraut in 1969 [220]. They called this mechanism "entero-insulin axis". In 1979, Creutzfeldt *et al.* [221] updated the model, suggesting that neural signals, food, and gut hormone are involved in regulating the function of the beta cell, and incretins have a major role in this mechanism. Creutzfeldt defined incretins as intestinal hormones that are released through the contact of nutrients with the intestinal mucosa and stimulate the release of insulin at physiological levels. Sirinek *et al.* 1986 [222] suggested that the entero-insulin axis changes hyperinsulinemia followed by gastric bypass in the morbidly obese.

GLP-1, one of the most studied incretins, has been reported as a potential mediator for the improvement in glucose tolerance due to its many benefits in the glucose metabolism [223,224]. It has also been shown that the weight loss observed by surgery is accompanied by an improved control of DM2 and increased levels of GLP-1 [225].

A dramatic improvement of DM2 in morbidly obese subjects after gastric bypass. has been confirmed by many other authors [226-230].

The β cells' responsiveness to GLP-1 action seems preserved in patients with diabetes mellitus type 2, because the intravenous infusion of 1 pmol.kg-1. min-1, GLP-1 has a rapid effect of normalizing the hyperglycemia [231]. Part of this effect may be due to inhibition of the stimulation of glucagon secretion, resulting in a decrease in hepatic glucose production. Although a large number of studies have examined the effect of GLP-1 in healthy volunteers and on others with Type 1 and Type 2 diabetes, the dose - response between the GLP-1 and secretion of insulin has not been established. Moreover, many studies have shown that the weight loss observed by surgery was accompanied by improved control of diabetes and increased levels of GLP-1 [225].

It is believed that this peptide enhances insulin secretion through mechanisms involving the regulation of ion channels (including sensitivity to ATP, the potassium channels and calcium channels as well as the regulation and homeostasis of intra - cell and exocytosis [232]. The sensitivity to insulin has been discussed for its performance enhancing glucose uptake in muscle and fat both in humans and in mice [233]. Weight loss through gastroplaty also enhances β-cell glucose sensitivity characterized by an increased acute insulin response after intravenous glucose stimulus [200]. The increased incretin effect after weight loss [220] can be one possible explanation for the improved β-cell glucose sensitivity [234].

4. CONCLUSION

The threat of starvation to survival has exerted greater influence than the long-term consequences of obesity. Humans and animals maintain the vital cellular functions consuming more calories than are required for immediate metabolic needs. Chronic positive energy balance leads to storage of excessive calories as glycogen in liver, protein in muscle and triglycerides in adipose tissue, particularly in adipocytes of white adipose tissue. Adipocytes physiology is regulated by a number of signals including nutrients, hormones and signals of central nervous system. The role of the adipocyte in metabolic homeostasis has long been known, however its role as an endocrine cell only recently has been recognized. Adipose tissue produces biologically active substances – the adipokines- with local/systemic actions. This adipokines are active in many body functions including glucose and lipid metabolism, vascular tone, immunity/ inflammation, steroid hormone production, angiogenesis and coagulation.

Obesity is characterized by chronic excessive accumulation of fat and, metabolically, by hyperinsulinemia and peripheral insulin resistance that occurs in skeletal muscle, liver, fat, pancreas and adipose tissue. It is associated with a low-grade inflammation process in adipose tissue, characterized by the activation of some pro-inflammatory signalling pathways, such as c-jun N-terminal kinase (JNK) and nuclear factor κB (NFκB), leading to increased expression of pro-inflammatory cytokines.

Furthermore it has been suggested that, in obesity, adipose tissue ER stress, oxygen species production and FFAs, can activate some pro-inflammatory signalling pathways which interfere with insulin signalling *via* serine/threonine inhibitory phosphorylation of IRS. Ultimately these mechanisms have been shown to be detrimental linking the obesity and the inflammation with numerous diseases, including insulin resistance, type 2 diabetes and cardiovascular disease.

Weight loss can improve fat function by promoting the reduction in size of dysfunctional fat cells. This goal can be achieved through hypocaloric diet, regular physical exercise and anti-obesity drugs.

New therapeutic approaches can be considered in order to improve adipose tissue functional capacity and adipose tissue-mediated nutrient metabolism, to reduce systemic inflammation and to correct the over or under production of adipocytes factors and thus, contribute to treatment of type 2 DM, hypertension, dyslipidemia and cardiovascular disease associated to obesity.

ACKNOWLEDGEMENT

We thank Stephen Shaw for help with the English revision of the manuscript.

REFERENCES

[1] Levin BE. Central regulation of energy homeostasis intelligent design: how to build the perfect survivor. Obesity (Silver Spring) 2006; 14 (Suppl 5): 1925-1965.
[2] Ogden CL, Yanovski SZ, Carroll MD, Flegal KM. The epidemiology of obesity. Gastroenterology 2007; 132: 2087-2102.
[3] Saris WH, Astrup A, Prentice AM, *et al.* Randomized controlled trial of changes in dietary carbohydrate/fat ratio and simple vs complex carbohydrates on body weight and blood lipids: the CARMEN study. The carbohydrate ratio management in European National diets. Int J Obes Relat Metab Disord 2000; 24: 1310-1318.
[4] Hull D, Segal M. Distinction of brown from white adipose tissue. Nature 1966; 21: 469-472.
[5] Cinti S. The adipose organ. Prostaglandins Leukot Essent Fatty Acids 2005; 73(1): 9-15.
[6] Oberkofler H, Dallinger G, Liu YM, Hell E, Krempler F, Patsch W. Uncoupling protein gene: Quantification of expression levels in adipose tissue of obese and non-obese humans. J Lipid Res 1997; 38: 2125-2133.
[7] Cinti S. The role of brown adipose tissue in human obesity. Nutr Metab Cardiovasc Dis 2006; 16: 569-574.
[8] Girardier L. The regulation of the biological furnace of warm blooded animals. Experientia 1977; 33: 1121-1131.
[9] Cannon B, Hedin A, Nedergaard J. Exclusive occurrence of thermogenic antigen in brown adipose tissue. FEBS 1982; 150: 129-132.
[10] Cannon B, Nedergaard J. Brown adipose tissue: function and physiological significance. Physiol Rev 2004; 84: 277-359.
[11] DiGirolamo M, Fine JB, Tagra K, Rossmanith R. Qualitative regional differences in adipose tissue growth and cellularity in male wistar rats fed ad libitum. Am J Physiol 1998; 274: R1460-R 1467.
[12] Weisberg SP, McCann D, Desai M, Rosenbaum M, Leibel RL, Ferrante AW. Obesity is associated with macrophage accumulation in adipose tissue. J Clin Invest 2003; 112: 1796-1808.
[13] Curat CA, Miranville A, Sengenes C, *et al.* From blood monocytes to adipose tissue-resident macrophages: Induction of diapedesis by human mature adipocytes. Diabetes 2004; 53: 1285-1292.
[14] Cinti S, Mitchel G, Barbatelli G, *et al.* Adipocyte death defines macrophage localization and function in adipose tissue of obese mice and humans. J Lipid Res 2005; 46: 2347-2355.
[15] Larson DR, Zipfel WR, Williams RM, *et al.* Water-soluble quantum dots for multiphoton fluorescence imaging *in vivo*. Science 2003; 300: 1434-1436.
[16] Bartness TJ, Bamshad M. Innervation of mammalian white adipose tissue: implications for the regulation of total body fat. Am Physiol 1998; 275: 1399-1411.
[17] Faust IM, Johnson PR, Stern JS, *et al.* Diet-induced adipocyte number increase in adult rats: a new model of obesity. Am J Physiol 1978; 235: E279-E286.
[18] Lafontan M. Fat cells: Afferent and efferent messages define new approaches to treat obesity. Ann Rev Pharmacol Toxicol 2005; 45: 119-146.
[19] Shrago E, Spennetta T, Gordon E. Fatty acid synthesis in human adipose tissue. J Biol Chem 1969; 244: 2761-2766.
[20] Kahn BB, Flier JS. Obesity and insulin resistance. J Clin Invest 2000; 106: 473-481.
[21] Berg J, Tymoczko J, Stryer L, Clarke ND. Biochemistry. New York: W.H. Freeman and Company 2002.
[22] Stralfros P, Bjorgell P, Belfrage P. Hormonal regulation of hormone-sensitive lipase in intact adipocytes: identification of phosphorylated sites and effects on the phosphorylation by lipolytic hormones and insulin. Proc Natl Acad Sci USA 1984; 81: 3317-3321.
[23] Anthonsen MW, Ronnstrand L, Wernstedt C, Degerman E, Holm C. Identification of novel phosphorilation sites in hormone-sensitive lipase that are phosphorylated in response to isoproterenol and govern activation properties *in vitro*. J Biol Chem 1998; 273: 215-221.
[24] Arner P, Langin D. The role of neutral lipase in human adipose tissue lipolysis. Curr Opin Lipidol 2007; 18: 246-250.
[25] Arner P. Human fat cell lipolysis: Biochemistry, regulation and clinical role. Best Pract Res Clin Endocrinol Metab 2005; 19: 471-482.
[26] Zhang Y, Proenca R, Maffei M, *et al.* Positional cloning of the mouse obese gene and its human homologue. Nature 1994; 372: 425-432.
[27] Fruhbeck G. Adipose tissue as an endocrine organ. Obesity 2001; 4: 16-19.
[28] Ahima RS, Flier JS. Adipose tissue as an endocrine organ. Trends Endocrinol Metab 2000; 11: 327-332.
[29] Trayhurn P, Beattie JH. Physiological role of adipose tissue: white adipose tissue as an endocrine and secretory organ. Proc Nutr Soc 2001; 60:329-339.
[30] Wiecek A, Kokot F, Chudek J, Adamczak M. The adipose tissue – a novel endocrine organ of interest to the nephrologists. Nephrol Dial Transplant 2002; 17: 191-195.
[31] Caspar-Bauguil S, Cousin B, Galinier A, *et al.* Adipose as an ancestral immune organ: Site-specific change in obesity. FEBS Lett 2005; 579: 3487-3492.
[32] Arner P. The adipocyte in insulin resistance: key molecules and the impact of the thiazolidinediones. Trends Endocrinol Metab 2003; 14:137-145.

[33] Suteri PK. Adipose tissue as a source of hormones. Am J Clin Nutr 1987; 47: 277-282.

[34] Halleux CM, Servais I, Reul BA, Detry R, Brichard SM. Multihormonal control of ob gene expression and leptin secretion from cultured human visceral adipose tissue: increased responsiveness to glucocorticoids in obesity. J Clin Endocrinol Metab 1998, 83: 902-910.

[35] Saad MF, Kahn A, Sharma A, *et al.* Physiological insulinemia acutely modulates plasma leptin. Diabetes 1998, 47: 544-549.

[36] Kirchgessner TG, Wysal T, Wiesbrock SM, Marino MW, Hotamisligil G. Tumor necrosis factor-alpha contributes to obesity-related hyperleptinemia by regulating leptin release from adipocytes. J Clin Invest 1997; 100: 2777-2782.

[37] Karlsson C, Lindell K, Ottoson M, *et al.* Human adipose tissue express angiotensinogen and enzymes required for its conversion to angiotensin II. J Clin Endocrinol Metab 1998; 83: 3925-3929.

[38] Arita Y, Kihara S, Ouchi N, *et al.* Paradoxal decrease of an adipose-specific protein, adiponectin, in obesity. Biochen Biophys Res Commun 1999; 257: 79-83.

[39] Fried SK, Bunkin DA, Greenberg AS. Omental and subcutaneous adipose tissues of obese subjects release interleukin-6: depot difference and regulation by glucocorticoid. J Clin Endocrinol Metab 1998; 83: 847-50.

[40] Bastard JP, Maachi M, Tran Van Nhieu J, *et al.* Adipose tissue IL-6 content correlates with resistance to insulin activation of glucose uptake both in vivo and in vitro. J Clin Endocrinol Metab 2002; 87: 2084-9

[41] Kamay Y, Mikawa S, Endo K, Sakai H, Komano T. Regulation of insulin-like growth factor-1 expression in mouse preadipocyte ob 1771. J Biol Chem 1996; 271: 9883-9886.

[42] Bastard JP, Jardel C, Bruckert E, *et al.* Elevated levels of interleukin 6 are reduced in serum and subcutaneous adipose tissue of obese women after weight loss. J Clin Endocrinol Metab 2000; 85: 3338-42.

[43] Mohamed-Ali V, Goodrick S, Rawesh A, *et al.* Subcutaneous adipose tissue releases interleukin-6, but not tumor necrosis factor-alpha *in vivo*. J Clin Endocrinol Metab 1997; 82(Suppl 12): 4196-4200.

[44] Kern RN, Ranganathan PA, Li S, Wool CL, Raganthan G. Adipose tissue tumor necrosis factor and interleukin-6 expression in human obesity and insulin resistance. Am J Physiol Endocrinol Metab 2001; 280(Suppl 5): E-745-51.

[45] Visser M. Higher levels of inflammation in obese children. Nutrition 2001; 17(Suppl 6): 480-481.

[46] Roytblat L, Rachinsky M, Fisher A, *et al.* Raised interleukin-6 levels in obese patients, Obes Res 2000; 8: 673-675.

[47] Straczkowski M, Dzienis-Straczkowska S, Stepien A, Kowalska I, Szelachowska M , Kinalska I. Plasma interleukin-8 concentrations are increased in obese subjects and related to fat mass and tumor necrosis factor-{alpha} system. J Clin Endocrinol Metab 2002; 87: 4602-4606.

[48] Hotamisligil GS, Spiegelman BM. Tumor necrosis factor alpha: a key component of the obesity-diabetes link. Diabetes 1994; 43(11): 1271-8.

[49] Sartipy P, Loskutoff DJ. Monocyte chemoattractant protein 1 in obesity and insulin resistance. Proc Natl Acad Sci USA 2003; 100 7265-7270.

[50] Hotamisligil GS, Arner P, Caro JF, Atkinson RL, Spiegelman BM. Increased adipose tissue expression of tumor necrosis factor-alpha in human obesity and insulin resistance. J Clin Inves 1995; 95: 2409-2415.

[51] Visser M, Bouter LM, McQuillan GM, Wener HM, Harris TB. Elevated C-reactive protein levels in overweight and obese adults. JAMA 1999; 282: 2131-2135.

[52] Seidell JC. Prevalence of obesity in Europe. Bibl Nutr Dieta 1989; 44: 1-7.

[53] Wang P, Mariman E Renes J, Keijer J. The secretory function of adipocytes in the physiology of white adipose tissue. J Cell Physiol 2008; 216: 3-13.

[54] World Health Organization. Obesity: preventing and managing the global epidemic. Report of a WHO consultation. World Health Organ Tech Rep Ser 2000; 894: i-xii, 1-253.

[55] World Health Organization. Fat sheet on obesity and overweight. Geneva: World Health Organization 2006.

[56] Goossens GH. The role of adipose tissue dysfunction in the pathogenesis of obesity-related insulin resistance. Physiol Behavior 2008; 94: 206-218.

[57] Ogden CL, Flegal KM, Carrol MD, Johnson CL. Prevalence and trends in overweight among US children and adolescents 1999 – 2000. JAMA 2002; 288: 1728-1732.

[58] Olshansky SJ, Hayflick L, Butler RN, Allison DB, Ludwig DS. A potential decline in life expectance in the United States in the 21st century. N Engl J Med 2005; 352: 1138-1145.

[59] Ashley FW, Kannel WB. Relation of weight change to changes in atherogenic traits: the Framingham study. J Chronic Dis 1974; 27: 103-114.

[60] Mokdad AH, Ford ES, Bowman BA, *et al.* Prevalence of obesity, diabetes and obesity-related health risk factor. JAMA 2003; 289(1):76-79.

[61] Bonadonna RC, Groop L, Kraemer N, Ferrannini E, Del Prato S, DeFronzo RA. Obesity and insulin resistance in humans: a dose-response study. Metabolism 1990; 39(5): 452-459.

[62] DeFronzo RA, Bonadonna RG, Ferrannini E. A balanced overview. Diabetes Care 1992; 151: 318-368.

[63] Hotamisligil GS. Molecular mechanisms of insulin resistance and the role of adipocyte. Int J Obes Relat Metab Disord 2000; 24: S23-S27.

[64] Hotamisligil GS, Shargill NS, Spiegelman BM. Adipose expression of tumor necrosis factor-alpha: direct role in obesity-linked insulin resistance. Science 1993; 259: 87-91.

[65] Das UN. Is metabolic syndrome X an inflammatory condition? Exp Biol Med (Maywood) 2002; 227: 989-97.

[66] Das UN. Obesity,metabolic syndrome X, and inflammation. Nutrition 2002; 18: 430-2.

[67] Ford ES. The metabolic syndrome and C-reactive protein, fibrinogen, and leukocyte count: findings from the Third National Health and Nutrition Examination Survey. Atherosclerosis 2003; 168: 351-8.

[68] Albert MA, Glynn RJ, Ridker PM. Plasma concentration of C-reactive protein and the calculated Framingham Coronary Heart Disease Risk Score. Circulation 2003; 108: 161-5.

[69] Luc G, Bard JM, Juhan-Vague I, *et al.* C-reactive protein, interleukin-6, and fibrinogen as predictors of coronary heart disease: the PRIME Study. Arterioscler Thromb Vasc Biol 2003; 23:1255-61.

[70] Ridker PM, Cushman M, Stampfer MJ, Tracy RP, Hennekens CH. Inflammation, aspirin, and the risk of cardiovascular disease in apparently healthy men. N Engl J Med 1997; 336: 973-9.

[71] Engstrom G, Hedblad B, Stavenow L, Lind P, Janzon L, Lindgarde F. Inflammation-sensitive plasma proteins are associated with future weight gain. Diabetes 2003; 52: 2097-101.

[72] Mosca L. C-reactive protein--to screen or not to screen? N Engl J Med 2002; 347: 1615-7.

[73] Moller DE. Potential role of TNF-α in the pathogenesis of insulin resistance and type 2 diabetes.Trends Endocrinol Meta 2000; 11: 212-217.
[74] Fernandez-Real JM, Vayreda M, Richart C, *et al*. Circulating interleukin 6 levels, blood pressure, and insulin sensitivity in apparently healthy men and women. J Clin Endocrinol Metab 2001; 86(Suppl 3): 1154-9.
[75] Weyer C, Yudkin JS, Stehouvwer CD, *et al*. Humoral markers of inflammation and endothelial dysfunction in relation to adiposity and *in vivo* insulin action in Pima Indians. Atherosclerosis 2002; 161: 233-242.
[76] Tchernof A, Nolan A, Sites CK, Ades PA, Poehlman ET. Weight loss reduces C-reactive protein levels in obese postmenopausal women. Circulation 2002; 105: 564-569.
[77] Straczkowski M, Lewczuk P, Dzienis-Straczkowska S, Kowalska I, Stepien A, Kinalska I. Elevated soluble intercellular adhesion molecule-1 levels in obesity: relationship to insulin resistance and tumor necrosis factor –α system activity. Metabolism 2002; 51: 75-78.
[78] Selvin E, Paynter NP, Erlinger TP. The effect of weight loss on C-reactive protein. Arch Intern Med 2007; 167: 31-39.
[79] Rosen BS, Cook KS, Yaglom J, *et al*. Adipsin and complement factor D activity: an immune-related defect in obesity. Science 1989; 244 (4911): 1483-7.
[80] Shi H, Kokoeva MV, Inouye K, Tzameli I, Yin H, Flier JS. TLR4 links innate immunity and fatty acid-induced insulin resistance J Clin Invest 2006; 116(Suppl 11): 3015-25.
[81] Cousin B, Munoz O, Andre M, *et al*. A role for preadipocytes as macrophage-like cells. FASEB J 1999; 13(2): 305-12.
[82] Charriere G, Cousin B, Arnaud E, *et al*. Preadipocyte conversion to macrophage. Evidence of plasticity. J Biol Chem 2003; 278(11): 9850-5.
[83] Fain JN, Madan AK, Hiler ML, Cheema P, Bahouth SW. Comparison of the release of adipokines by adipose tissue, adipose tissue matrix, and adipocytes from visceral and subcutaneous abdominal adipose tissues of obese humans. Endocrinology 2004; 145: 2273-82.
[84] Fain JN. Release of interleukins and other inflammatory cytokines by human adipose tissue is enhanced in obesity and primarily due to the nonfat cells. Vitam Horm 2006; 74: 443-77.
[85] Tontonoz P, Nagy L, Alvarez JG, Thomazy VA, Evans RM. PPARgamma promotes monocyte/ macrophage differentiation and uptake of oxidized LDL. Cell 1998; 93(2): 241-52.
[86] Nagy L, Tontonoz P, Alvarez JG, Chen H, Evans RM. Oxidized LDL regulates macrophage gene expression through ligand activation of PPARgamma. Cell 1998; 93(2): 229-40.
[87] Makowski L, Boord JB, Maeda K, *et al*. Lack of macrophage fatty-acid-binding protein aP2 protects mice deficient in apolipoprotein E against atherosclerosis. Nat Med 2001; 7(6): 699-705.
[88] Neels JG, Olefsky J. Inflammedd fat? What starts the fire? J Clin Invest 2006; 116: 33-35.
[89] Shoelson S, Lee J, Goldfine A. Inflammation and insulin resistance. J Clin Invest 2006; 116: 1793-1801.
[90] Ozcan U, Cao Q, Yilmaz E, *et al*. Endoplasmic reticulum stress links obesity, insulin action, and type 2 diabetes. Science 2004; 306(5695): 457-61.
[91] Ozawa K, Miyazaki M, Matsuhisa M, *et al*. The endoplasmic reticulum chaperone improves insulin resistance in type 2 diabetes. Diabetes 2005; 54(3): 657-63.
[92] Nakatani Y, Kaneto H, Kawamori D, *et al*. Involvement of endoplasmic reticulum stress in insulin resistance and diabetes. J Biol Chem 2005; 280(1): 847-51.
[93] Furukawa S, Fujita T, Shimabukuro M, *et al*. Increased oxidative stress in obesity and its impact on metabolic syndrome. J Clin Invest 2004; 114: 1752-61.
[94] Hotamisligil GS. Inflammation and metabolic disorders. Nature 2006; 444: 860-7.
[95] Gregor MG, Hotamisligil GS. Adipocyte stress: the endoplasmic reticulum and metabolic disease. J Lipid Res 2007; 48:1905-14.
[96] Aguirre V, Uchida T, Yenush L, Davis R, White MF. The c-Jun NH(2)-terminal kinase promotes insulin resistance during association with insulin receptor substrate-1 and phosphorylation of Ser(307). J Biol Chem 2000; 275: 9047-54.
[97] Hirosumi J, Tuncman G, Chang L, *et al*. A central role for JNK in obesity and insulin resistance. Nature 2002; 420: 333-6.
[98] Wellen KE, Hotamisligil GS. Inflammation, stress, and diabetes. J Clin Invest 2005; 115(Suppl 5): 1111-9.
[99] Vazquez LA, Pazos F, Berrazueta JR, *et al*. Effects of changes in body weight and insulin resistance on inflammation and endothelial function in morbid obesity after bariatric surgery. J Clin Endocrinol Metab 2005; 90(Suppl 1): 316-22.
[100] Kroder G, Bossenmaier B, Kellerer M, *et al*. Tumor necrosis factor-alpha- and hyperglycemia-induced insulin resistance. Evidence for different mechanisms and different effects on insulin signalling. J Clin Invest 1996; 97(6): 1471-7.
[101] Mooney RA, Senn J, Cameron S, *et al*. Suppressors of cytokine signaling-1 and -6 associate with and inhibit the insulin receptor. A potential mechanism for cytokine-mediated insulin resistance. J Biol Chem 2001; 276(28): 25889-93.
[102] Lagathu C, Bastard JP, Auclair M, Maachi M, Capeau J, Caron M. Chronic Interleukin-6 (IL-6) treatment increased IL-6 secretion and induced insulin resistance in adipocyte: Prevention by Rosiglitazone. Biochem Biophys Res Com 2003; 311(2): 372-9.
[103] Rieusset J, Bouzakri K, Chevillotte E, *et al*. SOCS (Suppressor of Cytokine Signaling)-3 Expression and insulin resistance in skeletal muscle of obese and type 2 diabetic patients. Diabetes 2004; 53(9): 2232-41.
[104] Hotamisligil GS, Peraldi P, Budavari A, Ellis R, White MF, Spiegelman BM. IRS-1-mediated inhibition of insulin receptor tyrosine kinase activity in TNF-alpha- and obesity-induced insulin resistance. Science 1996; 271(5249): 665-8.
[105] Grimble RF. Inflammatory status and insulin resistance. Curr Opin Clin Nutr Metab Care 2002; 5(5): 551-9.
[106] Dandona P, Weinstock R, Thusu K, Abdel-Rahman E, Aljada A, Wadden T. Tumor necrosis factor-α in sera of obese patients: fall with weight loss. J Clin Endocrinol Metab 1998, 83: 2907-10.
[107] Uysal KT, Wiesbrock SM, Marino MW, Hotamisligil GS. Protection from obesity-induced insulin resistance in mice lacking TNFalpha function. Nature 1997; 389(6651): 610-4.
[108] Liu LS, Spelleken M, Rohrig K, Hauner H, Eckel J. Tumor Necrosis factor alpha acutely inhibits insulin signalling in human adipocytes: implications of the p80 tumor necrosis factor receptor. Diabetes 1998; 47(4): 515-22.
[109] Kanety H, Feinstein R, Papa MZ, Hemi R, Karasik A. Tumor necrosis factor alpha induced phosphorylation of insulin receptor substrate-1 (IRS-1). Possible mechanism for suppression of insulin-stimulated tyrosine phosphorylation of IRS-1. J Biol Chem 1995; 270(40): 23780-4.
[110] Migrone G, Rosa G, Di Rocco P, *et al*. Skeletal muscle triglycerides lowering is associated with net improvement of insulin sensitivity, TNF-alfa reduction and GLUT4 expression enhancement. Int J Obes 2002; 26: 1165-1172.

[111] Ruan H, Hacohen N, Golub TR, Van Parijs L, Lodish HF. Tumor necrosis factor-alpha suppresses adipocyte-specific genes and activates expression of preadipocyte genes in 3T3-L1 adipocytes: nuclear factor-kappaB activation by TNF-alpha is obligatory. Diabetes 2002; 51: 1319-1336.
[112] Yudkin JS, Kumari M, Humphries SE, Mohamed-Ali V. Inflammation, obesity, stress and coronary heart disease: is interleukin-6 the link? Atherosclerosis 2000; 148(2): 209-214.
[113] Pradhan AD, Manson JE, Rifai N, Buring JE, Ridker PM. C-reactive protein, interleukin 6, and risk of developing type 2 Diabetes mellitus. JAMA 2001; 286(3): 327-334.
[114] Ridker PM. Clinical application of C-reactive protein for cardiovascular disease detection and prevention. Circulation 2003; 107(3): 363-369.
[115] Nonogaki K, Fuller GM, Fuentes NL, *et al.* Interleukin-6 stimulates hepatic triglyceride secretion in rats. Endocrinology 1995; 136(5): 2143-2149.
[116] Ihle JN, Witthuhn BA, Quelle FW, Yamamoto K, Silvennoinen O. Signaling through the hematopoietic cytokine receptors. Annu Rev Immunol 1995; 13: 369-398.
[117] Rieusset J, Bouzakri K, Cheviollotte E, *et al.* Suppressor of cytokine signaling 3 expression and insulin resistance in skeletal muscle of obese and type 2 diabetic patients. Diabetes 2004; 53: 2232-2241.
[118] Fasshauer M, Kralisch S, Klier M, *et al.* Adiponectin gene expression and secretion is inhibited by interleukin-6 in 3T3-L1 adipocytes. Biochem Biophys Res Commun 2003; 301: 1045-1050.
[119] Kim F, Tysseling KA, Rice J, *et al.* Free fatty acid impairment of nitric oxide production in endothelial cells is mediated by IKKbeta. Arterioscler Thromb Vasc Biol 2005; 25(5): 989-994.
[120] Lee JY, Hwang DH. The modulation of inflammatory gene expression by lipids: mediation through Toll-like receptors. Mol Cell 2006; 21: 174-185.
[121] Iwasaki A, Medzhitov R. Toll-like receptor control of the adaptive immune responses. Nat Immunol 2004; 5: 987-995.
[122] Trujillo ME, Scherer PE. Adiponectin—Journey from an adipocyte secretory protein to biomarker of the metabolic syndrome. J Intern Med 2005; 257: 167-175.
[123] Kadowaki T, Yamauchi T, Kubota N, Hara K, Ueki K, Tobe K. Adiponectin and adiponectin receptors in insulin resistance, diabetes, and the metabolic syndrome. J Clin Invest 2006; 116: 1784-1792.
[124] Guzik TJ, Mangalat D, Korbut R. Adipocytokines-Novel link between inflammation and vascular function? J Physiol Pharmacol 2006; 57: 505-528.
[125] Yokota T, Oritani K, Takahashi I, *et al.* Adiponectin, a new member of the family of soluble defense collagens, negatively regulates the growth of myelomonocytic progenitors and the functions of macrophages. Blood 2000; 96(5): 1723-1732.
[126] Weyer C, Funahashi T, Tanaka S, Hotta K, Matsuzawa Y, Pratlex RE. Hypoadiponetinemia in obesity and type 2 diabetes: close association with insulin resistance and hyperinsulinemia. J Clin Endocrinol Metabol 2001; 86(Suppl 5): 1930-1935.
[127] Stefan N, Vozarova B, Funahashi T, *et al.* Plasma adiponectin concentration is associated with skeletal muscle insulin receptor tyrosine phosphorylation, and low plasma concentration precedes a decrease in whole-body insulin sensitvity in humans. Diabetes 2002; 51: 1884-1888.
[128] Bruun JM, Lihn AS, Verdich C, *et al.* Regulation of adiponectin by adipose tissue-derived cytokines: *in vivo* and *in vitro* investigations in humans. Am J Physiol Endocrinol Metab 2003; 285(3): E527-E533.
[129] Szmitko PE, Teoh H, Stewart DJ, Verma S. Adiponectin and cardiovascular disease: state of the art? Am J Physiol Hear Circ Physiol 2007; 292: 1655-1663.
[130] Kadowaki T, Yamauchi T. Adiponectin and Adiponectin receptors. Endocrine Rev 2005; 26(3): 439-451.
[131] Kazumi T, Kawaguchi A, Sakai K, Hirano T, Yoshino G. Cdna cloning and expression of a novel adipose specific collagen-like factor, ap M 1. Biochem Biophys Res Commum 2002; 221: 286-289.
[132] Matsubara M, Maruoka S, Katayose S. Decreased plasma adiponectin concentrations in women with dyslipidemia. J Clin Endocrinol Metab 2002; 87: 2764-2769.
[133] Kershaw EE, Flier JS. Adipose tissue as an endocrine organ. J Clin Endocrinol Metab 2004; 89: 2548-2556.
[134] Nawrocki AR, Scherer PE. The delicate balance between fat and muscle: adipokines in metabolic disease and musculoskeletal inflammation. Curr Opin Pharmacol 2004; 4: 281-289.
[135] Havel PJ. Update on adipocyte hormones. Regulation of energy balance and carbohydrate/lipid metabolism. Diabetes 2004; 53: S143-S151.
[136] Shimada K, Miyazaki T, Daida H. Adiponectin and atherosclerotic disease. Clin Chim Acta 2004; 344: 1-12.
[137] Pischon T, Girman CJ, Hotamisligil GS, Rifai N, Hu FB, Rimm EB. Plasma adiponectin levels and risk of myocardial infarction in men. JAMA 2004; 291: 1730-1737.
[138] Maahs DM, Ogden LG, Kinney GL, *et al.* Low plasma adiponectin levels predict progression of coronary artery calcification. Circulation 2005; 111: 747-753.
[139] Coppack SW, Evans RD, Fisher RM, *et al.* Adipose tissue metabolism in obesity: lipase action in vivo before and after a mixed meal. Metabolism 1992; 41: 264-272.
[140] Jensen MD, Caruso M, Heiling V, Miles JM. Insulin regulation of lipolysis in nondiabetic and IDDM subjects. Diabetes 1989; 38: 1595-1601.
[141] Chan DC, Watts GF, Barrett PHR, Mamo JCL, Redgrave TG. Markers of triglyceride-rich lipoprotein remnant metabolism in visceral obesity. Clin Chem 2002; 48: 278-283.
[142] Chan DC, Barrett PHR, Watts GF. Dyslipidemia in visceral obesity: mechanisms, implications, and therapy. Am J Cardiovasc Drugs 2004; 4: 227-246.
[143] Riches FM, Watts GF, Naoumova RP, Kelly JM, Croft KD, Thompson GR. Hepatic secretion of very-low-density lipoprotein apolipoprotein B-100 studied with a stable isotope technique in men with visceral obesity. Int J Obes Relat Metab Disord 1998; 22: 414-423.
[144] Grundy SM. Obesity, metabolic syndrome, and cardiovascular disease. J Clin Endocrinol Metab 2004; 89: 2595-600.
[145] Despres JP. Dyslipidaemia and obesity. Baillieres Clin Endocrinol Metab 1994; 8: 629-60.
[146] Meier U, Gressner AM. Endocrine regulation of energy metabolism review of pathobiochemical and clinical chemical aspects of leptin, ghrelin, adiponectin, and resistin. Clin Chem 2004; 50: 1511-1525.
[147] Havel PJ. Update on adipocyte hormones: regulation of energy balance and carbohydrate/lipid metabolism. Diabetes 2004; 53: 143-151.

[148] Berg AH, Combs TP, Scherer PE. ACRP30/adiponectin: an adipokine regulating glucose and lipid metabolism. Trends Endocrinol Metab 2002; 13: 84-89.

[149] Hotta K, Funahashi T, Arita Y, Takahashi M, Matsuda M, Okamoto Y. Plasma concentrations of a novel, adipose-specific protein, adiponectin, in type 2 diabetic patients. Arterioscler Thromb Vasc Biol 2000; 20: 1595-1599.

[150] Baratta R, Amato S, Degano C, *et al.* Adiponectin relationship with lipid metabolism is independent of body fat mass: evidence from both cross-sectional and intervention studies. J Clin Endocrinol Metab 2004; 89: 2665-2671.

[151] Cnop M, Havel PJ, Utzschneider KM, *et al.* Relationship of adiponectin to body fat distribution, insulin sensitivity and plasma lipoproteins: evidence for independent roles of age and sex. Diabetologia 2003; 46: 459-469.

[152] Yamauchi T, Kamon J, Minokoshi Y, *et al.* Adiponectin stimulates glucose utilization and fatty-acid oxidation by activating AMP-activated protein kinase, Nat Med 2002; 8: 1288-1295.

[153] Combs TP, Pajvani UB, Berg AH, *et al.* A transgenic mouse with a deletion in the collagenous domain of adiponectin displays elevated circulating adiponectin and improved insulin sensitivity. Endocrinology 2004; 145: 367-383.

[154] Van Dielen FMH, Vant't Veer C, Schols AM, Soeters PB, Buurman WA, Greve JW. Increased leptin concentration correlate with increased concentrations of inflammatory markers in morbidly obese individuals. Int J obes Relat Metab Disord 2001; 25: 1759-1766.

[155] UK prospective diabetes study 7: Response of fasting plasma glucose to diet therapy in newly presenting type II diabetic patients. UKPDS Group. Metabolism 1990; vol. 39(9): 905-912.

[156] Sjöström CD, Lissner L, Wedel H, Sjöström L. Reduction in incidence of diabetes, hypertension and lipid disturbances after intentional weight loss induced by bariatric surgery: the SOS Intervention Study. Obes Res 1999; 7: 477-484.

[157] Dixon JB, O´Brien PE. Lipid profile in the severely obese: changes with weight loss after lap-band surgery. Obes Res 2002; 10(9): 903-910.

[158] St-Onge MP, Desmond R, Hunter G, Gower B. Baseline inflammatory markers do not modulate the lipid response to weight loss. Metabolism 2008; 57(5): 598-604.

[159] Reduction in the Incidence of Type2 Diabetes with Lifestyle Intervention or Metformin. Diabetes Prevention Program Research Group. N Engl J Med 2002; 346: 393-403.

[160] Toumilehto J, Lindstorm J, Eriksson JG, *et al.* Prevention of type 2 diabetes mellitus by changes in lifestyle among subjects with impaired glucose tolerance. N Engl J Med 2001; 344: 1343-1350.

[161] Ross R, Dagnone D, Jones PJ, *et al.* Reduction in obesity and related comorbid conditions after diet-induced weight loss in men. A randomized, controlled trial. Ann Intern Med 2000; 133: 92-103.

[162] Zamboni M, Armellini F, Turcato E, *et al.* Effect of weight loss on regional body fat distribution in premenopausal women. Am J Clin Nutr 1993; 58: 29 -34.

[163] Goodpaster BH, Kelley D, Wing RR, *et al.* Effects of weight loss on regional fat distribution and insulin sensitivity in obesity. Diabetes 1999; 48: 839-847.

[164] Pereira JA, Lararin MACT, Pareja JC, Souza AL, Muscelli E. Insulin resistance in nondiabetic morbidly obese patients: effect of bariatric surgery. Obes Res 2003; 11: 1495-1501.

[165] Korner J, Bessler M, Cirilo LJ, *et al.* Effects of Roux-en-Y Gastric Bypass Surgery on Fasting and Postprandial Concentrations of Plasma Ghrelin, Peptide YY, and Insulin. J Clin Endocrinol Metabol 2005; 90(1): 359-365.

[166] Shah M, Simha V, Garg A. Long-term impact of bariatric surgery on body weight, comorbidities and nutritional status. J Clin Endocrinol Metabol 2006; 91(11): 4223-4231.

[167] Madsen EL, Rissanen A, Bruun JM, *et al.* Weight loss larger than 10% is needed for general improvement of levels of circulating adiponectin and markers of inflammation in obese subjects: a 3-year weight loss study. Euro J Endocrinol 2008; 158: 179-187.

[168] Jazet IM, Schaart G, Gastaldelli A, *et al.* Loss of 50% of excess weight using a very low energy diet improves insulin-stimulated glucose disposal and skeletal muscle insulin signalling in obese insulin-treated type 2 diabetic patients. Diabetologia 2008; 51: 309-319.

[169] Bloem CJ, Chang AM. Short-term exercise improves β-cell function and insulin resistance in older people with impaired glucose tolerance. J Clin Endocrinol Metabol 2008; 93: 387-392.

[170] Wu T, Gao X, Chen M, van Dam RM. Long-term effectiveness of diet-plus-exercise interventions vs. diet-only interventions for weight loss: a meta-analysis. Obes Rev 2009; 10: 313-323.

[171] Mertens IL, Van Gaal LF. Overweight, obesity, and blood pressure: the effects of modest weight reduction. Obes Res 2000; 8: 270-278.

[172] Van Gaal LF, Wauters MA, De Leeuw IH. The beneficial effects of modest weight loss on cardiovascular risk factors. Int J Obes Relat Metab Disord 1997; 21(Suppl 1): S5-S9.

[173] Kolotkin RL, Crosby RD, Williams GR *et al.* The relationship between health-related quality of life and weight loss. Obes Res 2001; 9: 564-571.

[174] Felson DT, Zhang Y, Anthony JM, *et al.* Weight loss reduces the risk for symptomatic knee osteoarthritis in women. The Framingham Study. Ann Intern Med 1992; 116: 535-539.

[175] Lofgren IE, Herron KL, West KL, *et al.* Weight loss favorably modifies anthropometrics and reverses the metabolic syndrome in premenopausal women. J Am College Nutrit 2005; 24: 486-493.

[176] Esposito K, Pontillo A, Di Palo C, *et al.* Effect of weight loss and lifestyle changes on vascular inflammatory markers in obese women: a randomized trial. J Am Med Assoc 2003; 289: 1799-1804.

[177] Ryan AS, Nicklas BJ, Berman DM, Elahi D. Adiponectin levels do not change with moderate dietary induced weight loss and exercise in obese postmenopausal women. Int J Obes Relat Metab Disord 2003; 27(9): 1066-1071.

[178] Xydakis AM, Case CC, Jones PH, *et al.* Adiponectin, Inflammation, and the Expression of the Metabolic Syndrome in Obese Individuals: The Impact of Rapid Weight Loss through Caloric Restriction. J Clin Endocrinol Metabol 2004; 89: 2697-2703.

[179] Kopp CW, Kopp HP, Steiner S, *et al.* Weight loss reduces tissue factor in morbidly obese patients. Obes Res 2003; 11: 950-956.

[180] James WP, Astrup A, Finer N, *et al.* Effect of sibutramine on weight maintenance after weight loss: a randomized trial: STORM Study Group: Sibutramine Trial of Obesity Reduction and Maintenance. Lancet 2000; 356: 2119-2125.

[181] Malone DC, Raebel MA, Porter JA, *et al.* Cost-effectiveness of sibutramine in the LOSE Weight Study: evaluating the role of pharmacologic weight-loss therapy within a weight management program. J Manag Care Pharm 2005; 11(6): 458-468.

[182] Mohanty P, Aljada A, Ghanim H, *et al.* Evidence for a potent antiinflammatory effect of rosiglitazone. J Clin Endocrinol Metab 2004; 89: 2728-2735.
[183] Haffner SM, Greenberg AS, Weston WM, *et al.* Effect of rosiglitazone treatment on nontraditional markers of cardiovascular disease in patients with type 2 diabetes mellitus. Circulation 2002; 106: 679-684.
[184] Strandberg TE, Vanhanen H, Tikkanen MJ. Effect of statins on C-reactive protein in patients with coronary artery disease. Lancet 1999; 353: 118-119.
[185] Koh KK, Schenke WH, Waclawiw M, Csako G, Cannon RO III. Statin attenuates increase in C-reactive protein during estrogen re- placement therapy in postmenopausal women. Circulation 2002; 105: 1531-1533.
[186] Koh KK, Han SH, Quon MJ, Ahn JY, Shin EK. Beneficial effects of fenofibrate to improve endothelial dysfunction and raise adiponectin levels in patients with primary hypertriglyceridemia. Diabetes Care 2005; 28: 1419 -24.
[187] Wang T-D, Chen W-J, Lin J-W, *et al.* Efficacy of fenofibrate and simvastatin on endothelial function and inflammatory markers in patients with combined hyperlipidemia: relations with baseline lipid profiles. Atherosclerosis 2003; 170: 315-323.
[188] Koh KK, Quon MJ, Han SH, *et al.* Vascular and metabolic effects of combined therapy with ramipril and simvastatin in patients with type 2 diabetes. Hypertension 2005; 45: 1-6.
[189] Food and Drug Administration: Guidance for Industry Developing Products for Weight Management. Available at: http://www.fda.gov/ cder/guidance/7544dft.pdf (Accessed February 2007).
[190] Matfin G. Review: Challenges in developing therapies for the metabolic syndrome. Br J Diabetes Vasc Dis 2007; 7: 152.
[191] Nieuwenhuis-Ruifrok AE, Kuchenbecker WKH, Hoek A, Middleton P, Norman RJ. Insulin sensitizing drugs for weight loss in women of reproductive age who are overweight or obese: systematic review and meta-analysis. Hum Reprod Update 2009; 15: 57-68.
[192] Mason EC, Tang S, Renquist KE, *et al.* A decade of change in obesity surgery. National Bariatric Surgery Registry (NBSR) Contributors. Obes Surg 1997; 7(3): 189-197.
[193] Wardle J. Obesity and behavior change: matching problem to practice. Int J Obes Relat Metab Disord 1996; 20(1): 91-98.
[194] Toumilehto J, Lindstorm J, Eriksson JG, *et al.* Prevention of type 2 diabetes mellitus by changes in lifestyle among subjects with impaired glucose tolerance. N Engl J Med 2001; 344:1343-1350.
[195] Smith SC, Goodman GN, Edwards CB. Roux- en y gastric bypass: a 7-year retrospective review of 3855 patients. Obes Surg 1995; 5: 314-318.
[196] Kolanowski J. Surgical treatment for morbid obesity. Br Med Bul 1997; 53: 433-444.
[197] Linscheid P, Christ-Crain M, Stoeckli R, *et al.* Increase in high molecular weight adiponectin by bariatric surgery-induced weight loss. Diabetes Obes Metab 2008; 10(12): 1266-1270.
[198] Kopp HP, Krzyzanowska K, Mohlig M, Spranger J, Pfeiffer AF, Schernthaner G. Effects of marked weight loss on plasma levels of adiponectin, markers of chronic subclinical inflammation and insulin resistance in morbidly obese women. Int J Obes (Lond) 2005; 29(7): 766-771.
[199] Vilarrasa N, Vendrell J, Sanchez-Santos R, *et al.* Effect of weight loss induced by gastric bypass on proinflammatory interleukin-18, soluble tumour necrosis factor-alpha receptors, C-reactive protein and adiponectin in morbidly obese patients. Clin Endocrinol (Oxf) 2007; 67(5): 679-686.
[200] Marin DM, Monte Alegre S, Ortiz JNM, *et al.* Insulin secretion and β-cell glucose sensitivity in Severe Obesity: Effect of Weight Loss after Gastric bypass- unpublished data.
[201] Ortiz JNM, Monte Alegre S, Marin DM, Souza AL, Pareja JC, Muscelli E. The effect of insulin on serum adiponectin, IL-6, TNF-α and CRP in severely obese subjects with normal or impaired glucose tolerance - unpublished data.
[202] Yang WS, LEE WJ, Funahashi T, *et al.* Weight reduction increases plasma levels of an adipose-derived anti-inflammatory, adiponectin. J Clin Endocrinol Metabol 2001; 86: 3815-3819.
[203] Fruebis J, *et al.* Proteolytic cleavage product of 30-kDa adipocyte complement-related protein increases fatty acid oxidation in muscle and causes weight loss in mice. Proc Natl Acad Sci 2001; 98: 2005-2010.
[204] Carvalho CP, Marin DM, Souza AL, *et al.* GLP-1 and adiponectin: effect of weight loss after dietary restriction and gastric bypass in morbidly obese patients with normal and abnormal glucose metabolism. Obes Surg 2009; 19(3): 313-320.
[205] Bojanowska E. Physiology and patholphysiology and glucagons-like peptide-1(GLP-1): the role of GLP-1 in the pathogenesis of diabetes mellitus, obesity and stress. Med Sci Monit 2005; 11: RA 271-278.
[206] Gutzwiller JP, Degen L, Heuss L, *et al.* Glucagon-like peptide 1 (GLP-1) and eating. Physiol Behav 2004; 82: 17-19.
[207] Perfetti R, Zhoy J, Doyle ME, *et al.* Glucagon-like peptide-1 induces cell proliferation and pancreatic-duodenum home-obox-1 expression and increases endocrine cell mass in the pancreas of old, glucose-intolerant rats. Endocrinology 2000; 141: 4600-5b.
[208] Holz GG, Kuhtreiber WM, Habener JP. Pancreatic beta cells are rendered glucose-competent by the insulinotropic hormone glucagon-like peptide-1 (7-37). Nature 1993; 361: 362-365.
[209] Thorens B, Waeber G. Glucagon-like peptide 1 and the control of insulin secretion in the normal state and in NIDDM. Diabetes 1993; 42: 1219-1225.
[210] Heller RS, Keiffer TJ, Haberber JF. Insulinotropic glucagon-like peptide 1 receptor expression in glucagon-producing-cells of the rat endocrine pancreas. Diabetes 1997; 46: 785-791.
[211] Fehmann HC, Habener JF. Function receptors for the insulinotropic hormone glucagon-like peptide 1 9 7-37) on a somatostatin secretion cell line. FEBS Lett 1991; 279: 335-340.
[212] Willms B, Werner J, Host JJ, *et al.* Gastric emptying, glucose responses, and insulin secretion after a liquid test meal: effects of exogenous glucagon-like peptide-1 (GLP-1)-(7-36) amide in type 2 (non-insulin-dependent) diabetic patients. J Clin Endocrinol Metabol 1991; 81: 327-332.
[213] Schirra J, Katschinski M, Weidmann C, *et al.* Gastric emptying and release of incretin hormones after glucose ingestion in humans. J Clin Invest 1996; 97: 92-103.
[214] Flint A, Raben A, Aatrup A, *et al.* Glucagon-like peptide-1 promotes satiety and suppresses energy intake in humans. J Clin Invest 1998; 101: 515-520.
[215] Naslund E, Gryback P, Hellstrom PM. Gastrointestinal hormones and gastric empty 20 years after jejunoileal bypass for invasive obesity. Int J Obes Relat Metab Disord 1997; 21(5): 387-92.
[216] Kieffer TJ, Habener JF. The glucagon-like peptides. Endocrine Rev 1999; 20: 876-913.
[217] Redondo A, Trigo MV, Acitores A, *et al.* Cell signalling of teh GLP-1 action in rat liver. Mol Cell Endocrinol 2003; 204: 43-50.

[218] Trapote MA, Clemente F, Galera C, *et al.* Inositolphosfophoglycans are possible mediators of the glucagon-like peptide 1 (7-36) amide action in the liver. J Endocrinol Invest 1996; 19: 114-118.
[219] Luque MA, Gonzalez N, Marquez L, *et al.* Glucagon-like peptide-1 (GLP-1) and glucose metabolism in human myocytes. J Endocrinol 2002; 173: 465-473.
[220] Unger RH, Eisentraut AM. Entero-insular axis. Archives of Internal Medicine 1969; 123: 261-266.
[221] Creutzfeldt W. The incretin concept today. Diabetologia 1979; 16: 75-85.
[222] Sirinek KR, O'Dorisio TM, Hill D, *et al.* Hyperinsulinism, glucose-dependent insulinotropic polypeptide, and enteroinsular axis in morbidly obese patients before and after gastric bypass. Surgery 1986; 781-787.
[223] Host JJ. On the physiology of GIP and GLP-1. Horm Metab Res 2004; 34: 747-754.
[224] Vilsboll T, Host JJ. Incretins, insulin secretion and type 2 diabetes mellitus. Diabetologia 2004; 47: 357-366.
[225] Blandine L, Stanley H, Krystle W, *et al.* Incretin levels and effect are markedly enhanced 1 month after Roux-in –Y gastric bypass surgery in obese patients with type 2 diabetes. Diabetes Care 2007; 30: 1709-1716.
[226] Pories WJ, Macdonald KG, Morgan EJ, *et al.* Surgical treatment of obesity and its effects on diabetes: 10-y follow-up. Am J Clin Nutr 1992; 55: 582S-585S.
[227] Greenway SE, Greenway FL, Klein S. Effects of obesty surgery on non-insulin-dependent diabetes mellitus. Arch Surg 2002; 137: 1109-1117.
[228] Rubino F, Gagner M. Potential of surgery for curing type 2 diabetes mellitus. Ann Surg 2002; 236: 554-559.
[229] Patriti A, Facchiano E, Sanna A, Gulla N, Donini A. The enteroinsular axis and the recovery from type2 diabetes after bariatric surgery. Obes Surg 2004; 14: 840-848.
[230] Schauer PR, Burguera B, Ikramuddin S, *et al.* Effect of laparoscopic Roux- en Y gastric bypass on type 2 diabetes mellitus. Ann Surg 2003; 238: 467-84; discussion 484-65.
[231] Nauck A, Heinesaat MM, Orkor C, *et al.* Preserved incretin activity of synthetic human gastric inhibitory polypeptide in patients with type 2 diabetes. J Clin Invest 1993; 91: 301-307.
[232] MacDonald PE, Salapatek AM, Wheeler MB. Glucagon-like peptide-1 receptor activation antagonizes voltage-dependent repolarizing K(+) currents in beta-cells: a possible glucose-dependent insulinotropic mechanism. Diabetes 2002; 51 (Suppl 3): S443-S447.
[233] Perfetti R, Merkerl P. Glucagon-like peptide-1: a major regulator of pancreatic beta –cell function. Eur J Endocrinol 2000; 143: 717-725a.
[234] Ahren B, Holst JJ, Mari A. Characterization of GLP-1 effects on β-cell function after meal ingestion in humans. Diabetes Care 2003; 26: 2860-2864.

Pharmacological Approach for Obesity

Mohannad Kusti, Forrest Olgers and Ehab Akkary*

Department of Bariatric and Advanced Laparoscopic Surgery, Preston Memorial Hospital, Kingwood, West Virginia, USA

Abstract: Obesity has reached epidemic levels in the US and represents a major health and economic challenge. The weight loss process generally starts with behavioral modification and ends with surgical intervention in cases of severe or morbid obesity. Pharmacological therapies present a valid option for patients who are overweight or morbidly obese as an in addition to the role of behavioral modification, diet and exercise. This option should also be considered for post-operative patients with inadequate weight loss who are not candidates for revisional bariatric procedures. Weight loss medications (WLMs) can be divided into the following categories:

1. *Noradrenergic Appetite Suppressants (NASs):* more commonly used. Examples include phentermine, sibutramine, phendimetrazine, and diethylpropion.
2. *Pancreatic Lipase Inhibitors (PLIs):* examples include orlistat.
3. *Fat Substitutes (FSs):* examples include olestra which has been integrated into snack foods but not been studied as a formal weight loss medication.
4. *Cannabinoid Receptor Antagonists (CRAs):* examples include Rimonabant.
5. Thermogenics and Stimulators of Fat Mobilization.

There is multiple OTC and commercial brands, it is important to differentiate between the different types and their mechanism of action, for example Alli is the OTC version of orlistat with same mechanism and side effects.

Since the obesity "disease" is chronic, the medications have to be weighed carefully in terms of the risks and benefits for long term use.

Sibutramine, as a commonly used NAS, is a centrally acting serotonin/ noradrenaline reuptake inhibitor and increases thermogenesis. Studies showed weight reduction of 4.45 kg for sibutramine compared to placebo with overall improvement in the metabolic profile e.g. decreased triglycerides, increased HDL, and improved Hgb A1C. The main side effect is tachycardia; there is conflicting studies about the effect on blood pressure so overall NASs are not recommended in patients with uncontrolled hypertension, or in case of history of cardio- and cerebrovascular disease.

Orlistat, a PLI, blocks the lipolysis of dietary triglycerides. A recent meta-analysis showed mean weight loss of 2.89 kg with overall improvement of the metabolic profile especially diabetes parameters; however there was no effect on HDL and triglycerides. As mentioned, the side effects are mainly gastrointestinal but can cause considerable inconvenience for patients for example greasy diarrhea, incontinence, urgency and oily spotting. Overall it is not recommended for patients with malabsorption or cholestasis.

Rimonabant, as a CRA, inhibits the overactivation of the endocannabinoid system resulting in central anorexia. Rimonabant seems to have effects on the metabolism through the adipose tissue, liver, skeletal muscles and the pancreas. There are four published RIO trials (Rio-North America, RIO-Europe, RIO-Lipids, RIO-Diabetes), rimonabant decreased weight by 6.3-6.9 kg in the non-diabetic groups *vs.* placebo (-1.5-1.8 kg) ($p < 0.001$), whereas in the diabetic subjects enrolled in RIO-Diabetes, weight loss was 5.3 *vs.* 1.4 kg in the placebo group with overall improvement in the metabolic profile in diabetic and non-diabetic patients. Rimonabant is contraindicated in patients with history of depression, suicidal ideation or uncontrolled psychiatric disorder.

In spite of the fact that serotonergic agents (fenfluramine, dexfenfluramine) were withdrawn from the US market in the late 1990's secondary to their cardiovascular and pulmonary complications. At

*Corresponding author: Tel: 304-329-1400; E-mail: ehabakkary@yahoo.com

the present time, it is very important to assess the patient's history regarding their intake as this might result in further cardiac or pulmonary evaluations.

In conclusion, WLMs have shown decrease in body weight and improved metabolic and cardiovascular risk factors. Since, the weight loss is modest, they should be considered in overweight (BMI 25 – 29.9kg/m^2) or obese (BMI 30 – 34.9 kg/m^2) patients and should not be considered as an alternative for surgical intervention in patients with higher BMIs. Diet, exercise and behavioral modification should always be implemented regardless of the weight loss means being applied.

Keywords: Obesity, medical weight loss, appetite suppressants, lipase inhibitors, fat substitutes, cannabinoid.

INTRODUCTION

Obesity is an epidemic in today's society, and with the exponential increase, the development of methods to prevent, control, and treat this major epidemic is warranted. This need is justified by the co-morbidities associated with obesity including: cardiovascular, atherosclerosis, cancers, and several metabolic diseases and an increased risk of physical and cognitive disabilities [1]. Society has become obesogenic, this is mainly due the lifestyle and behavior of the community. Table **1** shows obesity rates state wide. In 2008, only one state (Colorado) had a prevalence of obesity less than twenty percent. Thirty-two states had prevalence equal to, or greater than twenty five percent. Six of these states (Alabama, Mississippi, Oklahoma, South Carolina, Tennessee, and West Virginia) had a prevalence of obesity equal to, or greater than thirty percent [This data is from the Center of Disease Control and Prevention (CDC) statistics data base]. Not only adults, but for children and adolescent a study showed that during the past three decades prevalence rates of childhood and adolescent obesity [defined as body mass index (BMI) above the ninety-fifth percentile for age and sex] have increased more than fifty percent in the United States [2]. Approximately one hundred and ten million children are now classified as overweight or obese [3]. Treatment for obesity has been the focus of research for the past twenty years. There are many drugs in the market, some are Food and Drug Administration (FDA) approved and some are not. Some people even use medications that are meant to treat other conditions to implement their possible weight loss side effect.

Table 1. Obesity Rates in all States 2008 - Centers for Disease Control and Prevention (CDC)

2008 State Obesity Rates							
State	**%**	**State**	**%**	**State**	**%**	**State**	**%**
Alabama	31.4	Illinois	26.4	Montana	23.9	Rhode Island	21.5
Alaska	26.1	Indiana	26.3	Nebraska	26.6	South Carolina	30.1
Arizona	24.8	Iowa	26.0	Nevada	25.0	South Dakota	27.5
Arkansas	28.7	Kansas	27.4	New Hampshire	24.0	Tennessee	30.6
California	23.7	Kentucky	29.8	New Jersey	22.9	Texas	28.3
Colorado	18.5	Louisiana	28.3	New Mexico	25.2	Utah	22.5
Connecticut	21.0	Maine	25.2	New York	24.4	Vermont	22.7
Delaware	27.0	Maryland	26.0	North Carolina	29.0	Virginia	25.0
Washington DC	21.8	Massachusetts	20.9	North Dakota	27.1	Washington	25.4
Florida	24.4	Michigan	28.9	Ohio	28.7	West Virginia	31.2
Georgia	27.3	Minnesota	24.3	Oklahoma	30.3	Wisconsin	25.4
Hawaii	22.6	Mississippi	32.8	Oregon	24.2	Wyoming	24.6
Idaho	24.5	Missouri	28.5	Pennsylvania	27.7		

In 2003-2004, 17.1% of American children and adolescents were overweight and 32.2% of adults were obese. Prevalence of morbid obesity (BMI $\geq$ 40) in 2003-2004 was 2.8% in men and 6.9% in women. Approximately thirty percent of Caucasian adults were obese as were 45.0% of African American adults, and 36.8% of Mexican American adults. Among adults aged twenty to thirty nine years old, 28.5% were obese while 36.8% of adults aged forty to fifty nine years old and 31.0% of those aged sixty years or older were obese in 2003-2004 [4].

Obesity was once considered a health problem only in rich countries and high socioeconomic areas of the world but now this epidemic is strikingly on the rise in low and middle income countries. The World Health Organization (WHO) report showed that globally in 2005 approximately 1.6 billion of the world adult populations were over weight, with at least 400 million adults suffering from clinical obesity. What this means is that more than one fifth of the world is overweight. WHO also predict in their report that by 2015, there will be 2.3 billion adult overweight with approximately 700 million suffering from obesity.

Now how much of this is genetic? Separating genetic factors from other factors is difficult. However; twin, adoption, and family studies have shown that genetic factors play a significant role in the pathogenesis of obesity. Rare mutations in humans and model organisms have provided insight into the pathways involved in body weight regulation. Many studies show a genetic contribution on many levels, and scientists have managed to attribute genetic factors as opposed to environmental factors (for Example: sidewalks, community design) or behavioral factors such as diet and exercise [5, 6].

Treatment of obesity starts with behavioral modifications (Such as: eating habits, physical activity and sleeping patterns). Medical and surgical therapies are also available. Medical therapy either targets the central nervous system, mainly the brain or peripherally affecting the GI Tract and/or the metabolism (Fig. **1**). Surgical treatment examples are laparoscopic adjustable gastric band, gastric bypass and gastric sleeve gastrectomy. However, patient must meet the National Institutes of Health' criteria (NIH' criteria) to qualify for weight loss surgery.

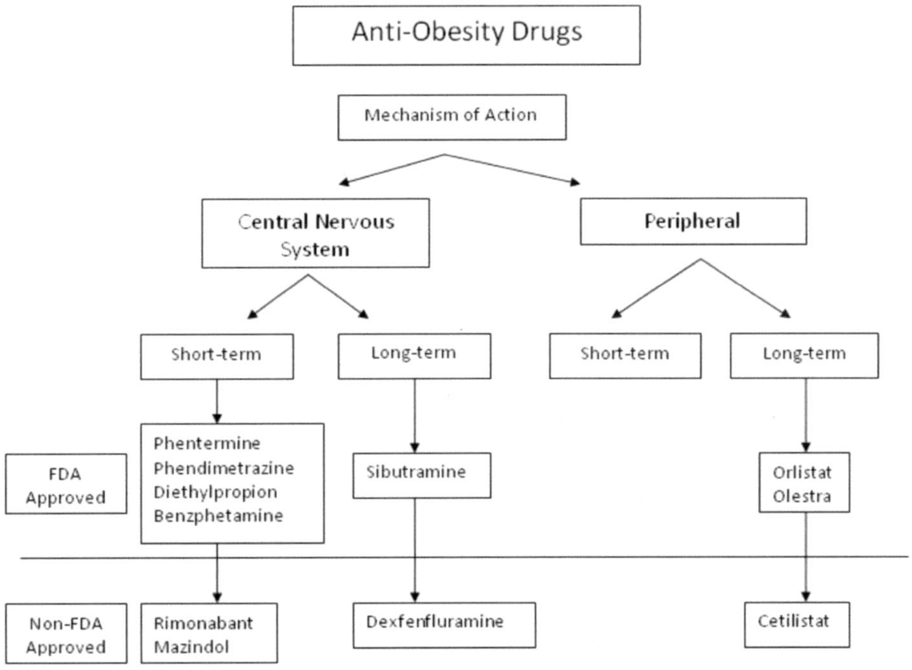

Fig. (1). Mechanisms of anti-obesity medications.

THE MECHANISM OF ANTI-OBESITY MEDICATIONS (AOM)

As mentioned, AOM works centrally or peripherally. CNS acting medications are classified into: Noradrenergic appetite Suppressants (NAS) and Cannabinoid Receptor Antagonist (CRA). Peripherally Acting medications include: Fat substitutes (FS) and Pancreatic Lipase Inhibitors (PLI), and Thermogenic drugs. Alternative medications used for weight loss are Metformin, Pralintide and GLP-1 derivative (used to treat type 2 Diabetes Mellitus [T2DM]), anti depressant medications such as Fluoxetine and Bupropoin, and anti epileptic medications such as Topiramate and Zonisamide (Fig. **2**). These medications are not approved for weight loss but some studies show positive results and it might be of some benefits for obese patients with those conditions. They are currently being investigated [7].

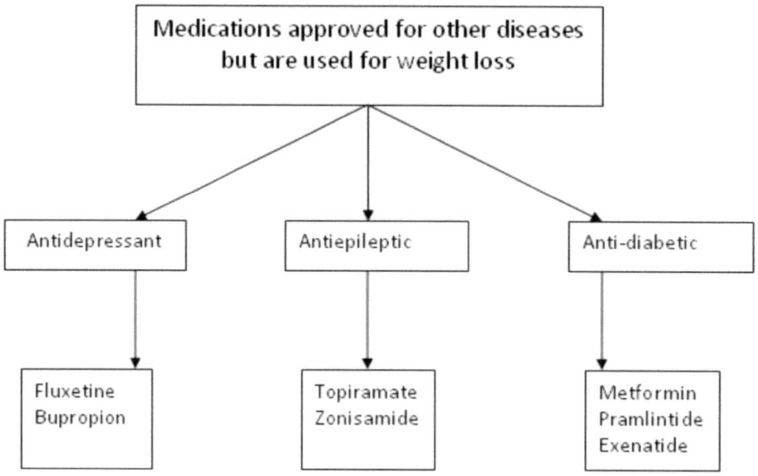

Fig. (2). Non-Approved medications commonly used.

MEDICATIONS WITH PRIMARY AFFECT ON CENTRAL NERVOUS SYSTEM

FDA Approved (Currently)

Noradrenergic appetite Suppressants (NAS) including: phentermine, sibutramine, phendimetrazine, diethylpropion, and benzphetamine

Non FDA Approved

- ∞ NAS: phenmetrazine: initially approved by the FDA in 1956 but was withdrawn for psychosis effects similar to amphetamines and was replaced by its analog “phendimetrazine”.
- ∞ Cannabinoid Receptor Antagonist (CRA) includes: Rimonabant.

NORADRENERGIC APPETITE SUPPRESSANTS (NAS)

Pharmacology and Efficacy of NAS

The mechanisms of action for this class of medication are sympathomimetic amines which have similar chemical structures as amphetamine which are Psychostimulants. *A*mphetamines effects are mediated by the action of norepinephrine centrally and peripherally, and appetite suppression activity is believed to be in the lateral hypothalamic feeding center. NAS exert its effects in the brain in a similar manner to amphetamine, stimulating the release, as well as inhibiting reuptake of neurotransmitters such as Dopamine (DA), Norepinephrine (NE), and Serotonin (5-HT) [8].

Safety and Monitoring

Amphetamines in general have a high potential for abuse and addiction. Amphetamines could also aggravate certain mental conditions such as nervousness or agitated behavior, psychosis, mania, and severe anxiety. Breast-feeding is not recommended while taking these medications because of unknown metabolites excretion in breast milk and possible complication to the infant. Amphetamines are category C for pregnant and breast feeding mothers.

Contraindications and Precautions

Advanced arteriosclerosis, congenital heart disease, symptomatic cardiovascular disease such as valve disease and arrhythmias, moderate to severe hypertension, hyperthyroidism, glaucoma, agitated states, history of drug abuse, and within 14 days of using monoamine oxidase (MAO) inhibitors. Due to the possible risk of hypertension crisis and sudden cardiac death, gradual discontinuation is highly recommended because abrupt discontinuation of phentermine after prolonged high doses may lead to severe mental depression and extreme fatigue; sleep electroencephalography (EEG) changes has been observed also. It is not recommend for patients with a history of eating disorders such as anorexia nervosa.

Patient should not use more than one centrally active AOM in the same time even if it was an over the counter or herbal preparation. Special cautions must be taken in patients with dental disease due to the decrease effect of salivary flow, which might contributing to the development of discomfort sensation, dental caries, periodontal disease, and oral candidiasis. There is an increased risk of Serotonin syndrome or neuroleptic malignant syndrome-like symptoms with the use alone or when used in combination with serotonergic drugs or medication that affects serotonin metabolism (such as MAO inhibitors), or antipsychotics or other DA antagonists.

Drug Interactions

These medications have many direct and indirect interactions with other medications. We describe some of the major interaction that should be looked after or avoided at best.

Atomoxetine	Potential for additive increases in blood pressure and heart rate.
Guanethidine	Amphetamines can decrease the antihypertensive effect of guanethidine.
Monoamine oxidase inhibitors	Can increase the pressor response to amphetamines.
Tricyclic antidepressants	Can decrease the effects of amphetamines.
Urinary acidifiers	Decrease the half-life, decrease the duration of action, and shorten the clinical effects of amphetamines.
Urinary alkalinizers	Increase the half-life, increase the duration of action, and prolong the clinical effects of amphetamines.

SHORT ACTING DRUGS

Phentermine

Phentermine was approved by the FDA in 1959 as an appetite suppressant to help reduce weight in obese patients when used short-term (8-12 weeks) in combinations with exercise, diet, and behavioral modification. Another preparation of Phentermine is Phentermine hydrochloride which is a salt preparation made as another brand was FDA approved in 1973. Phentermine is a schedule IV controlled substance.

Mechanism of Action

Like amphetamines, phentermine increases the release and inhibits the reuptake of norepinephrine and dopamine at the nerve terminals. For that reason, phentermine was classified as an indirect sympathomimetic. Clinically phentermine stimulates the central nervous system (CNS) and increases the blood pressure. Its appetite suppression effect is believed to be caused by direct stimulation of the satiety center in the hypothalamic and limbic region of the brain [9].

Tolerance to its anorexiant effects are most commonly seen within a few weeks of therapy. The tolerance appears to be pharmacodynamic in nature; higher doses of phentermine are required to produce the same response. When that occurs, it is recommended that phentermine be discontinued.

Pharmacokinetics

Phentermine is administrated orally, with greater absorption from the small intestine. The duration of action of the 8 mg capsules or tablets are approximately 4 hours after administration and 12—14 hours for higher doses. Primarily excreted is by renal. The estimated half-life (t½) for elimination ranges from 19 to 24 hours and is influenced by urine acidity. Because the pKa of phentermine is 9.84, the elimination t½ decreases to 7 or 8 hours under low urinary pH conditions.

Indications and Doses

Indications are severe obesity (BMI ≥ 30 kg/m^2) or obese patients (BMI ≥ 27 kg/m^2) with association of other risk factors including hypertension, diabetes mellitus, hyperlipidemia, etc.

Doses are 15 to 37.5 mg administered orally taken in the morning for adults, elderly and Adolescents >16 years of age. The max dose is 37.5mg per day, and drug should be taken before breakfast or up to 2 hours after; doses can be divided into two doses a day.

Doses may be adjusted for patients with reduced renal function such as patients with elevated plasma levels of blood urea nitrogen (BUN) and creatinine; it is recommended to monitor renal function at baseline and throughout therapy, if indicated.

Phendimetrazine

Phendimetrazine was FDA approved in 1961 to be used as an oral, indirect-acting, non-amphetamine sympathomimetic amine [9]. It is used as an appetite suppressant agent for short-term used between 8 to 12 weeks, as an adjunct to other obesity therapies. The pharmacologic effects of phendimetrazine are similar to amphetamines. It functions as a pro-drug to phenmetrazine, and approximately 30% of the oral dose is converted into Phenmetrazine. Phendimetrazine is virtually an extended release and a less abusable version of phenmetrazine and only indicated as a monotheraputic agent. Phendimetratizine is a schedule C-III controlled substance. There were also cases of cardiomyopathies related to phendimetrazine [10].

Mechanism of Action

The mechanism is similar to phentermine.

Pharmacokinetics

Phendimetrazine is absorbed mainly from the gastrointestinal tract. Its t½ is almost similar for both regular- and sustained-release preparations which showes similar onset of action for both dosage forms. The duration is prolonged for sustained-release formulations > 4 hours. In the circulation, part of the drug is metabolized to phenmetrazine and phendimetrazine-N-oxide [11]. The main route of elimination for the metabolites and non-metabolized medication is the kidneys. Average elimination t½ for regular- and sustained-release forms are approximately 1.9 hours and 9.8 hours respectively.

Indications and Doses

Phendimetrazine is indicated for the treatment of severe obesity (BMI ≥ 30) in a short-term period in association with a calorie restriction diet. It is recommended to discontinue the drug if satisfactory weight loss did not occur within the first 4 weeks of therapy (meaning a decrease of ≥ 4 lbs). This is to prevent the possibility of abuse [12, 13]. Dosage for regular capsules or tablets: Adults: 17.5—35 mg taken Orally 2—3 times a day, 1 hour before meals. And for extended-release formula: Adults: 105 mg orally once daily, 30min to 1 hr before breakfast. It is not recommended for ages < 16 years.

The Maximum Dosage for The Elderly, Adults and Adolescents ≥ 16 years is 210 mg/day orally for regular-release formulations. And since it has abuse potentials only 5 refills are allowed every 5 months.

Diethylpropion

It was approved by the FDA in 1959 for the use in the management of exogenous obesity as a short-term adjunct in a regimen of weight reduction based on caloric restriction. It is also known as Diethylcathinone or amfepramone. It is structurally, chemically and pharmacological effect is similarly related to the amphetamines. Diethylpropion induce – indirectly - the release as well as inhibit the reuptake of neurotransmitters such as a dopamine (DA) and norepinephrine (NE) [14]. A study showed significant weight reduction comparing with the placebo group which was most apparent in the first few month of use. After 6 months, the diethylpropion group lost an average of 9.8% (s.d. 6.9%) of initial body weight *vs.* 3.2% (3.7%) in the placebo group (P<0.0001). From baseline to month 12, the mean weight loss produced by diethylpropion was 10.6% (8.3%). Participants in the placebo group who were switched to diethylpropion after 6 months lost an average of 7.0% (7.7%) of initial body weight. The difference between groups at month 12 was not significant (P=0.07) [15]. Diethylpropion is only indicated for use as monotherapy (Fig. **3**).

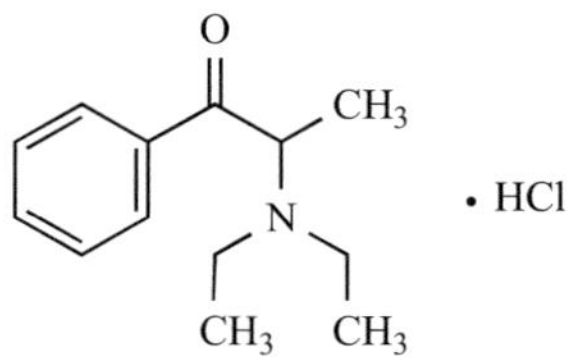

Fig. (3). Diethylpropion chemical structure.

Mechanism of Action

Similar to phentermine. But it is theorized that diethylpropion can raise levels of leptin. Principal biological effect of leptin in the central nervous system is the control of food intake and energy expenditure [16]. It is also theorized that increased levels of the catecholamines are partially responsible for halting another chemical messenger known as neuropeptide Y. This peptide initiates eating, decreases energy expenditure, and increases fat storage [17].

Pharmacokinetics

Diethylpropion is administered per oral. Chemically, it is the N,N-diethyl analog of cathinone. More gradual release properties are seen with the sustained-release tablets than three tablets given of the immediate-release in a single dose. This was based on studies of plasma levels obtained with each dosage form. Diethylpropion is rapidly absorbed from the GI tract and is extensively metabolized through a complex mechanism of N-dealkylation and reduction. N-dealkylation is thought to be responsible for metabolizing 45—55% of the dose whereas reduction accounts for 20—25% of the metabolic processes. Many of the diethylpropion metabolites are active.

Diethylpropion and/or its metabolites are believed to cross the blood-brain-barrier and the placenta. It is believed that it lacks any affinity for the monoamine transporters. Diethylpropion or Diethylcathinone functions as a prodrug to ethcathinone which is a low potent DA and 5-HT releasing agent. But is has 20 fold effect on NE and thereby can be considered a selective NE releasing agent [8].

The main route of excretion for diethylpropion and its metabolites is renal. More than 75% of the dose is recovered in the urine within 2 days after the initial does. Most of it is excreted as metabolites. The plasma t½ of the aminoketone metabolites is approximately between 4 to 6 hours.

Doses and Indications

This medication is indicated for the short-term management of obesity in adult patients with BMI of ≥ 30 kg/m^2 with a caloric restriction diet. It is administered as mentioned orally and the recommended dose for the immediate-release preparation is 25mg three times per day 1 hour before meals. It may also be taken in the mid-evening to suppress night time hunger. Meanwhile the dose for the sustained-release preparation is 75mg orally once a day in mid-morning time. It is not recommended for adolescents, children and pregnant or lactating ladies. The maximum daily dose is 75mg [18].

Contraindications and Precautions

Diethylpropion should be avoided in individuals who received anorexiant medications in the past 12 months. It should also be avoided in anorexia patients as stated earlier.

Contraindications are similar to other drugs in this class include preexisting arteriosclerosis disease, systemic or pulmonary hypertension. This is due its potential vasoconstriction effect. There has been a report of cardiac valvular disease associated with diethylpropion treatment but it is considered very rare. Nevertheless, it is recommended to be avoided in patient with cardiac arrhythmia, heart murmur or valvular heart disease. Other precautions were mentioned above. There was a case report indicating increase risk of developing pulmonary hypertension after short-term use [19].

Benzphetamine

This medication has a similar mechanism and effect as the previously mentioned short-term AOM. It was approved by the FDA in 1960.

Pharmacokinetics

Benzphetamine is taken per oral. Onset of action is within thirty minutes to one hour. The liver is where most of Benzphetamine metabolized to give out amphetamine and methamphetamine, as well as other metabolites (Fig. **4**). Elimination is mainly through the kidneys and maybe affected by changes in urine pH.

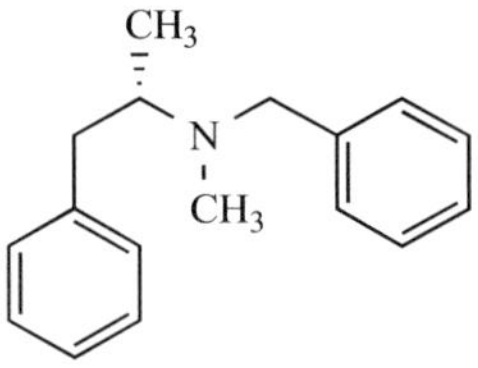

Fig. (4). Benzphetamine chemical structure.

Dosage

Benzphetamine is usually given 25—50 mg orally and only once daily. Preferred time for administration is during the day (In the mornings or afternoons). Dosage can then be titrated up to 50 mg three times daily. The maximum daily Dose is 150 mg.

Benzphetamine has the same recommendations and adverse effects as the other centrally acting AOM.

LONG ACTING DRUGS

Sibutramine

FDA Approved in 1997. Sibutramine is a serotonin-norepinephrine-Dopamine reuptake inhibitor. Patients taking sibutramine may achieve a 5—10% reduction from their baseline weight [20]. Another study found a dose-effect relationship in terms of weight loss. Sibutramine was also associated with better weight maintenance relative to placebo [21]. Additionally, sibutramine-mediated weight loss has been accompanied by reductions in serum uric acid and beneficial changes in serum lipids. A study done on female subjects showed Mean weight loss in Sibutramine group was 5.3 +/- 4.0% ($P < 0.001$) after 3 months and 10.5 +/- 4.4% ($P < 0.001$) after 12 months. The findings also demonstrated and decrease levels of leptin and C reactive protein and insulin resistance [22].

Another study done in Australia concluded that weight loss with sibutramine was associated with improvements in metabolic and body composition risk factors but not blood pressure or arterial stiffness. Improved insulin resistance was partly associated with reductions in liver fat and hypoxemia associated with sleep apnea. This conclusion was led to by the results at 6 months. They found that weight loss and improvements in obstructed sleep apnea were accompanied by improved insulin resistance checked by the Homeostatic Model Assessment (HOMA), increased HDL cholesterol, and reduced total cholesterol/ HDL ratio. There were also reductions in measures of visceral and subcutaneous abdominal fat and liver fat. Reductions in liver fat and sleep time spent below 90% oxyhemoglobin saturation partly explained the improvement in HOMA. In contrast, arterial stiffness (aortic augmentation index), heart rate, blood pressure, and total cholesterol did not change [23].

Mechanism of Action

Similar to other NASs, Sibutramine inhibits the central reuptake of dopamine, norepinephrine, and serotonin. These pharmacological actions are amphetamine like and are mediated by two active metabolites, M_1 and M_2. It is believed that the 5-HT mechanism enhances satiety and the NE mechanism raises the metabolic rate with higher affinity on NE and 5-HT than on DA reuptake.

Pharmacokinetics

Following oral administration, sibutramine is rapidly absorbed from the GI tract and undergoes extensive first-pass metabolism to two pharmacologically active metabolites, M1 and M2. More that 75% of an oral dose is absorbed. This medication and its metabolites reach peak plasma concentration at about 80 minutes and 3 to 4 hours, respectively. Sibutramine is rapidly and extensively distributed into tissues with the highest concentrations found in the kidney and liver where the drug is eliminated. The main organ to metabolize Sibutramine is the liver by cytochrome P450 3A4 (CYP3A4) isoenzyme to the active desmethyl metabolites (M1 and M2); these active metabolites are then hydroxylated and conjugated to inactive metabolites, M5 and M6. The t½ for Sibutramine and its metabolites are 60 – 70 minutes and 14 – 16 hours, respectively. Usually it takes about 4 days to reach steady-state. Excretion occurs via the feces, kidney, and liver. Almost 85% of a single radiolabeled oral dose is excreted in urine and feces over a 15-day collection period with the majority of the dose (≥75%) excreted in the urine. The liver is the main route of excretion for M1 and M2 (active) metabolites and renal for the inactive metabolites.

Contraindications and Precautions

Contraindications are similar to all centrally active AOM. Sibutramine is metabolized by CYP3A4 isoenzyme in the hepatic cells; it should be avoided in patient with hepatic impairment. There were also some reports of minor interactions with erythromycin, ketoconazole, and cimetidine. Special precaution for patients with preexisting neurological illnesses is recommended. Examples for neurological illnesses are major depression, epilepsy, migraines, Parkinson's disease, etc. This is because the risk of drug interactions with Sibutramine especially with MAO inhibitors due its effect on 5-HT uptake. A study done in New Zealand suggested an association between memory impairment and the use of Sibutramine [24]. Sibutramine might result in platelet serotonin depletion which might lead to impairment in platelet aggregation which will affect the platelet function. This will lead to an increase risk of bleeding especially in patient who are taking other anti-platelet or anti-coagulation medication. Because of the fact that Sibutramine metabolites are excreted through the kidneys; it should be used carefully in patient with renal impairment.

There were some reports about a possible association of acute myocardial infarction in a low atherosclerotic risk profile with the use of Sibutramine [25]. As all other centrally active AOM, it is not recommended to use them in patients with heart diseases [26]. Patients on Sibutramine might have discomfort oral sensation due its effect on salivary glands which might cause the development of caries, oral candidiasis, and periodontal disease. Other postmarketing adverse effects of sibutramine included abnormal ejaculation in men. A study investigates the effects of sibutramine on ejaculation and vas deferens and seminal vesicle contractility and showed delayed ejaculation observed with high doses of Sibutramine [27]. Sibutramine is classified as a schedule C-IV controlled substance by the DEA.

Doses and Indications

Sibutramine is indicated for treatment of adult patients with BMI of ≥ 30 kg/m^2 or BMI or ≥ 27 plus the preexisting of other risk factors such as DM, Hyperlipidemia, Hypertension, etc. Meridia recall has taken place recently secondary to cardiac events.

Rimonabant is made in the UK by Sanofi-Aventis as Acomplia.

If it had been approved in the United States, it was intended to be marketed under the name Zimulti.

Sibutramine is marketed under the name Meridia® which is made in North Chicago, IL: Abbott Laboratories; 2005 July. Initial dosage is 10 mg per day which can later be increased to 15 mg per day in patients who are not responding adequately [28]. If the 10 mg dose is not tolerated then the initial dose should be titrated down to 5 mg per day. The maximum dose is 15 mg per day. It is not recommended to go beyond that daily dose [29]. Sibutramine is not recommended for the use in children < 16 years of age, pregnant and lactating women.

Cannabinoid Receptor Antagonist (CRA)

Rimonabant: (also known as SR141716, Acomplia, Bethin, Monaslim, Riobant, Slimona, Rimoslim, and Zimulti, Riomont).

Cannabinoid receptor type 1 (CB_1) is a G protein-coupled cannabinoid receptor (Fig. **5**). It is found mainly in the brain and is stimulated by the psychoactive drug cannabis and its active compounds and also by a group of endocannabinoid neurotransmitters including anandamide. CB_1 is also found on the liver and GI Tract [30, 31]. The discovery of the endogenous cannabinoid system led to the development of CB_1 receptor antagonists.

The first cannabinoid receptor "antagonist", rimonabant, was described in 1994 (although it is technically an inverse agonist, not an antagonist). Rimonabant blocks the CB_1 receptor selectively and it has been shown to decrease food intake and regulate body-weight gain.

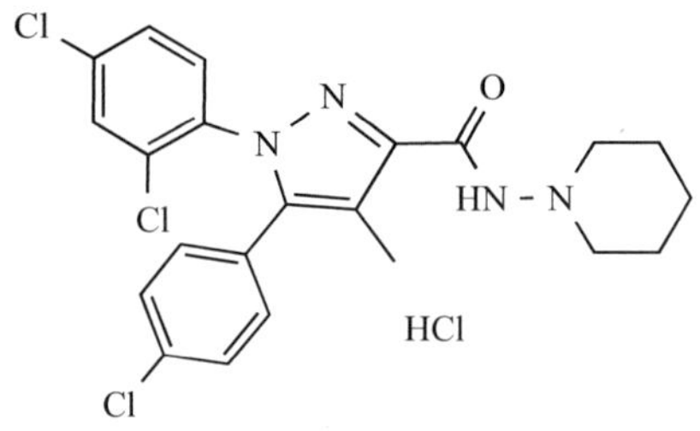

Fig. (5). Rimonabant chemical structure.

Doses and Indications

Initially it was under investigation for the treatment of obesity and smoking cessation. The dosage for adults is 20 mg once daily orally in addition to a mild hypocaloric diet (600 kcal/day deficit) for optimal results [32].

Pharmacology and Efficacy of CRA

Rimonabant, as a CRA, inhibits the overactivation of the endocannabinoid system resulting in central anorexia. Rimonabant seems to have effects on the metabolism through the adipose tissue, liver, skeletal muscles and the pancreas. There are four published RIO trials (Rio-North America, RIO-Europe, RIO-Lipids, RIO-Diabetes), Rimonabant decreased weight by 6.3-6.9 kg in the non-diabetic groups vs. placebo (-1.5-1.8 kg) ($p < 0.001$), whereas in the diabetic subjects enrolled in RIO-Diabetes, weight loss was 5.3 *vs.* 1.4 kg in the placebo group with overall improvement in the metabolic profile in diabetic and non-diabetic patients.

Safety and Monitoring

In June 2007, the FDA Endocrinologic and Metabolic Advisory Committee voted unanimously against the approval of rimonabant for the treatment of weight loss; they indicated that certain side effects mainly primarily psychiatric disturbances are increased in patients taking rimonabant compared to placebo [33-36]. In 2006, rimonabant was approved for use as an adjunct to diet and exercise in promoting weight loss in obese patients or overweight patients with risk factors such as diabetes mellitus type 2 or dyslipidemia in Europe and Mexico, respectively. The drug also received approval as an adjuvant treatment to diet and exercise to improve glycemic control in overweight patients with type 2 diabetes when used in combination with conventional therapies in Mexico. In Octobor 2008, rimonabant was pulled off the market in Europe because the risks of psychiatric effects outweigh any benefits [36].

Contraindications/Cautions

Rimonabant is contraindicated in patients with history of depression, suicidal ideation or uncontrolled psychiatric disorder.

Side Effects

Primarily psychiatric disturbances including depression, anxiety, changes in sleep patterns, and suicidal ideation, are increased in patients taking Rimonabant [33-36].

MEDICATIONS WITH PRIMARY AFFECT ON THE PERIPHERY AND METABOLISM

FDA Approved

Pancreatic Lipase Inhibitors (PLI) includes Orlistat.

Non FDA Approved

Other PLIs: Cetilistat

Pancreatic Lipase Inhibitors (PLI)

Orlistat: (also known as Xenical and Allī)

Initially approved by the FDA in 1999. In 2003, the FDA approved orlistat for use in obese adolescents 12 to 16 years of age and then it was approved by the FDA for over-the-counter sale in February 2007. Orlistat was approved for long-term use. Alli manufactured by Glaxosmithkline and Xenical made by Hoffmann La Roche.

Orlistat is indicated for obesity management, including weight loss and weight maintenance, when used in conjunction with a reduced-calorie diet. The first in a new class of drugs, Orlistat works non-systemically (locally) to block the absorption of dietary fat. It is classified as a gastrointestinal agent since that is where the mechanism of action occurs (Fig. **6**).

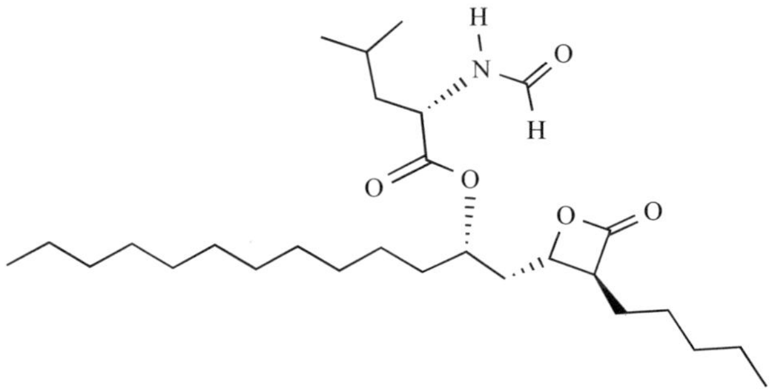

Fig. (6). Orlistat chemical structure.

Mechanism of Action

The weight loss is achieved via inhibiting absorption of nutrient in the intestine. In the stomach and small intestine, a covalent bond is formed with the active serine residue site of gastric and pancreatic lipases. These enzymes then become unavailable to hydrolyze dietary triglycerides into free fatty acids (FFA) and monoglycerides, less fat is absorbed by the body. This then results in less caloric intake that may lead to a negative energy balance and weight loss as per the weight change model. Therefore, the weight loss effect does not need a systemic absorption of the drug. At the recommended therapeutic dose, dietary fat absorption is inhibited by approximately 30%.

Pharmacokinetics

Orlistat is administered orally and seems to have minimal systemic absorption. Peak plasma concentrations (<5 ng/ml) occurred approximately 8 hours after a 360 mg dose. The effect of orlistat may be seen within 24 to 48 hours Based on fecal fat measurements. Orlistat is metabolized into weakly active and inactive metabolites, in which is believed to occur mainly within the gastrointestinal wall. The estimated half-life ($t\frac{1}{2}$) of the absorbed portion of orlistat is approximately 1 to 2 hours. Complete excretion of both urinary and fecal orlistat is reached within 3 to 5 days. Interestingly, 83% of a single oral dose is excreted unchanged in the feces with renal excretion of < 2% of the dose.

Doses and Efficacy

Oral doses: Adolescent's ≥ 12 of age and Adults: 120 mg per oral three times per day (120 mg capsules, e.g., Xenical®). A non-prescription (OTC) 60 mg capsules is also available as Alli. The maximum daily dose is 360 mg per day per oral for adults, elderly, and adolescents 12 years of age and above. It is not recommended to be used in children younger than the age of 12 years.

The manufacturer recommends that all patients should take a daily multivitamin that contains vitamins A, D, E, K, and beta-carotene; the supplement should be taken at least 2 hours before or after Orlistat [37].

Capsules are taken with fatty meals or 1 hour after at most. Doses greater than recommended did not increase weight loss. A multi-center clinical trial done from 1992 to 1995 showed that subjects treated with Orlistat, 120 mg 3 times a day, during year 1 and year 2 regained less weight during year 2 (3.2±0.45 kg; 35.2% regain) than those who received Orlistat, 60 mg (4.26±0.57 kg; 51.3% regain), or placebo (5.63±0.42 kg; 63.4% regain) in year 2 ($P<0.001$).

Treatment with Orlistat, 120 mg 3 times a day, was associated with improvements in fasting low-density lipoprotein cholesterol (LDL-C) and fasting insulin and concluded that treatment of obese adults with BMI's of 30—43 kg/m^2 with Orlistat plus diet significantly promotes weight loss, lessens weight regain, and improves some obesity-related disease risk factors [38]. Another clinical trial included patients (BMI 28-47 kg/m^2), recruited at 15 European centers found that the orlistat group lost, on average, more bodyweight than the placebo group (10.2% [10.3 kg] *vs.* 6.1% [6.1 kg]; [$p<0.001$] from randomisation to the end of year 1). During year 2, patients who continued with orlistat regained, on average, half as much weight as those patients switched to placebo ($p<0.001$). Patients switched from placebo to orlistat lost an additional 0.9 kg during year 2, compared with a mean regain of 2.5 kg in patients who continued on placebo ($p<0.001$). Total cholesterol, LDL-C, LDL/high-density lipoprotein (HDL) ratio, and concentrations of glucose and insulin decreased more in the orlistat group than in the placebo group. Gastrointestinal adverse events were more common in the orlistat group [39]. And in regards to reduction of cardiovascular risks, a study showed that orlistat-treated patients had significantly greater improvements than placebo-treated patients in several lipid parameters including total cholesterol, LDL-C, triglycerides (TG), and apolipoprotein B (Apo-B).

In addition, orlistat had a beneficial effect on oral glucose tolerance tests status, waist circumference and systolic and diastolic blood pressure [40]. When studied the effect on diabetes a study showed Orlistat treatment plus diet compared with placebo plus diet was associated with significant improvement in glycemic control, as reflected in decreases in HbA1c ($P < 0.001$) and fasting plasma glucose (FPG) ($P < 0.001$) and in dosage reductions of oral sulfonylurea medication ($P < 0.01$). Orlistat therapy also resulted in significantly greater improvements than placebo in several lipid parameters, namely, greater reductions in total cholesterol, ($P < 0.001$), LDL cholesterol ($P < 0.001$), TG ($P < 0.05$), Apo-B ($P < 0.001$), and the LDL-to-HDL cholesterol ratio ($P < 0.001$) [41]. And when given to obese adolescents a 21 day study; results demonstrated that orlistat reduced fat absorption by roughly 27%, but no significant changes were noted in the balance of calcium, phosphorus, magnesium, copper or zinc in the active *vs.* placebo groups [42].

Contraindications and Precautions

Orlistat is contraindicated for use in individuals with cholestasis, as may be present in cases of gallbladder disease. Cholecystokinin (CCK) stimulates contraction of the gallbladder, which depends on the presence of FFA in the intestinal lumen. Postprandial plasma concentrations of CCK decreased after multiple doses of Orlistat [43]. It is also contraindicated for use in patients with chronic malabsorption syndrome. Because orlistat can interfere with the absorption of fat-soluble vitamins, all patients should take a daily multivitamin that contains vitamins A, D, E, K, and beta-carotene; the supplement should be taken at least 2 hours before or after Orlistat [37].

Orlistat may interfere with the GI absorption of Warfarin, cyclosporine, amiodarone and levothyroxine.

Orlistat can affect patients who are on Warfarin therapy for anti coagulation since it can be affected by changes in dietary intake of vitamin K. The FDA has received reports of transplant recipients with subtherapeutic cyclosporine concentrations after the initiation of orlistat therapy. In a randomized, crossover study, all but 1 of 30 healthy adults had a decrease in steady state cyclosporine concentrations with concomitant orlistat administration with an average reduction in systemic cyclosporine exposure over 12 hours after dosing by 30% [44]. statistically significant number of obese, type 2 diabetics stabilized on sulfonylureas who received orlistat during a one-year double-blind, placebo-controlled study required a reduction in dose or discontinuation of drug therapy compared to the placebo group. Lower blood glucose may necessitate a dosage reduction of antidiabetic agents [41]. Orlistat produced additive lipid-lowering effects when used concomitantly with pravastatin. Serum concentrations of pravastatin increased by approximately 30% when administered with orlistat 120 mg three times per day for 10 days in a parallel study of 24 normal-weight, mildly hypercholesterolemic subjects [45]. Orlistat also reduces the absorption of amiodarone (and active metabolite) by about 25% [46] and with the absorption of levothyroxine from the gastrointestinal tract [47].

Side Effects

GI symptoms occurred at least twice that of placebo in ≥ 5% of patients taking Orlistat [38]. Mild to moderate and transient gastrointestinal events were reported with orlistat therapy, although their association with study withdrawal was low. Fat-soluble vitamin levels generally remained within the reference range, and vitamin supplementation was required in only a few patients [41].

Other rare adverse effects in ≤ 2% of patients taking olistat includes: hypersensitivity reactions, severe or prolonged abdominal pain and/or nausea and vomiting, dizziness, infectious diarrhea, rectal pain, gingival disorder, headache, menstrual irregularity, fatigue, anxiety/depression, rash, respiratory tract infection and many other general infections and musculoskeletal pain. In the 4-year XENDOS study, the general pattern of adverse events was similar to that reported for the 1- and 2-year studies with the total incidence of gastrointestinal-related adverse events occurring in year 1 decreasing each year over the 4-year period [37].

Cetilistat

Another PLI is Cetilistat is also treat obesity. In human trials, cetilistat was shown to produce similar weight loss to orlistat, but also produced similar side effects such as oily, loose stools, fecal incontinence, frequent bowel movements, and flatulence It is likely that the same precautions would apply in that absorption of fat-soluble vitamins and other fat-soluble nutrients may be inhibited, requiring vitamin supplements to be used to avoid deficiencies. Currently it is still in clinical trials which started in October of 2009.

FAT SUBSTITUTES

Olestra

Olestra is a fat substitute made from sucrose and vegetable oil. Olestra can not add calories or fat to the diet because it is neither digested nor absorbed in the GI tract nor is metabolized by the normal GI flora. After long-term exposure of the GI tract studies has shown no evidence that olestra causes injury to the GI mucosa. Olestra (also known by its brand name Olean) was approved by the FDA in 1996 as a food additive used in the preparation of high fat content food such as potato ships. Studies also showed no effect on stomach and intestinal motility. But they did demonstrate a decrease in the absorption of fat-soluble vitamins (Vitamins A, D, E, and K) which was dose-responsive. However, this effect is reversed by the adding of vitamins to olestra-containing foods which was a requirement by the FDA [40]. Olestra has no significant effect on bile acid absorption [49]. When consuming a large amount of olestra containing food; the occurrence of gastrointestinal symptoms, including diarrhea, loose stools, gas and abdominal cramping have been seen post marketing [50].

THERMOGENICS AND STIMULATORS OF FAT MOBILIZATION

There are many over the counter thermogenics pills sold in retail stores and many stimulators of fat metabolism that are even made into drinks and so called "Energy Drinks". Thee were many studies done to determine if they in fact do induce weight loss or at least increase the daily caloric burn. One study finding indicated that thermogenics increase resting energy expenditure and exercise oxygen consumption rate with only minimal effects on blood pressure and heart rate and no meaningful effects on respiratory exchange ratio or rating of perceived exertion. Their results suggested that combining of thermogenic ingredients in nutritional supplements may help maintaining a negative caloric balance [51]. Another study concluded that the consumption of a drink that contains green tea, catechins, caffeine, and calcium will increase the daily energy expenditure by only 4.8%. But they could not distinguish which of these individual ingredients has the most effect. And when consumed on regular bases as part of a diet and exercise program, these beverages might provide benefits for weight control [52].

MEDICATION WITHDRAWN FROM THE MARKET

In spite of the fact that serotonergic agents (fenfluramine, dexfenfluramine) were withdrawn from the US market in the late 1990's secondary to their cardiovascular and pulmonary complications. At the present time, it is very important to assess the patient's history regarding their intake as this might result in further cardiac or pulmonary evaluations.

The use of anorexic drugs (mainly derivatives of fenfluramine) was associated with an increased risk of primary pulmonary hypertension (odds ratio with any anorexic-drug use, 6.3; 95 percent confidence interval, 3.0 to 13.2). For the use of anorexic agents in the preceding year, the odds ratio was 10.1 (95 percent confidence interval, 3.4 to 29.9). When anorexic drugs were used to a total of more than three months, the odds ratio was 23.1 (95 percent confidence interval, 6.9 to 77.7).

Valvular heart disease has been reported in women receiving the combination of fenfluramine and phentermine (FDA Public Health Advisory, July 8, 1997). Primary pulmonary hypertension (PPH) has been reported to occur in patients receiving a combination of phentermine with fenfluramine or dexfenfluramine. The possibility of an association between the use of phentermine alone and PPH or valvular heart disease cannot be ruled out. The initial symptom of PPH is usually dyspnea. Other initial symptoms include: angina pectoris, syncope, or lower extremity edema.

CONCLUSION

A Pharmacological approach to treat obesity may be effective and should be considered in selected patients in addition to behavioral modification, diet and exercise. Only a few medications are approved by the FDA for weight loss. Others need more clinical studies to determine their efficacy, durability and side effects. Patients should follow up closely with their physician for signs of dependence, withdrawal and drug interactions. Surgical treatment for obesity must be considered when non-surgical methods fail.

REFERENCES

[1] Houston DK, Nicklas BJ, Zizza CA. Weighty Concerns: The Growing Prevalence of Obesity among Older Adults. J Am Diet Assoc 2009; 109(11): 1886-95.

[2] Ogden CL, Flegal KM, Carroll MD, Johnson CL. Prevalence and trends in overweight among US children and adolescents, 1999-2000. JAMA 2002 9; 288(14): 1728-32.

[3] Cali AM, Caprio S. Obesity in children and adolescents. J Clin Endocrinol Metab 2008; 93(11 Suppl 1): S31-6.

[4] Ogden CL, Carroll MD, Curtin LR, McDowell MA, Tabak CJ, Flegal KM. Prevalence of overweight and obesity in the United States, 1999-2004. JAMA 2006; 295(13): 1549-55.

[5] Newell A, Zlot A, Silvey K, Ariail K. Addressing the obesity epidemic: a genomics perspective. Prev Chronic Dis 2007; 4(2): A31.

[6] Loos RJ, Bouchard C. Obesity: is it a genetic disorder? J Intern Med 2003; 254(5): 401-25.

[7] Bray GA. Medications for obesity: mechanisms and applications. Clin Chest Med 2009; 30(3): 525-38.

[8] Rothman RB, Baumann MH. Therapeutic potential of monoamine transporter substrates. Curr Top Med Chem 2006; 6(17): 1845-59.

[9] Rothman RB, Baumann MH. Therapeutic potential of monoamine transporter substrates. Curr Top Med Chem 2006; 6(17): 1845-59.

[10] Landau D, Jackson J, Gonzalez G. A case of demand ischemia from phendimetrazine. Cases J 2008; 1(1): 105.

[11] Rothman RB, Katsnelson M, Vu N, *et al.* Interaction of the anorectic medication, phendimetrazine, and its metabolites with monoamine transporters in rat brain. Eur J Pharmacol 2002; 447(1): 51-7.

[12] Hoffmann M. Transient environmental dependency syndrome due to phendimetrazine tartrate. Eur Neurol 2007; 58(1): 49-50.

[13] Kwiker D, Godkar D, Lokhandwala N, Yakoby M. Rare case of rhabdomyolysis with therapeutic doses of phendimetrazine tartrate. Am J Ther 2006; 13(2): 175-6.

[14] Arias HR, Santamaría A, Ali SF. Pharmacological and neurotoxicological actions mediated by bupropion and diethylpropion. Int Rev Neurobiol 2009; 88: 223-55.

[15] Cercato C, Roizenblatt VA, Leança CC, *et al.* A randomized double-blind placebo-controlled study of the long-term efficacy and safety of diethylpropion in the treatment of obese subjects. Int J Obes (Lond) 2009; 33(8): 857-65.

[16] Antuna-Puente B, Feve B, Fellahi S, Bastard JP. Adipokines: the missing link between insulin resistance and obesity. Diabetes Metab 2008; 34(1): 2-11.

[17] BaryGA.Drug treatment of obesity. Baillieres Best Pract Res Clin Endocrinol Metab 1999; 13(1): 131-48.

[18] Wright GJ, Lang JF, Lemieux RE, Goodfriend MJ Jr. The objective and timing of drug disposition studies, appendix III. Diethylpropion and its metabolites in the blood plasma of the human after subcutaneous and oral administration. Drug Metab Rev 1975; 4(2): 267-76.

[19] Abramowicz MJ, Van Haecke P, Demedts M, Delcroix M. Primary pulmonary hypertension after amfepramone (diethylpropion) with BMPR2 mutation. Eur Respir J 2003; 22(3): 560-2.

[20] Lean ME. How does sibutramine work? Int J Obes Relat Metab Disord 2001; 25(Suppl 4): S8-11.

[21] Nisoli E, Carruba MO. A benefit-risk assessment of sibutramine in the management of obesity. Drug Saf 2003; 26(14): 1027-48.

[22] Sari R, Eray E, Ozdem S, Akbas H, Coban E. Comparison of the effects of sibutramine versus sibutramine plus metformin in obese women. Clin Exp Med 2010; 10(3): 179-84.

[23] Phillips CL, Yee BJ, Trenell MI, *et al.* Changes in regional adiposity and cardio-metabolic function following a weight loss program with sibutramine in obese men with obstructive sleep apnea. J Clin Sleep Med 2009; 5(5): 416-21.

[24] Clark DW, Harrison-Woolrych M. Sibutramine may be associated with memory impairment. BMJ 2004; 329(7478): 1316.

[25] Eroglu E, Gemici G, Bayrak F, Kalkan AK, Degertekin M. Acute myocardial infarction in a 24 year-old man possibly associated with sibutramine use. Int J Cardiol 2009; 137(2): e43-5.

[26] Sibutramine under FDA review for cardiovascular risk. Reactions Weekly; 11/28/2009, Issue 1280, p2-2, 1/4p.

[27] Nojimoto FD, Piffer RC, Kiguti LR, *et al.* Multiple effects of sibutramine on ejaculation and on vas deferens and seminal vesicle contractility. Toxicol Appl Pharmacol 2009; 239(3): 233-40.

[28] Poston WS, Foreyt JP. Sibutramine and the management of obesity. Expert Opin Pharmacother 2004; 5(3): 633-42.

[29] Park JY, Kim KA, Park PW, Suh KH, Lee GS. Relative bioavailability and pharmacokinetics of a new sibutramine formulation in healthy male subjects: A randomized, open-label, two-period, comparative crossover study. Clin Ther 2004; 26(12): 2092-101.

[30] Osei-Hyiaman D, DePetrillo M, Pacher P, *et al.* Endocannabinoid activation at hepatic CB1 receptors stimulates fatty acid synthesis and contributes to diet-induced obesity. J Clin Invest 2005; 115(5): 1298-305.

[31] Mathison R, Ho W, Pittman QJ, Davison JS, Sharkey KA. Effects of cannabinoid receptor-2 activation on accelerated gastrointestinal transit in lipopolysaccharide-treated rats. Br J Pharmacol 2004; 142(8): 1247-54.

[32] Van Gaal LF, Rissanen AM, Scheen AJ, Ziegler O, Rössner S; RIO-Europe Study Group. Effects of the cannabinoid-1 receptor blocker rimonabant on weight reduction and cardiovascular risk factors in overweight patients: 1-year experience from the RIO-Europe study. Lancet 2005; 365(9468): 1389-97.

[33] de Mattos Viana B, Prais HA, Daker MV. Melancholic features related to rimonabant. Gen Hosp Psychiatry 2009; 31(6): 583-5.

[34] Lee HK, Choi EB, Pak CS. The current status and future perspectives of studies of cannabinoid receptor 1 antagonists as anti-obesity agents. Curr Top Med Chem 2009; 9(6): 482-503.

[35] Moreira FA, Crippa JA. The psychiatric side-effects of rimonabant. Rev Bras Psiquiatr 2009; 31(2): 145-53.

[36] Johansson K, Neovius K, DeSantis SM, Rössner S, Neovius M. Discontinuation due to adverse events in randomized trials of orlistat, sibutramine and rimonabant: a meta-analysis. Obes Rev 2009; 10(5): 564-75. Epub 2009 May 12.

[37] Sjostrom L, Rissanen A, Andersen T, *et al.* Randomized placebo-controlled trial of orlistat for weight loss and prevention of weight regain in obese patients. European multicentre orlistat group. Lancet 1998; 352: 167-72.

[37] Xenical® (orlistat) package insert. Nutley, NJ: Roche Laboratories Inc.; 2009 Feb.

[38] Davidson MH, Hauptman J, Heymsfield SB, *et al.* Weight control and risk factor reduction in obese subjects treated for 2 years with orlistat: a randomized controlled trial. JAMA 1999; 281(3): 235-42.

[40] Zavoral JH. Treatment with orlistat reduces cardiovascular risk in obese patients. J Hypertens 1998; 16: 2013-7.

[41] Hollander PA, Elbein SC, Hirsch IB, *et al.* Role of orlistat in the treatment of obese patients with type 2 diabetes. A 1-year randomized double-blind study. Diabetes Care 1998; 21: 1288-94.

[42] Zhi J, Moore R, Kanitra L. The effect of short-term (21-day) orlistat treatment on the physiologic balance of six selected macrominerals and microminerals in obese adolescents. J Am Coll Nutr 2003; 22(5): 357-62.

[43] Froehlich F, Hartman D, Guezelhan C, *et al.* Influence of orlistat on the regulation of gallbladder contraction in man: a randomized double-blind placebo-controlled crossover study. Dig Dis Sci 1996; 41: 2404-8.

[44] Zhi J, Moore R, Kanitra L, *et al.* Pharmacokinetic evaluation of the possible interaction between selected concomitant medications and orlistat at steady state in healthy subjects. J Clin Pharmacol 2002; 42: 1011-19.

[45] Guerciolini R. Mode of action of orlistat. Int J Obes Relat Metab Disord 1997; (21 Suppl 3): S12-23.

[46] Zhi J, Moore R, Kanitra L, *et al.* Effects of orlistat, a lipase inhibitor, on the pharmacokinetics of three highly lipophilic drugs (amiodarone, fluoxetine, and simvastatin) in healthy volunteers. J Clin Pharmacol 2003; 43: 428-35.

[47] Filippatos TD, Derdemezis CS, Gazi IR, *et al.* Orlistat-associated adverse effects and drug interactions. A critical review. Drug Saf 2008; 31: 53-65.

[48] Prince DM, Welschenbach MA. Olestra: a new food additive. J Am Diet Assoc 1998; 98(5): 565-9.

[49] Thomson AB, Hunt RH, Zorich NL. Review article: olestra and its gastrointestinal safety. Aliment Pharmacol Ther 1998; 12(12): 1185-200.

[50] Freston JW, Ahnen DJ, Czinn SJ, *et al.* Review and analysis of the effects of olestra, a dietary fat substitute, on gastrointestinal function and symptoms. Regul Toxicol Pharmacol 1997; 26(2): 210-8.

[51] Ryan ED, Beck TW, Herda TJ, *et al.* Acute effects of a thermogenic nutritional supplement on energy expenditure and cardiovascular function at rest, during low-intensity exercise, and recovery from exercise. J Strength Cond Res 2009; 23(3): 807-17.

[52] Rudelle S, Ferruzzi MG, Cristiani I, Moulin J, Macé K, Acheson KJ, Tappy L. Effect of a thermogenic beverage on 24-hour energy metabolism in humans. Obesity (Silver Spring) 2007; 15(2): 349-55.

Omics Approaches to Obesity and Complex Disorders: Challenges and New Opportunities

Kyoungmi Kim* and Stanislav O. Zakharkin†

Division of Biostatistics, University of California Davis School of Medicine and Technology and Innovation, Solae, St. Louis, MO, USA

Abstract: Obesity is a complex disorder resulting from the interplay of genetic, environmental, behavioral factors and life style and has a significant impact on the public health. The complexity of the disorder entails multidisciplinary research efforts involving various research disciplines to enhance the understanding of the molecular mechanisms implicated in the development of the disease. The disruption of the balance between energy intake and energy expenditure which leads to obesity involves the action of many contributing factors and many molecular compounds, making high-dimensional profiling very attractive. Nonetheless, despite definite advances in omics research over the last decade, many challenges remain, including combining data from the heterogeneous sources, development of data mining tools, and integrative analysis methodologies to fully exploit various hypotheses. This review presents a brief overview of ongoing research, summarizes current methodologies, techniques, and challenges in omics approaches to obesity research, and identifies areas of further research.

Keywords: Omics, heterogeneous types of data, integrative approaches, statistical issues.

INTRODUCTION

Obesity is a multifactorial condition that results from the interactions among a variety of genetic, dietary, environmental, and lifestyle factors [1]. Obesity has become epidemic in the last decades primarily due to an increase in high-caloric food intake combined with a decrease in physical exercise since it is unlikely that genetic makeup has changed dramatically [2, 3]. The World Health Organization (WHO) estimates that worldwide approximately 1.6 billion adults are overweight (BMI > 25) and at least 400 million are obese (BMI > 30) [4]. Obesity is linked to increased morbidity due to cardiovascular diseases, to the development of insulin resistance and Type II diabetes mellitus, and to certain types of cancer [5].

The disruption of the balance between energy intake and energy expenditure which leads to the disease state arises from a contribution of many factors with relatively small effects rather than from fewer factors with strong effects [6-8]. Recent advances in omics technologies have rapidly enhanced the feasibility of high-throughput profiling of complex disorders. These approaches include, but are not limited to, the analysis of genetic variation (genomics), gene expression (transcriptomics), gene products (proteomics) and their end results, metabolites (metabolomics). When coupled with bioinformatics and biostatistics, omics approaches have proven to be successful in elucidating the molecular mechanisms of obesity [9], diabetes [10-12], hypertension and cardiovascular disease [13, 14]. The omics technologies permit high-throughput screening of molecular compounds (transcripts, proteins, and metabolites) and allow for the identification of a subset of the molecular markers that are critical for the responses at the whole organism level. Using these approaches, researchers have identified hundreds if not thousands of candidate molecular entities that may be involved in the development and progression of obesity [15-20]. Due to the complexity of the disorder, it is essential to develop integrative approaches to elucidate the pathophysiological mechanisms underlying the global obesity problem and related disorders. The integrative approaches attempt to combine multiple heterogeneous data extracted by different omics approaches.

Here, we review the current and potential applications of omics technologies and relevant statistical and bioinformatics methods of analysis, focusing on obesity and related complex disorders. The rest of this chapter is organized as follows: First, we give a brief overview of the current knowledge of molecular mechanisms related to development of obesity. Second, we outline available high-throughput technology

*Corresponding author: Tel: (530) 752-3422; Fax: (530) 754-6015; E-mail: kmkim@ucdavis.edu

†Currently at Science and Technology, Cadbury, Whippany, NJ, USA

Atta-ur-Rahman / M. Iqbal Choudhary (Eds.)

and statistical methodology for the analysis of high dimensional omics data. Third, we review the integration of various sources of data and discuss the challenges and perspectives of integrative approaches. Finally, we discuss limitations and challenges that future research will need to address.

OBESITY IS A COMPLEX DISEASE

Obesity has become a prominent public health problem affecting millions of people worldwide [2, 3, 21]. The Obesity Society estimates that approximately 31% of adults (59 million of people) in the United States are overweight [22]. Obesity is involved in the pathogenesis of major diseases, notably, hypertension, cardiovascular disease, and certain types of cancer [23, 24], and it is associated with a number of the cardiovascular risk factors which constitute the metabolic syndrome [25-27]. Systemic chronic inflammation has been proposed to have an important role in the pathogenesis of obesity-related insulin resistance insofar as experimental, epidemiological, and clinical evidence links obesity to inflammation and to the development of insulin resistance and Type II diabetes mellitus [28-30]. Moreover, effective management of overweight and obesity is crucial to the reduction of morbidity due to cardiovascular disease [31]. Studies have demonstrated that the etiology of obesity is complex and includes a combination of genetic and environmental factors that disrupt the balance between energy intake and energy expenditure [1, 32, 33]. There are tremendous efforts underway to better understand the complex genetics of human obesity and then to use the resulting knowledge about the metabolic and signaling pathways of obesity and weight regulation to design obesity drugs and novel therapies [34, 35].

Obesity appears to be under strong genetic control, with numerous genes, most with a modest effect, contributing to an individual's predisposition to obesity [36]. It is estimated that 40% to 70% of human fat mass is heritable [23, 37]. Genome-wide scans have led to the identification of several chromosome regions that are likely to harbor genes determining susceptibility [38, 39]. Extensive molecular studies using experimental animal models, "forward genetics" (e.g. generation of random mutations and screening for phenotypes of interest), and "reverse genetics" (e.g. generation mutations in a gene of interest and observing the resulting phenotypes) have helped establish critical pathways that regulate body fat and food intake [40, 41], such as the central melanocortin pathway that has a fundamental importance in mammalian energy balance [42]. As a result of these extensive efforts, human ortholog genes were identified as well [43].

White adipose tissue secretes a number of peptide hormones, including cytokines, adipsin and acylation-stimulating protein, angiotensinogen, plasminogen activator inhibitor 1, adiponectin, resistin, pro-omelanocortin and others [44, 45]. The fatty acids have an important role in regulation of homeostasis in liver, adipose tissue, and skeletal muscle and are critical in development of obesity and metabolic syndrome [46, 47]. Leptin is an adipose-derived protein hormone that plays a key role in regulation of energy balance. A total absence of leptin or a lack of signaling through the long isoform of a leptin receptor causes severe obesity [48, 49]. Neuropeptide Y, one of the most abundant peptides of the hypothalamus, can powerfully increase food intake [50, 51]. The peroxisome proliferator-activated receptors (PPARs) are nuclear fatty acid receptors that have been significantly implicated in obesity-related metabolic diseases such as hyperlipidemia, insulin resistance, and coronary artery disease [52-54]. The molecular mechanisms underlying metabolic abnormalities induced by visceral adiposity have yet to be fully elucidated; however, adipocytokines such as adiponectin, tumor necrosis factor-alpha, and resistin seem to play an important role in this process [33, 55-57].

In recent years our understanding how the physiological mechanisms that regulate body weight are perturbed in obesity has markedly increased [58, 59]. However, rigorous validation of previously identified pathways and additional research on the physiological and molecular mechanisms regulating body fat are necessary. Omics approaches can help in the experimental validation of suggestive pathways *in vitro* and *in vivo* and can further refine our understanding of those novel molecular pathways involved in energy homeostasis [60-62]. Multiple endocrine and neural pathways are simultaneously disturbed and can further modulate other signaling pathways (e.g. those related to certain types of cancer or cardiovascular diseases). When pathways are disturbed, other interconnected pathways also change and this process exacerbates the problem. For example, chronic inflammation has been linked to obesity via systemic inflammation markers, interleukins 6 and 8, and TNF-α [63, 64]. Many pathways and mediators are involved in other various diseases including tumors and autoimmune disorders [58]. The challenge is to determine which elements are disturbed and how such disturbances can be corrected without causing further problems [65, 66]. Addressing this challenge will require a detailed understanding of each system both in itself and in its interconnections with others.

OMICS APPROACHES IN OBESITY RESEARCH

In the last couple of decades, high-throughput technologies, commonly called omics approaches, have grown explosively [67, 68]. Although each of them has unique characteristics, all omics technologies use high-throughput analytical approaches to generate profiles (e.g. characteristic distributions) of molecular compounds (i.e., transcripts, proteins, metabolites). There are two general ways of profiling molecular compounds: a global approach to generate a hypothesis and a target-specific approach to test and validate a specific hypothesis.

The target-specific approach is intended to test a specific hypothesis and validate its plausibility. The hypothesis being tested relies on current findings of the biology and pathophysiology of obesity and related traits. Target-specific studies can be further refined by testing for associations with more detailed phenotypes. Eventually such testing can lead to development of experimental models that help elucidate the functional consequences of the identified molecules in cellular systems or in the whole organism [69].

By contrast, the global approach is data-driven and attempts to screen a set of compounds to generate new hypotheses and to identify new targets associated with a trait of interest without prior information. In addition, by documenting how multiple molecules interact with each other, the global profiling approach allows to develop a "big picture" view that provides a better understanding of dynamic changes at the level of molecular pathways and networks. The advantage of this approach is that it may help to identify completely new targets; the disadvantage is that many of the new targets are false-positives [70]. At initial screenings, global profiling studies typically examine hundreds or thousands of compounds. When strong evidence of association is found, selected candidates will be further examined in target-specific studies. This approach has proven successful in discovering new targets with large effects in diabetes and cardiovascular disease where obesity is involved in their pathogenesis [52, 71]; however, its success with targets that have modest effects is apparently limited.

Omics Studies Need Specific Objectives Beforehand

The profiling studies typically have one or several of the following objectives: (1) to identify individual molecular compounds whose levels are correlated with a phenotype of interest such as insulin resistance response to diet intervention or drug treatment; (2) to identify multiple molecular compounds forming pathways or regulatory networks and mediating biological phenomena or participating in a disease pathogenesis; (3) to discover potential molecular targets for drug development; and (4) to identify molecular markers for disease diagnosis and prognosis or as predictors of clinical outcomes. Regardless of the purpose of an omics study, there is one common underlying assumption - the primary end point of the study is associated with the expression or concentration levels of a number of compounds. For example, Kim *et al.* profiled genes from perioperative adipose tissue whose expression was associated with weight loss outcome following Roux-en-Y gastric bypass (RYGB) surgery [72]. Their results showed that genes for glycerolipid syntheses that are directly involved in regulating adipose tissue fat stores were significantly correlated with postoperative body weight loss. More interestingly, the network analysis demonstrated the unique impact of the regulation of the genes involved in lipid metabolism on weight loss (see Fig. **1**). Their gene expression profiling study has limited "generalizability" but is perfectly satisfactory to establish a 'proof of principle' and to provide the basis for later confirmatory (usually larger prospective) studies to assess the validity of gene expression profiles in obesity intervention. Clearly, it is possible for omics studies to yield clinically significant results, but it is also important to recognize first that different questions are addressed in different phases of research (feasibility, validation, confirmation, and proof of clinical merit) and second that the appropriate design and analysis strategy of an omic profiling study should be driven by a specific objective in the planning stage of each phase of research.

Genome-Wide Association Studies

Genome-wide association studies aim to examine genomic variation across the genome and to identify genetic polymorphisms associated with an increased risk for developing the disease. The human genome contains millions of Single Nucleotide Polymorphisms (SNPs) which may be associated with the disease directly through effects on gene expression or protein function, or indirectly through linkage disequilibrium [73]. The recent introduction of SNP genotyping methods has drastically increased the ability to assay hundreds of thousands of DNA sequence variants in a single experiment and has reduced the cost of genetic profiling, making such studies more affordable.

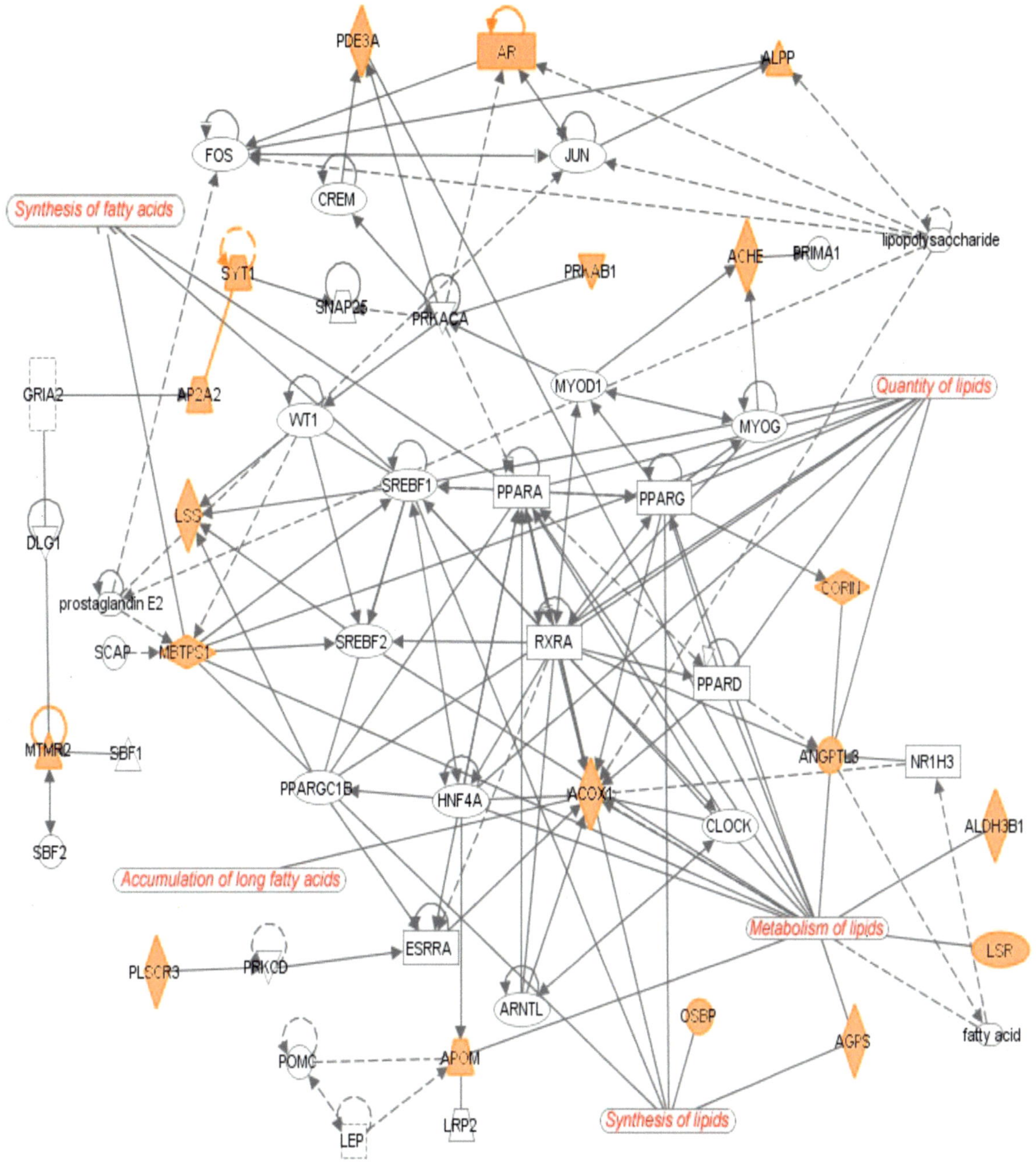

Fig. (1). Pathway Analysis: Gene networks grown from 19 genes involved in lipid metabolism and associated with weight reduction after RYGB (shown with a filled symbol). Solid lines represent direct interactions and dashed lines are indirect interactions (*Source: Kim et al. Int J Obes (Lond). 2008; 32(9): 1395-406 [72]*).

Association analyses and functional studies have demonstrated the contribution of polymorphisms of several candidate genes to obesity and related phenotypes [37, 74, 75]. Examples include INSIG2, a major obesity gene [76], TCF7L2, a transcription factor implicated in development of Type II diabetes [77], and ALOX5, a gene linked to susceptibility to obesity [78]. One of the most exciting findings from the genome-wide association studies was that the presence of certain fat mass and obesity associated (FTO) genotypes predisposed individuals to Type II diabetes by altering body mass index (BMI) [76]. The importance of this finding was that the association of FTO with increased BMI and risk of obesity was found in a large proportion of the general population [75, 79]. More interestingly, FTO's association with lean mass was found to be little to none in more than 5,000 children aged 9 years. Another important discovery is that the association of TCFL2 with Type II diabetes was replicated in several independent studies and gave support to the likelihood that TCFL2 is "truly" involved in the development of Type II diabetes [80-84].

A major limitation of genome-wide association studies is that they tend to lack reproducibility across multiple distinct cohorts and have a high potential for spurious associations and inconsistent findings [85]. For instance, several studies have generated extensive lists of candidate genes, but there is little overlap between these lists thus raising questions about reproducibility of results [69, 86-88]. In this context, the replication of involvement of TCFL2 to Type II diabetes in several independent studies is very important.

Transcriptional Profiling

Gene expression profiling, or transcriptomics, involves measurements of mRNA levels of many hundreds or thousands of genes simultaneously, typically comparing two or more treatments or conditions [89]. Transcriptomics attempts to explain the underlying biology using the patterns or profiles of gene expression [90, 91]. There is a variety of techniques used, including DNA microarray analysis and Serial Analysis of Gene Expression (SAGE) [92, 93]. The microarray profiling has become especially popular, and a number of different technologies for many different species are currently available. The RNA from samples is extracted, labeled, and hybridized to the probes immobilized on the array at specific locations. Then, the levels of fluorescence, which is proportional to the amounts of specific RNAs in the sample, can be measured and compared among different samples. Clearly, the microarray technology has many advantages. For instance, it makes it possible to monitor changes in the expression levels of specific transcripts or classes of genes and to detect novel gene targets. In obesity research, some expression studies have been directed toward understanding global changes in gene expression due to genetic knockouts or drug interventions, while others have attempted to characterize transcription profiles in individuals with changes in metabolic health [74, 94-102]. However, microarray technology also has certain limitations: changes in RNA may not correspond to changes in protein levels due to variable translation or protein degradation; post-translational modifications of proteins may affect their function but not register as a change in levels of corresponding mRNAs. In addition, genetic polymorphisms may cause important changes that are not detected by the microarrays (e.g. may affect post-transcriptional processing or protein stability). As with other high-throughput techniques, the majority of transcriptional variation may be just "physiological noise."

Proteomics

Proteomics examines the global expression of proteins and their changes in response to stimuli under different conditions [103]. The complexity of proteome is overwhelming; the human proteome is estimated at several hundreds of thousands of protein species with a variety of protein forms and variants due to splicing and post-translational modifications, such as phosphorylation, methylation, acetylation, glycosylation, and others [104]. The dynamic range of individual protein levels spans over several orders of magnitude over the body. The amounts of mRNA and corresponding protein do not always correlate; proteomics analysis confirms that specific proteins are present and measures their quantity. Two principal approaches exist to measure protein abundance: the "gel" approach and "shotgun" method. In the gel approach, proteins are separated on the two-dimensional gel by electrophoresis and by isoelectric point, followed by visualization and measurement of protein abundances in each spot. In the shotgun method, the protein mixture is digested and separated by mass-spectroscopy. Overall, two methods have been shown to be complementary conditions [103]. While proteomics profiling in obesity research is just getting popularity, there are several examples of the application of technology [105-107].

Metabolomics

Metabolomics characterizes and quantifies end results (i.e., metabolites) produced by an organism under certain conditions. Therefore, changes in metabolite levels represent the downstream changes in the genome, transcriptome, and proteome and are influenced by exogenous environmental factors. Small molecules or biochemical compounds are the end results of the entire chain of regulatory changes that occur in response to physiological stressors. Thus, profiling low molecular compounds through omics approaches can provide insights to metabolic physiology in the body. A number of studies have used metabolomics to map alterations in metabolite levels resulting from Type II diabetes, obesity, and the metabolic syndrome. Yang *et al.* employed metabolomics for the diagnosis of Type II diabetes and demonstrated that Type II diabetes patients could be distinguished from healthy control subjects based on the global profiles of fatty acid metabolites [108]. William *et al.* showed the feasibility of metabolomic techniques in the discovery of biomarkers of metabolic disease by comparing obese (*fa/fa*) Zucker and normal Wistar-derived rats [109]. Xu *et al.* studied hypoglycemia in the fasting *PPARα* null mouse related to impaired liver fatty acid β-oxidation [110, 111]. They showed that the PPARα receptor regulated hepatic glucose production in not only fasted but also fed states. Watkins *et al.* studied the effects of PPARγ agonist rosiglitazone on structural lipid metabolism in an obese mouse model of Type II diabetes using lipid metabolomic analysis [112]. They found that rosiglitazone induced *de novo* fatty acid synthesis, altered free fatty acid and cardiolipin metabolism in the heart and elicited an excessive accumulation of polyunsaturated fatty acids within adipose tissue, suggesting that agonist of rosiglitazone could mediate phenotypes by interacting with multiple metabolites in different tissues.

STATISTICAL ANALYSES

Given the abundance and complexity of data generated by omics technologies, it is crucial that statistical data analysis approaches be adequate and appropriate [113]. To obtain good quality data, careful planning and execution of experiments is required. Omics studies have design issues common to any experiment, but they also have their own peculiarities. When an omics study is proposed, it should have a clear goal and a specific biological hypothesis to test. In the design of an experiment, all potential sources of variation should be taken into account to avoid any systematic bias [114, 115]. When planning a study, researchers should adhere to sound principles of experimental design and should match the experimental variables of cases and controls to the fullest extent possible - selecting samples from biologically homogenous populations, balancing the design with respect to all factors that can confound results among the comparison groups, and handling samples uniformly through the course of the entire experiment. Randomization will assure baseline equality between the groups being compared. Violation of these principles will lead to biased results and can cause a loss in statistical power [116]. It should be pointed out that statistical analysis of data cannot solve fundamental flaws in the design of the study. Significantly, the validity of results depends on the characteristics of samples and selection bias, regarding all eligible criteria of participation and other confounding factors. As with all such studies, an adequate sample size is necessary to achieve sufficient statistical power to demonstrate the significance of findings, and this is particularly the case with omics studies where hundreds to thousands of variables (transcripts or compounds) are tested simultaneously. The sample size required for a study depends in part on methods of statistical or bioinformatics analysis.

Various statistical data analysis methods for profiling have been developed. Commonly used statistical methods can be classified as differential analysis (such as t-test, analysis of variance (ANOVA)), supervised classification methods (principal component analysis, linear discriminant analysis, support vector machines, etc), and unsupervised cluster analysis (hierarchical clustering, K-means clustering, etc). Differential analysis methods, often referred to as "group comparison" [117], are statistical tests for identifying differentially expressed variables (genes or proteins) by determining differences in mean values between different groups or between groups in different conditions. Classification and cluster analysis are statistical approaches that attempt to divide data into groups or classes.

One of the first things that researchers do is identify differentially expressed genes or compounds. For a two-group comparison, this is typically done using a series of t-tests. A number of other methods have also been proposed, including empirical Bayes, non-parametric tests, etc [56, 118]. Because analyses of global expression profiles involve multiple comparisons, they are typically accompanied by a multiple testing correction such as Benjamini-Hochberg's false discovery rate [36], the Westfall-Young step-down permutation correction [119], or the Bonferroni correction. The goal of multiple testing correction is to minimize the chance of false positives which is particularly important in global profiling studies whose goal is to generate a hypothesis for future downstream experiments. The general consensus is that the selection of differentially expressed genes or compounds should be based on the false discovery rate [3].

Cluster analysis is referred to as a class discovery method because no classes are predefined, and the procedure groups variables or samples into arbitrary classes based on their similarity/dissimilarity in expression or concentration levels. Cluster analysis is used to describe general gene expression (molecular concentration) patterns across the genome (proteome or metabolome) and may help investigators in formulating specific hypotheses for future research [120]. At the dawn of microarray era, clustering was considered as a method of choice, but later become increasingly criticized due to lack of stability and sensitivity to minor variations in the data [121, 122]. More robust alternatives are available, but they are typically more computationally intensive [123, 124].

Classification analysis differs from cluster analysis in the sense that it uses information on predefined classes. Unfortunately, in studies of class prediction which distinguish samples in one group from samples in the other group, a perfect discriminatory classifier can be found by chance, especially when assessing a large number of possible predictors. This problem is referred to 'overfitting.' Overfitting occurs when a classifier is made to perfectly fit the set of data that was used in the model development, but the classifier then has no discriminatory power when applied to a completely different sample set and the results of the model therefore cannot be reproduced.

There is a vast literature on the evaluation of the performance of different Machine Learning (ML) methods used for classification and in regard to overfitting issues [125, 126]. The main consensus points are that: (1) most of ML methods perform well in the presence of a small number of features, (2) all ML methods perform better with filter-based feature selection because irrelevant features are discarded prior to analysis, and (3) most ML methods show significant degradation in performance in the presence of noisy features [82, 127-129]. As a consequence, feature selection techniques have become a necessity in many high-dimensional applications because they allow to avoid overfitting, improve prediction performance, and provide more cost-effective predictive models. However, the advantages of feature selection techniques come at cost. Bias in feature selection could have a strong effect on results of downstream analyses, such as bioinformatics analysis. If certain features were selected due to sampling variation, the results could be skewed in favor of the certain pathways, even if they are not the relevant in the disease of interest. Hence the interpretation of this bias depends on the nature of how the features are selected upstream for downstream analysis, and, as one might expect, researchers have developed several feature-selection techniques including t-test feature selection, correlation-based feature selection [130], sequential selection [131], genetic algorithms [132], decision trees weighted naïve Bayes [44], feature selection using the weight vector of SVM [119, 133], and others.

Typically, omics studies have a small number of biological samples due to cost considerations or difficulties in obtaining the samples. Thus, combining several studies to increase statistical power got much attention [58, 79, 84]. There are two possible approaches to integrating multiple studies: meta-analysis of merged raw data which may be obtained in public repositories, such as GEO [26], or meta-review analysis of the published results (for example, to identify overrepresented pathways using the published gene and protein lists which resulted from the analyses of the raw data). Although meta-analysis of merged raw datasets from similar studies is most desirable, there are limitations to the approach. Meaningful raw data that can be used in meta-analysis may simply not be available for most studies, especially when combining different sources of data such as genomic and proteomic data. An alternative approach is a meta-review method that employs a vote-counting strategy in an analysis of published evidence [133]. The meta-review approach is built on the assumption that there are connections between molecular targets, pathways, cellular processes, and end points and the common process continues through the levels of cell, tissue, organ, and whole system - that one can think of the causative chain process from lower to higher levels of organization. The assumption can be satisfied when selected compounds extracted at different levels of the organism are consistently expressed and their expression is measureable. The potential of meta-analysis can improve when all prospective omics studies are considered in a "scheme" framework that integrates diverse approaches taken from different studies [134].

INTEGRATIVE APPROACH

As high-throughput technologies have continued to evolve, global scale profiling of omics data has become a routine method in various areas of biological research including obesity, diabetes, and cardiovascular diseases. With the significant advances and promises offered by the omics technologies, an integrated approach is needed for the meaningful and functional combining of data from heterogeneous sources [35, 135]. Each omics technology has its specific purposes, but it also complements the others as one type of data is simply not sufficient to understand a complex "big picture." For example, physiological responses to diet may be different in rats with the same genetic background, and this may be the case for human populations as well. Li *et al.* (2008) exposed a group of genetically identical rats to a high fat diet for 16 weeks and then selected "obesity-resistant" rats among them that had modest increases in body weight and "obesity-prone" rats that had significant changes in body weight [136]. The authors performed transcriptional and metabolic profiling of the two groups and used a combination of different sources of data in their analyses. As a result, they identified approximately 80 genes involved in lipid metabolism, lipid transport, and ketone body production. The integration of results revealed that altered metabolic pathways may involve the increased activity of sympathetic nervous system and the Krebs cycle. In another example, Mootha *et al.* (2003) demonstrated that a group of genes down-regulated in diabetes compared to controls was enriched for genes involved in oxidative phosphorylation [137]. The study illustrates how pathway analysis can lead to insights into altered metabolism in diabetes patients and can make possible novel therapies involving the modulation of oxidative phosphorylation pathways. Integrative approach allows one to increase confidence by assessing multiple genes or compounds in combination, ultimately enabling us to discover multiple physiological pathways that contribute to disease progression and can be used for diagnosis and prognosis [134].

Networks Structure Analysis

Omics techniques have the capacity to provide information about hundreds or thousands of individual molecular compounds. One way to summarize this overwhelming information is to use a network. The network - consisting of the nodes (e.g. genes or proteins) connected by the edges (lines or arrows) where edges indicate dependencies and possibly functional relations among nodes - provides a convenient framework to represent high-dimensional data [138]. There is a variety of molecular networks that include genomics, RNA (coding and non-coding), protein interactions, signaling networks and networks of metabolites. These networks do not act in isolation but interact with one another to form complicated web of interactions. Genetic variations and changes in the environment can disturb these networks in ways that eventually lead to physiological responses and may cause disease [35, 38, 139].

Biological networks are believed to have both hierarchical and scale-free properties [138, 140]. Hierarchical properties mean that there are clusters or modules of highly interconnected compounds that do not have many interactions outside the module [54, 141]. Functional units or modules of networks can be associated with pathways or certain subtypes of disease [122]. In contrast to cluster analysis that is commonly used to find compounds of similar profiles, networks provide better structured information on the connectivity among compounds. Scale-free properties mean that nodes have connections that extend outside the module, with a small number having many such connections. This has evolutionary implications - mutations in most of the nodes with a small number of connections may not affect the system as a whole, while vulnerability of hubs increases, since mutations in hubs are often lethal [135, 142]. Clearly, the transcription factors that regulate many genes may represent such hubs; but, complicating this research, the expres-sion levels of the transcription factors themselves may or may not change dramatically, and thus such hubs are difficult to identify from microarray studies alone [143].

Structural properties of networks inspire new strategies for exploring drug targets. One such property can be differential connectivity [144-146]. Genes may not be differentially expressed between two different conditions, yet connections between genes could be "wired" differently. For example, Dact 1 alters extracellular Wnt signals in preadipocytes and differentiating adipocytes. Deregulation and rewiring of this network may be a pathological basis leading to an altered balance between the processes of adipocyte growth and recruitment [59]. Though gene expression does not change, modulation of the network by Dact 1 may be of therapeutic value to improve the metabolic efficiency of the adipose tissue.

One significant challenge for researchers is to reconstruct network structure from available data. Many different methods for network inference have been proposed. In Boolean network models, each gene is considered to be either ON or OFF. If there are n genes, or variables, then there are total of 2n states. Each variable can be written as a function of others, for example: gene X will be expressed (i.e., will be ON), if genes Y and Z are currently expressed. Typically, one does not explicitly know all states of the system, and Boolean networks can provide a way to model states of all genes and find previously unknown interactions [147]. In kinetic logic models, which are extensions of Boolean models, the state of each gene is represented as a discrete value: not expressed, expressed at the low level, or expressed at the high level [148]. These models allow genes to change states at independent rates and predictions are more precise.

The more realistic and accurate approach is to transform the system of chemical reactions and physical constraints into a system of nonlinear ordinary differential equations, whose variables are concentrations of proteins and mRNA [44, 149]. A common problem of such models is exponential complexity: the number of unknown constants in equations increases exponentially with the number of variables. In addition, several hybrid approaches exist [150, 151].

Another class of models is Bayesian networks, graphical models that characterize conditional dependencies between variables [147]. Although Bayesian networks have been extensively used for data mining and classification, Friedman *et al.* (2000) may have been the first to apply this technique specifically to microarray data [143]. Bayesian networks have a number of properties that make them an attractive choice for such analysis. This approach allows compact and intuitive representation of data, has a concrete statistical foundation, and can handle missing data. Variables can be discrete, continuous, or hybrid; represent mRNA concentration, experimental conditions, or other information; and be informative (observable) or latent (unobservable). The original approach has been extended to incorporate latent variables [152-154]; use non-parametric models [72]; identify subnetworks [155]; and include relevant biological information, such as protein binding data [146, 156] or protein-protein interactions [157]. A similar methodology has been applied to combine gene ontology data with promoter and biochemical pathways information in order to identify network modules [158]. Dynamic Bayesian Networks, an extension of the method, allows modeling of time series and feedback loops [123, 159].

The limitation of the network inference methods is that many alternative and equally probable network structures may be constructed from a given dataset. In experimental biology, causal associations are being established using interventions such as genetic knockouts, RNAi, etc. Successful reconstruction of biological networks requires a systematic source of perturbation such as genetic variations or environmental changes which leads to changes in protein and metabolomic profiles [160]. Protein, genome data, and transcriptional and metabolomic profiles can be brought together into a single network in which DNA variations might serve as a "causal anchor". Integration of genetic and gene expression data has been successfully applied to identify a number of novel disease-related genes [80, 123, 161].

FUTURE DIRECTIONS

High-throughput omics methodologies have advanced significantly in the last decade and have been successfully utilized in the research of obesity and associated complex traits. However, there are several potential limitations that need to be acknowledged and overcome. First, systematic and integrated approaches have yet to be developed for the integration of heterogeneous data drawn from emerging studies in genetics, genomics, transcriptomics, proteomics, metabolomics, and other omics. Second, despite the progress in omics methods in biomarker or drug discovery and characterization, criticism has emerged against predictive models based on omic data. Researchers point out the complex relationships among genetic variation, environment, and disease, and the limited clinical validity and utility of genetic risk prediction in translational personalized and genomic medicine [36]. Quite often, claims are prematurely optimistic and may lead to unrealistic expectations. Ein-Dor *et al.* used a theoretical analysis to show that thousands of patients may be needed to obtain reliable gene lists [118]. Moreover, not only genetics but environment and lifestyle may have significant contribution to obesity and related disorders. The integration of genomics and other omics with clinical and environmental data, joining "nature and nurture," [162] will hopefully improve the robustness and practical impact of omic profiling studies for biomarker or drug development. Third, we have witnessed the explosive growth of data and available tools during the last decades. The January 2009 issue of *Nucleic Acids Research* includes descriptions of 179 biological databases, of which 95 are new. These databases (along with several molecular biology databases described in other journals) have been included in the Nucleic Acids Research online Molecular Biology Database Collection, bringing the total number of databases in the collection to 1170 [163]. Consequently, data management and handling become critical issues in any large scale omics project. Although each omics technology faces its own unique challenges, there are several common issues in omics fields. One of the serious problems historically has been a wide variety of data formats used in databases. There are ongoing efforts to develop a common standard for data input and reporting that could be shared among scientists in the field. For example, in 2001 the MGED created the Minimum Information About a Microarray Experiment (MIAME) guidelines which serve as a template for researchers to report an adequate description of how gene expression data were obtained. The Minimum Information About a Proteomic Experiment (MIAPE) documents describe information which should be given along with a proteomic experiment [164]. The Minimum Information About a METabolomics experiment (MIAMET) was proposed as an analogous standard adapted to the specifics of metabolomics [165]. Currently, many journals require these compliances as part of the manuscript submitting procedure. It is time to look forward to the development of a "universal" standard format that can be implemented in different omics technologies in order to share and integrate heterogeneous data among scientists from diverse disciplinary backgrounds [166].

Assuming researchers are able to effectively address these challenges, it appears that ultimately networks structure can provide a better understanding of the complexity of the molecular mechanisms involved in development and progression of obesity and associated disorders and can suggest points of interventions and search for drug targets [135, 167, 168]. Although omics techniques and applications have made great progress to prove its usefulness in finding drug targets and diagnostic biomarkers for obesity and other complex disorders, they are still in their infancy. The prospect of developing global approaches that integrate data collected at the genetic, transcript, protein, and metabolite levels is likely to provide the most comprehensive and informative views of biological mechanisms of the disease, ultimately bring us closer to understanding their nature.

ACKNOWLEDGEMENT

This work was supported in part by NIH/NIA grant P01AG025532 (KK).

REFERENCES

[1] Korner J, Woods SC, Woodworth KA. Regulation of energy homeostasis and health consequences in obesity. Am J Med 2009; 122 (4 Suppl 1): S12-8.
[2] Lewis CE, McTigue KM, Burke LE, Poirier P, *et al.* Mortality, health outcomes, and body mass index in the overweight range: a science advisory from the American Heart Association. Circulation 2009; 119(25): 3263-71.
[3] Allison DB, Cui C, Page PG, Sabripour M. Microarray data analysis: from disarray to consolidation and consensus. Nat Rev Genet 2005, 7: 55-65.
[4] Wolf G. Insulin resistance and obesity: resistin, a hormone secreted by adipose tissue. Nutr Rev 2004; 62(10): 389-94.
[5] Ginsberg HN, MacCallum PR. The obesity, metabolic syndrome, and type 2 diabetes mellitus pandemic: Part I. Increased cardiovascular disease risk and the importance of atherogenic dyslipidemia in persons with the metabolic syndrome and type 2 diabetes mellitus. J Cardiometab Syndr 2009; 4(2): 113-9.
[6] Phillips C, Lopez-Miranda J, Perez-Jimenez F, McManus R, Roche HM. Genetic and nutrient determinants of the metabolic syndrome. Curr Opin Cardiol 2006; 21(3): 185-93.
[7] Redinger RN. Fat storage and the biology of energy expenditure. Transl Res 2009; 154(2): 52-60.
[8] Ichihara S, Yamada Y. Genetic factors for human obesity. Cell Mol Life Sci 2008; 65(7-8): 1086-98.
[9] Chen X, Hess S. Adipose proteome analysis: focus on mediators of insulin resistance. Expert Rev Proteomics 2008; 5(6): 827-39.
[10] Franks PW, Jablonski KA, Delahanty LM, *et al.* Diabetes Prevention Program Research Group. Assessing gene-treatment interactions at the FTO and INSIG2 loci on obesity-related traits in the Diabetes Prevention Program. Diabetologia 2008; 51(12): 2214-23.
[11] Bougnères P, Valleron AJ. Causes of early-onset type 1 diabetes: toward data-driven environmental approaches. J Exp Med 2008; 205(13): 2953-7.
[12] Ng MC, So WY, Lam VK, Cockram CS, Bell GI, Cox NJ, Chan JC. Genome-wide scan for metabolic syndrome and related quantitative traits in Hong Kong Chinese and confirmation of a susceptibility locus on chromosome 1q21-q25. Diabetes 2004; 53(10): 2676-83.
[13] Edwards AV, White MY, Cordwell SJ. The role of proteomics in clinical cardiovascular biomarker discovery. Mol Cell Proteomics 2008; 7(10): 1824-37.
[14] Giovane A, Balestrieri A, Napoli C. New insights into cardiovascular and lipid metabolomics. J Cell Biochem 2008; 105(3): 648-54.
[15] Belacel N, Wang Q, Cuperlovic-Culf M. Clustering methods for microarray gene expression data. OMICS 2006; 10(4): 507-31.
[16] Burton GR, McGehee RE Jr. Identification of candidate genes involved in the regulation of adipocyte differentiation using microarray-based gene expression profiling. Nutrition 2004; 20(1): 109-14.
[17] Cawthorn WP, Sethi JK. TNF-alpha and adipocyte biology. FEBS Lett 2008; 582(1): 117-31.
[18] Damcott CM, Feingold E, Moffett SP, *et al.* Variation in the FABP2 promoter alters transcriptional activity and is associated with body composition and plasma lipid levels. Hum Genet 2003; 112(5-6): 610-6.
[19] Ghosh D, Poisson LM. "Omics" data and levels of evidence for biomarker discovery. Genomics 2009; 93(1):13-6.
[20] Hartemink AJ, Gifford DK, Jaakkola TS, Young RA. Using graphical models and genomic expression data to statistically validate models of genetic regulatory networks. Pac Symp Biocomput 2001: 422-33.
[21] Fontaine KR, Redden DT, Wang C, Westfall AO, Allison DB. Years of life lost due to obesity. JAMA 2003; 289(2): 187-93.
[22] The Obesity Society. What is Obesity. Available at http://www.obesity.org/information/ what_is_obesity.asp [Accessed September 23, 2009].
[23] Andreasen CH, Andersen G. Gene-environment interactions and obesity--further aspects of genomewide association studies. Nutrition 2009; 25(10): 998-1003.
[24] LeRoith D, Novosyadlyy R, Gallagher EJ, Lann D, Vijayakumar A, Yakar S. Obesity and type 2 diabetes are associated with an increased risk of developing cancer and a worse prognosis; epidemiological and mechanistic evidence. Exp Clin Endocrinol Diabetes 2008; 116 (Suppl 1): S4-6.
[25] Huang PL. A comprehensive definition for metabolic syndrome. Dis Model Mech 2009; 2(5-6): 231-7.
[26] Barrett T, Troup DB, Wilhite SE, *et al.* NCBI GEO: mining tens of millions of expression profiles--database and tools update. Nucleic Acids Res 2007; 35: D760-5.
[27] Reisin E, Jack AV. Obesity and hypertension: mechanisms, cardio-renal consequences, and therapeutic approaches. Med Clin North Am 2009; 93(3): 733-51.
[28] Ginsberg HN, MacCallum PR. The obesity, metabolic syndrome, and type 2 diabetes mellitus pandemic: Part I. Increased cardiovascular disease risk and the importance of atherogenic dyslipidemia in persons with the metabolic syndrome and type 2 diabetes mellitus. J Cardiometab Syndr 2009; 4(2): 113-9.
[29] Hebebrand J, Hinney A. Environmental and genetic risk factors in obesity. Child Adolesc Psychiatr Clin N Am 2009; 18(1): 83-94.

[30] Rocha VZ, Libby P. Obesity, inflammation, and atherosclerosis. Nat Rev Cardiol 2009; 6(6): 399-409.

[31] Isomaa B, Almgren P, Tuomi T, *et al.* Cardiovascular morbidity and mortality associated with the metabolic syndrome. Diabetes Care 2001; 24(4): 683-9.

[32] Schoeller DA. The energy balance equation: looking back and looking forward are two very different views. Nutr Rev 2009; 67(5): 249-54.

[33] Roche HM, Phillips C, Gibney MJ. The metabolic syndrome: the crossroads of diet and genetics. Proc Nutr Soc 2005; 64(3): 371-7.

[34] Chakrabarti R. Pharmacotherapy of obesity: emerging drugs and targets. Expert Opin Ther Targets 2009; 13(2): 195-207.

[35] Schadt EE, Zhang B, Zhu J. Advances in systems biology are enhancing our understanding of disease and moving us closer to novel disease treatments. Genetica 2009; 136(2): 259-69.

[36] Bell CG, Walley AJ, Froguel P. The genetics of human obesity. Nat Rev Genet 2005; 6(3): 221-34.

[37] Herbert A. The fat tail of obesity as told by the genome. Curr Opin Clin Nutr Metab Care 2008; 11(4): 366-70.

[38] Chen Y, Zhu J, Lum PY, Yang X, *et al.* Variations in DNA elucidate molecular networks that cause disease. Nature 2008; 452(7186): 429-35.

[39] Ng MC, So WY, Lam VK, *et al.* Genome-wide scan for metabolic syndrome and related quantitative traits in Hong Kong Chinese and confirmation of a susceptibility locus on chromosome 1q21-q25. Diabetes 2004; 53(10): 2676-83.

[40] Blakemore AI, Froguel P. Is obesity our genetic legacy? J Clin Endocrinol Metab 2008; 93(11 Suppl 1): S51-6.

[41] Lee YS. The role of genes in the current obesity epidemic. Ann Acad Med Singapore 2009; 38(1): 45-3.

[42] Garfield AS, Lam DD, Marston OJ, Przydzial MJ, Heisler LK. Role of central melanocortin pathways in energy homeostasis. Trends Endocrinol Metab 2009; 20(5): 203-15.

[43] Blüher S, Mantzoros CS. Leptin in humans: lessons from translational research. Am J Clin Nutr 2009; 89(3): 991S-7S.

[44] Adeghate E, Ponery A. Diabetes mellitus influences the degree of colocalization of calcitonin gene-related peptide with insulin and somatostatin in the rat pancreas. Pancreas 2004; 29(4): 311-9.

[45] Antuna-Puente B, Feve B, Fellahi S, Bastard JP. Adipokines: the missing link between insulin resistance and obesity. Diabetes Metab 2008; 34(1): 2-11.

[46] Brookheart RT, Michel CI, Schaffer JE. As a matter of fat. Cell Metab 2009; 10(1): 9-12.

[47] Roche HM. Fatty acids and the metabolic syndrome. Proc Nutr Soc 2005; 64(1): 23-9.

[48] Farooqi IS, O'Rahilly S. Leptin: a pivotal regulator of human energy homeostasis. Am J Clin Nutr 2009; 89(3): 980S-4S.

[49] Soukas A, Cohen P, Socci ND, Friedman JM. Leptin-specific patterns of gene expression in white adipose tissue. Genes Dev 2000 15; 14(8): 963-80.

[50] Kamiji MM, Inui A. Neuropeptide y receptor selective ligands in the treatment of obesity. Endocr Rev 2007; 28(6): 664-84.

[51] Valassi E, Scacchi M, Cavagnini F. Neuroendocrine control of food intake. Nutr Metab Cardiovasc Dis 2008; 18(2): 158-68.

[52] Conner SC, Wu W, Sweatman BC, *et al.* Effects of feeding and body weight loss on the 1H-NMR-based urine metabolic profiles of male wistar han rats: implications for biomarker discovery. Biomarkers 2004, 9: 156-79.

[53] Desvergne B, Feige JN, Casals-Casas C. PPAR-mediated activity of phthalates: A link to the obesity epidemic? Mol Cell Endocrinol 2009 25; 304(1-2): 43-8.

[54] Lee HK, Hsu AK, Sajdak J, Qin J, Pavlidis P. Coexpression analysis of human genes across many microarray data sets. Genome Res 2004; 14(6): 1085-94.

[55] Hotamisligil GS, Arner P, Caro JF, Atkinson RL, Spiegelman BM. Increased adipose tissue expression of tumor necrosis factor-alpha in human obesity and insulin resistance. J Clin Invest 1995; 95(5): 2409-15.

[56] Hotamisligil GS, Arner P, Caro JF, Atkinson RL, Spiegelman BM. Increased adipose tissue expression of tumor necrosis factor-alpha in human obesity and insulin resistance. J Clin Invest 1995; 95(5): 2409-15.

[57] Pradhan AD, Manson JE, Rifai N, Buring JE, Ridker PM. C-reactive protein, interleukin 6, and risk of developing type 2 diabetes mellitus. JAMA 2001; 286(3): 327-34.

[58] DeConde RP, Hawley S, Falcon S, Clegg N, Knudsen B, Etzioni R. Combining results of microarray experiments: a rank aggregation approach. Stat Appl Genet Mol Biol 2006; 5: Article 15.

[59] Lagathu C, Christodoulides C, Virtue S, *et al.* Dact1, a nutritionally regulated preadipocyte gene, controls adipogenesis by coordinating the Wnt/beta-catenin signaling network. Diabetes 2009; 58(3): 609-19.

[60] Lenard NR, Berthoud HR. Central and peripheral regulation of food intake and physical activity: pathways and genes. Obesity (Silver Spring) 2008; 16 (Suppl 3): S11-22.

[61] McMillen IC, Rattanatray L, Duffield JA, *et al.* The early origins of later obesity: pathways and mechanisms. Adv Exp Med Biol 2009; 646: 71-81.

[62] Raghow R, Yellaturu C, Deng X, Park EA, Elam MB. SREBPs: the crossroads of physiological and pathological lipid homeostasis. Trends Endocrinol Metab 2008; 19(2): 65-73.

[63] Ozcan U, Cao Q, Yilmaz E, Lee AH, *et al.* Hotamisligil GS. Endoplasmic reticulum stress links obesity, insulin action, and type 2 diabetes. Science 2004; 306(5695): 457-61.

[64] Van Guilder GP, Hoetzer GL, Greiner JJ, *et al.* Desouza CA. Influence of metabolic syndrome on biomarkers of oxidative stress and inflammation in obese adults. Obesity (Silver Spring) 2006; 14(12): 2127-31.

[65] Fischer HP. Towards quantitative biology: integration of biological information to elucidate disease pathways and to guide drug discovery. Biotechnol Annu Rev 2005; 11: 1-68.

[66] Zhu J, Zhang B, Smith EN, *et al.* Integrating large-scale functional genomic data to dissect the complexity of yeast regulatory networks. Nat Genet 2008; 40(7): 854-61.

[67] Mariman EC. Nutrigenomics and nutrigenetics: the 'omics' revolution in nutritional science. Biotechnol Appl Biochem 2006; 44(Pt3): 119-28.

[68] Zhang X, Yap Y, Wei D, *et al.* Novel omics technologies in nutrition research. Biotechnol Adv 2008; 26(2): 169-76.

[69] Ghosh D, Poisson LM. "Omics" data and levels of evidence for biomarker discovery. Genomics 2009; 93(1): 13-6.

[70] Ioannidis JP. Why most published research findings are false. PLoS Med 2005; 2(8): e124.

[71] Jones GL, Sang E, Goddard C, *et al.* A functional analysis of mouse models of cardiac disease through metabolic profiling. J Bio Chem 2005, 280: 7530-9.

[72] Kim K, Perroud B, Espinal G, *et al.* Genes and networks expressed in perioperative omental adipose tissue are correlated with weight loss from Roux-en-Y gastric bypass. Int J Obes (Lond) 2008; 32(9): 1395-406.

[73] Rankinen T, Zuberi A, Chagnon YC, *et al.* The human obesity gene map: the 2005 update. Obesity (Silver Spring) 2006; 14(4): 529-644.
[74] Damcott CM, Feingold E, Moffett SP, *et al.* Variation in the FABP2 promoter alters transcriptional activity and is associated with body composition and plasma lipid levels. Hum Genet 2003; 112(5-6): 610-6.
[75] Loktionov A. Common gene polymorphisms and nutrition: emerging links with pathogenesis of multifactorial chronic diseases (review). J Nutr Biochem 2003; 14(8): 426-51.
[76] Franks PW, Jablonski KA, Delahanty LM, *et al.* Diabetes Prevention Program Research Group. Assessing gene-treatment interactions at the FTO and INSIG2 loci on obesity-related traits in the Diabetes Prevention Program. Diabetologia 2008; 51(12): 2214-23.
[77] Grant SF, Thorleifsson G, Reynisdottir I, *et al.* Variant of transcription factor 7-like 2 (TCF7L2) gene confers risk of type 2 diabetes. Nat Genet 2006; 38(3): 320-3.
[78] Lyons MA. Arachidonate 5-lipoxygenase variants in atherosclerosis, obesity, and bone traits. Circ Res 2006; 98(8): e66.
[79] Sohal D, Yeatts A, Ye K, *et al.* Meta-analysis of microarray studies reveals a novel hematopoietic progenitor cell signature and demonstrates feasibility of inter-platform data integration. PLoS One 2008; 3(8): e2965.
[80] Saxena R, Gianniny L, Burtt NP, *et al.* Common single nucleotide polymorphisms in TCF7L2 are reproducibly associated with type 2 diabetes and reduce the insulin response to glucose in nondiabetic individuals. Diabetes 2006; 55(10): 2890-5.
[81] Scott LJ, Mohlke KL, Bonnycastle LL, *et al.* A genome-wide association study of type 2 diabetes in Finns detects multiple susceptibility variants. Science 2007; 316(5829): 1341-5.
[82] Sima C, Dougherty ER. What should be expected from feature selection in small-sample settings. Bioinformatics 2006; 22(19): 2430-6.
[83] Steinthorsdottir V, Thorleifsson G, Reynisdottir I, *et al.* A variant in CDKAL1 influences insulin response and risk of type 2 diabetes. Nat Genet 2007; 39(6): 770-5.
[84] Yu T, Ye H, Chen Z, *et al.* Dimension reduction and mixed-effects model for microarray meta-analysis of cancer. Front Biosci 2008; 13: 2714-20.
[85] Wang WY, Barratt BJ, Clayton DG, Todd JA. Genome-wide association studies: theoretical and practical concerns. Nat Rev Genet 2005; 6(2): 109-18.
[86] Büettner R, Schäffler A, Arndt H, *et al.* The Trp64Arg polymorphism of the beta 3-adrenergic receptor gene is not associated with obesity or type 2 diabetes mellitus in a large population-based Caucasian cohort. J Clin Endocrinol Metab 1998; 83(8): 2892-7.
[87] Endo K, Yanagi H, Hirano C, *et al.* Association of Trp64Arg polymorphism of the beta3-adrenergic receptor gene and no association of Gln223Arg polymorphism of the leptin receptor gene in Japanese schoolchildren with obesity. Int J Obes Relat Metab Disord 2000; 24(4): 443-9.
[88] Kurokawa N, Nakai K, Kameo S, *et al.* Association of BMI with the beta3-adrenergic receptor gene polymorphism in Japanese: meta-analysis. Obes Res 2001; 9(12): 741-5.
[89] Sun G. Application of DNA microarrays in the study of human obesity and type 2 diabetes. OMICS 2007; 11(1): 25-40.
[90] Segal E, Friedman N, Kaminski N, *et al.* From signatures to models: understanding cancer using microarrays. Nat Genet 2005; 37 (Suppl): S38-45.
[91] van Steensel B. Mapping of genetic and epigenetic regulatory networks using microarrays. Nat Genet 2005; 37 (Suppl): S18-24.
[92] Anisimov SV. Serial Analysis of Gene Expression (SAGE): 13 years of application in research. Curr Pharm Biotechnol 2008; 9(5): 338-50.
[93] Takamura T, Misu H, Yamashita T, *et al.* SAGE application in the study of diabetes. Curr Pharm Biotechnol 2008; 9(5): 392-9.
[94] Baranova A, Schlauch K, Gowder S, *et al.* Microarray technology in the study of obesity and non-alcoholic fatty liver disease. Liver Int 2005; 25(6): 1091-6.
[95] Burton GR, McGehee RE Jr. Identification of candidate genes involved in the regulation of adipocyte differentiation using microarray-based gene expression profiling. Nutrition 2004; 20(1): 109-14.
[96] Gómez-Ambrosi J, Catalán V, Diez-Caballero A, *et al.* Gene expression profile of omental adipose tissue in human obesity. FASEB J 2004; 18(1): 215-7.
[97] Henegar C, Tordjman J, Achard V, *et al.* Adipose tissue transcriptomic signature highlights the pathological relevance of extracellular matrix in human obesity. Genome Biol 2008; 9(1): R14.
[98] Linder K, Arner P, Flores-Morales A, *et al.* Differentially expressed genes in visceral or subcutaneous adipose tissue of obese men and women. J Lipid Res 2004; 45(1): 148-54.
[99] Patti ME, Butte AJ, Crunkhorn S, *et al.* Coordinated reduction of genes of oxidative metabolism in humans with insulin resistance and diabetes: Potential role of PGC1 and NRF1. Proc Natl Acad Sci USA 2003; 100(14): 8466-71.
[100] Permana PA, Del Parigi A, Tataranni PA. Microarray gene expression profiling in obesity and insulin resistance. Nutrition 2004; 20(1): 134-8.
[101] Sreekumar R, Halvatsiotis P, Schimke JC, *et al.* Gene expression profile in skeletal muscle of type 2 diabetes and the effect of insulin treatment. Diabetes 2002; 51(6): 1913-20.
[102] von Eyben FE, Kroustrup JP, Larsen JF, *et al.* Abdominal Obesity Study Group. Comparison of gene expression in intra-abdominal and subcutaneous fat: a study of men with morbid obesity and nonobese men using microarray and proteomics. Ann N Y Acad Sci 2004; 1030: 508-36.
[103] Kussmann M, Affolter M, Fay LB. Proteomics in nutrition and health. Comb Chem High Throughput Screen 2005; 8(8): 679-96.
[104] Sanchez JC, Chiappe D, Converset V, *et al.* The mouse SWISS-2D PAGE database: a tool for proteomics study of diabetes and obesity. Proteomics 2001; 1(1): 136-63.
[105] Chen X, Hess S. Adipose proteome analysis: focus on mediators of insulin resistance. Expert Rev Proteomics 2008; 5(6): 827-39.
[106] Højlund K, Mogensen M, Sahlin K, Beck-Nielsen H. Mitochondrial dysfunction in type 2 diabetes and obesity. Endocrinol Metab Clin North Am 2008; 37(3): 713-31.
[107] Pérez-Pérez R, Ortega-Delgado FJ, García-Santos E, *et al.* Differential proteomics of omental and subcutaneous adipose tissue reflects their unalike biochemical and metabolic properties. J Proteome Res 2009; 8(4): 1682-93.

[108] Yang J, Xu G, Hong Q, *et al.* Discrimination of Type 2 diabetic patients from healthy controls by using metabonomics method based on their serum fatty acid profiles. J Chromatogr B Analyt Technol Biomed Life Sci 2004; 813(1-2): 53-8.
[109] Williams RE, Lenz EM, Evans JA, *et al.* A combined (1)H NMR and HPLC-MS-based metabonomic study of urine from obese(fa/fa) Zucker and normal Wistar-derived rats. J Pharm Biomed Anal 2005; 38(3): 465-71.
[110] Xu J, Chang V, Joseph SB, Trujillo *et al.* Peroxisomal proliferator-activated receptor alpha deficiency diminishes insulin-responsiveness of gluconeogenic/glycolytic/pentose gene expression and substrate cycle flux. Endocrinology 2004; 145(3): 1087-95.
[111] Xu J, Xiao G, Trujillo C, *et al.* Peroxisome proliferator-activated receptor alpha (PPARalpha) influences substrate utilization for hepatic glucose production. J Biol Chem 2002; 277(52): 50237-44.
[112] Watkins SM, Reifsnyder PR, Pan HJ, *et al.* Lipid metabolome-wide effects of the PPARgamma agonist rosiglitazone. J Lipid Res 2002; 43(11): 1809-17.
[113] Mehta TS, Zakharkin SO, Gadbury GL, *et al.* Epistemological issues in omics and high-dimensional biology: give the people what they want. Physiol Genomics 2006; 28(1): 24-32.
[114] Knapen D, Vergauwen L, Laukens K, *et al.* Best practices for hybridization design in two-colour microarray analysis. Trends Biotechnol 2009; 27(7): 406-14.
[115] Page GP, Edwards JW, Barnes S, *et al.* A design and statistical perspective on microarray gene expression studies in nutrition: the need for playful creativity and scientific hard-mindedness. Nutrition 2003; 19(11-12): 997-1000.
[116] Jafari P, Azuaje F. An assessment of recently published gene expression data analyses: reporting experimental design and statistical factors. BMC Med Inform Decis Mak 2006; 6: 27.
[117] Simon R. Diagnostic and prognostic prediction using gene expression profiles in high-dimensional microarray data. Br J Cancer 2003; 89: 1599-604.
[118] Efron B, Tibshirani R. Empirical bayes methods and false discovery rates for microarrays. Genet Epidemiol 2002; 23(1): 70-86.
[119] Efron B, Tibshirani R. Empirical bayes methods and false discovery rates for microarrays. Genet Epidemiol 2002; 23(1): 70-86.
[120] Belacel N, Wang Q, Cuperlovic-Culf M. Clustering methods for microarray gene expression data. OMICS 2006; 10(4): 507-31.
[121] Gana Dresen IM, Boes T, Huesing J, *et al.* New resampling method for evaluating stability of clusters. BMC Bioinformatics 2008; 9: 42.
[122] Garge NR, Page GP, Sprague AP, *et. al.* Reproducible clusters from microarray research: whither? BMC Bioinformatics 2005; 6 (Suppl 2): S10.
[123] Datta S, Datta S. Evaluation of clustering algorithms for gene expression data. BMC Bioinformatics 2006; 7 (Suppl 4): S17.
[124] Zhu Y, Wang Z, Miller DJ, *et al.* A ground truth based comparative study on clustering of gene expression data. Front Biosci 2008; 13: 3839-49.
[125] Plewczynski D, Spieser SA, Koch U. Performance of machine learning methods for ligand-based virtual screening. Comb Chem High Throughput Screen 2009; 12(4): 358-68.
[126] Schwaighofer A, Schroeter T, Mika S, *et al.* How wrong can we get? A review of machine learning approaches and error bars. Comb Chem High Throughput Screen 2009; 12(5): 453-68.
[127] Ancona N, Maglietta R, Piepoli A, *et al.* On the statistical assessment of classifiers using DNA microarray data. BMC Bioinformatics 2006; 7: 387.
[128] Judson R, Elloumi F, Setzer RW, *et al.* A comparison of machine learning algorithms for chemical toxicity classification using a simulated multi-scale data model. BMC Bioinformatics 2008; 9: 241.
[129] Statnikov A, Aliferis CF, Tsamardinos I, *et al.* A comprehensive evaluation of multicategory classification methods for microarray gene expression cancer diagnosis. Bioinformatics 2005; 21(5): 631-43.
[130] Wang Y, Tetko IV, Hall MA, *et al.* Gene selection from microarray data for cancer classification--a machine learning approach. Comput Biol Chem 2005; 29(1): 37-46.
[131] Inza I, Larrañaga P, Blanco R, *et al.* Filter versus wrapper gene selection approaches in DNA microarray domains. Artif Intell Med 31: 91-103.
[132] Vohradsky J. A parallel genetic algorithm for single class pattern classification and its application for gene expression profiling in Streptomyces coelicolor. BMC Genomics 2007; 8: 49.
[133] Griffith OL, Melck A, Jones SJ, Wiseman SM. Meta-analysis and meta-review of thyroid cancer gene expression profiling studies identifies important diagnostic biomarkers. J Clin Oncol 2006; 24(31): 5043-51.
[134] Cahan P, Rovegno F, Mooney D, *et al.* Meta-analysis of microarray results: challenges, opportunities, and recommendations for standardization. Gene 2007; 401(1-2): 12-8.
[135] Zhu J, Zhang B, Schadt EE. A systems biology approach to drug discovery. Adv Genet 2008; 60: 603-35.
[136] Li H, Xie Z, Lin J, *et al.* Transcriptomic and metabonomic profiling of obesity-prone and obesity-resistant rats under high fat diet. J Proteome Res 2008; 7(11): 4775-83.
[137] Mootha VK, Lindgren CM, Eriksson KF, *et al.* PGC-1alpha-responsive genes involved in oxidative phosphorylation are coordinately downregulated in human diabetes. Nat Genet 2003; 34(3): 267-73.
[138] Barabási AL, Oltvai ZN. Network biology: understanding the cell's functional organization. Nat Rev Genet 2004; 5(2): 101-13.
[139] Park J, Lee DS, Christakis NA, *et al.* The impact of cellular networks on disease comorbidity. Mol Syst Biol 2009; 5: 262.
[140] Ravasz E, Somera AL, Mongru DA, *et al.* Hierarchical organization of modularity in metabolic networks. Science 2002; 297(5586): 1551-5.
[141] Stuart JM, Segal E, Koller D, *et al.* A gene-coexpression network for global discovery of conserved genetic modules. Science 2003; 302(5643): 249-55.
[142] Mehrabian M, Allayee H, Stockton J, *et al.* Integrating genotypic and expression data in a segregating mouse population to identify 5-lipoxygenase as a susceptibility gene for obesity and bone traits. Nat Genet 2005; 37(11): 1224-33.
[143] Friedman N, Linial M, Nachman I, *et al.* Using Bayesian networks to analyze expression data. J Comput Biol 2000; 7(3-4): 601-20.
[144] Luscombe NM, Babu MM, Yu H, *et al.* Genomic analysis of regulatory network dynamics reveals large topological changes. Nature 2004; 431(7006): 308-12.

[145] Pinto S, Roseberry AG, Liu H, *et al.* Rapid rewiring of arcuate nucleus feeding circuits by leptin. Science 2004; 304(5667): 110-5.
[146] Wang Y, Zhang XS, Xia Y. Predicting eukaryotic transcriptional cooperativity by Bayesian network integration of genome-wide data. Nucleic Acids Res 2009.
[147] Smyth P, Heckerman D, Jordan MI. Probabilistic independence networks for hidden Markov probability models. Neural Comput 1997; 9(2): 227-69.
[148] Thomas R, Thieffry D, Kaufman M. Dynamical behaviour of biological regulatory networks--I. Biological role of feedback loops and practical use of the concept of the loop-characteristic state. Bull Math Biol 1995; 57(2): 247-76.
[149] Napoletani D, Sauer T, Struppa DC, *et al.* Augmented sparse reconstruction of protein signaling networks. J Theor Biol 2008; 255(1): 40-52.
[150] Bosl WJ. Systems biology by the rules: hybrid intelligent systems for pathway modeling and discovery. BMC Syst Biol 2007; 1: 13.
[151] Chiang JH, Chao SY. Modeling human cancer-related regulatory modules by GA-RNN hybrid algorithms. BMC Bioinformatics 2007; 8: 91.
[152] Hartemink AJ, Gifford DK, Jaakkola TS, *et al.* Combining location and expression data for principled discovery of genetic regulatory network models. Pac Symp Biocomput 2002; 437-49.
[153] Lin K, Husmeier D. Modelling transcriptional regulation with a mixture of factor analyzers and variational bayesian expectation maximization. EURASIP J Bioinform Syst Biol 2009; 601068.
[154] Yoo C, Thorsson V, Cooper GF. Discovery of causal relationships in a gene-regulation pathway from a mixture of experimental and observational DNA microarray data. Pac Symp Biocomput 2002; 498-509.
[155] Hofman JM, Wiggins CH. Bayesian approach to network modularity. Phys Rev Lett 2008; 100(25): 258701.
[156] Hartemink AJ, Gifford DK, Jaakkola TS, *et al.* Using graphical models and genomic expression data to statistically validate models of genetic regulatory networks. Pac Symp Biocomput 2001: 422-33.
[157] Nariai N, Kim S, Imoto S, *et al.* Using protein-protein interactions for refining gene networks estimated from microarray data by Bayesian networks. Pac Symp Biocomput 2004: 36-47.
[158] Segal E, Shapira M, Regev A, *et al.* Module networks: identifying regulatory modules and their condition-specific regulators from gene expression data. Nat Genet 2003; 34(2): 166-76.
[159] Luna IT, Huang Y, Yin Y, *et al.* Uncovering gene regulatory networks from time-series microarray data with variational bayesian structural expectation maximization. EURASIP J Bioinform Syst Biol 2007: 71312.
[160] Yang X, Deignan JL, Qi H, *et al.* Validation of candidate causal genes for obesity that affect shared metabolic pathways and networks. Nat Genet 2009; 41(4): 415-23.
[161] Zhu J, Wiener MC, Zhang C, *et al.* Increasing the power to detect causal associations by combining genotypic and expression data in segregating populations. PLoS Comput Biol 2007; 3(4): e69.
[162] Ridley M. Nature via nurture: genes, experience, and what makes us human. HarperCollins, USA 2003; p. 336.
[163] Galperin MY, Cochrane GR. Nucleic Acids Research annual Database Issue and the NAR online Molecular Biology Database Collection in 2009. Nucleic Acids Res 2009; 37: Database issue D1-D4.
[164] Taylor CF, Paton NW, Lilley KS, *et al.* The minimum information about a proteomics experiment (MIAPE). Nat Biotechnol 2007; 25(8): 887-93.
[165] Bellazzi R, Zupan B. Predictive data mining in clinical medicine: current issues and guidelines. Int J Med Inform 2008; 77(2): 81-97.
[166] Sieberts SK, Schadt EE. Moving toward a system genetics view of disease. Mamm Genome 2007; 18(6-7): 389-401.
[167] Schadt EE, Lamb J, Yang X, *et al.* An integrative genomics approach to infer causal associations between gene expression and disease. Nat Genet 2005; 37(7): 710-7.
[168] Schadt EE, Lum PY. Reverse engineering gene networks to identify key drivers of complex disease phenotypes. J Lipid Res 2006; 47(12): 2601-13.

The Search for New Anti-Obesity Agents to Reduce Cardiometabolic Risk

Cynthia Arbeeny*

Vice President Endocrine and Metabolic Diseases, Genzyme Corporation, 49 New York Ave., Framingham MA 01701-9322, USA

Abstract: The global epidemic of obesity is rapidly accelerating in both industrialized and developing countries, and has raised significant healthcare concerns worldwide. Obesity leads to numerous co-morbidities, including cardiovascular diseases (CVD), type 2 diabetes (T2D), hypertension, certain cancers, and sleep apnea. Obesity is considered an independent risk factor for CVD, and is associated with dyslipidemia, hypertension, glucose intolerance and inflammatory markers; all of which contribute to CV risk. The benefits of weight reduction to decrease cardiometabolic risk are well-documented, yet long term weight loss has been difficult to achieve. This has lead to intense efforts within the pharmaceutical industry to develop agents that result in weight loss and prevent weight regain. Numerous strategies have been directed toward decreasing food intake and/or increasing energy expenditure, yet this has met with limited success in developing a safe and effective drug. This review summarizes the underlying mechanisms contributing to CV risk in obesity, and discusses the targets that may result in novel pharmacological agents that can sustain weight loss and reduce cardio-vascular morbidity and mortality.

Keywords: Obesity, weight loss, adipose tissue, metabolic syndrome, cardiovascular disease.

INTRODUCTION

Obesity is a complex metabolic disease that reduces the quality of life and is associated with serious diseases and to greater mortality [1]. The rampant obesity epidemic continues to escalate worldwide and has raised serious healthcare concerns on a global level [2]. Obesity contributes to chronic and debilitating diseases, and increases the risk of T2D and CV morbidity and mortality [3, 4]. Once considered a problem of industrialized countries, obesity is now a problem in low- and middle- income countries, where the population generally has limited access to healthcare [5]. The excess accumulation of body fat results from an energy imbalance between calories consumed and calories expended, which is influenced by both genetic and environmental factors. The global increase in overweight and obesity is due to a shift in diet towards increased intake of energy-dense foods lacking macronutrients, and a trend towards decreased physical activity. Up to 80% of the global burden of T2D is attributed to excess body weight and is preventable by adopting a healthy diet and physical activity [6]. Overweight and obesity, as well as their related chronic diseases, are largely preventable by limiting energy intake and increasing energy expenditure. A modest weight loss of 5 to 10% has significant impact on preventing progression to T2D [7-9] and improving CV risk factors [10].

In adults, calculation of body mass index (BMI) is a simple measure to classify overweight and obesity, although this method has its limitations [11]. BMI is calculated from the patient's weight in kilograms divided by the square of the height in meters (kg/m^2). The World Health Organization (WHO) defines "overweight" as a BMI equal to or more than 25, and "obese" as a BMI equal to or more than 30. Obesity and overweight in children has been difficult to classify and a standard definition of childhood obesity has not been established. Currently, assessment of childhood obesity is based on growth charts.

In 2005, the WHO estimated that over 1.6 billion adults worldwide were overweight and 400 million adults were obese [2]. Furthermore, by 2015, projections indicate that approximately 2.3 billion adults will be overweight, and more than 700 million will be obese. In the United States, obesity prevalence doubled among adults between 1980 and 2004, and has now plateaued at levels where two-thirds of American adults are overweight and one-third are obese [11, 12]. The personal, social and economic consequences for

*Corresponding author: Tel: 508-271-3057, Cell: 508-685-7846; Fax: 508-661-8725; E-mail: cynthia.arbeeny@genzyme.com

Atta-ur-Rahman / M. Iqbal Choudhary (Eds.)

the obese are significant [13]. In the US, annual expenditures for obesity and obesity-related conditions, including heart disease and T2D, cost $62.7 billion in doctors' visits and $39.3 billion in lost workdays.

The prevalence of childhood obesity represents one of the most serious problems of the new millennium. In the US, childhood obesity has doubled over the past two decades. The most recent NHANES data (2003–2006) showed that for children and adolescents aged 6 – 11 years and 12–19 years, the prevalence of overweight was 17.0% and 17.6% respectively [12]. In 2007, an estimated 22 million children under the age of 5 years were overweight throughout the world [14]. The additional concerns for the rise in overweight and obesity in children and adolescents is that they are likely to remain obese as adults, and are more likely to develop non-communicable diseases such as diabetes and CVD at a younger age.

OBESITY AND CARDIOMETABOLIC RISK

Obesity Increases CV Risk Factors

Overweight and obesity are positively associated with diabetes and CVD, and leads to the increased risk of overall mortality and death from ischemic heart disease and stroke [3, 15-17]. CV risk versus BMI is shown in Fig. (**1**).

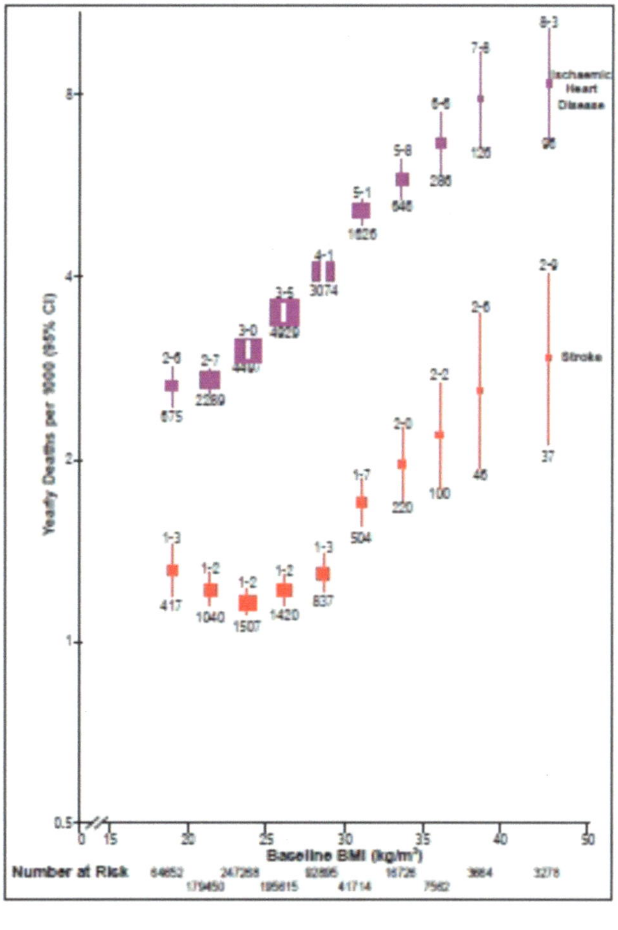

Fig. (1). Ischemic heart disease and stroke mortality *versus* BMI. Relative risks at ages 35-89 years, adjusted for age at risk, sex, smoking and study, were multiplied by a common factor (floated) to make the weighted average match the PSC mortality rate at ages 35-79. Floated mortality rates shown above each square and numbers of deaths below. Area of square is inversely proportional to the variance of the log risk. Boundaries of BMI groups are indicated by tick marks. 95% CIs for floated rates reflect uncertainty in the log risk for each single rate. *Reproduced from [17] with permission from Elsevier.*

For the US population, cardiovascular risk factors versus BMI have been tracked and reported by National Health Examination Survey (1960-1962); National Health and Nutrition Examination Survey (NHANES) I (1971-1975), II (1976-1980), and III (1988-1994); and NHANES 1999-2000. Of interest is the decline in the prevalence of high cholesterol and high blood pressure in all BMI groups over the past 30-40 years, which is related to the use of lipid-lowering and anti-hypertensive drugs, and to the decline in smoking [16]. Shown in Fig. (**2**) is the prevalence of CV risk factors (diagnosed and total diabetes, hypertension and high cholesterol) for the US population versus BMI category, based on NHANES 1999-2000.

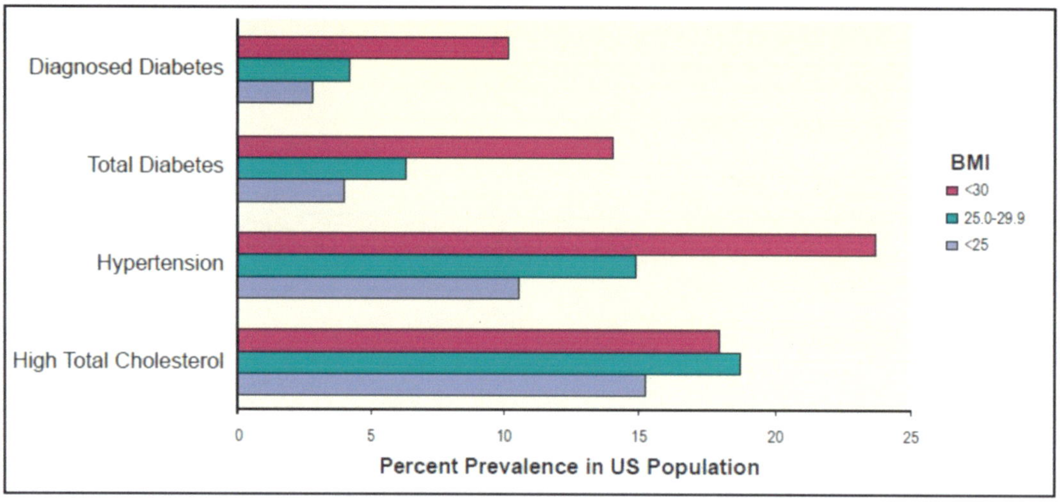

Fig. (2). Prevalence of diagnoses and total diabetes, hypertension and high cholesterol in the US population aged 20-74 years, *versus* BMI categories for lean (<25), overweight (25.0-29.9) and obese (≥30). *Data is from NHANES (1999-2000)[16].*

The recent NHANES data indicate that there have been greater absolute reductions in the prevalence of high total cholesterol in overweight and obese subjects versus lean subjects, when compared to recent surveys. This is largely due to the greater use of lipid-lowering agents in this group, resulting in the narrowing the difference between lean versus obese by only 2.7 percentage points. However, the prevalence of hypertension in obese individuals was at least twice that of the lean population. In contrast to the decline in prevalence of high cholesterol and high blood pressure over the past four decades, the prevalence of diagnosed diabetes has doubled over this period, and the prevalence of total diabetes (diagnosed and undiagnosed) increased by 55% between 1976-2000. Increasing BMI was positively correlated with increase in diabetes prevalence. Since diabetes is a known risk factor for CVD [18, 19], the increase in diabetes among obese patients may be the key driver of CV risk in this patient population. Of particular concern is an abdominal distribution of body fat, which is highly correlated with insulin resistance, dyslipidemia, inflammation and CVD [20, 21]. A reduction in abdominal fat decreases insulin resistance, reduces inflammation, improves the atherogenic lipid profile, and decreases blood pressure; thereby decreasing CV risk [22, 23].

"Metabolic Syndrome" *versus* "Cardiometabolic Risk"

Obesity, hypertension and dyslipidemia are considered separate diseases, but often cluster within patients. This has lead to the concept of "The Metabolic Syndrome", in order to identify patients who are at an increased risk of CVD and T2D. Numerous organizations have developed definitions of the Metabolic Syndrome. The most widely utilized are from The WHO, The American Heart Association (AHA)/National Cholesterol Education Program-Adult Treatment Panel (NCEP-ATP) and The International Diabetes Federation (IDF), which are compared in [24]. Each definition includes traditional risk factors: obesity and an abdominal fat distribution, insulin resistance, diabetes, dyslipidemia (high TG, low HDL) and hypertension, but differ in the importance of each risk factor to overall CV risk. The organizations are currently working toward harmonizing criteria [25]. Currently there are a plethora of drugs, which are often used in combination, to reduce risk factors for diabetes and CVD [26]. However, the management of multiple risk factors remains challenging, and some drugs improve one risk factor and exacerbate another.

LIMITATIONS OF THE METABOLIC SYNDROME

There are several limitations and concerns with utilizing The Metabolic Syndrome as a simple diagnostic tool. The Metabolic Syndrome does not predict CVD as well as the Framingham Risk Score [27] and is a stronger predictor of the development of T2D rather than CVD. The clinical significance of the metabolic syndrome came into question by The American Diabetes Association (ADA) and the European Association for the Study of Diabetes (EASD). They questioned the clinical value of diagnosing the metabolic syndrome, since treatment of the syndrome is no different than the treatment for each of its components [28]. The multiple organizations and agencies are working toward understanding the relationships of the multiple risk factors for CVD [29], but recognize abdominal obesity as a key risk factor for CVD.

COMMON PATHOPHYSIOLOGY LINKING OBESITY, DIABETES AND CVD

Obesity, diabetes and CVD share common pathophysiologcal mechanisms and are considered as low grade, chronic inflammatory diseases [30-32]. Their common features include: the activation of innate and adaptive immunity, cellular lipid accumulation and. lipotoxicity, inflammatory cell infiltration and cytokine production, oxidative stress, altered cellular signaling and cell dysfunction, and ultimately cell death.

ADIPOSE TISSUE INFLAMMATION

The adipose tissue is not only the normal depot for fat storage, but is a critical endocrine organ that regulates the synthesis and secretion of adipokines (such as leptin, adiponectin) that are involved in nutrient homeostasis, growth, energy expenditure, bone mass, reproductive function, and the immune response [33, 34]. In obesity, the accumulation of excess lipid within adipocytes leads to a pro-inflammatory state [31, 32, 34, 35], with increased secretion of pro-inflammatory factors (including TNF-α, IL-6, MCP-1 and PAI-1), and reduced secretion of anti-inflammatory factors (including adiponectin). The secretion of large amounts of MCP-1 [36], leads to the infiltration of macrophages into adipose tissue [37, 38] which further exacerbates the inflammatory response in adipose tissue. Key adipokines and regulatory factors that are dysregulated in obesity are shown in Table **1**.

Table 1. Alterations in Adipokines, Cytokines and Inflammatory Proteins in Obesity and the Metabolic Consequences

Regulatory Factor	Metabolic Consequence
Leptin	∞ Leptin is secreted by adipocytes and circulating levels parallel adipose mass. Leptin decreases appetite by action on the hypothalamus, and stimulates energy expenditure by central and peripheral actions [39]. Peripheral target tissues include adipose tissue, pancreas, liver, and immune system. Leptin stimulates lipolysis and fatty acid oxidation, reduces lipogenesis, and improves insulin sensitivity. ∞ Obesity leads to increased leptin secretion by adipocytes but also results in leptin resistance in the CNS and in the periphery, which impairs its regulation of food intake and metabolism [40].
Adiponectin	∞ Adiponectin is secreted by adipocytes and improves insulin sensitivity [41]. It acts *via* AMPK signaling [42], to stimulate fatty acid oxidation and glucose utilization in skeletal muscle, and to increase fatty acid oxidation and to decrease glucose output in liver. Adiponectin acts on the hypothalamus leading to increased energy expenditure. Anti-inflammatory and anti-atherosclerotic effects in the vasculature [43]. ∞ Levels are decreased in obesity and result in insulin resistance and loss of adiponectin's protective effect on peripheral tissues.
Resistin	∞ Resistin is expressed by adipocytes in rodents and by macrophages in humans. Resistin promotes insulin resistance in rodents [44], but its role in humans is unclear. ∞ In rodents, resistin is increased by obesity. In humans, resistin is correlated with other markers of inflammation [45], and is associated with endothelial cell activation [46].
TNF-α	∞ TNF-α is a cytokine that is secreted by immune cells and adipocytes. ∞ TNF-α is increased in obesity and induces insulin resistance [47, 48]. It has pro-atherosclerotic effects in the vasculature, and enhances monocyte recruitment and accumulation of LDL into atherosclerotic lesions [49].
IL-6	∞ IL-6 is secreted by adipocytes and is linked to inflammation [50] . ∞ It increased in obesity and is associated with a decrease in insulin and leptin signaling and insulin resistance.
MCP-1	∞ MCP-1 is a chemo-attractant that recruits immune cells to sites of inflammation. ∞ In obesity, MCP-1 is secreted by hypertrophied adipocytes and enhances macrophage infiltration into adipose tissue [37]. MCP-1 expression in adipocytes leads to systemic insulin resistance [36] .
PAI-1	∞ PAI-1 inhibits plasminogen activator and α-thrombin, and is the primary inhibitor of fiibrinolysis. ∞ PAI-1 is increased in obesity and is linked to insulin resistance [51], and has prothrombotic and pro-atherosclerotic effects [52].

Chronic inflammation in adipose tissue activates several serine/threonine kinases, including inhibitor of kappa B kinase (IKK) [53] and c-jun N-terminal kinase (JNK) [54]. The activation of nuclear factor kappa-B (NFκB) (by inhibition of IKK) and JNK signaling pathways results in adipose tissue dysfunction by impairing insulin receptor signaling and insulin-stimulated glucose uptake, decreasing triglyceride (TG) deposition and enhancing lipolysis. The increased free fatty acid flux from adipose tissue contributes to the deposition of fat in non-adipose tissues (referred to as "ectopic fat"). This has serious adverse metabolic consequences [35, 40, 55-57], which are described in more detail below. Thus, dysfunctional adipose tissue is the trigger for damage to the pancreatic β-cell, liver, muscle and vasculature, and is the link between obesity, diabetes and CVD [58-61]. The contribution of adipose tissue inflammation to insulin resistance and atherosclerosis is shown in Fig. (**3**).

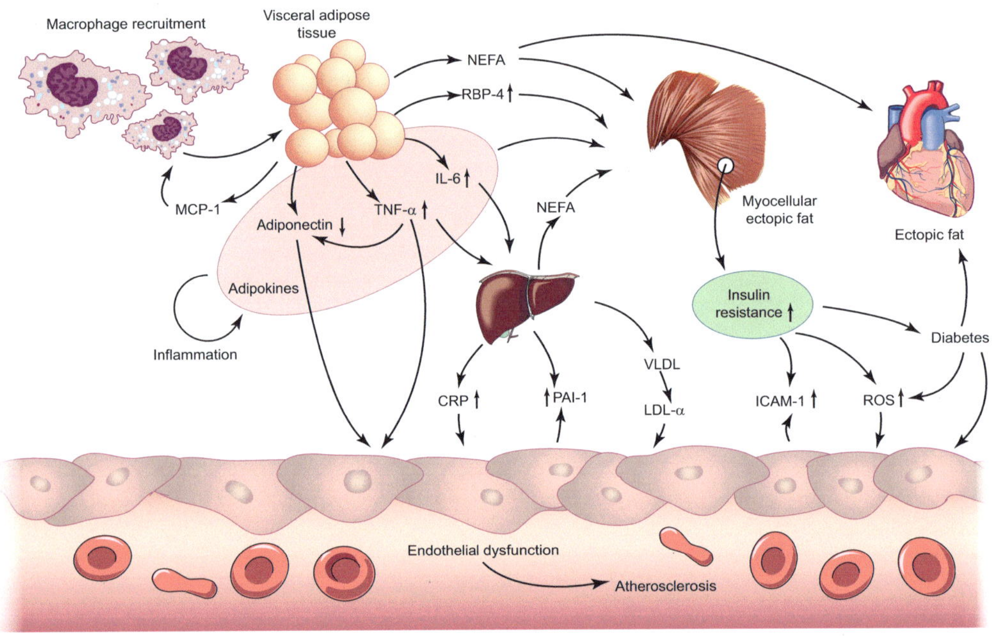

Fig. (3). The relationship between adipose tissue inflammation, insulin resistance and atherosclerosis. Obesity leads to adipose tissue inflammation and macrophage recruitment (mediated by MCP-1), which further exacerbating the inflammatory process. The release of non-esterified/free fatty acids (NEFA) and pro-inflammatory adipokines (including IL-6, TNFα) and reduction of anti-inflammatory cytokines (adiponectin) from "inflamed" adipose tissue results in ectopic fat, impaired skeletal muscle and liver function, insulin resistance, dyslipidemia and the production of atherogenic lipoproteins (including oxidized LDL), a procoagulant state (mediated by PAI-1) and further inflammation. This whole-body metabolic imbalance contributes to diabetes, endothelial dysfunction and atherosclerosis. *Reproduced from [60] with permission from Nature Publishing Group.*

ABNORMAL METABOLISM IN SKELETAL MUSCLE AND LIVER

The inflammatory mileau and increased flux of fatty acids from dysfunctional adipose tissue and intracellular accumulation of lipid metabolites (such as long chain fatty acyl CoA, diacylglycerol, and ceramide), contribute to impaired insulin action in skeletal muscle and liver [53, 54, 62, 63]. In these tissues, inflammatory cytokines, adipokines and lipid mediators activate a number of serine/threonine kinases, including protein kinase C (PKC) isoforms [64] in addition to IKK [53, 64] and JNK [54]. In skeletal muscle, insulin resistance leads to impaired insulin-stimulated glucose transport and decreased glycogen synthesis, resulting in impaired glucose uptake and utilization [57, 65]. In the liver, glycogen synthesis is decreased and gluconeogenesis is stimulated, leading to increased hepatic glucose output and hyperglycemia.

The altered metabolic mileau in obesity also drives hepatic lipid synthesis and secretion of TG-rich VLDL [55, 66]. This often leads to hypertriglyceridemia, small, dense and modified LDL, Lp(a) and low HDL; all of which exacerbate the risk for CVD [67, 68]. In response to pro-inflammatory state, the liver also secretes high sensitivity C-reactive protein (hsCRP) which is a validated biomarker for inflammation. hsCRP is correlated with BMI [69] and is an independent predictor of CV events [70].

β-CELL COMPENSATION VERSUS FAILURE

Although obesity and T2D are characterized by insulin resistance, and obesity is a key risk factor for T2D, not all obese patients become insulin resistant [35] and not all obese/insulin resistant patients develop diabetes [71, 72] which is defined as a fasting plasma glucose above 126 mg/dL. Genetic factors appear to play a key role in determining the patient's susceptibility to insulin-resistance and progression to T2D. In obese patients who become insulin-resistant but who do not have a genetic predisposition to develop T2D, the metabolic mileau (principally increased circulating FFAs) leads to β-cell hypertrophy and increased insulin secretion. The elevated insulin levels compensate for the insulin resistance, and therefore blood glucose remains in the normal range. In obese patients who are genetically predisposed to develop T2D, insufficient compensation occurs which leads to relative insulin deficiency, glucose intolerance and eventually T2D. Hyperglycemia results in "glucotoxicity" [73] which further impairs β-cell function and contributes to apoptosis. Adipose-derived factors, including FFAs (resulting in "lipotoxicity"), elevated pro-inflammatory adipokines (IL-6, TNF-α leptin, and resistin), and reduced adiponectin levels are also detrimental to β-cells [72, 73].

VASCULATURE ALTERATIONS

Obesity results in stimulation of the renin-angiotensin-aldosterone-system (RAAS) and sympathetic nervous system (SNS), which drive endothelial dysfunction, hypertension and vascular damage [74-76]. "Inflamed" adipose tissue secretes vasoactive factors (including free fatty acids, angiotensinogen and prostaglandins) which strongly activate RAAS. Furthermore, obesity leads to hyperleptinemia and leptin-resistance, which stimulates the central nervous system and increases SNS activity. Activation of RAAS and SNS and physical compression of the kidney in obesity contribute to renal impairment, sodium reabsorption and hypertension.

Nutrient excess and inflammation also generate reactive oxygen species (ROS), which results in protein modifications and cellular dysfunction [77]. Generation of ROS is particularly damaging to the vasculature, since it depletes nitric oxide (NO), which maintains vascular tone [78]. Obesity and insulin resistance result in defective insulin signaling in the endothelial cell leading to an imbalance between the vasodilating agent NO and the vasoconstricting agent endothelin-1 (ET-1), resulting in additional endothelial dysfunction and hypertension.

Dysfunctional endothelium is susceptible to damage by inflammatory cytokines, activated platelets, adhesion molecules, and lipids; all of which contribute to the atherosclerotic process [79-81]. Obesity also leads to the secretion of PAI-1 and fibrinogen, which is associated with a pro-coagulant and pro-thrombotic state, which exacerbates endothelial damage and increases CV risk [82]. When obese patients progress to overt diabetes, the hyperglycemic environment results in further damage to the vasculature. This involves the production of nonenzymatic glycosylation of proteins and lipids, forming advanced glycation endproducts (AGEs) which can interfere with normal cellular function. AGEs also induce oxidative and nitrosative stress which further drive the inflammatory response [83-85]. These abnormalities lead to platelet activation, which could result in arterial thrombosis, and consequently myocardial infarction and stroke [86].

MARKETED TREATMENTS THAT CAUSE WEIGHT LOSS

Although modest weight loss of 5-10 kg reduces diabetes and CV risk [7-10], most obese patients require substantial weight loss, which has been difficult to achieve and to sustain by non-surgical methods. Diet and exercise lead to an average weight loss of less than 5 kg after 2 years [87, 88]. Currently available oral anti-obesity agents, when used in conjunction with limiting caloric intake are associated with 5-10% weight loss in 1-2 years [23, 88-90]. There are few pharmacological agents on the market that are approved for weight loss, which is attributed to the hurdles in developing weight loss drugs. Large placebo-controlled trials, which are lengthy and expensive, are required. Some drugs fail due to issues of long-term safety in obese patients, many of whom have a number of other health conditions. Difficulties are also encountered in demonstrating efficacy, since the placebo group (which is given a low caloric diet) also shows weight loss, the treatment group shows a variable response, and there are a significant number of non-responders.

Approved weight loss treatments (sibutramine, orlistat, rimonabant) also improve metabolic risk factors [23, 89-91] but each drug is associated with side effects which limit usage. In addition, antidiabetic agents (metformin, exenatide and pramlintide) are also associated with weight reduction and improvement in cardiometabolic risk [92-96] Bariatric surgery is also another option to treat obesity, and can result in significant weight loss and improvement in metabolic risk factors [97, 98]. However, this is not an option for most obese patients because of the health risks and costs associated with this procedure.

The characteristics of approved weight-loss drugs and anti-diabetic agents that induce weight loss are presented below.

SIBUTRAMINE

Sibutramine inhibits the reuptake of norepinepherine, serotonin and dopamine; leading to appetite suppression and increased energy expenditure [89, 91]. Sibutramine causes weight loss, improves lipid profile and increases insulin sensitivity. Controlled clinical trials showed that at 2 years of treatment, 67% of sibutramine-treated patients and 49% of placebo-treated patients lost ≥5% of their body weight. Drug usage may increase blood pressure and heart rate, which limits usage in obese patients with hypertension or heart problems.

ORLISTAT

Ingested fat is mostly TG and requires lipolysis by pancreatic lipase, an enzyme that is present in the GI tract, in order to be absorbed by the body. By inhibiting this enzyme, fat cannot be absorbed and is excreted in the feces, leading to a decrease in caloric intake. Orlistat is the "first-in-class" pancreatic lipase inhibitor that results in weight loss and improves lipid profile and insulin sensitivity [90, 91]. The results from clinical trials showed that at 1 year of treatment, 57% of the orlistat-treated patients and 31% of the placebo-treated patients lost ≥5% of their body weight; weight loss was maintained at 2 years of treatment. Side effects include oily spotting, abdominal pain and fecal urgency. Recently, the Food and Drug Administration (FDA) announced that it is reviewing new safety information regarding reports of liver-related adverse events in patients taking orlistat [99]. Another novel pancreatic lipase inhibitor is in clinical development.

RIMONABANT

Rimonabant is an inverse agonist for the cannabinoid receptor 1 (CB1) that reduces appetite and improves metabolism [23, 91]. Rimonabant causes weight loss, improves lipid profile, blood pressure and insulin sensitivity. At 1 year of treatment, 75% of rimonabant-treated patients and 28% of placebo-treated patients lost ≥5% of their body weight. The drug may cause nausea, dizziness, and severe depression. It is not approved for use in the US. Recently, the European Medicine Agency's Committee for Medical Products for Human Use (CHMP) authorized suspension of rimonabant across the European Union, since review of the safety data indicated that risks of treatment outweigh the clinical benefits [100]. Additional CB1 receptor agonists are in development, but they might also be associated with risks and therefore may not be approvable.

METFORMIN

Metformin decreases hepatic glucose output, but also regulates other pathways that improve glycemic control [93, 101]. The drug is considered safe and effective, and recommended as the first line drug therapy for treating T2D [102]. GI tract problems are the most common side effects, and usage can lead to lactic acidosis, but this is rare. Metformin has additional metabolic benefits in that it results in weight loss and an improvement in lipid profile [92]. Treatment of hyperinsulinemic obese children and adolescents with metformin reduces BMI and insulin resistance [103].

EXENATIDE

Exenatide is a glucagon-like peptide 1 (GLP-1) analog and is a new class of incretin-based antidiabetic therapies [94]. The mechanism of action of GLP-1 is described in more detail in the next section. Exenatide is a long acting GLP-1 analog which improves glycemic control, decreases triglyceride and increases HDL, and causes weight loss [95]. It is an injectable protein which limits usage and may be associated with GI problems. The development of novel GLP-1 agonists is an active area within the biotech and pharmaceutical industry.

PRAMLINTIDE

Pramlintide is a synthetic analog of the hormone amylin, and is approved for use as an anti-diabetic agent in T1D and in T2D patients who require insulin [96]. Pramlintide delays gastric emptying lowers postprandial glucose levels and decreases postprandial glucagon secretion. Usage is often accompanied by weight loss and favorable effects on blood lipids but usage is associated with GI problems. Additional amylin analogs are in clinical development.

COMBINATION THERAPIES

The failure of anti-obesity drugs to achieve significant and sustained weight loss is due, in part, to compensatory mechanisms, which may overcome a drug's effect. Use of combination therapies could achieve greater efficacy by additive or synergistic effects. Combination therapies currently in development for weight loss include naltrexone and bupropion, zonisamide and bupropion, topiramate and phentermine (reviewed in [104]). However, long term efficacy and safety remain key factors.

FUTURE TREATMENT STRATEGIES

Considerable progress has been made to understand the complex signaling pathways between the GI tract, peripheral tissues (adipose, pancreas, liver and muscle) and the CNS which regulate energy homeostasis [105]. Signaling between the peripheral tissues and brain is shown in Fig. (**4**).

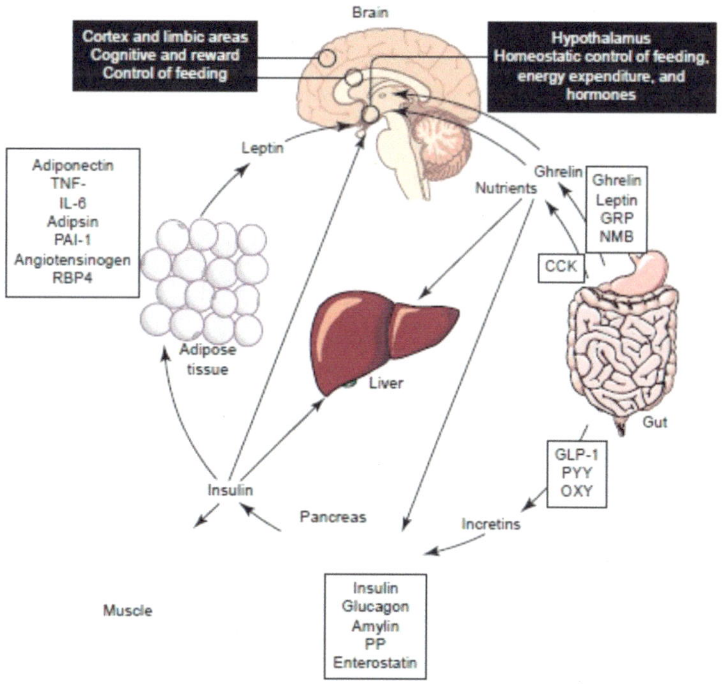

Fig. (4). Integration of metabolic signals in the control of energy balance. Peptides and nutrients provide signals to the CNS and peripheral tissues to regulate food intake, energy expenditure and energy storage. *Reproduced from [105], with permission from The American Society for Clinical Investigation.*

In the fasting state, the initiation of feeding involves secretion of ghrelin from the gut, which signals in the hypothalamus resulting in the initiation of feeding. The cortex and limbic areas of the brain also provide cognitive and reward control of feeding behavior. Ingestion of food triggers the secretion of gut peptides, which act in concert with ingested nutrients (glucose and fatty acids) to regulate signaling in the hypothalamus to halt feeding, and also signal the peripheral tissues to facilitate nutrient metabolism [106-108]. The key metabolic regulators which are targets for development of effective weight loss therapies have been recently reviewed [109, 110], and are described below. A more comprehensive list of development candidates is shown in the Appendix Table **2**.

STIMULATING FAT LOSS

In addition to inhibiting pancreatic lipase to prevent fat absorption, another strategy is to inhibit intestinal microsomal triglyceride transfer protein (MTP), another enzyme that plays a key role in lipid absorption. After a meal, dietary TG is cleaved by pancreatic lipase the intestinal lumen into fatty acids and monoglycerides for absorption. The products of lipolysis enter the intestinal mucosal cells and are then reformed into intracellular TG. Intracellular lipids (TG, cholesterol and phospholipid) are then incorporated into chylomicrons and secreted into the bloodstream. Most of the absorbed lipid of dietary origin enters the bloodstream as chylomicrons, since it is an efficient means by which lipids can be effectively "packaged" for transport in an aqueous environment. The assembly of triglyceride-rich lipoproteins, i.e., chylomicrons by the intestine and VLDL by the liver requires microsomal triglyceride transfer protein (MTP) [111]. In T2D patients, intestinal MTP is elevated and is positively associated with increased post-prandial lipid [112]. Inhibiting this enzyme prevents chylomicron formation and consequently the absorption of lipid into the bloodstream. The lipid remains within the intestinal cells which rapidly turn-over and are sloughed-off into the feces. An intestinally active (non-absorbable) MPT inhibitor is in clinical development for lipid lowering and anti-obesity indications [113].

TARGETING THE GUT-BRAIN AXIS

Control of energy homeostasis involves signaling between the GI tract, brain and peripheral tissues [106-108]. An understanding of this signaling network has provided targets for therapeutic intervention.

After a meal, the GI tract secretes a number of signaling peptides, including cholecystokinin (CCK) glucagon-like peptide (GLP-1) and peptide-tyrosine-tyrosine (PYY). These signals act locally in the GI tract and are conveyed to the brain *via* the vagus nerve to produce a satiety signal, thereby decreasing food intake. CCK receptor agonism was initially a promising approach for a weight loss treatment, since orally active small molecule receptor agonists could be identified. However, these compounds failed in clinical trials because of side-effects. Mimicking GLP-1 and PYY action is being pursued by the pharmaceutical industry to induce weight loss and to improve additional metabolic parameters. In addition, ghrelin antagonists have emerged as a promising new anti-obesity treatment.

GLP-1 acts locally, peripherally and centrally to regulate insulin sensitivity and body weight [94]. GLP-1 is a cleavage product of proglucagon [114], and is synthesized by intestinal L-cells which are most prevalent in the ileum and colon. GLP-1(7-36) amide is the active secreted form, which is rapidly inactivated by the ubiquitous enzyme, serine protease dipeptidyl peptidase (DPPT-IV). Since GLP-1 is secreted from the distal intestine shortly after a meal, this suggests that signaling from the proximal small intestine is involved. GLP-1 acts locally as the "ileal brake" to slow the GI tract motility and centrally to reduce food intake. GLP-1 regulates glucose metabolism by stimulating insulin secretion and inhibiting glucagon secretion by the pancreas. GLP-1 also passes the blood brain barrier and has central effects to inhibit food intake. GLP-1 levels are reduced in obese patients and are increased with weight loss [115]. Thus, GLP-1 represents a good therapy for diabetes and obesity. However, the naturally occurring peptide has a short half-life of 1-2 minutes, so long-acting formations are required to achieve clinical efficacy. Exenatide is the "first in class" GLP-1 mimetic to be marketed; and is effective in diabetes control, weight loss and shows improvement in cardiovascular risk factors [116]. Another long acting GLP-1 analog has been shown to block the induction of TNFα, the glucose-mediated induction of PAI-1, and vascular adhesion molecule expression in cultured human endothelial cells [117], which could reduce vascular damage in obese, insulin resistant patients. Limitations to current GLP-1 analog approaches are that the current and future therapies are peptides that require parenteral administration. The search for small molecule agonists for the GLP-1 receptor has not been successful, and more research is needed to understand GLP-1 receptor(s) pharmacology.

PYY is a member of a super-family of peptides that include pancreatic polypeptide (PP) and neuropeptide-Y (NPY). PYY shares a number of characteristics with GLP-1 [106]. PYY is secreted as PYY(1-36) and is metabolized by DPP-IV, resulting in the active form, PYY3-36. It is synthesized and secreted by L cells in the distal ileum and colon after a meal, and acts locally within the GI tract as an "ileal brake". PYY also acts centrally to reduce food intake. The PYY, PP and NPY super-family act on the Y family of G-protein coupled receptors (Y1, Y2, Y4 and Y5) that are expressed in the hypothalamus [118]. The integration of signaling of gut peptides and neurotransmitters in the brain is described below and is reviewed in more detail elsewhere [106, 107]. NPY is believed to act *via* Y1 and Y5 to stimulate appetite ("orexigenic effect"). PYY 3-36 acts on Y2 to inhibit appetite ("anorectic effect") [119], while PP acts on Y4 receptor resulting in an anorectic effect. Since PYY exerts an anoretic effect, PYY mimetics are an active area in the development of anti-obesity drugs.

Ingestion of a meal also triggers peripheral signals, resulting in secretion of leptin by adipocytes and insulin by pancreatic β-cells [107, 120]. Secretion of these hormones is directly related to the amount of body fat. These hormones are secreted into the blood and act on peripheral tissue metabolism, and also pass the blood brain barrier and act on hypothalamic neurons to regulate energy balance. An understanding of hypothalamic signaling in body energy balance has identified novel targets for treating obesity and its co-morbidities.

In the hypothalamus, leptin stimulates pro-opiomelanocortin (POMPC) and cocaine and amphetamine-regulated transcript (CART) neurons and inhibits NPY/agouti-related peptide (AgRP) neurons (reviewed in [107, 108]). Stimulation of POMPC/CART neurons in the arcuate nucleus stimulates secretion of αMSH, which activates melanocortin receptor 3 and 4 (MC3/4) receptors. This leads to a decrease in appetite, an increase in thermogenesis and increased peripheral metabolism. NPY/AgRP opposes POMP/CART signaling and promotes food intake and weight gain. Leptin inhibits NPY/AgRP neurons with consequent inhibition of the activation of NPY1 and 5 receptors. Inhibition of NPY/AgRP also blocks the inhibitory effect of NPY/AgRP on MC3/4R. Obesity is associated with insulin and leptin resistance both in the CNS and periphery. An approach has been to target the CNS directly with small molecules. Since NPY/AgRP increases appetite and decreases energy expenditure, NPY1 and NPY5 antagonists are in development as anti-obesity agents. In addition, stimulation of MC3/4R has also been an approach for weight loss. A problem with targeting specific neuropeptide signaling as an anti-obesity approach is that there are redundancies in the control of feeding behavior and other areas of the brain are involved [108].

Ghrelin is the only known circulating peptide that increases food intake [121]. It is a 28-amino acid peptide that is cleaved from preproghrelin. This peptide undergoes posttranslational modification by covalent attachment of medium chain fatty acids, which is required for activity [122]. Ghrelin is secreted principally by the X/A endocrine cells of the stomach, but is also secreted by other areas of the GI tract and the periphery. The acylated peptide is an endogenous ligand for the growth hormone secretagogue receptor (GHS-R1a) which is widely expressed throughout the body. In the brain, GHS-R1a is found in areas that regulate appetite and energy balance, including the hypothalamus, dorsal vagal complex and mesolimbic system. Ghrelin's orexigenic effect is believed to be growth hormone independent, and is mediated by stimulation of NPY and AgRP [123]. GHS-R1a receptors are also found in the pituitary, myocardium, stomach, pancreas, adipose tissue, liver, placenta, and T-cells; contributing to the diverse functions of ghrelin on glucose homeostasis, gut motility, cardiovascular function, immunity and inflammation [124]. However, the principal role of ghrelin is believed to be in the regulation of preprandial hunger. Ghrelin antagonists are under development as weight loss agents.

TARGETING FATTY ACID METABOLISM

Fatty acid synthesis and oxidation are regulated by a complex signaling system to meet the needs of the body. During nutrient excess, fat is stored in adipose tissue, which can be rapidly mobilized and oxidized during physical activity or during starvation. Adenosine 5'-monophosphate-activated protein kinase (AMPK) is the master switch in fat metabolism [125, 126]. It integrates signals between the periphery and hypothalamus, and mediates the signaling of leptin and adiponectin, leading to regulation of food intake, energy expenditure, and insulin sensitivity. AMPK is phosphorylated by several upstream kinases, including the tumor suppressor, LKB1, leading to activation [127]. Exercise and the marketed anti-diabetic drug metformin stimulate AMPK activity [101]. AMPK is present in all tissues, but it plays a critical role in nutrient metabolism in the liver, adipose tissue, pancreatic β-cells and skeletal muscle. In liver, AMPK activation stimulates hepatic fatty acid oxidation and ketogenesis and inhibits cholesterol synthesis, lipogenesis, and triglyceride synthesis. In adipocytes, AMPK activation inhibits lipolysis and lipogenesis.

AMP kinase activation also modulates insulin secretion by pancreatic β-cells and stimulates fatty acid oxidation and glucose uptake in skeletal muscle. A model for the stimulatory effect of AMPK on fatty acid oxidation in skeletal muscle is shown in Fig. (**5**).

Exercise, adipokines (leptin, adiponectin) and hypothalamic-sympathetic nervous system stimulation lead to the phosphorylation and activation of AMK, which phosphorylates and inhibits acetyl CoA carboxylase (ACC), the rate limiting step in fatty acid synthesis. Inhibition of ACC decreases malonyl CoA levels, leading to stimulation of carnitine palmitoyl transferase (CPT-1) and transport of fatty acids into the mitochondria for oxidation. In times of caloric abundance, excess fatty acid and carbohydrate stimulate ACC, resulting in an increase in malonyl CoA and fatty acid synthesis, and a decrease in fat oxidation. In obese patients, the excess caloric intake and a sedentary lifestyle leads to defective AMPK action, excessive accumulation of fat in adipose tissue, inflammatory adipokines and cytokines, ectopic fat and consequently insulin resistance and impaired β-cell function.

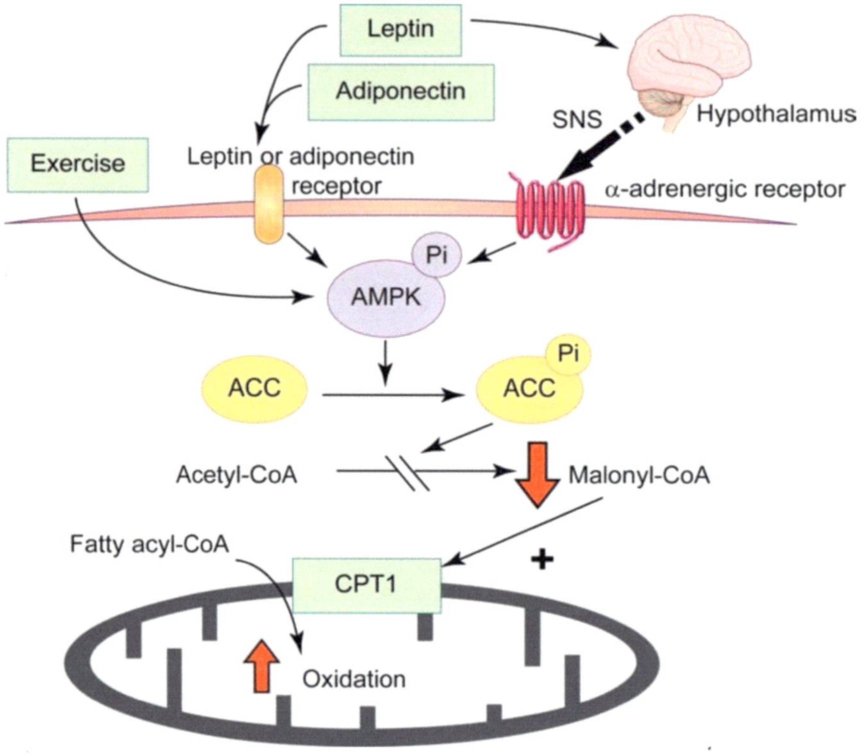

Fig. (5). AMPK intergrates metabolic signaling in skeletal muscle. Exercise, leptin, and adiponectin convey signals that stimulate AMPK activation, leading to increased fatty acid oxidation and decrease lipogenesis. *Reproduced from [126] with permission from Elsevier*.

Pharmacological activation of AMPK may be an effective treatment for treating obese patients in order to restore metabolic homeostasis, improve insulin sensitivity and decrease body weight. Other strategies which might induce weight loss are focused on inhibiting enzymes involved in lipogenesis, including ACC and stearoyl CoA desaturase (SCD).

ACC is a biotin-dependent enzyme that catalyzes the irreversible carboxylation of acetyl-CoA to produce malonyl-CoA. Malonyl CoA is the substrate for the biosynthesis of fatty acids, and also prevents fatty acid oxidation by inhibiting CPT-1. In humans there are two ACC isoforms with different tissue distributions. ACC1 is found lipogenic tissues such as adipose tissue, and ACC2 is found in oxidative tissues such as skeletal muscle and heart. The liver expresses both isoforms. A dual acting inhibitor of both isoforms has been shown to inhibit fatty acid synthesis and promote weight loss in animals [128], but currently no ACC inhibitors are in pharmaceutical development. SCD is the rate-limiting enzyme in monounsaturated fatty acid synthesis, and recent data from animals studies indicate that it is another key regulatory point in lipid metabolism [129]. Stimulation of SCD-1 leads to hepatic lipogenesis and decreased lipid oxidation. SCD-1 knockout mice have increased fatty acid oxidation and increased energy expenditure, decreased lipid synthesis and reduced body adiposity, and increased insulin sensitivity [130].

These mice are also resistant to diet-induced obesity and liver steatosis, indicating that pharmacological inhibition of this enzyme would result in weight loss and improvement in metabolic risk factors. Small molecule SCD-1 inhibitors are in early stage development.

CLOSING REMARKS

An understanding of the processes, which regulate food intake, energy expenditure and energy storage has provided novel targets for body weight regulation. A focus for new anti-obesity approaches has been to target the gut-brain axis to regulate feeding behavior and energy expenditure and to modulate peripheral metabolism. Since obesity is strongly linked to T2D and CVD, effective weight loss therapies should also be effective in treating these co-morbidities. However, it has been difficult to target feeding behavior, since there are considerable redundancies in the regulation of food intake, and behavioral factors may over-ride metabolic signals. The development of new compounds that target peripheral metabolism has been hampered by the lack of predictive animal models, and in some cases, risk benefit concerns.

The pharmaceutical industry also faces challenges in developing safe and effective weight loss therapies. The clinical development for new weight-loss treatments is a significant hurdle, and weight-regain following weight-loss is still another hurdle that needs to be overcome for long-term weight reduction. However, there is clearly an unmet medical need for safe and effective weight-loss therapies to combat the twin epidemics of obesity and T2D. Recent advances have been made by the scientific community to unravel the metabolic networks that contribute to obesity, and these new findings hold promise for novel approaches to treat obesity and reduce cardiometabolic risk.

ABBREVIATIONS

ACC = Acetyl CoA carboxylase

AGE = Advanced glycation endproducts

AgRP = Agouti-related protein

AMPK = AMP-activated protein kinase

βAR = Beta adrenergic receptor

BMI = Body mass index

CB1 = Canabinoid receptor 1

CCK = Cholecystokinin

CPT-1 = Carnitine palmitoyl transferase 1

CVD = Cardiovascular disease

CRP = C-reactive protein

ET-1 = Endothelin 1

FFA = Free fatty acid

GHS-R1a = Growth hormone secretagogue receptor 1a

GLP-1 = Glucagon-like protein 1

HDL = High density lipoprotein

IL-6 = Interleukin-6

IKK = Inhibitor of kappa B kinase

JNK = c-jun N-terminal kinase

LDL = Low density lipoprotein

Lp(a) = Lipoprotein "little" a

MCP-1 = Monocyte chemoattractant protein-1

MSH-R	=	Melanocyte stimulating hormone receptor
MTP	=	Microsomal triglyceride transfer protein
NFκB	=	Nuclear factor kappa B
NO	=	Nitric oxide
NPY	=	Neuropeptide Y
PAI-1	=	Plasminogen activator inhibitor
PKC	=	Protein kinase C
PYY	=	Peptide-tyrosine-tyrosine
RAAS	=	Renin, angiotensin, aldosterone system
ROS	=	Reactive oxygen species
SCD-1	=	Stearoyl-CoA desaturase 1
TG	=	Triglyceride
TNF-α	=	Tumor necrosis factor alpha
T2D	=	Type 2 diabetes mellitus
VLDL	=	Very low density lipoprotein

Appendix

Table 2. Therapeutic Candidates that are in Development for the Treatment of Obesity. Source: Company Websites and Press Releases (Disclaimer: List Might Not Cover all Candidates that are in Development)

Development Phase	Therapeutic Candidate, Route of Administration	Company	Target
Phase III	Cetilistat, oral	Alizyme	pancreatic lipase inhibitor
	Locaserin, oral	Arena	Serotonin 2CR agonist
	Naltrexone/bupropion formulation, oral	Orexigen	multiple
	Phemtermine/topiramate formulation, oral	Vivus	multiple
Phase II	Velneperit (S-2367)	Shionogi	NPY5R antagonist
	Obinepitide, subcutaneous	7TM Pharma	NPY2R and NPY4R agonist
	TM 30339, sucutaneous	7TM Pharma	NPY4 R agonist
	Betahistine, oral	Obecure	Histamine H1R agonist, H3R antagonist
	Davalintide (AC2307), subcutaneous	Amylin Pharma	Amylin receptor agonists
	Pramlintide/metleptin combination	Amylin Pharma	Amylin and leptin receptor agonists
	N 5984, oral	Kyorin Pharma/ Nisshin Pharma	β_3-AR agonist
	Tesofensine, oral	NeuroSearch	Norepinephrine, serotonin and dopamine re-uptake inhibitor

(Appendix Table 2) Contd…..

Development Phase	Therapeutic Candidate, Route of Administration	Company	Target
Phase II	TTP-435, oral	TransTech Pharma	AgRP inhibitor
	SLx 4090, oral	Surface Logix	Intestinal MTP inhibitor
Phase I	AP 1030, oral	Action Pharma	MC1R and MC4R agonist
	Diazoxide choline controlled release, oral (in Phase II for TG lowering indication)	Essentialis	ATP sensitive, K-channel agoinst
	DOV 21947, oral (in Phase II for depression indication)	DOV Pharma	Norepinephrine, serotonin and dopamine re-uptake inhibitor
	BVT 74316, oral	Biovitrum	Serotonin 6R (5-HT_6R) antagonist
	PRX 07034, oral	EPIX Pharma	Serotonin 6R (5-HT_6R) antagonist
	GSK 1521498, oral	Glaxo Smith Kline	mu-opioid receptor (MOR) antagonist
	PYY3-36 formulation, oral	Emisphere Technologies	PYY3-36 action
	PSN 602, oral	Prosidion (OSI)	Dual monoamine reuptake inhibitor and serotonin 1A agonist
	PSN 821, oral	Prosidion (OSI)	GPR119 agonist
	Delta-9-tetrahydrocannabivarin, oral	GW Pharma	Cannabinoid type 1 (CB1) receptor antagonist
Preclinical R&D	EX-1350, oral	Elixir	GhrelinR antagonist
	AEZS-123	Aeterna Zentaris	GhrelinR antagonist
	NOX-B11	Noxxon	Ghrelin antagonist
	PT-15	AstraZeneca/Palatin	MC4R agonist
	Research program	Amura	MC4R agonist
	Research program	Ipsen	MC4R agonist
	Debio-0930 (T2D indication)	Mercury/Debiopharm	AMPK activator
	Research program	TransTech Pharma	AMPK activator
	Research program	FasGen/P&G	FASyn inhibitor
	GRC-9332	Glenmark Pharma	SCD inhibitor
	Research program	iNovacia	SCD inhibitor
	Leptin mimetics, oral	Cambridge Biotechnology (Biovitrum)	Leptin mimetic

REFERENCES

[1] Allison DB, Downey M, Atkinson RL, *et al.* Obesity as a disease: a white paper on evidence and arguments commissioned by the Council of The Obesity Society. Obesity 2008; 16(6): 1161-77.

[2] World Health Organization: Obesity, http: //www.who.int/topics/obesity/en/ (accessed on Oct 1, 2009).

[3] Must A, Spadano J, Coakley EH, Field AE, Colditz G, Dietz WH. The disease burden associated with overweight and obesity. JAMA 1999; 282(16): 1523-9.

[4] Mokdad AH, Ford ES, Bowman BA, *et al.* Prevalence of obesity, diabetes, and obesity-related health risk factors, 2001. JAMA 2003; 289(1): 76-9.

[5] Popkin BM. Global nutrition dynamics: the world is shifting rapidly toward a diet linked with noncommunicable diseases. Am J Clin Nutr 2006; 84(2): 289-98.
[6] International Diabetes Federation (IDF): Diabetes facts and figures, http: //www.idf.org/home/ index.cfm?unode=3B96906B-C026-2FD3-87B73F80BC22682A (accessed Oct 1, 2009).
[7] Williamson DF, Thompson TJ, Thun M, Flanders D, Pamuk E, Byers T. Intentional weight loss and mortality among overweight individuals with diabetes. Diabetes Care 2000; 23(10): 1499-504.
[8] Tuomilehto J, Lindstrom J, Eriksson JG, *et al.* Prevention of type 2 diabetes mellitus by changes in lifestyle among subjects with impaired glucose tolerance. N Engl J Med 2001; 344(18): 1343-50.
[9] Diabetes Prevention Program: Reduction in the incidence of type 2 diabetes with lifestyle intervention or metformin. N Engl J Med 2002; 346(6): 393-403.
[10] Poirier P, Giles TD, Bray GA, *et al.* Obesity and cardiovascular disease: Pathophysiology, evaluation, and effect of weight loss: An Update of the 1997 American Heart Association Scientific Statement on Obesity and Heart Disease from the Obesity Committee of the Council on Nutrition, Physical Activity, and Metabolism. Circulation 2006; 113(6): 898-918.
[11] Centers for Disease Control (CDC): Overweight and obesity, http: //www.cdc.gov/nccdphp/dnpa/obesity/ (accessed Oct 1, 2009).
[12] Ogden CL, Carroll MD, Curtin LR, McDowell MA, Tabak CJ, Flegal KM. Prevalence of overweight and obesity in the US, 1999-2004. JAMA 2006; 295(13): 1549-55.
[13] Runge CF. Economic consequences of the obese. Diabetes 2007; 56(11): 2668-72.
[14] World Health Organization (WHO): Childhood overweight and obesity. http: //www.who.int/dietphysicalactivity/childhood/ en/ (accessed Oct 1, 2009).
[15] Lewis CE, McTigue KM, Burke LE, *et al.* Mortality, health outcomes, and body mass index in the overweight range: A science advisory from the American Heart Association. Circulation 2009; 119(25): 3263-71.
[16] Gregg EW, Cheng YJ, Cadwell BL, *et al.* Secular trends in cardiovascular disease risk factors according to body mass index in US adults. JAMA 2005; 293(15): 1868-74.
[17] Perspective Studies Collaboration: Body-mass index and cause-specific mortality in 900000 adults: collaborative analyses of 57 prospective studies. Lancet 2009; 373(9669): 1083-96.
[18] Fox CS, Coady S, Sorlie PD, *et al.* Increasing cardiovascular disease burden due to diabetes mellitus: The Framingham Heart Study. Circulation 2007; 115(12): 1544-50.
[19] Haffner SM, Lehto S, Ronnemaa T, Pyorala K, Laakso M. Mortality from coronary heart disease in subjects with type 2 diabetes and in nondiabetic subjects with and without prior myocardial infarction. N Engl J Med 1998; 339(4): 229-34.
[20] Després J. Health consequences of visceral obesity. Ann Med 2001; 33(8): 534-41.
[21] Zhang C, Rexrode KM, van Dam RM, Li TY, Hu FB. Abdominal obesity and the risk of all-cause, cardiovascular, and cancer mortality: Sixteen years of follow-up in US women. Circulation 2008; 117(13): 1658-67.
[22] Kopp HP, Kopp CW, Festa A, *et al.* Impact of weight loss on inflammatory proteins and their association with the insulin resistance syndrome in morbidly obese patients. Arterioscler Thromb Vasc Biol 2003; 23(6): 1042-7.
[23] Scheen AJ, Finer N, Hollander P, Jensen M, Van Gaal L. Efficacy and tolerability of rimonabant in overweight or obese patients with type 2 diabetes: a randomised controlled study. Lancet 2006; 368(9548): 1660-72.
[24] Rana JS, Nieuwdorp M, Jukema JW, Kastelein JJP. Cardiovascular metabolic syndrome - an interplay of, obesity, inflammation, diabetes and coronary heart disease. Diabetes Obes Metab 2007; 9(3): 218-32.
[25] Assmann GGR, Fox G, Cullen P, Schulte H, Willett D, Grundy SM. Harmonizing the definition of the metabolic syndrome: comparison of the criteria of the Adult Treatment Panel III and the International Diabetes Federation in United States American and European populations. Am J Cardiol 2007; 99(4): 541-8.
[26] Grundy SM, Hansen B, Smith SC, Jr, Cleeman JI, Kahn RA. Clinical management of metabolic syndrome: Report of the American Heart Association/National Heart, Lung, and Blood Institute/American Diabetes Association Conference on Scientific Issues Related to Management. Circulation 2004; 109(4): 551-6.
[27] Wannamethee SG, Shaper AG, Lennon L, Morris RW. Metabolic syndrome *vs.* Framingham risk score for prediction of coronary heart disease, stroke, and type 2 diabetes mellitus. Arch Int Med 2005; 165(22): 2644-50.
[28] Kahn R, Buse J, Ferrannini E, Stern M. The metabolic syndrome: time for a critical appraisal: joint statement from the American Diabetes Association and the European Association for the Study of Diabetes. Diabetes Care 2005; 28(9): 2289-304.
[29] Buse JB, Ginsberg HN, Bakris GL, *et al.* Primary prevention of cardiovascular diseases in people with diabetes mellitus: A scientific statement from the American Heart Association and the American Diabetes Association. Circulation 2007; 115(1): 114-26.
[30] Ross R. Atherosclerosis - An inflammatory disease. N Engl J Med 1999; 340(2): 115-26.
[31] Wellen KE, Hotamisligil G. Obesity-induced inflammatory changes in adipose tissue. J Clin Invest 2003; 112(12): 1785-8.
[32] Shoelson SE, Herrero L, Naaz A. Obesity, inflammation, and insulin resistance. Gastroenterology 2007; 132(6): 2169-80.
[33] Ahima RS. Adipose tissue as an endocrine organ. Obesity 2006; 14(S8): 242S-9S.
[34] Lago F, Dieguez C, Gomez-Reino J, Gualillo O. Adipokines as emerging mediators of immune response and inflammation. Nat Clin Pract Rheum 2007; 3(12): 716-24.
[35] Guilherme A, Virbasius JV, Puri V, Czech MP. Adipocyte dysfunctions linking obesity to insulin resistance and type 2 diabetes. Nat Rev Mol Cell Biol 2008; 9(5): 367-77.
[36] Sartipy P, Loskutoff DJ. Monocyte chemoattractant protein 1 in obesity and insulin resistance. Pro Natl Acad Sci 2003; 100(12): 7265-70.
[37] Weisberg SP, McCann D, Desai M, Rosenbaum M, Leibel RL, Ferrante AW. Obesity is associated with macrophage accumulation in adipose tissue. J Clin Invest 2003; 112(12): 1796-808.
[38] Xu H, Barnes GT, Yang Q, *et al.* Chronic inflammation in fat plays a crucial role in the development of obesity-related insulin resistance. J Clin Invest 2003; 112(12): 1821-30.
[39] Bjorbaek C, Kahn BB. Leptin signaling in the central nervous system and the periphery. Recent Prog Horm Res 2004; 59(1): 305-31.
[40] Attie AD, Scherer PE. Adipocyte metabolism and obesity. J Lipid Res 2009; 50(Suppl): S395-9.
[41] Kadowaki T, Yamauchi T, Kubota N, Hara K, Ueki K, Tobe K. Adiponectin and adiponectin receptors in insulin resistance, diabetes, and the metabolic syndrome. J Clin Invest 2006; 116(7): 1784-92.

[42] Yamauchi TKJ, Minokoshi Y, Ito Y, *et al.* Adiponectin stimulates glucose utilization and fatty-acid oxidation by activating AMP-activated protein kinase. Nat Med 2002; 8(11): 1288-95.
[43] Ouchi NWK. A novel role for adiponectin in the regulation of inflammation. Arterioscler Thromb Vasc Biol 2008; 28(7): 1219-21.
[44] Steppan CM, Bailey ST, Bhat S, *et al.* The hormone resistin links obesity to diabetes. Nature 2001; 409(6818): 307-12.
[45] Bokarewa M, Nagaev I, Dahlberg L, Smith U, Tarkowski A. Resistin, an adipokine with potent proinflammatory properties. J Immunol 2005; 174(9): 5789-95.
[46] Verma S, Li S-H, Wang C-H, *et al.* Resistin promotes endothelial cell activation: Further evidence of adipokine-endothelial interaction. Circulation 2003; 108(6): 736-40.
[47] Hotamisligil GS. Inflammatory pathways and insulin action. Int J Obes Relat Metab Disord 2003; 27(S3): S53-S5.
[48] Steinberg GR, Michell BJ, van Denderen BJW, *et al.* Tumor necrosis factor [alpha]-induced skeletal muscle insulin resistance involves suppression of AMP-kinase signaling. Cel Metabol 2006; 4(6): 465-74.
[49] Niemann-Jonsson A, Dimayuga P, Jovinge S, *et al.* Accumulation of LDL in rat arteries is associated with activation of Tumor Necrosis Factor-{alpha} expression. Arterioscler Thromb Vasc Biol 2000; 20(10): 2205-11.
[50] Eder K, Baffy N, Falus A, Fulop A. The major inflammatory mediator interleukin-6 and obesity. Inflam Res 2009; 58(11): 727-36.
[51] Alessi M-C, Juhan-Vague I. PAI-1 and the metabolic syndrome: Links, causes, and consequences. Arterioscler Thromb Vasc Biol 2006; 26(10): 2200-7.
[52] Trost S, Pratley R, Sobel B. Impaired fibrinolysis and risk for cardiovascular disease in the metabolic syndrome and type 2 diabetes. Curr Diab Rep 2006; 6(1): 47-54.
[53] Shoelson SE, Lee J, Yuan M. Inflammation and the IKK[beta]//I[kappa]B//NF-[kappa]B axis in obesity- and diet-induced insulin resistance. Int J Obes Relat Metab Disord 2003; 27(S3): S49-S52.
[54] Hirosumi J, Tuncman G, Chang L, *et al.* A central role for JNK in obesity and insulin resistance. Nature 2002; 420(6913): 333-6.
[55] James R, Brulhart-Meynet M, Lehmann T, Golay A. Lipoprotein distribution and composition in obesity: Their association with central adiposity. Int J Obes 1999; 21(12): 1115-20.
[56] Boden G, Carnell LH. Nutritional effects of fat on carbohydrate metabolism. Best Prac Res Clin Endocrinol Metab 2003; 17(3): 399-410.
[57] Savage DB, Petersen KF, Shulman GI. Disordered lipid metabolism and the pathogenesis of insulin resistance. Physiol Rev 2007; 87(2): 507-20.
[58] Hotamisligil GS. Inflammation and metabolic disorders. Nature 2006; 444(7121): 860-7.
[59] Kahn SE, Hull RL, Utzschneider KM. Mechanisms linking obesity to insulin resistance and type 2 diabetes. Nature 2006; 444(7121): 840-6.
[60] Van Gaal LF, Mertens IL, De Block CE. Mechanisms linking obesity with cardiovascular disease. Nature 2006; 444(7121): 875-80.
[61] Rocha VZ, Libby P. Obesity, inflammation, and atherosclerosis. Nat Rev Cardiol 2009; 6(6): 399-409.
[62] Yu C, Chen Y, Cline GW, *et al.* Mechanism by which fatty acids inhibit insulin activation of insulin receptor substrate-1 (IRS-1)-associated phosphatidylinositol 3-kinase activity in muscle. J Biol Chem 2002; 277(52): 50230-6.
[63] Summers SA. Ceramides in insulin resistance and lipotoxicity. Prog Lipid Res 2006; 45(1): 42-72.
[64] Itani SIRN, Schmieder F, Boden G. Lipid-induced insulin resistance in human muscle is associated with changes in diacylglycerol, protein kinase C, and IkappaB-alpha. Diabetes 2002; 51(7): 2005-11.
[65] Boden G. Pathogenesis of type 2 diabetes. Insulin resistance. Endocrinol Metab Clin North Am 2001; 30(4): 801-15.
[66] Bamba V, Rader DJ. Obesity and atherogenic dyslipidemia. Gastroenterology [Obesity review] 2007; 132(6): 2181-90.
[67] Szapary PO, Rader DJ. The triglyceride-high-density lipoprotein axis: An important target of therapy? Am Heart J 2004; 148(2): 211-21.
[68] Moon JY, Kwon HM, Kwon SW, *et al.* Lipoprotein(a) and LDL particle size are related to the severity of coronary artery disease. Cardiology 2007; 108(4): 282-9.
[69] Visser M, Bouter LM, McQuillan GM, Wener MH, Harris TB. Elevated C-reactive protein levels in overweight and obese adults. JAMA 1999; 282(22): 2131-5.
[70] Ridker PM. C-reactive protein and the prediction of cardiovascular events among those at intermediate risk: Moving an inflammatory hypothesis toward consensus. J Am Col Cardiol 2007; 49(21): 2129-38.
[71] Kahn SE. The relative contributions of insulin resistance and beta-cell dysfunction to the pathophysiology of Type 2 diabetes. Diabetologia 2003; 46(1): 3-19.
[72] Maedler K. Beta cells in type 2 diabetes - a crucial contribution to pathogenesis. Diab Obesity Metab 2008; 10(5): 408-20.
[73] Robertson R, Harmon J, Tran P, Poitout V. Beta-cell glucose toxicity, lipotoxicity, and chronic oxidative stress in type 2 diabetes. Diabetes 2004; 53(Suppl 1): S119-24.
[74] Engeli S, Sharma A. Role of adipose tissue for cardiovascular-renal regulation in health and disease. Horm Metab Res 2000; 32(11-12): 485-99.
[75] Wofford M, Hall J. Pathophysiology and treatment of obesity hypertension. Curr Pharm Des 2004; 10(29): 3621-37.
[76] Narkiewicz K. Obesity and hypertension--the issue is more complex than we thought. Nephrol Dial Transplant 2006; 21(2): 264-7.
[77] Furukawa S, Fujita T, Shimabukuro M, *et al.* Increased oxidative stress in obesity and its impact on metabolic syndrome. J Clin Invest 2004; 114(12): 1752-61.
[78] Jansson PA. Endothelial dysfunction in insulin resistance and type 2 diabetes. J Int Med 2007; 262(2): 173-83.
[79] John S, Schmieder RE. Potential mechanisms of impaired endothelial function in arterial hypertension and hypercholesterolemia. Curr Hypertens Rep 2003; 5(3): 199-207.
[80] Wilkinson IB, McEniery CM. Arterial stiffness, endothelial function and novel pharmacological approaches. Clin Exp Pharm Physiol 2004; 31(11): 795-9.
[81] Libby P. Inflammation and cardiovascular disease mechanisms. Am J Clin Nutr 2006; 83(2): 456S-60.
[82] Goldberg RB. Cytokine and cytokine-like inflammation markers, endothelial dysfunction, and imbalanced coagulation in development of diabetes and its complications. J Clin Endocrinol Metab 2009; 94(9): 3171-82.
[83] Brownlee M. Biochemistry and molecular cell biology of diabetic complications. Nature 2001; 414(6865): 813-20.

[84] Aronson D. Hyperglycemia and the pathobiology of diabetic complications. Adv Cardiol 2008; 45: 1-16.
[85] Gao L, Mann GE. Vascular NAD(P)H oxidase activation in diabetes: a double-edged sword in redox signalling. Cardiovasc Res 2009; 82(1): 9-20.
[86] Schäfer AJB. Endothelial dysfunction, impaired endogenous platelet inhibition and platelet activation in diabetes and atherosclerosis. Curr Vasc Pharmacol 2008; 6(1): 52-60.
[87] Curioni CC, Lourenco PM. Long-term weight loss after diet and exercise: a systematic review. Int J Obes Relat Metab Disord 2005; 29(10): 1168-74.
[88] Douketis JD, Macie C, Thabane L, Williamson DF. Systematic review of long-term weight loss studies in obese adults: clinical significance and applicability to clinical practice. Int J Obes Relat Metab Disord 2005; 29(10): 1153-67.
[89] Arterburn DE, Crane PK, Veenstra DL. The Efficacy and Safety of Sibutramine for Weight Loss: A Systematic Review. Arch Intern Med 2004; 164(9): 994-1003.
[90] Henness S, Perry C. Orlistat: a review of its use in the management of obesity. Drugs 2006; 66(12): 1625.
[91] Souzana C, Angeliki AM, Constantinos CF, Eleni Th P, Stella SD. Effect of antiobesity medications in patients with type 2 diabetes mellitus. Diab Obesity Metab 2009; 11(7): 641-64.
[92] UK Prospective Diabetes Study (UKPDS) Group: Effect of intensive blood-glucose control with metformin on complications in overweight patients with type 2 diabetes (UKPDS 34). Lancet 1998; 352(9131): 854-65.
[93] Hundal RS IS. Metformin: new understandings, new uses. Drugs 2003; 63(18): 1879-94.
[94] Baggio LL, Drucker DJ. Biology of incretins: GLP-1 and GIP. Gastroenterology 2007; 132(6): 2131-57.
[95] Norris SL, Lee N, Thakurta S, Chan BKS. Exenatide efficacy and safety: a systematic review. Diabet Med 2009; 26(9): 837-46.
[96] Hoogwerf BJDK, Diab D. Pramlintide, the synthetic analogue of amylin: physiology, pathophysiology, and effects on glycemic control, body weight, and selected biomarkers of vascular risk. Vasc Health Risk Manag 2008; 4(2): 355-62.
[97] National Institute for Diabetes and Digestive and Kidney Diseases (NIDDK): Bariatric surgery for severe obesity, http: //win.niddk.nih.gov/publications/gastric.htm (accessed Oct 1, 2009).
[98] Trakhtenbroit M, Leichman J, Algahim M, *et al.* Body weight, insulin resistance, and serum adipokine levels 2 years after 2 types of bariatric surgery. Am J Med 2009; 122(5): 435-42.
[99] Lang LH. FDA issues early communication about ongoing safety review of weight loss drug Orlistat. Gastroenterology 2009; 137(5): 1546-7.
[100] The European Medicines Agency (EMEA): Oct 23, 2008 press release, http: //www.emea.europa.eu.humandocs/PDFs/EPAR/accomplia/53777708en.pdf (accessed Oct 1, 2009).
[101] Zhou G, Myers R, Li Y, *et al.* Role of AMP-activated protein kinase in mechanism of metformin action. J Clin Invest 2001; 8: 1167-74.
[102] Nathan DM, Buse JB, Davidson MB, *et al.* Management of hyperglycemia in type 2 diabetes: a consensus algorithm for the initiation and adjustment of therapy: update regarding thiazolidinediones: a consensus statement from the American Diabetes Association and the European Association for the Study of Diabetes. Diabetes Care 2008; 31(1): 173-5.
[103] Park MH KS, Ward KJ, White B, Viner RM. Metformin for obesity in children and adolescents: A systematic review. Diabetes Care 2009; 32(9): 1743-5.
[104] Gadde KM, Allison DB. Combination therapy for obesity and metabolic disease. Curr Opin Endocrinol Diabetes Obes 2009; 16(5): 353-8.
[105] Ahima RS. Revisiting leptin's role in obesity and weight loss. J Clin Invest 2008; 118(7): 2380-3.
[106] Wren AM, Bloom SR. Gut hormones and appetite control. Gastroenterology 2007; 132(6): 2116-30.
[107] Woods SC, D'Alessio DA. Central control of body weight and appetite. J Clin Endo Metab 2008; 93(11(Suppl1): S37-50.
[108] Obici S. Molecular targets for obesity therapy in the brain. Endocrinology 2009; 2512-7.
[109] Aronne LJ, Thornton-Jones ZD. New targets for obesity pharmacotherapy. Clin Pharmacol Ther 2007; 81(5): 748-52.
[110] Chakrabarti R. Pharmacotherapy of obesity: emerging drugs and targets. Exper Opin Ther Targets 2009; 13(2): 195-207.
[111] Gordon D, Wetterau J, Gregg R. Microsomal triglyceride transfer protein: a protein complex required for the assembly of lipoprotein particles. Trends Cel Biol 1995; 5(8): 317-21.
[112] Catherine P, Karen M, Daphne O, Gerald HT. Intestinal microsomal triglyceride transfer protein in type 2 diabetic and non-diabetic subjects: The relationship to triglyceride-rich postprandial lipoprotein composition. Atherosclerosis 2006; 187(1): 57-64.
[113] Sweetnam P, Kim E, Yang Y, Campbell S. SLx-4090: A novel, intestinal-specific MTP inhibitor for lowering plasma triglyceride and cholesterol levels in dyslipidemia. Am J Gastroenterol 2005; 100 (Suppl) (9): 58-9.
[114] Sinclair EM, Drucker DJ. Proglucagon-derived peptides: Mechanisms of action and therapeutic potential. Physiology 2005; 20(5): 357-65.
[115] Verdich C, Toubro S, Buemann B, Lysgård Madsen J, Juul Holst J, Astrup A. The role of postprandial releases of insulin and incretin hormones in meal-induced satiety-effect of obesity and weight reduction. Int J Obes Relat Metab Disord 2001; 25(8): 1206-14.
[116] Mafong DD HR. Exenatide as a treatment for diabetes and obesity: implications for cardiovascular risk reduction. Curr Atheroscler Rep 2008; 10(1): 55-60.
[117] Liu H, Dear A, Knudsen L, Simpson R. A long-acting GLP-1 analogue attenuates induction of PAI-1 and vascular adhesion molecules. J Endocrinol 2009; 201(1): 59-66.
[118] Larhammar D. Structural diversity of receptors for neuropeptide Y, peptide YY and pancreatic polypeptide. Regul Pept 1996; 65(4): 165-75.
[119] Batterham RL, Cohen MA, Ellis SM, *et al.* Inhibition of food intake in obese subjects by Peptide YY3-36. N Engl J Med 2003; 349(10): 941-8.
[120] Badman MK, Flier JS. The adipocyte as an active participant in energy balance and metabolism. Gastroenterology 2007; 132(6): 2103-15.
[121] Wren AM, Seal LJ, Cohen MA, *et al.* Ghrelin enhances appetite and increases food intake in humans. J Clin Endocrinol Metab 2001; 86(12): 5992-5.
[122] Date Y, Kojima M, Hosoda H, *et al.* Ghrelin, a novel growth hormone-releasing acylated peptide, is synthesized in a distinct endocrine cell type in the gastrointestinal tracts of rats and humans. Endocrinology 2000; 141(11): 4255-61.

[123] Chen HY, Trumbauer ME, Chen AS, *et al.* Orexigenic action of peripheral ghrelin is mediated by neuropeptide Y and agouti-related protein. Endocrinology 2004; 145(6): 2607-12.
[124] van der Lely AJ, Tschop M, Heiman ML, Ghigo E. Biological, physiological, pathophysiological, and pharmacological aspects of ghrelin. Endocr Rev 2004; 25(3): 426-57.
[125] Winder WW, Hardie DG. AMP-activated protein kinase, a metabolic master switch: possible roles in type 2 diabetes. Am J Physiol Endocrinol Metab 1999; 277(1): E1-10.
[126] Kahn BB, Alquier T, Carling D, Hardie DG. AMP-activated protein kinase: ancient energy gauge provides clues to modern understanding of metabolism. Cell Metabol 2005; 1(1): 15-25.
[127] Hawley S, Boudeau J, Reid J, *et al.* Complexes between the LKB1 tumor suppressor, STRAD alpha/beta and MO25 alpha/beta are upstream kinases in the AMP-activated protein kinase cascade. J Biol 2003; 2(4): 1-16.
[128] Harwood HJ, Petras SF, Shelly LD, *et al.* Isozyme-nonselective N-substituted bipiperidylcarboxamide acetyl-CoA carboxylase inhibitors reduce tissue malonyl-CoA concentrations, inhibit fatty acid synthesis, and increase fatty acid oxidation in cultured cells and in experimental animals. J Biol Chem 2003; 278(39): 37099-111.
[129] Dobrzyn A, Ntambi JM. Stearoyl-CoA desaturase as a new drug target for obesity treatment. Obes Rev 2005; 6(2): 169-74.
[130] Ntambi JM, Miyazaki M, Stoehr JP, *et al.* Loss of stearoyl CoA desaturase-1 function protects mice against adiposity. Proc Natl Acad Sci USA 2002; 99(17): 11482-6.

Anti-Obesity Drug Discovery and Development, **2011**, *1*, 114-130

Monoaminergic Systems and Anti-Obesity Drug Discovery: Chronic Administration of Sympathicomimetic Amines, Re-Uptake Inhibitors, or Amine Oxidase Inhibitors?

Christian Carpéné[*,1,2] and Zsuzsa Iffiú-Soltész[2,3]

[1]*INSERM, U858, Institut de Médecine Moléculaire de Rangueil, Toulouse, France*

[2]*Université de Toulouse III, UPS, IFR 150, Toulouse, France*

[3]*Department of Pharmacodynamics, Semmelweis University, Budapest, Hungary*

Abstract: The concept that monoamines related to the sympathetic nervous system can act as slimming agents is very well-known. The utmost interest in this approach followed the β3-adrenergic receptor discovery and the impressive lipolytic capacities of its agonists in rodent adipocytes. However, the clinical trials using β3-adrenergic agonists have led to a very limited anti-obesity clinical application. The differences between species regarding expression level and pharmacology of β3-adrenoceptors may be the cause of this missed extrapolation. In this review, the interests and limits of cultured adipocytes *vs.* animal models in the discovery of anti-obesity drugs are discussed. Nevertheless, biogenic amines that share β3-adrenoceptor agonist properties, are used via self-prescription to promote weight loss. The effects of one of them, octopamine is discussed in this chapter, focusing on the large species-differences that exist regarding its action on adipocytes. Even older is the wish to use of monoamine oxidase (MAO) inhibitors in the treatment of obesity. Reduction of body weight gain has been observed in rodents, but negative side-effects, such as increased aggressiveness, mouth dryness and hypertensive crises, seriously limit their anti-obesity utilisation in overweight patients. More recent is the observation of the limitation of fat development by agents that inhibit amine oxidases distinct from MAO, especially the semicarbazide-sensitive amine oxidase (SSAO) highly expressed in fat cells. The impairment of adipose tissue extension induced by semicarbazide is mirroring the insulin-like actions of SSAO and MAO substrates that activate lipogenesis and inhibit lipolysis in adipocytes. Nevertheless, another mode of action cannot be eliminated. Since combined inhibition of MAO and SSAO affects adipose tissue extension, phenelzine, which inhibits MAO and SSAO, has been tested recently. *In vitro*, it impairs adipogenesis, and *in vivo*, it decreases the adiposomatic index in obese rats. Taken together, the reduction of adipose tissue development by catecholaminergic amines or by amine oxidase inhibitors warrants further studies and can prompt the search for new anti-obesity drugs.

Keywords: Adipocytes, lipolysis, amine uptake inhibitors, monoamine oxidases, copper-containing amine oxidases.

BODY WEIGHT LOSS *VS.* REDUCED ADIPOSITY

The potential pharmacological strategies to facilitate weight loss can be conceptually separated in two aspects: on the one hand, agents that reduce energy intake, by stimulating anorexigenic signals or by blocking orexigenic signals or even factors impairing nutriment absorption during digestive processes; on the other hand, agents that increase energy expenditure. However these two aspects are not always completely separated and many experimental slimming agents or numerous candidates for managing obesity act on both of them. Nevertheless, the two weight-loss drugs currently approved for long-term treatment of obesity in many countries, namely Sibutramine and Orlistat, essentially belong to the first class of pharmacological agents. By contrast, the majority of the weight-loss supplements, marketed on the Internet and/or available without medical prescription, belong to the second class: they are currently sold as "fat burning factors" while they actually contain ingredients which potentially have more adverse effects on the heart than beneficial stimulating properties on lipid mobilization and fat oxidation.

Based on our experience in adipose tissue physiology, we will present these two aspects and focus interest on several members of the monoaminergic pharmacology promoting weight loss rather than discussing all the current and promising anti-obesity strategies (reviewed elsewhere, *e.g.* [1, 2]).

*Corresponding author: Tel: (33) (0)5 61 32 56 36; Fax: (33) 5 61 32 56 22; E-mail: Christian.Carpene@inserm.fr

Atta-ur-Rahman / M. Iqbal Choudhary (Eds.)

Before focusing on monoaminergic systems, it is worth mentioning that although obesity is obviously an excess of adipose tissue, the various recent transgenic mouse models with genetic ablation of adipose tissue have brought evidence that the total lack of adipose tissue is even more deleterious than its excess. Any design of an anti-obesity drug would therefore be intended to limit fat deposition but not to entirely obliterate adipose tissue. In many pharmacological studies, it has appeared so difficult to reduce fat mass without altering lean mass, especially when energy intake is reduced, that both the European Medicines Evaluation Agency and the US Food and Drug Administration nowadays ask that the weight-loss induced by a given anti-obesity strategy reaches an "appropriate" loss of fat. This safety consideration facilitates the interest to present below the advantages and disadvantages of the investigations that should be performed *in vitro* with cultured preadipocytes and *in vivo* using obese rodents, before evidencing a probe-of-concept for any novel anti-obesity approach.

EVIDENCING ANTI-OBESITY EFFECTS: FROM *IN VITRO* TO *IN VIVO* APPROACHES AND VICE VERSA

The recommended use of alternative investigations or substitution models aiming at limiting the sacrifice of laboratory animals has increased the usage of preadipocyte cell lines (*e.g.* murine 3T3L1 and 3T3F442A, human SGBS...) in the screening and development of anti-obesity drugs. It is in agreement with the paradigm that (directly or indirectly) fat cells are targets of anti-obesity pharmacology. This can be supported by the piece of evidence that leptin, one of the most important keys in food intake and metabolic rate regulation, is acting on the hypothalamus and is produced by the adipocytes themselves. Of course, limiting adipose tissue extension is a major goal for anti-obesity strategies, but the simple observation of an inhibition of lipid accumulation in cultured adipocytes is not a sufficient probe of anti-obesity action, regardless of which drug candidate tested. The increasingly used expression "anti-obesity effect of a given agent on cultured adipose cells" is misleading as an anti-obesity effect should be demonstrated both *in vivo* and *in vitro*. Instead, the far clearer "anti-adipogenic effect on cultured adipose cells" should be used. Only several of the numerous factors reported to hamper *in vitro* adipogenesis of cultured preadipocytes have also been shown to alter lipid deposition *in vivo*. As definitively accepted examples, we will choose the following substances, as listed below:

- Tumor necrosis factor-alpha (TNF-alpha) is a cytokine involved in the loss of body fat in the course of wasting diseases and is a potent inhibitor of adipose differentiation [3].
- Ciliary neurotrophic factor (CNTF) is a cytokine with neuroprotective effects that has been experimentally used to treat neurodegenerative diseases and found to induce weight loss. CNTF also exerts anti-adipogenic effects in adipocytes [1].
- Leukemia inhibitory factor (LIF) belongs to the same family of gp130 receptor ligands and shares the same receptor complex with CNTF; it has been reported to inhibit the sterol regulatory element binding protein-1 (SREBP1) implicated in lipogenic pathway. However its effects on adipose conversion depends on the model studied [4, 5].
- Efavirenz is an antiretroviral drug that induces lipodystrophy when used in therapy for HIV-infected patients, and which has been reported to alter triglyceride accumulation in cultured adipocytes, also by impairing the SREBP1-dependent lipogenic pathway [6].

Taken together, these examples illustrate that relationships exist between anti-adipogenic and anti-obesity actions. However they are sometimes complicated and "anti-obesity" should be used only when *in vivo* studies have been achieved. Therefore, developments at pre-clinical stage of novel anti-obesity strategies (reviewed elsewhere: [1]) definitely need both animal and cellular models.

So, the use of animal models remains mandatory for unravelling the complex aspects of fattening. The mouse constitutes an invaluable model since the spontaneous obese diabetic (ob/ob, db/db and KKAy) mice have helped a lot in discovering the disorders related to obesity. Moreover, the increasing number of transgenic mice (essentially knock-out strains), characterized by monogenic obesity, has improved the identification of mechanisms underlying the development of obesity [7]. Nevertheless the use of rats, especially when individually housed, remains of non-negligible interest. In spite of a limited number of genetically obese strains, each rat model offers advantages: the Zucker rat (fa/fa), is obese with hyperinsulinemia but without diabetes and allows us to detect anti-obesity drugs which do not need an intact leptin system to function; the spontaneous hypertensive/NIH corpulent rat (SHR/N-*cp*) is clearly obese and diabetic, therefore useful for studying various features of the metabolic syndrome [8]. Lastly, the cafeteria rat remains an excellent model of diet-induced obesity.

While we heartily recommend the use of animal models, we do not ban the use of freshly isolated or cultured adipocytes in the screening and development of novel anti-obesity drugs. All the recently approved anti-obesity drugs (see Table **1** for chemical structures) show direct effects on adipocytes *in vitro*, even when their primary target was considered to be in the central nervous system or in peripheral tissues other than adipose tissue:

- Sibutramine, the racemate mixture of (N-{1-[1-(4-chlorophenyl)cyclobutyl]-3-methylbutyl}-N,N-dimethylamine hydrochloride monohydrate) is a monoamine re-uptake inhibitor having hypophagic effects [9] and is transformed into metabolites once administered *in vivo*. One of them has been reported to activate *in vitro* lipolysis in isolated human or mouse adipocytes [10].

- Orlistat, a general lipase inhibitor shown to inhibit the gastrointestinal digestion of ingested lipids, reduces by one third the fat absorption, hence contributing to a negative energy balance. In spite of being poorly absorbed *in vivo* at therapeutic doses, the *in vitro* addition of Orlistat to 3T3-L1 adipocytes inhibits lipolysis [11].

- Rimonabant, an antagonist of endocannabinoid receptors of the CB1R type expressed in both the brain and peripheral tissues, has been definitively demonstrated to reduce food intake and body mass by a "reward inhibition" mechanism. This antagonist also directly inhibits lipogenesis in adipose tissue [12]. So, Rimonabant decreases adiposity by complementing in the adipose tissue its central inhibitory effect on food intake. Because monoamine oxidase inhibitors, antidepressant drugs and anorectic inhibitors of norepinephrine/serotonin re-uptake will be considered in the following chapters, it is worth mentioning here that, while the monoamine re-uptake inhibitor sibutramine is related to the family of antidepressants, rimonabant exerts depressant effects, which is a concern regarding its use as an anti-obesity agent.

ANIMAL MODELS: REDUCTION OF BODY WEIGHT GAIN *VS*. REDUCTION OF ADIPOSITY

As mentioned above, a good candidate for being an anti-obesity drug is one which promotes a substantial fat loss in obese patients. This is valid for man, but more difficult to obtain in laboratory rodents, since rats and mice have a continuous growth during the studied period of their life. For instance, a Wistar male rat generally gains around 4 g of body mass daily when weighing between 200 and 350 g and an obese Zucker rat can gain up to 8 g daily. Thus, there is a daily increase of 2-3 % of body mass that hardly occurs in obese patients even those with non-stabilized body weight (bw). Therefore, most of the pharmacological agents tested on rats slow down the spontaneous weight gain during their prolonged administration rather than promoting weight loss. Even more, decreases in body mass make us suspect a toxicological action in these models. Therefore, the restriction of weight gain by a given factor, found in a relatively short period in rodent models, requires that extrapolation as potential slimming action in man must be done with caution. Routinely, it is worth traducing "slimming" action or agent into growth retardation or reduction of body weight gain (bw-gain) when the reported findings have been observed in rodents. Weight loss is achievable in rodents, for instance after prolonged fasting, as reported in Table **2** (where it is expressed as negative values of bw-gain).

Furthermore, a given anti-obesity pharmacological drug ideally reduces fat deposits more than any other tissue in the body. Indeed, there is a myriad of agents lowering bw-gain without especially reducing white adipose tissue (WAT) mass. The use of an "adiposomatic index" is strongly recommended: it is defined as the ratio of fat depot mass/whole body mass. The bottom line is that fat is not only stored in WAT, but also is present in other tissues. In spite of several differences that cannot be rejected under special conditions (lipodystrophies, fat liver...), it can be asserted that the percentage of fat mass relative to body mass varies in parallel with the percentage of WAT mass relative to body mass. The former percentage (% fat/body) can be investigated nowadays in a non-invasive manner owing to the use of Nuclear Magnetic Resonance, since there are devices adapted for the measurement of fat and water mass in living small animals. By using an EchoMRI-100TM apparatus in accordance with the manufacturer's instructions (Echo Medical Systems, Houston, USA), we have observed that, at the age of ten weeks, the fat mass is 13 ± 2 % in lean male mice while it rises up to 45 ± 4 % in the obese and diabetic db/db mice ($n = 10$, $p<0.001$). A good anti-obesity drug should delay this increase when administered in young animals or should normalize it in older mice.

Table 1. Main Effects and Molecular Structure of the Base of Recently used Anti-Obesity Drugs

Name and Chemical Structure	Mode of Action	Effects
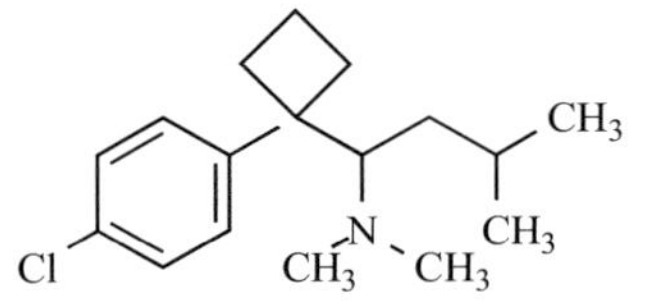 Sibutramine	Monoamine (serotonin dopamine, norepineohrine) re-uptake inhibitor	Antidepressant Hypophagic
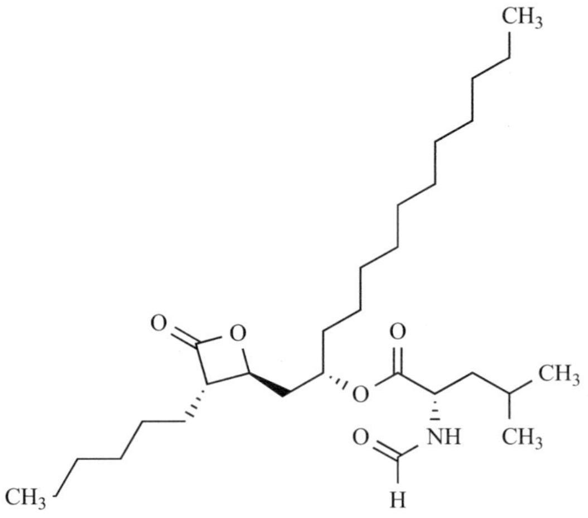 Orlistat	General lipase inhibitor	Reduction of fat absorption
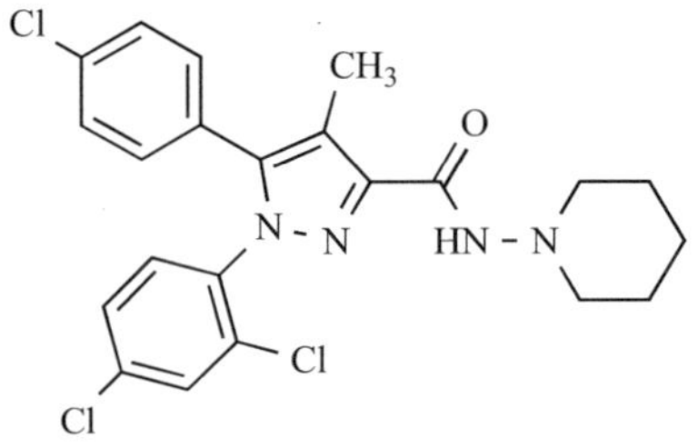 Rimonabant	Antagonist of the endocannabinoid receptors CB1R	Hypophagic, depressant

Nevertheless, the % of WAT/bw is more informative than the % fat mass because WAT is constituted by numerous fat pads located in different anatomical regions and a current paradigm associates insulin resistance and other deleterious complications of obesity with excess visceral rather than subcutaneous fat. In our studies, we have considered that, in rats as well as in mice, the sum of the easily dissectible fat depots located in perigonadal (epididymal in males, or parametrial in females), perirenal and retroperitoneal regions constitutes a good estimate of visceral fat. We have called this sum of WATs as internal or intra-abdominal adipose tissue (INWAT) to distinguish it from the subcutaneous WAT (SCWAT), mainly located in the inguinal areas in rodents (while it is mainly located in the umbilical region in man). However, the sum of these three main locations does not encompass the omental fat depot (anatomically more distinguishable in man or dog [13] than in rodents) and the mesenteric fat that develops in creeping fat in massive obesity. As a consequence of the detrimental nature of the visceral fat, suspected to increase features of the metabolic syndrome via adiposopathy [14], we have proposed the calculation of % INWAT/bw as a definition of adiposomatic index [15]. Of course, the % SCWAT/bw and the percentage of all the dissectible fat pads/bw could also be used. In this context, Table **2** shows that %SCWAT/bw remains intact under several conditions, even during complete starvation.

The comparison of all these percentages between treated rodents and an adequate control group (constituted at the start of treatment by weight- and age-matched animals) is undoubtedly informative during the pre-clinical study of new anti-obesity drugs. When they are not reduced, these percentages indicate that the tested agent has retarded the whole growth, rather than impeded specifically the lipid deposition in fat stores. Such absence of decreased adiposomatic index occurs even when the absolute mass of INWAT is lower in the treated group than in the control group: this occurs in several of the treatments reported in Table **2**. In these conditions, the treatment has impeded fat stores enlargement, but has also altered similarly the lean mass. Obviously, any treatment that does modify both bw gain and adiposomatic index has not altered enough the balance between energy intake and expenditure. False positive observations for a decreased adiposomatic index could be made when the lean mass has increased considerably or when experimental events have modified the growth curve (*e.g.* tissue graft or surgical ablation). However, such observations can be securely distinguished from the real positive tests. More interestingly, any clear-cut activation of lipid mobilisation and reduced fat accretion will decrease adiposomatic index, indicating that the slow down of bw-gain, if any, was concomitant with a specific loss of fat mass. Such real decrease of adiposity has to be obtained by the design and development of anti-obesity drugs. Unfortunately, at this experimental stage, the best candidates for further development are still years away from clinical use.

IMPORTANCE OF INTERSPECIES DIFFERENCES: THE CASE OF β3-AR-AGONISTS

The concept that the monoamines related to the sympathetic nervous system constitute a family of slimming of agents has been proposed several decades ago. The pioneering demonstration of the impressive lipolytic capacities of "atypical" β-adrenergic agonists in rodent adipocytes [16] greatly renewed the interest for this old concept. The mechanism of action of these agonists, which were more potent than endogenous catecholamines, was explained by discovery of the β3-adrenergic receptor (β3-AR) [17].

In fact, the "atypical" beta-adrenergic agonists are the activators of the β3-AR and were seen by independent research teams to increase lipolysis and fat oxidation, two aspects of energy expenditure activation. Alongside their attractive properties regarding the treatment of obesity, they also revealed antidiabetic properties. Despite their lead to glycemic improvements in rodent models of diabetes and obesity, the β3-AR agonists were shown to favour glucose utilization in muscle [18] while they reduced the capacity of white adipocytes to take up glucose in response to insulin [19, 20]. The resulting balance between fat depletion and muscle accretion did not impair the treatment of obesity since fat was replaced by muscle. However, this balance has resulted, in some models, in an absence of weight loss after treatment, as it is reported in Table **2**, for non-obese [21], non-diabetic rats [22, 23]. Accordingly, several β3-AR agonist treatments have resulted in conserved - or even increased - lean mass depending on the dose and model [24]. Furthermore, "atypical" beta-adrenergic agonists and/or poorly selective β2-AR agonists are used for enhancing anabolism in muscle [25], and in a clinical study, the β3-AR agonist BRL 26830 has been proven to limit nitrogen excretion in obese men [24].

In keeping with this, Table **2** shows that the bw-gain was not altered in rats treated with β3-AR agonists and with free access to food. In spite of being in apparent disagreement with the anti-obesity potential of such agents, these observations exemplify the well-recognized lipid mobilizing effect of such agonists when one considers the reported adiposity indexes (given as % of bw). The bw-gain did not change after one week of treatment by either the β3-AR agonist CL-316243 (5-[(2R)-2-[[(2R)-2- (3-chlorophenyl)-2-hydroxyethyl] amino] propyl]-1,3-benzodioxole-2,2-dicarboxylic acid), or by BRL 35135 [methyl 4-[2-[2-hydroxy-2-(3-chlorophenyl)ethyl-amino]propyl]phenoxyacetate] (a precusor of β3-AR agonist); but the percentage of visceral fat (estimated as shown above) was dramatically reduced. Our observations, therefore, agree with the lipolytic properties attributed to such atypical agonists in various rodents [24] and even in dogs [13] but not in guinea pigs [22, 23] or in man [26]. It can be supposed that the lost fat mass was "replaced" by another tissue, which was probably skeletal muscle, according to the anabolic effect of β-AR agonists [24].

Of note, the impressive reduction in the percentage of visceral fat, found in β3-AR agonist-treated rats, weighing approx. 310 g at the start of the treatments, was not obtained in mature rats subjected to a prolonged 4-day calorie starvation (with same strain and initial bw). The latter animals experienced a clear depletion of their fat stores, but the proportion of visceral fat depots relative to body mass was not reduced. In other words, although totally lacking of energy intake, the fasting mature rats lost fat mass, but also lost weight in other tissues of their body, the brain being likely the least affected. Their adiposity was hardly reduced although they tended to normalize their fat/lean ratio. Only younger rats (initial bw around 210 g) experienced a dramatic emaciation during prolonged fasting and could not spare their fat stores: the relative proportion of visceral fat being reduced by one half and that of subcutaneous fat being reduced by one third. The low dosage of BRL 35135 also induced a greater mobilization in visceral than in subcutaneous fat (Table **2**), a finding that has been hardly shown during the intensive studies of the promising anti-obesity effects of β3-AR agonism [24].

Table 2. Body Mass Gain and Adiposity in Rats Subjected to Fasting or to β3-AR Agonist Treatment

Model and Treatment	Control	Treated
Young Wistar male rats fasted for 4 days (n = 5)		
body weight gain, g	18.0± 2.5	-43.2 ± 1.5 ***
Visceral fat, % bw	2.6 ± 0.1	1.3 ± 0.1 ***
Subcutaneous fat, % bw	4.6 ± 0.3	3.1 ± 0.2 ***
Mature Wistar male rats fasted for 4 days (n = 3)		
Body weight gain, g	16.0± 2.0	-36.0 ± 4.6 ***
Visceral fat, % bw	3.5 ± 0.3	3.0 ± 0.2 NS
Subcutaneous fat, % bw	5.4 ± 0.6	5.2 ± 0.3 NS
Mature Wistar male rats treated by CL 316243 1 mg/kg/d for 7 days (n = 9)		
Body weight gain, g	28.1± 4.7	33.3 ± 3.7 NS
Visceral fat, % bw	2.5 ± 0.1	1.0 ± 0.1 ***
Subcutaneous fat, % bw	2.7 ± 0.1	1.9 ± 0.1 ***
Mature Wistar male rats treated by BRL 35135 0.6 mg/kg/d for 7 days (n = 5)		
Body weight gain, g	36.7± 4.4	35.5 ± 1.2 NS
Visceral fat, % bw	2.0 ± 0.2	1.3 ± 0.2 *
Subcutaneous fat, % bw	3.1 ± 0.2	2.3 ± 0.3 NS

Negative values of body weight (bw) gain correspond to weight loss; n = number of rats in each group. NS: non significantly different from control. Difference statistically significant at: * $p<0.05$; *** $p<0.001$.

The chemical structures of the above mentioned β3-AR agonists are reported in Table **3**. It can be noted that all the three adrenergic stimulators contain an aromatic cycle and a secondary amine moiety more or less resembling to adrenaline, one of the physiological catecholamines activating β3-ARs.

The apparent contradiction between bw-gain and percentage of dissectible fat in β3-AR agonist-treated rats seems unimportant when one considers that several pharmaceutical problems have hampered the development of β3-AR agonists as therapeutic agents in humans. For several investigators, it is the considerable pharmacological differences between the rodent and the human β3-AR that have been an obstacle for such development.

Fig. (**1**) shows that the binding of labelled iodocyanopindol is lower in human than in rodent white fat cells, especially at high concentration, near the KD towards β3-ARs [24]. Thus, a reduced expression of target receptors could also probably explain the poor lipolytic effect of β3-AR agonists in man [26]. However, the cultured 3T3F442A adipose cells, or L6E9 muscle cells, also possess a weak specific binding capacity for iodocyanopindol (Fig. **1**) while they are somewhat responsive to β3-AR agonists. Thus, the concern was probably both the number and efficacy of the β3-ARs present in human fat cells [27].

Fig. (**1**) also shows the huge expression of iodocyanopindol binding sites in CHO cells transfected with human β3-AR gene, which has sometimes led to overestimated interpretations of their coupling capacity and was not representative of what happened (or did not happen) in human adipocytes. Certainly, the β3-ARs found in human, lipid-laden, white adipocytes were limited in their expression and in their functionality because their agonists have never been able to clearly activate lipolysis, while β1-AR (and β2-AR activation to a lesser extent) was fully active, at least in our hands [26].

Table 3. Chemical Structure of the Molecules Studied for their Possible Anti-Obesity Action

Name	Chemical Structure	Mode of Action
BRL 26830	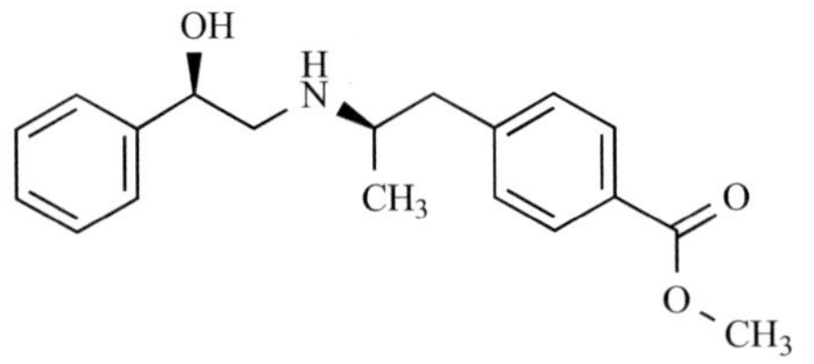	β3-AR agonist
CL 316243	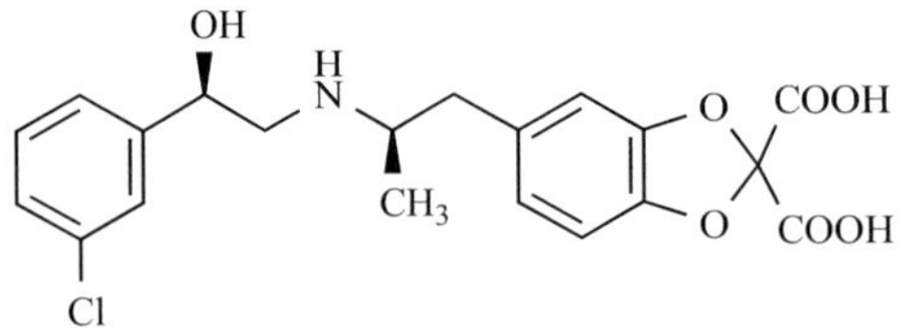	β3-AR agonist
BRL 35135	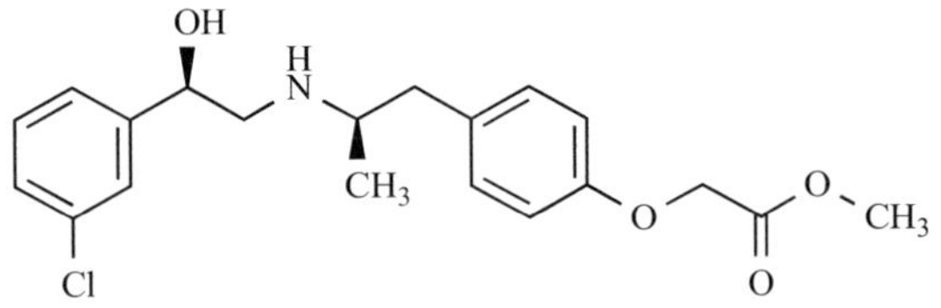	β3-AR agonist
Octopamine	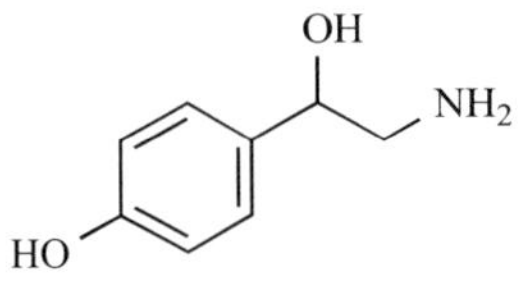	Natural biogenic amine false neurotransmitter in mammals β3-AR agonist MAO and SSAO substrate
Pargyline	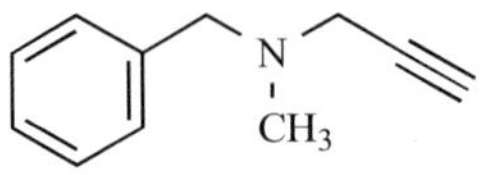	Irreversible inhibitor of MAO
Moclobemide	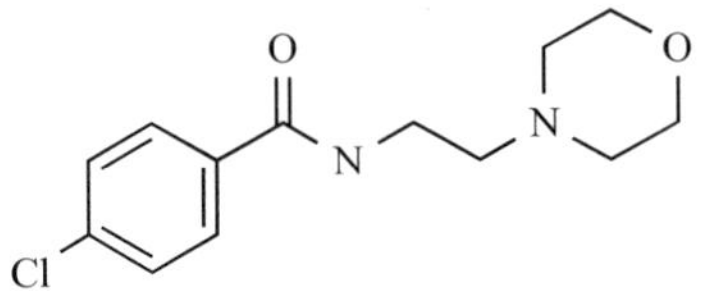	Reversible inhibitor of MAO-A
Clorgyline	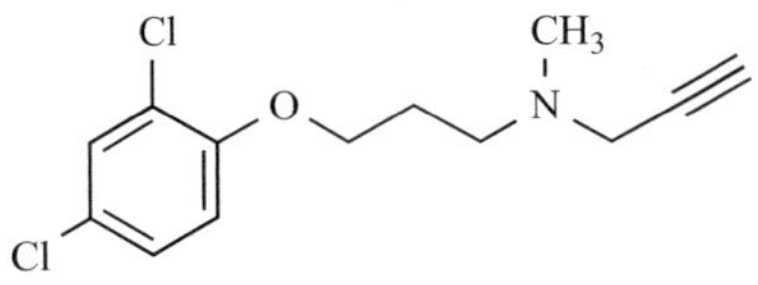	Irreversible inhibitor of MAO-A
R-deprenyl	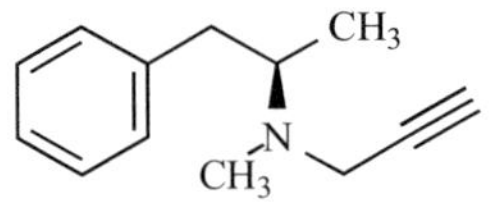	Irreversible inhibitor of MAO-B also known as selegiline
BFI	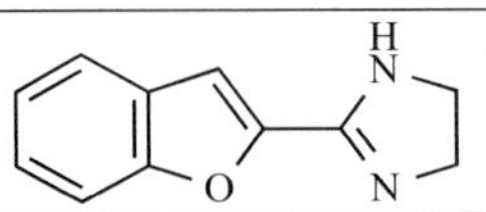	Ligand of imidazoline receptors MAO inhibitor
BU 224	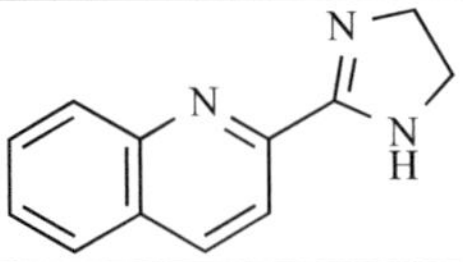	Ligand of imidazoline receptors MAO inhibitor

(Table 3) Contd…..

Name	Chemical Structure	Mode of Action
Phenelzine	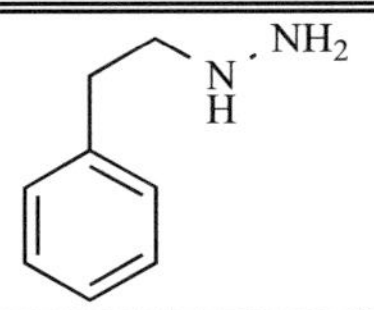	MAO and SSAO inhibitor
Semicarbazide	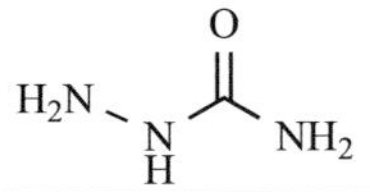	Irreversible inhibitor of LO, SSAO, diamine oxidase
Aminoguanidine	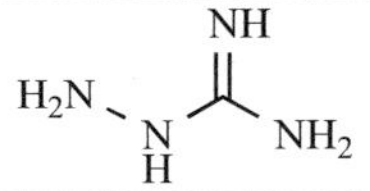	Irreversible inhibitor of LO, SSAO, diamine oxidase and NOS
β-APN	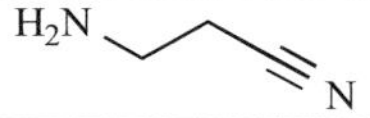	Inhibitor of LO

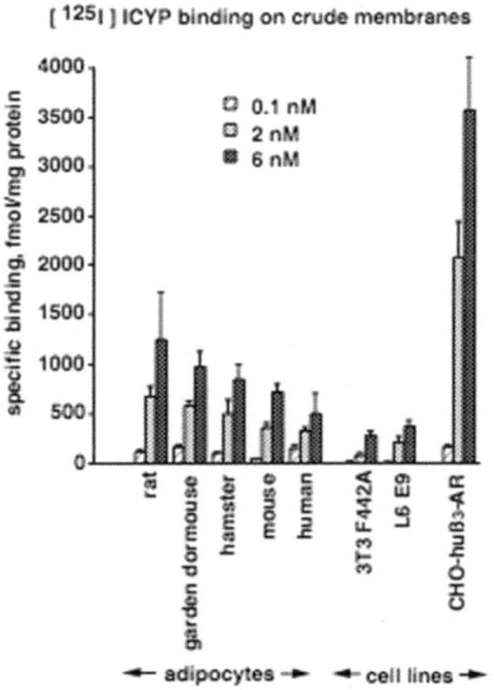

Fig. (1). [^{125}I]-Iodocyanopindolol binding to crude membrane preparations from white adipocytes of different species and from cultured cells. The indicated concentrations of [^{125}I]-Iodocyanopindolol were incubated for 60 min with thawed membranes (approx. 75 μg protein/ml). Non-specific binding was defined by using 0.1 mM bupranolol. Binding experiments and cell culture conditions were performed as described in [28].

Besides lipolysis, thermogenesis was a primary response in rodent brown adipocytes, and the increase of uncoupling proteins was of paramount importance in the whole response to β3-AR agonist treatment. That has prevented β3-AR agonists from being anti-obesity drugs in humans since the most expressed uncoupling protein in the brown fat is UCP1, and since this pivotal step of mitochondrial response to β3-AR activation was even more lacking in humans than their poorly functional adipose β3-ARs. The physiological relevance of brown fat is of borderline interest in humans (even when considering recent findings [29]) when compared to laboratory rodents or wild animals, especially the hibernators, but allows a line of ongoing investigations aimed at reactivating UCPs to mitigate obesity. Definitively, guinea-pigs were not responsive to β3-AR-agonists, regarding fat deposition (Table **4**) while their adipocytes lacked lipolytic response to β3-AR agonists [22, 23]. Since the guinea pig is closer to man in evolutionary terms, any "last chance" to increase UCPs or β3-AR functionality deserves to be tested in this model. This does not imply that guinea pig must be used as a mandatory model during the design of other new anti-obesity drugs, but taken as a whole, the "β3-AR agonist story" tells us that it is of great importance to verify the effects of the drug candidates on human adipose cells or at least on other laboratory models than rat or mouse, even when the candidates are believed to act directly on targets other than the fat cells themselves.

Table 4. CL 316243 Chronic Treatment Does Not Reduce Adipose Tissue Mass in Guinea Pigs

Species:	Rats		Guinea pigs	
Treatment	**Control**	**CL-Treated**	**Control**	**CL-Treated**
INWAT mass, g	5.0 ± 0.3	3.3 ± 0.3 ***	2.3 ± 0.5	1.7 ± 0.3
SCWAT mass, g	3.3 ± 0.2	2.6 ± 0.1 *	1.4 ± 0.2	1.8 ± 0.1

Means ± SEM of 9 rats and 3 guinea pigs one-week treated with CL 316243 at 1 mg/kg/d (CL-treated) or receiving saline (control). Significant effect of treatment at: * $P< 0.05$; *** $P< 0.01$

ADDITION OF EXOGENOUS AMINES: THE CASE OF OCTOPAMINE

The use of products containing ephedrine that were marketed without approval to promote weight-loss have experienced market recalls in several developed countries less than a decade ago. In the subsequent search for substitutive agents that was prompted, *Citrus Aurantium*, believed to increase lipid mobilization, has been considered as a good candidate for such slimming factors. Since *Citrus Aurantium* was demonstrated to be rich in synephrine and octopamine and since we were studying the effect of octopamine on adipocytes [28], we have contributed without any disclosure in comparing its *in vitro* and *in vivo* effects as detailed above. We observed that octopamine, which corresponds to dehydroxylated and demethylated adrenaline (see Table **3**), was able, *in vitro*, to activate lipolysis by activation of β3-ARs. In accordance with the findings exposed above for synthetic agonists it was fully lipolytic in rodent fat cells, not in human adipocytes [28]. Our *in vivo* pilot experiment consisted of treating daily obese Zucker rats with i.p. injection of octopamine (81 μmol/kg) during 25 days. Since octopamine is spontaneously present in mammals at very low levels, it belongs to the family of trace amines, and we hypothesized that exogenous addition would be effective.

The treated rats exhibited a significant decrease of bw-gain at the end of treatment (Fig. **2**). A group of rats was food-restricted (receiving only 23 g/day, *i.e.* 83 % of the rodent chow consumed by the obese controls) since we expected an anorectic effect of the monoamine. At the end of treatment the mean

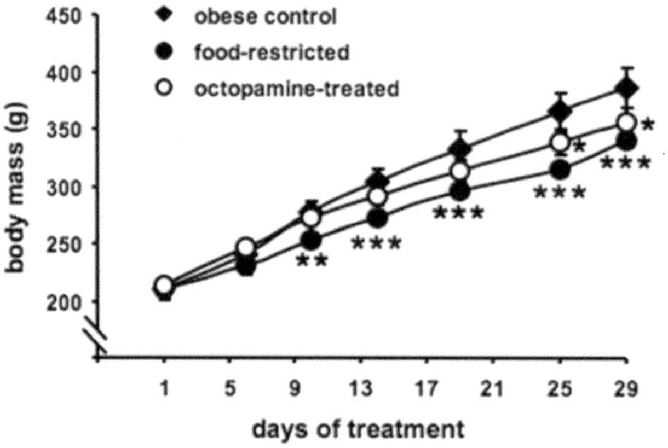

Fig. (2). Influence of octopamine administration on body mass in male Zucker obese rats. Body mass of control obese rats (closed diamonds), food-restricted (receiving 83 % of the calorie intake of untreated obese, closed circles), and obese rats treated daily with i.p. injection of octopamine (81 μmol/kg/day, open circles). Mean ± SEM of five rats. Different from untreated obese at: * $p < 0.05$; ** $p < 0.02$; *** $p < 0.01$. *Redrawn from [30].*

cumulative food consumption was 777 ± 20 g in control, 638 ± 9 g ($p<0.01$) and 697 ± 16 g ($p<0.05$) in food-restricted and in octopamine-treated rats, respectively. Therefore, the anorectic action of i.p. octopamine was confirmed. The bw-gain was 176 ± 12 g in control rats while it was 131 ± 2 g in food-restricted ($p<0.01$) and 143 ± 6 g in octopamine-treated ($p<0.05$), respectively. Thus, octopamine administration in the obese, hyperphagic, Zucker rat was significantly lowering bw-gain. However, octopamine prolonged administration was not producing a specific loss of fat mass since the adiposomatic index was not reduced, when using the visceral fat mass for calculations. Either the percentage of subcutaneous fat or even the percentage of all the dissectible fat depots were not decreased by chronic octopamine. Interestingly, the food restriction did not provoke a significant decrease of the adiposomatic index in young obese rats (as it is the case for starved mature Wistar rats, see Table **2**). In other terms, only a minor part of the 30 to 40 g "lost" in food-restricted or in octopamine-treated rats, when compared to control, could be attributed to WAT. This can be explained by the fact that many "lean" tissues, such as skeletal muscles contain more hidden fat in the obese than in the lean rat.

Thus, in response to the lowered energy intake and to the lipolytic stimulus, the oxidation of endogenous lipids has been performed with fuel mobilized not only from dissectible WAT but also from other smaller depots as well as from skeletal muscles and liver. The WAT is probably more recruited only when the latter origins reach a threshold. Such situation has to be safely facilitated by anti-obesity drugs. It can be concluded that octopamine induced a somewhat general growth retardation, roughly as effective as a 18 % reduction in energy intake, leading to animals having the same fatness but being less heavy than the control rats. In this context, qualifying octopamine as a "slimming agent" is overestimating its properties on energy balance. Whether this more or less slimming action could be extrapolated into a safe method to produce weight loss in obese individuals chronically ingesting octopamine remains to be demonstrated. To our knowledge, the only link found in the medical literature between octopamine ingestion and energy balance is related to the influence of the dietary supplement "Meltdown", the significant effect of which has been recently demonstrated on catecholamine secretion, lipolysis, and metabolic rate in young men and women in a randomized, placebo controlled, cross-over study [31]. It must be specified that octopamine is only one of the numerous components found in the non-completely elucidated composition of the dietary supplement "Meltdown". Moreover, such dietary supplement also increased blood pressure, no more than with a little bout of mild physical exercise, but sufficiently for it to be cautiously considered as a putative adverse effect.

Of note, the extremely elevated plasma insulin levels of obese rats were reduced by one third in the octopamine-treated rats, in spite of an increase of circulating free fatty acids [30]. This led us to suspect an insulin-sensitizing action of the trace amine, which is known to have, like tyramine, its own receptors in insects (for a recent review, consult: [32]).

Octopamine, suspected to be a false neurotransmitter in mammals, shares with other biogenic amines, the property to be a substrate of monoamine oxidases (MAO) involved in the catabolism of monoaminergic neurotransmitters, dietary amines and several xenobiotics. Octopamine is also a substrate for semicarbazide-sensitive amine oxidase (SSAO), a member of the family of copper-containing amine oxidases. Since we previously found that such substrates were able to increase glucose uptake in rodent adipocytes [33], we have verified whether octopamine could also exhibit such insulin-like properties. This functioned only in β3-AR KO mice because octopamine has a dual effect on glucose uptake into adipocytes. On the one hand, its inhibits the effect of insulin, via β3-AR activation [19, 20, 34], on the other hand it activates uptake via the hydrogen peroxide it generates when oxidized by MAO or SSAO [35].

Based on the octopamine's *in vitro* activation of glucose transport in β3-AR KO mouse adipocytes, or on its *in vivo* improvement of circulating insulin in obese Zucker rats, we still need to establish whether octopamine could improve glucose tolerance or mitigate insulin resistance rather than "fat burning" in obese men who are devoid of functional adipose β3-ARs in their WAT [26].

INCREASING AMINE AVAILABILITY BY RE-UPTAKE INHIBITION OR BY OXIDATION INHIBITION

A common way to increase monoamines in the brain and eventually in the body is to use monoamine re-uptake inhibitors. They belong to a large family that encompasses norepine-phrine re-uptake inhibitors (NRIs, reboxetine, mazindol), selective serotonin re-uptake inhibitors (SSRIs, fluoxetine, paroxetine), serotonin-norepinephrine re-uptake inhibitors (SNRIs, duloxetine) and norepinephrine-dopamine re-uptake inhibitors (NDRIs, bupropion).

In this family, there are at least three members that have been used to treat obese patients: sibutramine, fenfluramine, and dexfenfluramine. All increase the levels of the neurotransmitter serotonin (5-hydroxytryptamine; 5-HT) and therefore amplify its action on the 5-HT receptors which exist under the form of more than a dozen subtypes. Sibutramine also inhibits the re-uptake of norepinephrine and that of dopamine, to a lesser extent.

One can reasonably suppose that directly activating the corresponding receptors with exogenous agonists may reproduce the anti-obesity effect of the above-mentioned re-uptake inhibitors. Unfortunately, the complicated serotonergic and adrenergic pharmacology has not facilitated the emergence of a subtype specific agonist that clearly reproduces the effects of sibutramine, fenfluramine, or dexfenfluramine on appetite suppression. Such a challenge had led to drug development strategies in diverse pharmaceutical companies, the results of which have not been entirely published. Indeed, selective serotonin receptor activation is perhaps not the way to substantially reproduce the anorectic effects of the SSRIs/SNRIs without promoting their cardiovascular adverse effects because 5-HT has multifaceted effects involving different 5HT-subtypes and possibly other targets too (idem for adrenergic agonists). Discussing the available results of these investigations is out of the scope of the present review. To summarize, sibutramine one of the utmost important marketed anti-obesity drugs, raises the level of multiple biogenic amines and the sympathetic activity [36]. This prompts us to ask whether other modes of sympathetic activation could help in safely fighting obesity.

Part of the answer was already given in the 80s since many of the antidepressants tested by Dulloo and Miller in animal models of obesity were able to stimulate the activity of the sympathetic nervous system, either by an inhibition of noradrenaline re-uptake (butriptyline) or by inhibiting MAOs (tranylcypromine), and simultaneously increased thermogenesis and energy expenditure [37, 38]. In fact, another way to elevate the above mentioned biogenic amines/neurotransmitters is to protect them from catabolism by amine oxidases. Thus, it has been tested more recently whether other agents inhibiting MAO were able to modify bw-gain in non-obese rats. Fig. (**3**) shows that classical MAO inhibitors reduced bw-gain when repeatedly s.c. administered during two weeks in rats. Under these conditions, the irreversible MAO-A inhibitor clorgyline was more efficient than deprenyl (irreversible MAO-B inhibitor) or than moclobemide

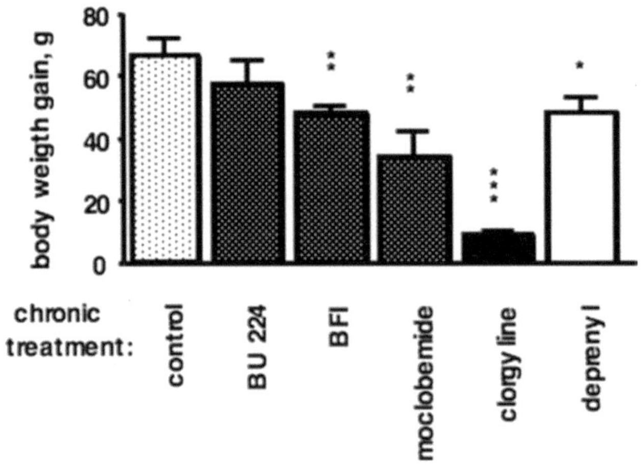

Fig. (3). Body mass gain in control and in rats treated with classical or novel MAO inhibitors. The reversible MAO-inhibitors BU 224, BFI or moclobemide (shaded columns) were administred s.c. at 20 mg/kg/d during 15 days to male Wistar rats of 250 g bw; the irreversible inhibitors of MAO-B (deprenyl) or MAO-A(clorgyline) were administered at 6 mg/kg/d. Mean ± sem of 5 rats per group. Different from control at * p<0.05, ** p<0.01, *** p< <0.001.

(reversible MAO inhibitor). Among the imidazoline compounds, elsewhere shown to inhibit MAO [39], the derivative 2-(2-benzofuranyl)2-imidazoline, named BFI, was able to slow down bw-gain, but not BU 224 (see chemical structures in Table **3**). We have thereafter verified whether such imidazoline derivatives can mitigate obesity in the Zucker obese rat model. The results we saw with BFI (15 mg/kg/d during 3 weeks) showed only a tendency to reduce bw-gain (136 ± 6 *vs.* 123 ± 3 g, n = 4, p>0.09). When chronically administered to lean or obese animals, the I2-ligand BFI was unable to change adiposity and fat cell metabolism [40]. Our data obtained with clorgyline experiments have never been published, in spite of the impressive reduction of bw-gain induced by the irreversible MAO-A inhibitor (control: 91 ± 3 *vs.* 70 ± g in female Zucker obese rats treated for two weeks at 6 mg/kg/d, n = 5, p<0.02) since clorgyline was provoking an exacerbated aggressive behaviour in the treated rats, which led to the cessation of treatment. Increased impulsive aggressiveness is a common feature of MAO-A blockade and has allowed the initial detection of the invalidation of MAO-A in several MAO-A-KO mouse lineages [41].

When studying different dosages of the MAO-A and -B irreversible inhibitor pargyline in obese Zucker rats, we observed that it was without effect on bw-gain at 20 µmol/kg/d but was limiting the growth of male rats (bw-gain: 177 ± 12 *vs.* 135 ± 4, $p<0.01$) or female rats (142 ± 10 *vs.* 117 ± 7, $p<0.05$) when used at around 60 µmol/kg/d. In parallel, we found in isolated adipocytes that the insulin-like effects of various amines were more clearly impaired by the inhibition of both MAO and SSAO than with the separate use of selective inhibitors. Therefore, although SSAO is absent from neurones, it appeared attractive to study not only the influence of MAO inhibitors on obesity but also that of SSAO inhibitors.

INHIBITORS OF AMINE OXIDASES AND BODY WEIGHT REGULATION

Semicarbazide is the reference agent for inhibiting SSAO (see Table **3**); it has been reported that it reduces body weight in at least 4 independent studies:

- The most recent, performed by Takahashi and co-workers [42], showed that when added to the food at 1000 ppm, semicarbazide hydrochloride dramatically reduces bw-gain from the first week of treatment until the end of the experiment 12 weeks later. If one considers that the treated rats weighed 200-300 g and were eating daily 20-25 g/animal of semicarbazide-containing chow depending on their age or sex, then the spontaneous consumption of such food brings an average daily intake of 75-110 mg/kg bw, *i.e.* the equivalent of 700 to 1000 µmol/kg bw/d. At this high dose, many toxicological effects were observed, mainly deformation of connective tissues and articular cartilage, together with loss of bone mass.
- Mercier and colleagues recently reported that the daily i.p. administration of semicarbazide at 900 µmol/kg bw/d (*i.e.* similar dose as above) to Brown Norway rats induced a similar body wt loss [43]. However, this strain presents spontaneous arterial defects that have been seriously increased by the 12-week treatment. The treated animals exhibited decreased resistance of arteries to pressure as a consequence of arterial extracellular matrix disorganization, and inhibition of SSAO and LOX in vascular tissues.
- We observed that, at 900 µmol/kg bw/d, semicarbazide decreased both bw-gain and adiposomatic index in mice (Table **5**). Formerly, we observed under similar conditions a reduced bw-gain in the Sprague Dawley rats [15], together a significant decrease of adiposomatic index (Table **5**). However, a three-fold lower dose of semicarbazide did not provoke such growth retardation and WAT decline in rats (Table **5**). This 300 µmol/kg/d dose was accompanied with fewer deleterious effects than in the two studies above. However it was devoid of slimming action while it completely inhibited SSAO activity, at least in WAT [15].
- In obese (Zucker) [44], as well as in lean (Wistar) [15] rats, a chronic treatment with the low dose semicarbazide together with pargyline induced a significant reduction of bw-gain and of adiposity without detectable side-effects, indicating that the combined inhibition of several amine oxidases should be more effective than the inhibition of SSAO.

Table 5. Effect of Semicarbazide Treatments on Body Weight Gain and Visceral Adiposity in Different Animal Models

Condition/Model	Control	Semicarbazide-Treated
Sprague-Dawley male rats treated 7 weeks with i.p. 900 mmol/kg/d (n = 11)		
body weight gain, g	296.5 ± 10.5	248.1 ± 2.3 **
adiposomatic index, %	1.7 ± 0.1	1.3 ± 0.1 ***
FVB/n male mice treated during 8 weeks with p.o. 900 µmol/kg/d (n = 9)		
body weight gain, g	6.9 ± 0.7	2.0 ± 0.6 ***
adiposomatic index, %	3.0 ± 0.2	2.1 ± 0.2 ***
Wistar male rats treated during 4 weeks with i.p. 300 µmol/kg/d (n = 5)		
body weight gain, g	152.9 ± 9.6	150.6 ± 9.4 NS
adiposomatic index, %	3.6 ± 0.4	2.9 ± 0.2 NS
Zucker male rats treated during 4 weeks with i.p. 300 µmol/kg/d (n = 5)		
body weight gain, g	176.5 ± 11.8	174.2 ± 10.4 NS
adiposomatic index, %	3.3 ± 0.1	3.3 ± 0.2 NS

Adiposomatic index is % INWAT/bw. Different from control at: ** $p < 0.01$; *** $p < 0.001$.

From these observations, it could be concluded that SSAO inhibition is necessary but not sufficient to assign anti-obesity properties to chronically administered semicarbazide. Two other findings support this point of view. Firstly, P. Yu and colleagues serendipitously observed that fluorophenetyl-fluoroallylamine, a SSAO- and MAO-inhibitor, produces a slimming effect in obese and diabetic KKAy mice [45]. Secondly, aminoguanidine (a multipotent drug able to irreversibly block copper-containing amine oxidases, including SSAO, but also nitric oxide synthases) slightly reduces fat deposition in obese rats [46].

In this context, a comparison between semicarbazide and other inhibitors of copper-containing amine oxidases was performed regarding their inhibitory action of fat depot enlargement. The results reported in Table **6** show that only the complete inhibition of SSAO activity in intra-abdominal fat depot, obtained with the high dose of semicarbazide, was concomitant with an impairment of body weight and fat deposition. Since we have already reported that fat depot mobilization is not accompanied by a decrease in SSAO activity in rats subjected to prolonged fasting [47], one can suppose that the fat depletion observed in the semicarbazide-treated rats was not the cause of the SSAO inhibition. On the contrary, it might be suspected that the fat depletion was a consequence of the irreversible SSAO blockade by semicarbazide. Even if semicarbazide was also inhibiting Lysyl oxidase (LO), this latter action was not necessary or sufficient to induce fat mass loss since beta-aminopropionitrile (beta-APN), a well-recognized LO-inhibitor, which did not impair SSAO activity, did not significantly limit fat enlargement. So, LO inhibition was not sufficient to reduce bw-gain (Table **6**) but was likely implied in the adverse effects of semicarbazide on conjonctive tissues and bones, The combination of beta-APN and semicarbazide resulted in reduction of visceral fat but concomitantly with considerable growth retardation (reduced nose-rump length), probably resulting from the toxicity of this combination [43]. The comparison between semicarbazide and beta-APN allows to propose that SSAO has a role in WAT development, but did not rule out semicarbazide acting on other targets than this copper-containing amine oxidase highly expressed in adipose tissue. In fact, semicarbazide has been reported as inhibiting glutamic acid decarboxylase [48] or sphingosine-1-phosphate lyase [49].

Table 6. Body Mass, Mass and SSAO Activity in Epididymal (EPI WAT) and Perirenal (PERI WAT) Adipose Tissues of Rats Treated with Semicarbazide and Beta-APN

Treatment:	Control	Semicarbazide	Beta-APN	Semi + Beta-APN
		Mass at sacrifice, g		
Body	260 ± 12	217 ± 10 *	243 ± 7	155 ± 7***
EPI WAT	2.03 ± 0.13	1.65 ± 0.17	1.95 ± 0.20	1.27 ± 0.21 *
PERI WAT	0.86 ± 0.22	0.35 ± 0.10 *	0.82 ± 0.17	0.23 ± 0.08 *
		SSAO activity, nmol benzylamine oxidized/mg protein/min		
EPI WAT	2.22 ± 0.33	0.04 ± 0.01 ***	1.36 ± 0.46	0.05 ± 0.01 ***
PERI WAT	2.63 ± 0.20	0.06 ± 0.01 ***	2.34 ± 0.54	0.09 ± 0.01 ***

Weight-matched groups of male Brown-Norway rats daily received i.p. injection of semicarbazide at 900 μmol/kg (Semi), beta-aminopropionitrile at 710 μmol/kg (beta-APN), or both for 8 weeks before sacrifice. Mean ± SEM of five rats. Different from control at: * $p < 0.05$, *** $p < 0.001$.

Certainly, SSAO inhibition was probably not the sole mechanism underlying the slim-ming effects of high doses of semicarbazide administered in young rats or mice. The genetic invalidation of SSAO has not the same inhibitor effect on adipose tissue development as the pharmacological inhibitors. The mice deficient in AOC3, a gene encoding for SSAO, have several vascular troubles; such as enlarged aortas [50], present less infiltrated leukocytes in their tissues, including WAT [51] and other defects that are analyzed by ongoing research, but they are far from being less fat than their wild-type controls since they exhibit an overweight occurring with ageing [51]. Whether AOC3-KO mice, lacking functional SSAO, respond to semicarbazide treatment remains to be determined.

The above comparison between beta-APN and semicarbazide argued that the inhibition of SSAO, highly expressed in adipocytes, was probably more implied in adiposity alteration than that of LO, mainly present in the blood vessels. The difference between semicarbazide treated animals and AOC3 KO mice, also observed at the vascular level [50, 52], allows us to suppose that semicarbazide was not solely inhibiting SSAO. Moreover caution is warranted regarding SSAO inhibition, because the enzyme highly expressed in WAT [53] is also present in vascular smooth muscle cells, and involved in cell matrix regulation [54]. SSAO is also present at the endothelium surface and involved in leukocyte migration [55]. Since MAO was also present in adipocytes, and since both MAO and SSAO substrates can elicit short- and long-term insulin-like effect on cultured adipocytes [56], attention was focused on MAO-and SSAO-combined treatments.

EFFECTS OF COMBINED INHIBITION OF MAO AND SSAO ON BODY WEIGHT REGULATION

We observed that the combination of pargyline and semicarbazide led to complete inhibition of MAO and SSAO in the INWAT of non obese rats receiving respectively 60 and 300 μmol inhibitor/kg/d [15]. The *in vitro* insulin-like effects of tyramine and benzylamine (inhibition of lipolysis and stimulation of hexose transport) were deeply impaired in the adipocytes isolated from the treated animals. This could partly explain the limited fat accretion after MAO- and SSAO-blockade. Fig. (**4**) shows the effects of pargyline plus semicarbazide in the male obese Zucker rats. Again, complete inhibition of both MAO and SSAO was reached only with the combination of both inhibitors in the hyperphagic, hyperinsulinemic model [44]. Regarding food intake, the fact that combined SSAO and MAO inhibition down-regulates food intake in the Zucker obese rats indicates that the implied mechanism does not require intact leptin signalling and therefore can be extrapolated to man, since most of the obese patients are leptin-resistant. Regarding body weight gain, the reduction obtained with pargyline plus semicarbazide was similar to that observed in pair-fed animals (corresponding to a 17% reduction relative to the *ad libitum* intake of control group). Fat accretion was more reduced in the inhibitor-treated than in the pair-fed group while they shared similar growth retardation and calorie restriction (Fig. **4**). Thus MAO and SSAO inhibition was probably impairing fat accumulation in a more pronounced manner than the simple calorie restriction.

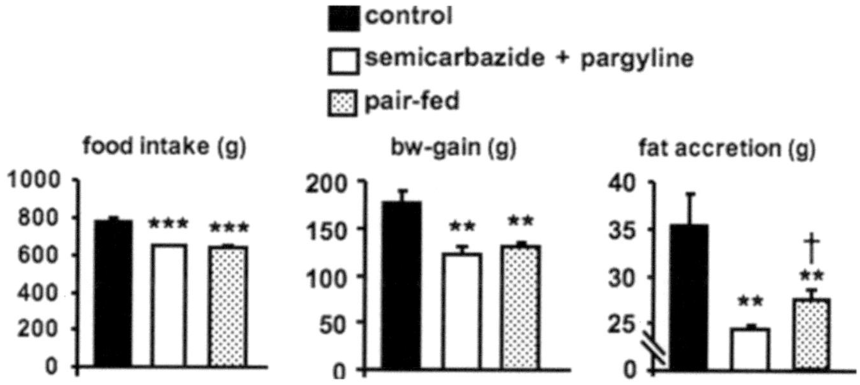

Fig. (4). Influence of 4-week treatment by amine oxidases inhibitors on cumulative food intake, weight gain and fat accretion in obese rats. Fat accretion in WAT was estimated by subtracting to the WAT mass at sacrifice a reference value of 25 g, *i.e.* the average WAT mass in age- and weight-matched rats at the beginning of the treatment. Mean ± sem of 5 male Zucker rats per group. Different from control at: ** $p < 0.01$; *** $p < 0.001$. Difference between pair-fed and semicarbazide (300 μmol/kg/d) + pargyline (60 μmol/kg/d) treated at: † $p < 0.05$.

Similar observations were made when female obese rats were treated with MAO plus SSAO inhibitors [44]. The bw-gain was reduced from 114 ± 6 to 86 ± 7 g in control and pargyline plus semicarbazide-treated rats, respectively (n = 5-6, $p<0.01$). The percentage of INWAT + SCWAT relative to bw was also reduced from 18.5 ± 0.4 to 16.7 ± 0.3 % ($p<0.01$), indicating that, as in males, a specific lipid mobilization was participating in the reduction of bw-gain. So, the female obese rats receiving pargyline plus semicarbazide were less heavy and slimmer than their controls. The combined inhibition appeared to be necessary to protect amines from catabolic pathways and to influence body weight regulatory systems. However, there is little motivation for pharmaceutical companies to develop cocktails of multiple agents. As several molecules are known to inhibit both MAO and SSAO, we studied whether one of them, phenelzine was exhibiting anti-obesity properties.

On the one hand, as recommended above, *in vitro* studies on both murine and human cultured preadipocytes showed that phenelzine inhibited triacylglycerol accumulation mainly by impairing the action of the lipogenic transcription factor SREBP1 [57]. On the other hand, phenelzine was tested *in vivo* at the dose of 17 μmol/kg/d on obese Zucker rats. An inhibitory effect on body weight of female Zucker rats appeared after the second week of i.p. treatment, and at the end of 3-week treatment, the bw-gain was

116 ± 2 and + 102 ± 4 g for control and phenelzine-treated obese rats, respectively ($n = 5$, $p<0.05$). Phenelzine treatment altered by only less than 2 % the cumulative food consumption over the same period. At sacrifice, INWAT was significantly smaller in phenelzine-treated rats. Consequently, their adiposomatic index was reduced from 7.1 ± 0.2 to 6.3 ± 0.2 % ($p<0.02$) but SCWAT mass did not exhibit any significant change (14.8 ± 0.4 *vs.* 13.8 ± 1.1 %). As expected, both MAO and SSAO activities were strongly inhibited in adipose tissues. Thus, phenelzine clearly limited body weight gain in obese rats and did specifically reduce their visceral adiposity. Very recently, we observed that phenelzine impairs *in vitro* the lipogenic response to insulin in rodent adipocytes (Carpéné C., unpublished data). These observations bring novel insight into an old drug used for its antidepressive properties from long ago. However, there is a discrepancy with numerous clinical observations that generally report a bw-gain promoted by antidepressant drugs [58], including MAO inhibitors, and less often a weight loss. In the case of phenelzine, weight gain is a common side effect observed in clinical use [59], even in young patients [60]. This weight gain has been reported as reaching an extent comparable to tricyclic antidepressants, even if the contribution of increased adiposity remains unknown. This apparent discrepancy between clinical observations and our experimental data must be analyzed cautiously. Firstly, many psychiatric disorders are associated *per se* with weight changes, most often with weight loss. Thus, it was thought that drug-induced weight gain merely reflects the restoration of normal body weight. Secondly, the production of dry mouth and thirst by psychotropic drugs appears to contribute to weight gain, due to consumption of high-calorie beverages. Otherwise, the general mechanisms influencing body weight during treatment for mental disorders are still far from clear, and will probably include disease-related, improvement-related, and drug-related factors. This still open debate will not prevent to further study into the putative anti-obesity effects of phenelzine in other obesity models or in clinical trials.

CONCLUSION

In conclusion, several molecules belonging to the major classes of antidepressants, such as monoamine re-uptake inhibitors, but also MAO inhibitors employed to treat severe depression, may represent similar usefulness for pharmacological treatment of alterations of food intake and/or energy expenditure. However, their effect in peripheral tissues may be revealed in the future to be as important as their well-recognized actions on the central nervous system. In this way, the inhibition of peripheral SSAO, which is not expressed in neurones, but which is abundant in fat cells, represents a fascinating novel approach to modulate adipose tissue physiology. However, such approach requires further experimental studies before being applied in the field of anti-obesity drug discovery.

ACKNOWLEDGEMENTS

The authors wish to express their gratitude to V. Visentin, S. Bour, X. Brenachot, J. Mercader and D. Prévot, for invaluable help, and to A. Desquesnes and S. Le Gonidec for biochemical analyses at ANEXPLO platform, as well as to the staff of animal unit of I2MR, Toulouse, for animal handling. Thanks to N. Mercier (Inserm U961, Nancy) for providing us with biological material and advices related to the experiments reported in Table **6**. The expertise of P. Valet and all members of his Adipolab team regarding adipose tissue physiology is gratefully acknowledged. Some of the studies reported were supported by grants facilitating Franco-Hungarian (Balaton) and Franco-Spanish (CTP network) exchanges and by INTERREG IVB-SUDOE-FEDER project (DIOMED, SOE1/P1/E178).

REFERENCES

[1] Foster-Schubert KE, Cummings DE. Emerging therapeutic strategies for obesity. Endocr Rev 2006; 27: 779-93.

[2] Vincent RP, le Roux CW. New agents in development for the management of obesity. Int J Clin Pract 2007; 61: 2103-12.

[3] Hube F, Hauner H. The role of TNF-alpha in human adipose tissue: prevention of weight gain at the expense of insulin resistance? Horm Metab Res 1999; 31: 626-31.

[4] Aubert J, Dessolin S, Belmonte N, Li M, McKenzie FR, Staccini L, *et al.* Leukemia inhibitory factor and its receptor promote adipocyte differentiation via the mitogen-activated protein kinase cascade. J Biol Chem 1999; 274: 24965-72.

[5] Hogan JC, Stephens JM. Effects of leukemia inhibitory factor on 3T3-L1 adipocytes. J Endocrinol 2005; 185: 485-96.

[6] El Hadri K, Glorian M, Monsempes C, *et al. In vitro* suppression of the lipogenic pathway by the nonnucleoside reverse transcriptase inhibitor efavirenz in 3T3 and human preadipocytes or adipocytes. J Biol Chem 2004; 279: 15130-41.

[7] Valet P, Tavernier G, Castan-Laurell I, Saulnier-Blache JS, Langin D. Understanding adipose tissue development from transgenic animal models. J Lipid Res 2002; 43: 835-60.

[8] Atgié C, Hadj-Sassi L, Bukowiecki L, Mauriège P. High lipolytic activity and dyslipidemia in a spontaneous hypertensive/NIH corpulent (SHR/N-*cp*) rat: a genetic model of obesity and type 2 diabetes mellitus. J Physiol Biochem 2009; 65: 33-42.

[9] Heal DJ. Sibutramine: a novel anti-obesity drug. A review of the pharmacological evidence to differentiate it from d-amphetamine and d-fenfluramine. Int J Obes 1998; 22(suppl 1): S18-S28.

[10] Richardson DK, Jones RB, Bailey CJ. The primary amine metabolite of sibutramine stimulates lipolysis in adipocytes isolated from lean and obese mice and in isolated human adipocytes. Horm Metab Res 2006; 38: 727-31.

[11] Gauthier MS, Miyoshi H, Souza SC, *et al.* AMP-activated protein kinase is activated as a consequence of lipolysis in the adipocyte: potential mechanism and physiological relevance. J Biol Chem 2008; 283: 16514-24.

[12] Lafontan M, Piazza PV, Girard J. Effects of CB1 antagonist on the control of metabolic functions in obese type 2 diabetic patients. Diabetes Metab 2007; 33: 85-95.

[13] Wanecq E, Bour S, Verwaerde P, Smih F, Valet P, Carpéné C. Increased monoamine oxidase and semicarbazide-sensitive amine oxidase activities in white adipose tissue of obese dogs fed a high-fat diet. J Physiol Biochem 2006; 62(2): 113-23.

[14] Bays H, Ballantyne C. Adiposopathy: why do adiposity and obesity cause metabolic disease? Future Lipidol 2006; 1: 389-420.

[15] Carpéné C, Abello V, Iffiú-Soltész Z, Mercier N, Fève B, Valet P. Limitation of adipose tissue enlargement in rats chronically treated with semicarbazide-sensitive amine oxidase and monoamine oxidase inhibitors. Pharmacol Res 2008; 57: 426-34.

[16] Arch JRS, Ainsworth AT, Cawthorne MA, *et al.* Atypical β-adrenoceptor on brown adipocytes as target for anti-obesity drugs. Nature 1984; 309: 163-5.

[17] Emorine LJ, Marullo S, Briend-Sutren MM, *et al.* Molecular characterization of the human β3-adrenergic receptor. Science 1989; 245: 1118-21.

[18] Liu YL, Cawthorne MA, Stock MJ. Biphasic effects of the beta-adrenoceptor agonist, BRL 37344, on glucose utilization in rat isolated skeletal muscle. Br J Pharmacol 1996; 117: 1355-61.

[19] Carpéné C, Chalaux E, Lizarbe M, *et al.* β_3-adrenergic receptors are responsible for the adrenergic inhibition of insulin-stimulated glucose transport in rat adipocytes. Biochem J 1993; 296: 99-105.

[20] Yen ST, Li MH, Hsu CT, Lee TL, Cheng JT. Stimulatory effect of octopamine on β3-adrenoceptors to lower the uptake of [14C]-deoxy-D-glucose into rat adipocytes *in vitro* J Autonomic Pharmacol 1998; 18: 13-9.

[21] El-Khatib AS, Moustafa AM, Abdel-Aziz A-AH, Al-Shabanah OA, El-Kashef HA. Effects of aminoguanidine and desferrioxamine on some vascular and biochemical changes associated with streptozotocin-induced hyperglycaemia in rats. Pharmacol Res 2001; 43: 233-40.

[22] Ferrand C, Redonnet A, Prévot D, Carpéné C, Atgié C. Prolonged treatment with the β3-adrenergic agonist CL 316243 induces adipose tissue remodeling in rat but not in guinea pig: 1) fat store depletion and desensitization of β-adrenergic responses. J Physiol Biochem 2006; 62: 89-100.

[23] Duffaut C, Bour S, Prévot D, *et al.* Prolonged treatment with the β3-adrenergic agonist CL 316243 induces adipose tissue remodeling in rat but not in guinea pig: 2) modulation of glucose uptake and monoamine oxidase activity. J Physiol Biochem 2006; 62: 101-12.

[24] Arch JRS. The discovery of drugs for obesity, the metabolic effects of leptin and variable receptor pharmacology: perspectives from β3-adrenoceptor agonists. Naunyn-Schmiedebergs Arch Pharmacol 2008; 378: 225-40.

[25] Ngala RA, O'Dowd J, Wang SJ, Agarwal A, Stocker C, Cawthorne MA, *et al.* Metabolic responses to BRL37344 and clenbuterol in soleus muscle and C2C12 cells via different atypical pharmacologies and beta2-adrenoceptor mechanisms. Br J Pharmacol 2008; 155: 395-406.

[26] Carpéné C, Bousquet-Mélou A, Galitzky J, Berlan M, Lafontan M. Lypolytic effects of $beta_1$-,$beta_2$-, and $beta_3$-adrenergic agonists in white adipose tissue of mammals. Ann N Y Sci 1998; 839: 186-9.

[27] Emorine L, Blin N, Strosberg AD. The human β3-adrenoceptor: the search for a physiologic function. Trends Pharmacol Sci 1994; 15: 3-6.

[28] Carpéné C, Galitzky J, Fontana E, Atgié C, Lafontan M, Berlan M. Selective activation of $beta_3$-adrenoceptors by octopamine: comparative studies in mammalian fat cells. Naunyn-Schmiedebergs Arch Pharmacol 1999; 359: 310-21.

[29] Nedergaard J, Bengtsson T, Cannon B. Unexpected evidence for active brown adipose tissue in adult humans. Am J Physiol Endocrinol Metab 2007; 293: E444-52.

[30] Bour S, Visentin V, Prévot D, Carpéné C. Moderate weight-lowering effect of octopamine treatment in obese Zucker rats. J Physiol Biochem 2003; 59: 175-82.

[31] Bloomer RJ, Canale RE, Blankenship MM, Hammond KG, Fisher-Wellman KH, Schilling BK. Effect of the dietary supplement meltdown on catecholamine secretion, markers of lipolysis, and metabolic rate in men and women: a randomized, placebo controlled, cross-over study. Lipids Health Dis 2009; 8: 32.

[32] Lange AB. Tyramine: from octopamine precursor to neuroactive chemical in insects. Gen Comp Endocrinol 2009; 162: 18-26.

[33] Enrique-Tarancon G, Castan I, Morin N, Marti L, Abella A, Camps M, *et al.* Substrates of semicarbazide-sensitive amine oxidase cooperate with vanadate to stimulate tyrosine phosphorylation of IRS proteins, phosphatidylinositol 3-kinase activity and GLUT4 translocation in adipose cells. Biochem J 2000; 350: 171-80.

[34] Fontana E, Morin N, Prévot D, Carpéné C. Effects of octopamine on lipolysis, glucose transport and amine oxidation in mammalian fat cells. Comp Biochem Physiol C 2000; 125: 33-44.

[35] Visentin V, Morin N, Fontana E, *et al.* Dual action of octopamine on glucose transport into adipocytes: inhibition via β_3-adrenoceptor activation and stimulation via oxidation by amine oxidases. J Pharmacol Exp Ther 2001; 299: 96-104.

[36] Hirsch J, Mackintosh RM, Aronne LJ. The effects of drugs used to treat obesity on the autonomic nervous system. Obes Res 2000; 8: 227-33.

[37] Dulloo AG, Miller DS. Thermogenic drugs for the treatment of obesity: sympathetic stimulants in animal models. Br J Nutr 1984; 52: 179-96.

[38] Dulloo AG, Miller DS. Screening of drugs for thermogenic anti-obesity properties: antidepressants. Ann Nutr Metab 1987; 31: 69-80.

[39] Holt A. Imidazoline binding sites on receptors and enzymes: emerging targets for novel antidepressant drugs? J Psychiatry Neurosci 2003; 28: 409-14.

[40] Bour S, Iglesias-Osma MC, Marti L, Duro P, Garcia-Barrado M, Pastor M-F, *et al.* The imidazoline I2-site ligands BU 224 and 2-BFI inhibit MAO-A and MAO-B activities, hydrogen peroxide production, and lipolysis in rodent and human adipocytes. Eur J Pharmacol 2006; 552: 20-30.

[41] Scott AL, Bortolato M, Chen K, Shih JC. Novel monoamine oxidase A knock out mice with human-like spontaneous mutation. Neuroreport 2008; 19: 739-43.

[42] Takahashi M, Yoshida M, Inoue K, Morikawa T, Nishikawa A. A ninety-day toxicity study of semicarbazide hydrochloride in Wistar Hannover GALAS rats. Food Chem Toxicol 2009; 47: 2490-8.

[43] Mercier N, Kakou A, Challande P, Lacolley P, Osborne-Pellegrin M. Comparison of the effects of semicarbazide and β-aminopropionitrile on the arterial extracellular matrix in the Brown Norway rat. Toxicol Appl Pharmacol 2009; 239: 258-67.

[44] Carpéné C, Iffiú-Soltesz Z, Bour S, Prévot D, Valet P. Reduction of fat deposition by combined inhibition of monoamine oxidases and semicarbazide-sensitive amine oxidases in obese Zucker rats. Pharmacol Res 2007; 56: 522-30.

[45] Yu PH, Wang M, Fan H, Deng Y, Gubisne-Haberle D. Involvement of SSAO-mediated deamination in adipose glucose transport and weight gain in obese diabetic KKAy mice. Am J Physiol Endocrinol Metab 2004; 286: E634-E41.

[46] Prévot D, Soltesz Z, Abello V, *et al.* Prolonged treatment with aminoguanidine strongly inhibits adipocyte semicarbazide-sensitive amine oxidase and slightly reduces fat deposition in obese Zucker rats. Pharmacol Res 2007; 56: 70-9.

[47] Iffiú-Soltész Z, Prévot D, Carpéné C. Influence of prolonged fasting on monoamine oxidase and semicarbazide-sensitive amine oxidase activities in rat white adipose tissue. J Physiol Biochem 2009; 65: 11-23.

[48] Borelli KG, Ferreira-Netto C, Brandao ML. Distribution of Fos immunoreactivity in the rat brain after freezing or escape elicited by inhibition of glutamic acid decarboxylase or antagonism of GABA-A receptors in the inferior colliculus. Behav Brain Res 2006; 170: 84-93.

[49] Bandhuvula P, Fyrst H, Saba JD. A rapid fluorescence assay for sphingosine-1-phosphate lysase enzyme activity. J Lipid Res 2007; 48: 2769-78.

[50] Mercier N, Osborne-Pellegrin M, El Hadri K, *et al.* Carotid arterial stiffness, elastic fibre network and vasoreactivity in semicarbazide-sensitive amine-oxidase null mouse. Cardiovasc Res 2006; 72: 349-57.

[51] Bour S, Caspar-Bauguil S, Iffiú-Soltész Z, *et al.* Semicarbazide-sensitive amine oxidase/vascular adhesion protein-1 deficiency reduces leukocyte infiltration into adipose tissue and favors fat deposition. Am J Pathol 2009; 174: 1075-83.

[52] Mercier N, El Hadri K, Osborne-Pellegrin M, *et al.* Modifications of arterial phenotype in response to amine oxidase inhibition by semicarbazide. Hypertension 2007; 50: 234-41.

[53] Bour S, Daviaud D, Gres S, *et al.* Adipogenesis-related increase of semicarbazide-sensitive amine oxidase and monoamine oxidase in human adipocytes. Biochimie 2007; 89: 916-25.

[54] Conklin DJ, Langford SD, Boor PJ. Contribution of serum and cellular semicarbazide-sensitive amine oxidase to amine metabolism and cardiovascular toxicity. Toxicol Sci 1998; 46(2): 386-92.

[55] Jalkanen S, Karikoski M, Mercier N, *et al.* The oxidase activity of vascular adhesion protein-1 (VAP-1) induces endothelial E- and P-selectins and leukocyte binding. Blood 2007; 110: 1864-70.

[56] Carpéné C, Daviaud D, Boucher J, *et al.* Short-and long-term insulinlike effects of substrates of monoamine oxidases and semicarbazide-sensitive amine oxidases in cultured adipocytes. Metabolism 2006; 55: 1397-405.

[57] Chiche F, Le Guillou M, Chetrite G, *et al.* The antidepressant phenelzine alters differentiation of cultured human and mouse preadipocytes. Mol Pharmacol 2009; 75: 1052-61.

[58] Fava M. Weight gain and antidepressants. J Clin Psychiatry 2000; 61 (Suppl 11): 37-41.

[59] Bernstein JG. Induction of obesity by psychotropic drugs. Ann N Y Acad Sci 1987; 499: 203-15.

[60] Golwyn DH, Sevlie CP. Phenelzine treatment of selective mutism in four prepubertal children. J Child Adolesc Psychopharmacol 1999; 9: 109-13.

Rimonabant for Obesity

Cintia Curioni[*,1], Cintia Azara[2] and Jane Capelli[3]

[1]*Departamento de Nutrição Social, Universidade do Estado do Rio de Janeiro, Rua S Francisco Xavier, 524 – Maracanã, Rio de Janeiro - RJ, 20550-900, Brazil*

[2]*Faculdade Arthur Sá Earp Neto, Av. Barão do Rio Branco 1003, Centro Petrópolis/RJ, 25680-120, Brazil*

[3]*Universidade Federal do Rio de Janeiro, Campus Macaé – Curso de Nutrição, Rua Aluísio da Silva Gomes, 50, Granja dos Cavaleiros – Macaé – RJ, CEP: 27930-560, Brazil*

Abstract: According to the World Health Organization, obesity is a multifactorial disease with increasing frequency in many countries that can be characterized as an epidemic of major public health concern. Recognized since 1985 as a chronic disease, obesity is the second leading cause of preventable death, exceeded only by cigarette smoking. Obesity has been established as a major risk factor for diabetes, hypertension, cardiovascular disease and some cancers in both men and women. The general goals of obesity treatment are to reduce body weight, to maintain a lower body weight over the long term or to prevent further weight gain. Traditional methods to promote weight loss focus on reducing energy intake through low-calorie or low-fat diets, increasing energy expenditure by increase in physical activity, and behavioral modification. Numerous other weight loss interventions are available including pharmacotherapy, surgery to reduce food consumption and alternative therapies. Although the pharmacological treatment of obesity should not be the first therapeutic option, its use is now fully approved. Rimonabant is a selective cannabinoid-1 receptor antagonist that has been suggested to reduce hunger and consumption by affecting the endocannabinoid system. Rimonabant has entered the market in some countries as a promising new drug for obesity. However, although effective as an anti-obesity drug, rimonabant also causes serious adverse side-effects, thus is being doubted and denied for medical usage. This chapter focuses on the role of rimonabant as anti-obesity drug, elucidating the mechanisms of action, the main results of clinical trials, FDA and EMEA recommendations, and the future perspectives.

Keywords: Obesity, endocannabinoid system, rimonabant.

INTRODUCTION

The introduction of modern culture brings with it a change to subsistence patterns. A significant change has occurred in lifestyle in contemporary society. Changes in the food consumed and in the patterns of eating behavior associated with decreased levels of physical activity may have contributed to increasing risk of obesity. Furthermore, increasing prevalence of obesity in a population is an early indicator of emerging health burden due to non-communicable chronic diseases such as cardiovascular diseases, hypertension and diabetes. Not only this, obesity also has drastic social, economic and psychological consequences.

Obesity is a complex, multifactorial chronic disease that develops from an interaction of genotype and the environment. Worldwide, the prevalence of obesity and overweight is increasing at an alarming rate and according to World Health Organization (WHO), more than 1 billion adults are overweight - and at least 300 million of them are clinically obese [1].

Obesity is prevalent in both developed and developing countries, particularly those in rapid transition, and is affecting both children and adults. Indeed, it is now so common that is replacing the more traditional public health concerns, as one of the most significant contributors to ill health [1].

In the USA, adult obesity rates rose from 14.25% in 1978 to 31% in 2000. In the UK, adult obesity rates rose from 6% of men and 8% of women in 1980, to 21% of men and 23.5% of women in 2001. The World Health Report 2002 estimated that worldwide >2.5 million deaths per year are weight related – 220,000 per year in Europe and >300,000 per year in USA [2]. Obesity accounts for 2-6% of total health care costs in

*Corresponding author: Tel: +55 24 22446464; Fax: +55 24 22446464; E-mails: c_curioni@uol.com.br, c_curioni@hotmail.com

several developed countries; some estimates put the figure as high as 7%. The true costs are undoubtedly much greater as not all obesity-related conditions are included in the calculations.

Obesity is seen as a disease, which requires treatment. Treatment means, first of all, weight reduction. The general goals of weight loss and management are to reduce body weight; and to maintain a lower body weight over the long term; or at a minimum, to prevent further weight gain. There is strong evidence that weight loss (5% to 15% of the body weight) in obese individuals reduces risk factors associated with obesity [3].

Traditional methods to promote weight loss focus on reducing energy intake through low-calorie or low-fat diets, increasing energy expenditure by increase in physical activity, and behavioral modification. The inclusion of exercise in a weight reduction program is supposed to make the weight loss easier, compared with food restriction alone. However, the effectiveness of these weight reduction methods is limited; with an overall pattern of moderate weight loss followed by gradual weight regain [4]. Numerous other weight loss interventions are available including pharmacotherapy, surgery to reduce food consumption and alternative therapies.

Rimonabant is a selective cannabinoid-1 receptor antagonist that has been investigated for its efficacy in reducing body weight and associated risk factors in obese people [5]. The cannabinoid-1 receptor plays a role in the regulation of appetite and body weight.

The purpose of this chapter is to discuss the role of rimonabant as anti-obesity drug, elucidating the mechanisms of action, the main results of clinical trials, the position of drug agencies and the future perspectives. Given the prevalence of overweight and obesity, it is important to assess the possible impact of rimonabant in people suffering from these conditions.

OBESITY

Obesity has been classified into two types, accordingly with genetic and environmental aspects: endogenous, secondary to genetic syndromes and endocrinopathies, and exogenous, caused by excessive energy intake compared to energy expenditure. Currently, exogenous obesity is supposed to account for around 95% of cases of obesity [6].

Obesity occurs when adipose cells increase excessively in size (hypertrophy) and/or number (hyperplasia). Obesity that results from an increase in the size of fat cells is hypertrophic, obesity that results from an increase in the number of fat cells is hyperplastic, and obesity that results from an increase in both is hypertrophic/hyperplastic. Adipose cells follow a normal pattern of growth and development [7].

In children, obesity typically involves both hyperplasia and hypertrophy of adipocytes, whereas in the adult, obesity is mainly caused by adipocyte hypertrophy [8]. The increased adipocyte number in obese children may predispose them to lasting obesity or may even be causative because childhood obesity frequently persists into adulthood. In extreme forms of adult-onset obesity, adipocyte hyperplasia can occur secondary to adipocyte hypertrophy, possibly due to a critical increase in the adipocyte size leading to production of growth factors that induce adipocyte hyperplasia [9]. Clinical studies indicate that extreme obesity is rarely treated successfully, suggesting that the adipocyte hyperplasia in the severely obese may strongly predispose them to continued obesity. Also, the rising incidence and severity of obesity seen in older individuals may be due to increased adipocyte number during aging [10]. Therefore, it is suggested that adipocyte hyperplasia could be a factor in the development and subsequent clinical manifestations of some types of obesity. However, little is known about the mechanisms for this hyperplasia or for the regulation of fat cell number in general [11].

According to the body fat distribution, obesity can still be classified into four different types [12]: Type I - characterized by excess total body fat without any particular concentration of fat in a given area of the body. Type II – defined as excess of subcutaneous fat on the trunk, particularly in the abdominal area, and is equivalent to the so-called android (apple shape) or male type of fat deposition. Obesity type II is a public health concern because of its association with hypertension, insulin resistance, diabetes and cardiovascular diseases. Type III - characterized by an excessive amount of fat in the abdominal visceral area and can be labeled abdominal visceral obesity. This type is also associated to cardiovascular disease and insulin resistance. Type IV - defined as gluteo-femoral obesity and is observed primarily in women. It is equivalent to the so-called gynoid obesity (pear shape).

OBESITY: MULTICAUSALITY

Clinical studies suggest interactive influences of numerous factors that might be involved in the development of obesity – genetic, environmental, hormonal, occupational, psychological, and others [13]. The environment is considered as a major determinant of obesity. Environmental influences on obesity are primarily related to food intake and physical activity behaviors, which, associated with genetic factors, would explain the accumulation of excess body fat in the world population [14].

Genetic influences are difficult to elucidate and the contribution to human body weight has been established through family studies, investigations of parent–offspring relationships, and the study of twins and adopted children [15, 16]. Studies demonstrate that identical twins have similar body mass index even being raised in separate environments. Furthermore, whatever the influence the genotype has on the etiology of obesity, it is generally attenuated or exacerbated by non-genetic factors [3].

The contribution of genetic factors to obesity can be either a single, dysfunctional gene (monogenic obesity) or, as in the case of common (polygenic) obesity, numerous genes that make up minor contributions in determining the phenotype. Currently, several genes with a possible role in weight regulation have been isolated and more than 400 genes or markers are associated with obesity. Some genetic research gives us a sight of the complex relationships between gene variants, genes and age, and genes and environment. Changes in gene expression that result from epigenetic influences (modifications of DNA structure rather than DNA sequence) were also explored because of their potential role in obesity and associated chronic diseases. Associations between fetal environment (undernourishment or exposure to maternal hyperglycemia) and adult-onset obesity may be due to epigenetic influences that promote fat storage, but possible mechanisms are not well understood [17, 18].

In modern societies of affluence, high palatability and orosensory properties of certain foods, in combination with environmental influences that promote a sedentary way of life, promote a positive energy balance and development of obesity [19]. In countries like the United States, there is an overall abundance of palatable, calorie-dense food. In addition, aggressive and sophisticated food marketing in the mass media, supermarkets, and restaurants, and the large portions of food served outside the home, promote high calorie consumption [3].

Among several environmental factors, probably associated to the development of obesity, the "metabolic imprinting" - the effects of diet during pregnancy and infant feeding on the development of chronic diseases in later life - is suggested to influence ('imprint'/'program') the development of diseases such as obesity, diabetes, metabolic syndrome, atherosclerosis, hypertension, cancer, mental disorder, food allergy and intolerance [17, 20, 21].

Food intake has been related to obesity not only in terms of the volume of food ingested, but also in terms of the composition and quality of the diet. Furthermore, eating habits have also changed including the low consumption of fruits, greens and milk, increasing consumption of tidbits/goodies (cookies with fillings, salty industrialized snacks, and sweets) and soft drinks, as well as not having breakfast [22-24].

For many people, even when caloric intake is not above the recommended level, the number of calories expended in physical activity is insufficient to offset consumption. Mechanization limits the necessity of physical activity required to function in society [3]. Diminished physical activity has been shown in the population to be associated with an intensified risk of cardiovascular disease.

The prevalence of sedentary people has increased specially due to remarkable technological developments that came to facilitate the life of man. Many people are entrenched in sedentary daily routines consisting of sitting at work, sitting in traffic, and sitting in front of a television or a computer monitor for most of their waking hours [3].

Data from several countries indicate that physical activity significantly declines as adolescents transition into adulthood, and evidence suggest that the developmental transitions of this phase in life may be an important aspect in understanding the age-related decline in physical activity. Particularly in developing countries, such transitions during youth (15-24 years) include concurrent pressures such as: economic demands to be in the workforce, the desire to seek college education; getting married; in addition to the lack of information, time or opportunities for a healthier lifestyle [25-27].

Hormonal system is also enrolled in the development of obesity. Hormones serve as peripheral signals to CNS to provide information regarding energy storage and metabolic state. These hormones deriving mainly from the adipose tissue, the gastrointestinal tract, and the pancreas contribute to the homeostatic control system for the regulation of food intake and energy balance [19].

Leptin is expressed predominantly in adipocytes but has also been found in the hypothalamus, pituitary, placenta, skeletal muscle, and the gastrointestinal tract [28, 29]. Leptin levels decrease in response to caloric restriction and they increase in response to overfeeding irrespective of adipose tissue mass [30]. The majority of obese individuals are characterized by high levels of leptin, suggesting leptin insensitivity or resistance [31]. In rodent models leptin resistance exacerbates diet-induced obesity [32].

While leptin and ghrelin are produced peripherally, they control appetite through their actions on the central nervous system [33, 34]. In particular, they and other appetite-related hormones act on the hypothalamus, a region of the brain central to the regulation of food intake and energy expenditure. There are several circuits within the hypothalamus that contribute to its role in integrating appetite. The circuit begins with an area of the hypothalamus, the arcuate nucleus that has outputs to the lateral hypothalamus (LH) and ventromedial hypothalamus (VMH), the brain's feeding and satiety centers, respectively [35].

Ghrelin is mainly expressed in stomach but may also be expressed centrally in the hypothalamus [33, 34]. Plasma ghrelin levels are regulated both by food intake and by endogenous diurnal rhythms [36]. In normal humans, ghrelin levels rise before meals and in response to diet-induced weight loss, whereas they fall acutely after feeding [37].

The levels of ghrelin are correlated with adiposity in humans, with an inverse relationship between plasma ghrelin levels and body mass index [38]. Obese individuals show reduced levels of plasma ghrelin, which rise to normal after diet-induced weight loss [37]. Furthermore, in obese individuals the postprandial regulation of ghrelin seems to be altered, which may be related to continuous food intake or obesity [39]. Studies demonstrated that ghrelin antagonizes leptin action and promotes the production of orexigenic neuropeptides, such as neuropeptide Y, resulting in an increase in feeding and body weight [40]. Indeed, peripheral infusion of ghrelin stimulates food intake in both rats and humans [41].

Cholecystokinin (CCK) is a peptide that is released by the duodenum and jejunum in response to nutrient ingestion (protein and fatty acid), and by acting via specific receptors, it slows gastric emptying and stimulates gastric distension, intestinal motility, gall bladder contraction, and pancreatic enzyme secretion [42]. Antagonists of these receptors increase food and energy intake in rodents and in human subjects [43, 44].

Neuropeptide Y (NPY) is one of the most abundant and widely distributed peptides in the central nervous system. Within the hypothalamus, NPY plays an essential role in the control of food intake and body weight. Centrally administered NPY causes robust increases in food intake and body weight and, with chronic administration, can eventually produce obesity [45].

Several other hormonal mechanisms have been described to participate in the regulation of appetite and food intake including adiponectin, and interleukin-6, insulin, peptide YY, and glucagon-like peptide 1.

ASSESSMENT AND CLASSIFICATION OF OBESITY

For population studies, the World Health Organization defines cut-off values for obesity based on the body mass index (BMI). It is a simple index of weight-for-height that is commonly used to classify underweight, overweight and obesity in adults. It is defined as the weight in kilograms divided by the square of the height in meters (kg/m^2). BMI values are age-independent and the same for both sexes [13].

According to BMI, obesity in adults is defined as a BMI greater than or equal 30 kg/m^2. However, if the BMI is between 30 and 34.9 kg/m^2 can be classified as obesity class I, BMI between 35 and 39.9 kg/m^2 obesity class II and BMI between 40 and 44 kg/m^2 obesity class III [13].

BMI correlates well with directly measured body fat, and large-scale epidemiological studies have demonstrated that the inflection point at which mortality rates start to rise more sharply corresponds to a BMI of about 30 kg/m^2 [46].

Other methods in addition to the measurement of BMI are valuable for identifying individuals at increased risk for obesity-related illness due to abdominal fat accumulation. Waist circumference and waist-to-hip circumference ratio (WHR) provide a useful estimation of the proportion of abdominal or upper-body fat [47-49]. A WHR greater than 1.0 in men and 0.85 in women indicates abdominal fat accumulation; a high-risk waist circumference is thought to be 88 cm or greater for women and 102 cm or greater for men [3].

Waist circumference is a common measure used to assess abdominal fat content. The presence of excess body fat in the abdomen, when out of proportion to total body fat, is considered an independent predictor of risk factors and ailments associated with obesity [3].

OBESITY TREATMENT

Since obesity is a result of an imbalance between energy income and energy expenditure, the global approach to its treatment must be directed toward correcting this imbalance, trying both to reduce energy intake and to increase energy expenditure. A number of approaches have been and continue to be used to treat obesity. These include diet, exercise, drugs, surgery, and behavior modification.

Despite the numerous health and social problems associated with obesity, as well as the physical limitations it imposes, the treatment of obesity, mostly, is frustrating and usually unsuccessful.

The World Health Organization indicates a moderate weight-loss associated with changes in lifestyle such as healthy eating habits and regular physical activity [13]. However, for many people a reduction in weight is difficult to achieve and appropriate pharmacological therapy can augment diet, physical activity, and behavior therapy in weight loss.

Pharmacotherapy should be considered in overweight and obese patients with a BMI greater than 27 kg/m^2, particularly in the presence of comorbidities or an increased waist circumference, when conservative measures such as behavior therapy, diet and exercise have not resulted in the desired weight loss [3]. Drugs should always be used in conjunction with non-pharmacological therapy, though.

Pharmacotherapy for the management of obesity is primarily aimed at weight loss, weight loss maintenance and improvement of associated morbidities. Importantly, it should be observed if adverse effects are tolerable or transient, efficacy and safety in long-term. Finally, it should be available and affordable for most individuals needing weight loss [50].

Primary endpoints used to evaluate anti-obesity drugs most frequently include mean weight loss and percentage weight loss of initial body weight. Secondary endpoints may include reduction in body fat, risk factors for cardiovascular disease and the incidences of diseases such as diabetes mellitus [51]. Pharmacotherapy should be discontinued if patients demonstrate insufficient weight-loss (so called 'therapeutic hurdles') [52].

The criteria used to evaluate the efficacy of anti-obesity treatments vary. The United States Food and Drug Administration (US FDA) recommends loss of at least 5% of initial weight as the criterion for efficacy, whereas the European Medicines Evaluation Agency (EMEA) suggest a body weight loss of >10% as significant [53,54].

Body weight is regulated through a series of feedback systems that provide targets for effective drug treatment and strategies for drug development. An anti-obesity drug can reduce food intake either by amplifying anorexigenic (anti-appetite) signals or blocking orexigenic (pro-appetite) factors, and increase energy expenditure by uncoupling fuel metabolism from the generation of ATP. It is also possible to modulate fat metabolism by regulating fat synthesis or lipolysis or by moderating the fixed 'internal reference point' maintained by the central controller of body weight [55]. An effective anti-obesity treatment must target a number of these regulatory points.

Most of the anti-obesity drugs are approved for short-term use. Sibutramine and orlistat are weight-loss medications approved for long-term use in patients who are significantly obese. Their safety and effectiveness have not been established for use beyond 2 years, however. Rimonabant was previously approved in Europe and never receive approval in the US due to concerns of psychiatric side effects, which will be discussed in detail later.

Medications approved for the short-term (up to 12 weeks) treatment of obesity include diethylpropion, phentermine, benzphetamine, and phendimetrazine. These medications release dopamine and noradrenaline centrally. The dopamine release is related to their addictive potential, whereas the release of noradrenaline is related to the stimulatory side effects [56]. All of these drugs have the potential for CNS stimulation, increased pulse rate, increased blood pressure and increased release of glycerol and free fatty acids. Beyond increased blood pressure and heart rate, these drugs also are related to dizziness, headache, insomnia, nervousness and other adverse effects [57].

Sibutramine is a noradrenaline and serotonin re-uptake inhibitor, having been approved in 1997. Sibutramine produces an increase in serotonin and noradrenaline at the synapse when these transmitters are normally released by inhibiting their re-uptake [57]. It seems to increase satiety and result in early termination of the meal, in contrast to noradrenergic releasers that generally decrease appetite [58]. In addition to the effect sibutramine has in decreasing food intake, it also has an effect on increasing metabolic rate [59].

Results of a meta-analysis of long-term pharmacotherapy for obesity demonstrate that patients receiving sibutramine lost 3.6 kg to 4.7 kg more weight than those taking placebo [60]. Related to adverse effects, compared with placebo, sibutramine increased systolic and diastolic blood pressure and pulse rate. Insomnia, nausea, dry mouth, and constipation were more common in patients receiving sibutramine, occurring at frequency rates of 7-20%.

Due to sibutramine's known side effects to reasonably increase heart rate and blood pressure, these parameters should be monitored after initiation of therapy. Sibutramine is contraindicated in patients receiving monoamine oxidase inhibitors or serotonergic agents or those with coronary artery disease, congestive heart failure, poorly controlled hypertension, arrhythmias, stroke, or severe liver failure [61].

Orlistat was brought to market in the end of 1998. It is an inhibitor of pancreatic and gastrointestinal lipases, preventing the absorption of approximately 30% of dietary fat and, consequently, preventing a portion of energy ingested from being absorbed. Results of a meta-analysis with 15 studies assessing orlistat treatment demonstrate an average weight-loss of 2.9 kg, comparing with placebo [60].

The adverse effects are almost entirely related to the intestinal tract. The anal sphincter cannot detect oil as well as it can gas, solids or liquids. Therefore, orlistat can be associated with loose stools, the passage of oil, leaking of oil from the rectum, fecal urgency and fecal incontinence. The passage of oil in the stool also has the potential for dissolving fat-soluble vitamins, increasing their loss in the stool and putting those using this drug at risk of fat-soluble vitamin deficiency [57]. Less than 1% of an oral dose of orlistat is absorbed systemically, and therefore, it is relatively safe with few contraindications to use except for chronic malabsorption and cholestasis [61].

There are several medications approved for other uses, mainly psychiatric and neurologic, that have been found to be associated with weight loss. These drugs include the antidepressants fluoxetine and bupropion, the anticonvulsants topiramate and zonisamide and a drug used for the treatment of amyotrophic lateral sclerosis - ciliary neurotrophic factor [57].

A number of anti-obesity drugs are currently undergoing clinical development. These include CB1 receptor antagonists (e.g., CP-945,598), CB1 receptor inverse agonists (taranabant), other lipase inhibitors (Cetilistat and GT-389255), selective 5-HT 2C receptor agonists (APD356 and WAY-163909), a combined low-dose phentermine and topiramate agent (Qnexa), a combined bupropion and naltrexone agent (Contrave), an orally available lipolytic domain of human growth hormone (AOD9604) and others [61,62].

Rimonabant is an anti-obesity medication with a novel mechanism of action as a selective antagonist of the CB1 cannabinoid receptor. The next section will discuss the mechanisms of action, clinical effectiveness, safety and positioning of drug agencies.

ENDOCANNABINOID SYSTEM

The discovery of endocannabinoid system began several centuries ago, when the psychotropic and medicinal actions of the plant *Cannabis sativa* (marijuana) were first documented in India [63]. Cannabis is the most widely produced plant-based illicit drug worldwide and the illegal drug most frequently used in the Western world. Since 300 AD, it has been observed that Cannabis is able to stimulate appetite [64]. However, only a few years ago this phenomenon was seriously taken into consideration in research.

The historical reports have provided the rationale for introducing the natural compounds derived from Cannabis or its synthetic analogues in clinical trials, in the eighties, in order to stimulate appetite and to reduce the weight loss in cachectic states associated with AIDS or malignant tumors [65, 66]. Cannabinoid research received a crucial advance from the characterization of the chemical structure of Δ^9-tetrahydrocannabinol (THC), the main psychoactive constituent of marijuana [67]. This finding covered the way to the understanding of marijuana's mechanisms of action and to the cloning of the two receptor subtypes that are able to bind exogenous cannabinoids, named cannabinoid receptor type 1 (CB_1 receptor) and type 2 (CB_2 receptor), respectively, and to the identification of their endogenous ligands: the endocannabinoids [68-70].

CB1 receptors are expressed predominantly in several areas of the brain and in peripheral organs, including the autonomic nervous system, liver, muscle, gastrointestinal tract, and adipose tissue, while the CB2 receptors are located mainly in the immune and blood cells, where they may participate in regulating immune responses – see table 1 [71]. Pharmacological evidence exists for the presence of other cannabinoid receptors, which, however, have not yet been cloned [72].

Table 1. Human Tissues and Organs Expressing the CB_1 and CB_2 Receptor

CB_1 Receptor	Central Nervous System	Brain
		Spinal Cord
	Genitourinary/ Reproductive	Kidney
		Placenta
		Prostate
		Testis and sperm
		Uterus
	Gastrointestinal	Ileum
		Liver
		Stomach
		Pancreas
	Other	Adipose
		Lung
		Skeletal muscle
		Spleen
CB_2 Receptor	Immune System	T Cells
		B Cells
		Macrophages
		Activated Microglial cell

Three types of endocannabinoids have been identified. The first endocannabinoid to be discovered, arachidonoyl ethanolamide (anandamide), is the most widely investigated representative of the class of endocannabinoid polyunsaturated fatty acid ethanol amides [69]. The two further types are represented by 2-arachidonoylglycerol (2-AG) [70,73] and 2-arachidonyl glyceryl ether (Noladin ether) [74].

The endocannabinoid system consists of cannabinoid receptors, their endogenous ligands - endocannabinoids and the proteins involved in endocannabinoid synthesis and inactivation, as well as the intracellular signaling pathways affected by endocannabinoids [75].

The endocannabinoid system seems to be involved in many different physiologic processes, including nociception (pain sense), motor control, memory and learning, appetite, food intake, and energy balance [76-78]. Other functions of the endocannabinoid system in normal physiology may be related to endocrine functions, vascular responses, immune modulation, neuroprotection, and bone turnover [79].

UNDERSTANDING THE ENDOCANNABINOID SYSTEM

The endocannabinoids are lipophilic and cannot be stored in vesicles like other neurotransmitters. Therefore, tight regulation of endocannabinoid signaling is apparent at the level of synthesis, release, uptake and degradation, respectively [80]. They are produced where and when necessary, are metabolized immediately after their action is finalized. Because of their lipophilic nature and the mechanism of their synthesis and release, endocannabinoids are considered to be local neurotransmitters.

Stimuli such as membrane depolarization, increased intracellular Ca^{2+} and/or receptor stimulation may induce cleavage of membrane phospholipids and the synthesis of endocannabinoids [80]. Within the brain, endocannabinoids are released from postsynaptic membranes [81]. Postsynaptic depolarization opens voltage-dependent Ca^{2+} channels; postsynaptic Ca^{2+} then activates enzymes that synthesize endocannabinoids from lipid precursors. Endocannabinoids leave the postsynaptic cells and activate presynaptic CB_1 receptors. CB1 receptors are typically coupled to G proteins. A change in the conformation of the receptor-coupled G protein directly inhibits presynaptic Ca^{2+} influx channels, and thus decreases the release of a neurotransmitter vesicle [81]. Endocannabinoids are then rapidly inactivated via cellular uptake and enzymatic hydrolysis [82]. In general, the ECS is characterized by rapid endocannabinoid synthesis, receptor activation, and endocannabinoid degradation, with tightly regulated spatial and temporal selectivity [67].

PROPOSED ROLE OF THE ENDOGENOUS CANNABINOID SYSTEM IN THE REGULATION OF FOOD INTAKE AND APPETITE

The cannabinoid system seems to have a role in several processes. Although the distribution of receptors in the body is becoming clearer and their putative ligands becoming more fully characterized, the correlation between pathophysiological responses and the production and activation of these ligands is still unknown. Nevertheless, from the existing data, it is possible to suggest a widespread modulatory role for the cannabinoid system, responsible for regulating a number of functions, such as, food intake and appetite, memory and learning, pain, fertility, immune system, neuroprotection, and others. This system is not limited to the central nervous system but is also concerned with peripheral processes and could act to modulate neurotransmitter release and action from autonomic and sensory nerve fibers.

The ability of cannabis to stimulate hunger and increase appetite, especially for sweet and palatable food, has been known about since ancient times [83]. The ECS is postulated to connect the physical and emotional responses to stress with appetite and energy regulation [78, 83].

Appetite regulation and food intake are complex physiologic processes involving interactions among multiple neuromodulatory systems in the brain [84]. The hypothalamus and hindbrain are the key areas of the brain that regulate food intake, energy homeostasis, and body weight, while the limbic system is believed to contain the neuronal circuitry that determines perceptions of food palatability [83, 85].

The state of the relative energy balance coming from a variety of signals of peripheral origin is known to modulate the neurochemical activation of the hypothalamic neurons [86]. Several signals arising from the periphery include signals represented by hormones released by the gastrointestinal tract, like the hormone cholecystokinin, with a short-term action that are released concomitantly with the meal and help limit further ingestion of food (signals related to satiety); and signals including hormones such as leptin and insulin, which inform the brain about the amount and distribution of fat in the body (signals related to adiposity) [87]. The second category of signals has direct access to neuronal circuits within the hypothalamus and other brain regions, and thereby directly influences energy-balance regulation [87, 88].

The endocannabinoid system appears to be involved in energy balance regulation. Anandamide and 2-AG, as well as the cannabinoid CB1 receptor, are present in the hypothalamus, a brain area known to be associated with feeding. Δ9-THC, the major active component of the marijuana plant, stimulates eating in people [89]. Studies demonstrated that the drug significantly increased intake, elevated hunger ratings, and enhanced food appreciation [90, 91]. It was also observed that after cannabis smoke inhalation, a caloric intake occurred, primarily through an increase in the frequency and consumption of snack foods, such as candy bars, cookies, and cakes [92, 93].

The action of Δ9-THC has been shown to be mediated by central-type CB1 cannabinoid receptors [94]. The hyperphagic effect of THC in rats is remarkably potent, stimulating animals to eat even when satiated [94, 95]. The hyperphagic actions of Δ9-THC have been replicated following administration of the endocannabinoids anandamide and 2-AG. These substances increase intake in rodents following systemic or central injection, and their actions are CB1 receptor-mediated [96-99]. Moreover, anandamide and 2-AG promote feeding when administered into hypothalamic nuclei and into the shell region of the nucleus accumbens. Both the hypothalamus and the nucleus accumbens are brain regions that are tightly associated with eating motivation and their sensitivity to the hyperphagic actions of anandamide and 2-AG strongly supports an important role for endocannabinoids in the control of eating [100, 101]. In addition, CB1 receptor antagonism reverse the 2-AG effect on food intake, suggesting that CB1 receptor activity in both the hypothalamus and the limbic system is essential to induce feeding in response to cannabinoids [97].

The endocannabinoid system appears to regulate the expression and/or action of several hypothalamic anorectic and orexigenic mediators [67]. CB1 receptors colocalize with corticotrophin-releasing hormone (CRH) in the paraventricular nucleus, with melanin-concentrating hormone (MCH) in the lateral hypothalamus, and with pre-pro-orexin in the ventromedial hypothalamus [102].

There is also evidence for functional interaction between endocannabinoids and orexin A, an orexigenic peptide that has been linked to the stimulation of feeding. Indeed, evidence for hypersensitization of the orexin 1 receptor by the CB1 receptor (cross-talk) has been reported [103]. Additionally, CB1 receptor knockout mice (which are characterized by hypophagia, reduced body weight, and reduced fat mass) show higher levels of RNA for the anorexigen CRH [102].

Neuropeptide Y (NPY) is a very potent orexigenic neuropeptide that stimulates feeding when administered to wild-type mice [88]. However, NPY fails to induce food intake when administered to CB1 receptor knockout mice [104]. This indicates that the induction of food intake by endocannabinoids is not mediated by NPY [67]. Therefore, whereas NPY does not seem to be essential for the endocannabinoid modulation of food intake, the CB1 receptor is necessary for the orexigenic action of NPY.

Regarding the mesolimbic system, evidence supports the hypothesis that endocannabinoids increase the drive to eat by enhancing dopamine release in the nucleus accumbens shell or by synergizing with opioids through as yet undefined mechanisms [105-107].

Another pathway at which the endocannabinoid system acts on food intake occurs in the vagus nerve that connects the gastrointestinal tract with medulla and brainstem nuclei involved in control of satiety [67]. Cholecystokinin (anorexigenic peptide produced in gall bladder, pancreas, and stomach and concentrated in the small intestine) is secreted during a meal, and interacts with specific receptors located on the afferent terminals of the vagus nerve. From there, information is transmitted via vagal axons and ultimately relayed to the hypothalamus, where it is integrated with other signals to decrease food intake [83]. It is therefore noteworthy that gastric and intestinal vagal afferents that express CCK receptors also express CB1 receptors. CCK administration reduces food intake and also decreases CB1 receptor expression in vagal afferent neurons. These data suggest that the endocannabinoid system may influence food intake by a gastroduodenal cross-talk with CCK signalling [108].

Concerning the peripheral regulation of energy balance, CB1 receptors are expressed in adipocytes from white adipose tissue, and their expression is increased in adipocytes of rats that have hypertrophied in response to a high fat diet [109]. In the white adipocytes, stimulation of CB1 leads to activation of lipoprotein lipase, whereas its blockade causes up-regulation both *in vitro* and *in vivo* of adiponectin, a hormone crucial in reducing the expression of enzymes involved in lipogenesis [102, 110]. There is evidence that adipose tissue inflammation, as shown by elevated levels of tumor necrosis factor (TNF) alpha, is associated with activation of the endocannabinoid system [111]. In studies comparing lean subjects with subcutaneously obese and viscerally obese subjects, circulating levels of 2-AG were significantly correlated with body fat and visceral fat mass [112]. Endocannabinoids have a role in channeling excess energy into fat cells. It has been demonstrated that the endocannabinoid agonist administration, increases glucose uptake by 50% in human adipocytes, as a result of increased translocation of glucose transporter 4 as well as intracellular calcium [113]. Stimulation of CB1 receptors stimulates lipoprotein lipase and is thought to cause proliferation and differentiation of adipocytes resulting in triglyceride accumulation and reduced adiponectin production and secretion. Low adiponectin levels are strongly associated with increased insulin resistance, increased hepatic glucose production and a proatherogenic state, thereby increasing the likelihood of the metabolic syndrome and cardiovascular disease [114].

Other peripheral organs and tissues, in particular the liver, pancreas and skeletal muscles might also be involved in the control of energy balance by endocannabinoids. Indeed, stimulation of CB1 receptors in the liver and hepatocytes increases once again fatty acid biosynthesis by increasing the expression of the lipogenic transcription factor sterol response element-binding protein 1c and two of its targets, acetyl-CoA carboxylase-1 and fatty acid synthase [115]. The finding that a CB1 agonist enhances the expression of the later enzyme also in the hypothalamus, together with the discovery of adiponectin receptors in the paraventricular nucleus, supports the concept the endocannabinoid control of energy balance at the hypothalamic and peripheral level are likely to be related, cross-talking phenomena [116].

In summary, obesity may result from an overactive endocannabinoid system. The ubiquitous role of the endocannabinoid system in food intake and energy metabolism is now established. Drugs that manipulate different aspects of this system may benefit subjects with the metabolic and cachectic syndromes.

Because of the recently understood role of the endocannabinoid system in promoting obesity, CB1 antagonists have been developed to block the effects of endocannabinoids [85, 117]. Cannabinoid receptor 1 antagonists have been shown to have multiple central and peripheral effects in laboratory animals. The activation of CB1 receptors in the hypothalamus mediates food-deprived hunger, whereas CB1 agonism in the nucleus accumbens shell mediates the hedonically driven motivation to consume highly palatable foods, such as fats and sweets [117]. One clinical implication for inhibiting the central effects of endocannibinoids with CB1 antagonists is decreased food consumption, particularly the cravings that may be associated with obesity.

In terms of peripheral effects, Cannabinoid receptor 1 antagonism in adipocytes leads to increased adiponectin production and decreased lipogenesis. Clinically, these effects translate into an improvement in dyslipidemia, a decrease in insulin resistance, and a decrease in cardiometabolic risk [117, 118].

The blockade of CB1 in muscle tissue results in increased glucose uptake and decreased insulin resistance [119]. In the liver, cannabinoid receptor 1 has been shown to mediate the degradation of FAAH. Cannabinoid receptor 1 antagonists can reverse this effect, blocking the pathway to hepatic lipogenesis. Thus, CB1 antagonists may ultimately lead to reversal of hepatic steatosis, resulting in an improvement in dyslipidemia and insulin resistance [115].

RIMONABANT – ANTAGONIST OF THE ENDOCANNABINOID SYSTEM

General Characteristics

Rimonabant is a selective cannabinoid-1 receptor antagonist that has been investigated for its efficacy in reducing body weight and associated risk factors in obese people [5]. Rimonabant (SR-141716A; 5-[4-chlorophenyl]-1-(2,4-dichlorophenyl)-4-methyl-N-[piperidin-1-yl]-1H-pyrazole-3-carboxamide) was synthesized and described in 1994 by Rinaldi-Carmona *et al.* [120].

Rimonabant analogs have recently been described by several groups, leading to a good understanding of the structure-activity relationship within this chemical group. While most compounds described are less potent than SR141716, two of them are worth mentioning, SR147778 and AM251 [121]. The Fig. (**1**) shows the chemical structure of rimonabant, SR147778 and AM251.

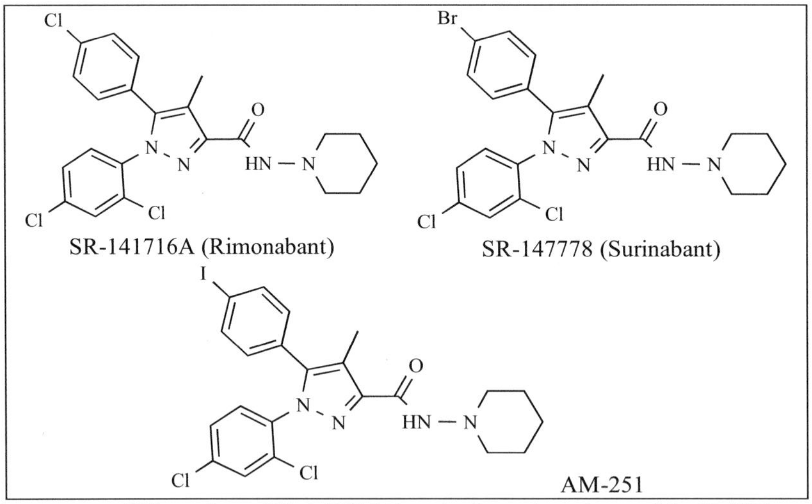

Fig. (1). Chemical structure of Rimonabant (SR-141716A) and other selected cannabinoid CB1 antagonists acting on food intake.

It is the first known substance to block CB1 receptors and is 99% linked to plasma proteins. It is metabolized by cytochrome P450 in the liver and is almost completely expelled in the feces. It may interact with other drugs metabolized by cytochrome P450, especially those biotransformed by isoforms CYP 2A6, 2C9, 2C19, and 3A4 [122]. Some CYP3A4 inhibitors, like ketoconazole, lead to an increase in rimonabant blood levels, while CYP3A4 inductors decrease plasma concentrations and consequently lead to loss in rimonabant effectiveness [123].

Functional *in vitro* and *in vivo* studies showed that rimonabant is able to antagonize the pharmacologic effect induced by cannabinoid receptor agonists. Rimonabant antagonizes anandamide-, 2-AG-, and THC-induced hyperphagia [124]. It selectively decreases the intake of savory drink and food (products that are rich in carbohydrates and lipids), the intake of which are generally increased in obese patients, which indicates that central cannabinoid system blockage can alter the pleasure response induced by food intake and, therefore, reduce the quantity of ingested food [117].

An overall profile of the central and peripheral activities of rimonabant is summarized in Fig. (**2**).

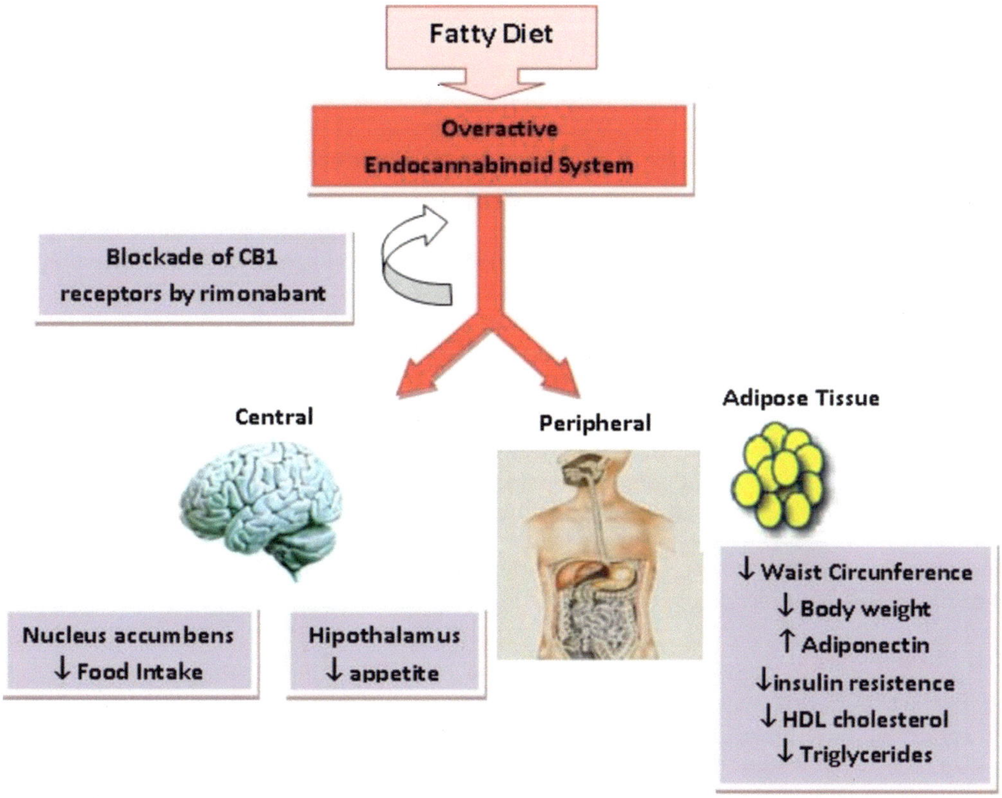

Fig. (2). Central and peripheral effects of CB1 blockade with rimonabant.

Pre-Clinical Studies

The rimonabant effect on food intake occurs in humans as well as in animals, reason why the use of rats and mice in the test phase was considered an appropriate experimental model. A number of preclinical trials have been conducted on the effect of rimonabant in rodent models. One of the earliest studies was in Wistar and Sprague-Dawley mice and rats to determine the effect of rimonabant on appetite behavior, specifically palatable sucrose intake [125]. The results demonstrated that, in food restricted rats, rimonabant produced a dose-dependent reduction in spontaneous sucrose eating without altering regular food intake. Additionally, they noted that tolerance for the suppression of sucrose ingestion did not develop. In non-food-restricted and sucrose-addicted rats, particularly, the intensity of sucrose seeking was dose dependently reduced by rimonabant. Therefore, the inhibition of endocannabinoid system with rimonabant treatment was associated with a reduction in intake of highly palatable foods [125].

Another study was undertaken to determine the effect of rimonabant treatment in rodents fed with normal food. The administration of rimonabant produced a dose-dependent decrease in rates of responding for normal food. This demonstrated that intake of normal food is sensitive to cannabinoid receptors blockade. Moreover, the dose range used did not disrupt other normal behaviors. This study, consequently, suggest that high palatability is not required to observe an appetite suppressant effect with administration of rimonabant [126].

Studies assessing the effect on body weight were also carried out in rodent models. The effect of rimonabant on food intake and body weight in non-obese rats was evaluated. It was found that food intake was quickly decreased with rimonabant compared with placebo treated rats. However, as treatment continued, tolerance to the suppressant effect of rimonabant developed. Overall body weigh decreased in the treatment group. While there was a rapid return to baseline levels of food intake after rimonabant was no longer administered, body weight in rimonabant treated rats grew consistently slower than that of placebo-treated throughout the entire treatment period. These results suggest that tolerance to the anoretic effect of rimonabant developed over time, but weight loss persisted well beyond the effect of the drug on food intake [127].

The results of other study demonstrated that treatment with rimonabant was associated with a reduction in food intake and a 4% loss of body weight in wild-type mice, but not in CB1 receptor-deficient mice [128]. In another study, rodents were put on a high fat diet to develop obesity by an increase in energy intake and insulin resistance. During a five-week treatment period, rimonabant resulted in 48% reduction of food and 20% reduction in body weight. In addition, it helped in correcting insulin resistance [129].

Recent studies also undertaken with rodents have helped to understand the mechanisms of action of the endocannabinoid system and should be pointed out. It has showed elevated levels of free fatty acids postprandially after treatment with rimonabant, demonstrating that rimonabant could induce lipolysis. The weight-reducing effect of rimonabant was thus determined to be due to continuously elevated energy expenditure based on increased fat oxidation driven by lipolysis from fat tissues as long as fat stores were elevated. When the amount of endogenous fat stores declined, the rimonabant-induced increased energy expenditure was maintained by a re-increase in food intake [130].

The results from another study exhibited the liver protecting effect of rimonabant and its potential clinical use in obesity-related liver disorders. Obese mice were treated daily with rimonabant (30 mg/kg) over a period of 8 weeks. Treatment reduced hepatomegaly, the plasma levels of markers of liver damage (alanine aminotransferase, gamma-glutamyl transferase, and alkaline phosphatase), and the high levels of TNF-α associated with steatohepatitis. The effects on the lipid profile were demonstrated by improvements in dyslipidemia through the decrease of triglyceride, free fatty acid and total cholesterol levels, and the increase of the HDL/LDL ratio [131].

Phase I/II Studies

Some phase I/II clinical trials have been completed with rimonabant. However, limited information is available regarding these trials. In a short-term double-bind placebo-controlled crossover study, the effect of seven-day repeated oral administration of rimonabant was evaluated. The treatment group received 20mg of rimonabant once daily. Participants were then crossed over after 28-day wash-out period and all subjects received seven days of placebo. The results showed that participants decreased hunger when taking rimonabant. In addition, the caloric intake over one week showed a consistent reduction with rimonabant with all kind of food. The body weight also showed a significant reduction over one week treatment [132].

In a randomized, controlled 16-week Phase II study, the effect of rimonabant on body weight and waist circumference was tested in 287 subjects whose BMI values were between 29 and 41 kg/m^2 and who followed a mildly hypocaloric diet. Rimonabant in doses of 5, 10 or 20 mg/day lowered body weight and waist circumference measurements compared with placebo. Notably, the decreases in body weight and waist circumference were maintained at a follow-up visit 4 weeks after the end of treatment [133].

Phase III Studies

Based on the animal data and phase II studies, phase III clinical trials of rimonabant were initiated in 2001. The Rimonabant in Obesity (RIO) phase III program consists of four randomized double-blind placebo-controlled clinical trials in humans. The purpose was to assess the role of rimonabant in obesity management, weight loss maintenance, weight regain prevention after initial weight loss, and improvement of obesity-related risk factors in 6600 obese patients. The methodology used in RIO studies – RIO-Lipids, RIO-North America, RIO-Europe, and RIO-Diabetes – was the same, differing only in number and type of patients studied.

The first of the four Phase III trials was the RIO-Lipids which enrolled over 1000 overweight and obese patients with untreated dyslipidemia. The study was a multicenter, randomized, double-blind, placebo-controlled, parallel group, fixed-dose, which compared treatments of 20 mg/day or 5 mg/day of rimonabant to placebo during one year of treatment. The results showed that patients treated with one daily dose of 20 mg of rimonabant exhibited a significant weight and waist circumference reduction and also a decrease in many cardiometabolic risk factors, such as, triglyceride level reduction and HDL cholesterol increase, abdominal, glucose tolerance improvement, and blood pressure decrease. Other important findings were also observed regarding emerging risk markers, including an increase in adiponectin, a protein associated with a reduced risk of diabetes and heart disease and a decrease in C-reactive protein (CRP), an inflammation marker associated with cardiovascular risks [134].

Concurrently with RIO-Lipids, a similarly sized RIO-Europe trial enrolled obese subjects with either hypertension or hyperlipidaemia. Patients were advised to follow a hypocaloric diet and were randomized to rimonabant 20 or 5 mg, or placebo. The on-treatment analysis of its results showed that following a full year of therapy, treatment with either rimonabant 5 or 20 mg/day was associated with significantly greater waist circumference reduction than placebo. There were favorable changes in the lipid profile of subjects in both rimonabant groups: triglyceride levels decreased and high-density lipoprotein (HDL) levels increased, which may have been mediated by increased levels of adiponectin [135]. The 2-year results from RIO-Europe were recently presented and demonstrate a substantial decrease in the proportion of subjects with metabolic syndrome with the combination of a hypocaloric diet and rimonabant 20 mg/day: 42.2% at baseline, 19.6% at 1 year and 21.5% at 2 years [136].

The RIO-North America was a randomized, double-blind, placebo controlled trial enrolled over 3000 overweight and obese patients with treated or untreated hypertension or dyslipidemia. After a 4-week single-blind placebo plus diet run-in period, patients were randomized to receive placebo, 5 mg/d of rimonabant, or 20 mg/d of rimonabant for 1 year. Rimonabant-treated patients were re-randomized to receive placebo or continued to receive the same rimonabant dose while the placebo group continued to receive placebo during year 2. Similar results of Rio-Lipids trial were encountered. The patients treated with 20mg/day rimonabant showed significant weight and waist circumference reduction, as well as decrease in many cardiometabolic risk factors. Patients who were switched from the 20 mg of rimonabant group to the placebo group during year 2 experienced weight regain while those who continued to receive 20 mg of rimonabant maintained their weight loss and favorable changes in cardiometabolic risk factors [137].

Finally, the RIO-Diabetes trial enrolled over 1000 overweight or obese patients with type 2 diabetes mellitus. Again, subjects were randomized to receive rimonabant 20 mg/day, rimonabant 5 mg/day, or placebo for one year. All patients were also treated with an oral hypoglycemic drug, as prescribed by their treatment physician. At the end of one year, therapy with rimonabant 20 mg was associated with a clinically meaningful reduction in body weight and improved glycosylated hemoglobin levels and a number of cardiovascular and metabolic risk factors [138].

A meta-analysis evaluating the joined effect of rimonabant in the four RIO-studies showed that patients receiving rimonabant lost 4.7 kg (4.1 kg to 5.3 kg) more weight than those taking placebo. Rimonabant treatment also significantly increased the placebo subtracted absolute percentage of 5% and 10% responders by 33% (51% *vs.* 18%; 29% to 37%). During the weight maintenance phase of the rimonabant in obesity-North America study, patients treated with rimonabant maintained the weight differential observed in the weight loss phase of the study [60].

Clinical trials have revealed that rimonabant may promote weight loss and improve cardiovascular and metabolic risk factors in obese patients, although it may also induce important adverse effects.

In the RIO-Europe Study, the authors described psychiatric side-effects as detected by the Hospital Anxiety and Depression Scale (HAD) – which may be acceptable to screen for depression and anxiety in non-psychiatric patients, but it is not suitable as a primary outcome measure for depression – employed to evaluate mood. In some cases, the effects were severe, leading patients to abandon the trial. An analysis of the second year of this study has been published with similar outcomes [136]. Concerns on the safety of rimonabant have further increased after the RIO-Lipids Study. As in the RIO-Europe Study, the most common symptoms leading patients to drop out of the study were depression and anxiety. Although the percentage of patients leaving the trial was similar among the groups, those taking 20mg attributed it more to adverse events, essentially anxiety and depression [134]. In the RIO-North America Study the same side-effects present in the former studies were reported. Actually, the trial was limited by a high dropout rate. The authors stated that the overall incidence of adverse events leading to withdrawal was greater with 20mg, mainly due to anxiety and depression [137]. Finally, in the RIO-Diabetes Study, discontinuation due to adverse effects was more common in rimonabant-treated patients, mainly due to depressed mood disorders. However, the authors concluded that no serious adverse events linked to psychiatric disorders occurred [138].

It should be mentioned that the average attrition rates were approximately 40% to 50% in the RIO-Studies, similar to the studies assessing sibutramine or orlistat treatment for obese people [139].

Therefore, studies with different populations of obese subjects demonstrated that rimonabant has a potential to induce anxiety and depression. Since psychiatric patients were not included, these trials do not entirely mimic the clinical practice and underestimate the potential problems to be found with this drug, which might eventually be prescribed for patients already suffering from anxiety or depression, disorders commonly associated with obesity that could be aggravated by such compounds [140, 141].

Efficacy and safety were further analyzed pooling data obtained from a total of 5,580 non-diabetic and 1,047 diabetic patients from the RIO-Studies. The group treated with rimonabant 20mg (2,503 patients) was associated with a higher discontinuation due to depressive disorders (1.9%) and anxiety (1.0%) as compared to those receiving placebo (1,602 patients), whose rates of discontinuation were 0.8 and 0.3% for depressive and anxiety disorders, respectively [136].

Although rimonabant increases the likelihood of depressive episodes, this effect is more pronounced in patients with a history of depression, suggesting that blocking CB1 receptor is more likely to exacerbate existing conditions rather than producing them in healthy individuals [142].

EMEA AND FDA RECOMMENDATIONS

In April 2005 the Sanofi-Aventis submitted to the European Medicines Agency (EMEA) an application for marketing authorization for Acomplia® and Zimuti® (brand name of rimonabant), which did not yet have trading license in any country.

The application submitted was a complete file composed of administrative information, full quality data, non-clinical and clinical data based on applicants' own tests and studies. After submission - which has the legal basis of the application according to Article 8.3 of Directive 2001/83/EC- the Committee for Medicinal Products for Human Use (CHMP) of the EMEA has issued a positive opinion recommending approval of marketing authorization for rimonabant in June 2006.

Rimonabant has been marketed in 18 EU countries, besides America, Asia and others, with more than 700 thousand users in the world. The information disclosed by research showed rimonabant as one of the biggest promises of the pharmaceutical industry in combating obesity and associated risk factors, but later studies showed caution in administering to patients with a history of psychiatric illness and subsequent suspension of the marketing by the EMEA.

In the first studies used as basis for approval of the drug by the EMEA, a higher incidence of dizziness, anxiety and depressive disorders in the group that used 20mg of rimonabant comparing with placebo has been observed [134]. Therefore, contraindication to individuals with a history of depressive disorders has been included. Moreover, it has been recommended to pharmaceutical industry producing strategies to minimize risks and support the patients treated with rimonabant.

According to Periodic Safety Update Report (PSUR 3), the occurrence of depressive disorders had significantly increased during the six months after the end of first year of the study used for approval. The incidence was 24 cases per 10,000 individuals using the drug for 13 in the first year of study [138]. The reports of aggressive behavior and suicide also increased during this period of study. Concerns over the safety of using rimonabant increased after publication of a study that demonstrated the absolute rate of reporting psychiatric adverse events was higher compared to previous studies (43.4% *vs.* 28.4%, for rimonabant and placebo, respectively) [143].

In July 2008 the CHMP wondered about the risk / benefit of rimonabant and requested the marketing authorization holder (MAH) further analysis on security-related issues regarding medication treatment time and side-effects. Prescribers were advised to monitor patients for signs and symptoms of psychiatric disorders, particularly depression, after the start of treatment. The CHMP concluded that depression may occur as a side effect of Acomplia® in patients who had no obvious risk factors, apart from obesity itself. More than half of the patients, who developed depression, did after one month of treatment, and approximately 80% did after three months [144].

The Commission examined all available information on the benefits and risks of Acomplia®. In clinical studies in which patients were treated for more than one year, the effect of weight reduction was moderate and clinically relevant in 20-30% of treated patients, as reflected by a 10% response rate. The Committee found that rimonabant also had moderate beneficial effects in the modulation of HDL-cholesterol, triglycerides and HbA1c [130]. However, since the available data indicate that patients use the drug for short periods of time, there is currently no evidence of cardiovascular disease prevention by rimonabant [136].

The new data from clinical studies post-marketing showed that in clinical practice, psychiatric disorders such as depression, anxiety, sleep disorders and aggressive behavior are more common in relation to what had been at the time of approval. Furthermore, reports of suicide cases in the course of clinical trials are of great concern [134, 136, 138].

According to Article 20 of Regulation (EC) No 726/2004 of March 31, 2004, the European Commission requested on 20 October 2008, the CHMP opinion on necessary measures to ensure the safety and the use of rimonabant due to great concerns about psychiatric adverse events.

Given the available data, it has been concluded that the risks associated with the use of rimonabant for treating obesity and associated factors outweigh the benefits, considering thus, the risk / benefit ratio is not positive. Furthermore, the Committee considered that the current proposals for activities to minimize the risks of developing side effects to patients treated with medication were not sufficient to reduce risk to an acceptable level, or to predict which patients may be at risk. The CHMP recommended the suspension of the marketing authorization for Acomplia on 16 January 2009, and the European Commission issued a decision to withdraw the marketing authorization for Acomplia® and Zimulti® [144, 145].

It is noteworthy that on 5 December 2008, the marketing authorization holder (MAH), responsible for Acomplia®, Sanofi-Aventis, notified the European Commission of its decision to voluntarily withdraw its marketing authorization. The MAH stated that no additional clinical data will now be available to lift the suspension of the marketing authorization for Acomplia following its decision to discontinue the ongoing rimonabant clinical development program in all indications.

In relation to the Food and Drug Administration (FDA), the request for marketing authorization was made in 2007. A thorough review of rimonabant carried out by the Cochrane Database of Systematic Reviews concluded that the average weight loss was moderate and also suggested the need of more rigorous studies evaluating the efficacy and safety to fully estimate the risk /benefit ratio of this drug. Additional studies evaluated by FDA concluded that the incidence of suicidality – specifically suicidal ideation – was higher for 20 mg rimonabant compared to placebo. Similarly, the incidence of psychiatric adverse events, neurological adverse events and seizures were consistently higher for 20 mg rimonabant compared to placebo. Thus, these data lead to rejection of the approval of rimonabant because of lack of ability to fully evaluate the risk/benefit ratio of this new drug [146].

CONCLUSION

Rimonabant, perhaps the most anxiously awaited drug in years, has been successful in randomized clinical trials in promoting weight loss and, as well as improving cardiometabolic risk factors. However, in the rimonabant studies the number of discontinuation due to adverse effects was greater when compared with placebo. Based on safety concerns, mainly related to psychiatric disorders, the FDA in 2007 rejected the approval of rimonabant as a drug to treat obesity. In 2008 EMEA concluded that the benefits of rimonabant did not outweigh its risk and recommended the suspension of the drugs's marketing authorization across the EU. Therefore, Sanofi-Aventis discontinued all ongoing trials with rimonabant.

It is noteworthy that therapeutic approaches are needed to promote weight loss safely and effectively in obese patients and to prevent or ameliorate many obesity-related conditions. Advances in our understanding of the complex systems regulating energy balance, the genetic determinants of obesity, and the environmental factors that promote obesity should lead to the development of more effective and targeted treatments in the future.

From a clinical perspective, the advantages and restrictions of rimonabant must be critically inquired, although the study and development of new compounds targeting the endocannabinoid system for the treatment of obesity would be necessary and opportune.

REFERENCES

[1] World Health Organization. Obesity: Preventing and Managing the Global Epidemic. Technical Report Series 894. WHO: Geneva; 2000.

[2] World Health Organization. World Health Report 2002: reducing risks, promoting healthy life. Geneva: WHO Available from URL: http://www.who.int/peh/burden/ globalestim.htm [Accessed 2009 Jul 20].

[3] National Institutes of Health. National Heart, Lung, and Blood Institute (NIHLBI). Clinical Guidelines on the identification, evaluation, and treatment of overweight and obesity in adults – the evidence report (Clinical Gdlns). Obes Res 1998; 6: 51S-209S.

[4] Curioni CC, Lourenço PM. Long-term weight loss after diet and exercise - a systematic review. Int J Obes 2005; 29: 1168-74.

[5] Bonner TI. Structure of a cannabinoid receptor and functional antagonist. Ann Pharmacother 2005; 39: 684-90.

[6] Rodrigues L. Obesidade Infantil. In: Accioly E, Saunders C, Lacerda EMA, Eds. Nutrição em Obstetrícia e Pediatria. Rio de Janeiro, Cultura Médica, 2009; pp. 449-89.

[7] Pi-Sunyer FX. Obesity. In: Shils ME, Olson JA, Shike M, Eds. Modern nutrition in health and disease. Lea and Febiger, Philadelphia 1994; pp. 984-1006.

[8] Hager A, Sjostrm L, Arvidsson B, Björntorp P, Smith U. Body fat and adipose tissue cellularity in infants: a longitudinal study. Metabolism 1997; 26: 607-14.

[9] Marques BG, Hausman DB, Martin RJ. Association of fat cell size and paracrine growth factors in development of hyperplastic obesity. Am J Physiol 1998; 275: R1898-908.

[10] Kirkland JL, Hollenberg CH, Gillon WS. Age, anatomic site, and the replication and differentiation of adipocyte precursors. Am J Physiol 1990; 258: C206-10.

[11] Ro HS, Zhang L, Majdalawieh A, *et al.* Adipocyte enhancer-binding protein 1 modulates adiposity and energy homeostasis. Obesity 2007; 15: 288-302.

[12] Bouchard C. Genetic determinants of regional fat distribution. Hum Reprod 1997; 12(1): 1-5.

[13] WHO Consultation on Obesity. Preventing and managing the global epidemic. Geneva: World Health Organization, 1998.

[14] James WP. A public health approach to the problem of obesity. Int J Obes Relat Metab Disord 1995; 19 (3): S37-45.

[15] Sorensen TI. The genetics of obesity. Metabolism 1995; 44: 4-6.

[16] Maes HH, Neale MC, Eaves LJ. Genetic and environmental factors in relative body weight and human adiposity. Behav Genet 1997; 27: 325-51.

[17] Waterland RA, Garza C. Potential mechanisms of metabolic imprinting that lead to chronic disease. Am J Clin Nutr 1999; 69(2): 179-197.

[18] Gillman MW. Epidemiological challenges in studying the fetal origins of adult chronic disease. Int J Epidemiol 2002; 31: 294-9.

[19] Kelesidis T, Kelesidis I, Mantzoros CS. Environmental inputs, intake of nutrients, and endogenous molecules contributing to the regulation of energy homeostasis. In: Mantzoros CS, Ed. Nutrition and metabolism: underlying mechanisms and clinical consequences. Boston: Humana Press 2009; pp. 41-76.

[20] Waterland RA, Garza C. Potential for metabolic imprinting by nutritional perturbation of epigenetic gene regulation. Public Health Issues Infant Child Nutr 2002; 48: 317-33.

[21] Morley R, Dwyer T. Early exposures and later health and development. Public Health Issues Infant Child Nutr 2002; 48: 257-78.

[22] Hanley JG, Hamis SB, Gittelsohn J, Wolever Ms, Saksvig B, Zinman B. Overweight among children and adolescents in a Native Canadian community: prevalence e associated factors. Am J Clin Nutr 2000; 71: 693-700.

[23] Harnack L, Stang J, Story M. Soft drink consumption among US children and adolescents: nutritional consequences. J Am Diet Assoc 1999; 99: 436-41.

[24] Nicklas TA, Baranowsky T, Cullen KW, Berenson G. Eating patterns, dietary quality and obesity. J Am Coll Nutr 2001; 20: 599-608.

[25] Gordon-Larsen P, Nelson M, Popkin B. Longitudinal physical activity and sedentary behavior trends: adolescent to adulthood. Am J Prev Med 2004; 27: 277-83.

[26] Sallis JF, Porchaska JJ, Taylor WC. A review of correlates of physical activity of children and adolescents. Med Sci Sports Exerc 2000; 32: 963-75.

[27] Zick CD, Smith KR, Brown BB, Fan JX, Kowaleski-Jones L. Physical activity during the transition from adolescence to adulthood. J Phys Act Health 2007; 4 (2): 125-37.

[28] Zhang Y, Proenca R, Maffei M, Barone M, Leopold L, Friedman JM. Positional cloning of the mouse obese gene and its human homologue. Nature 1994; 372 (6505): 425-32.

[29] Moschos S, Chan JL, Mantzoros CS. Leptin and reproduction: a review. Fertil Steril 2002; 77 (3): 433-44.

[30] Mantzoros CS, Flier JS. Editorial: leptin as a therapeutic agent – trials and tribulations. J Clin Endocrinol Metab 2000; 85: 4000-2.

[31] Considine RV, Sinha MK, Heiman ML, *et al.* Serum immunoreactive-leptin concentrations in normal-weight and obese humans. N Engl J Med 1996; 334 (5): 292-5.

[32] Scarpace PJ, Zhang Y. Leptin resistance: a prediposing factor for diet-induced obesity. Am J Physiol Regul Integr Comp Physiol 2009; 296 (1): R493-500

[33] Kojima M, Hosoda H, Date Y, Nakazato M, Matsuo H, Kangawa K. Ghrelin is a growth-hormone releasing acylated peptide from stomach. Nature 1999; 402 (6762): 656-60.

[34] Toshinai K, Date Y, Murakami N, *et al.* Ghrelin-induced food intake is mediated via the orexin pathway. Endocrinology 2003; 144(4): 1506-12.
[35] Coll AP, Farooqi IS, O'Rahilly S. The Hormonal Control of Food Intake. Cell 2007; 129(2): 251-62
[36] Cummings DE, Purnell JQ, Frayo RS, Schmidova K, Wisse BE, Weigle DS. A preprandial rise in plasma ghrelin levels suggests a role in meal initiation in humans. Diabetes 2001; 50(8): 1714-9.
[37] Cummings DE, Weigle DS, Frayo RS, *et al.* Plasma ghrelin levels after diet-induced weight loss or gastric bypass surgery. N Engl J Med 2002; 346 (21): 1623-30.
[38] Tschop M, Weyer C, Tataranni PA, Devanarayan V, Ravussin E, Heiman ML. Circulating ghrelin levels are decreased in human obesity. Diabetes 2001; 50(4): 707-9.
[39] English PJ, Ghatei MA, Malik IA, Bloom SR, Wilding JP. Food fails to suppress ghrelin levels in obese humans. J Clin Endocrinol Metab 2002; 87(6): 2984.
[40] Nakazato M, Murakami N, Date Y, *et al.* A role for ghrelin in the central regulation of feeding. Nature 2001; 409: 194-8.
[41] Wren AM, Seal LJ, Cohen MA, *et al.* Ghrelin enhances appetite and increases food intake in humans. J Clin Endocrinol Metab 2001; 86: 5992-5
[42] Kissileff HR, Carretta JC, Geliebter A, Pi-Sunyer FX. Cholecystokinin and stomach distension combine to reduce food intake in humans. Am J Physiol Regul Integr Comp Physiol 2003; 285(5): R992-8.
[43] Corp ES, Curcio M, Gibbs J, Smith GP. The effect of centrally administered CCK-receptor antagonists on food intake in rats. Physiol Behav 1997; 61(6): 823-7.
[44] Beglinger C, Degen L, Matzinger D, D'Amato M, Drewe J. Loxiglumide, a CCK-A receptor antagonist, stimulates calorie intake and hunger feelings in humans. Am J Physiol Regul Integr Comp Physiol 2001; 280 (4): R1149-54.
[45] Kamiji MM, Inui A. Neuropeptide y receptor selective ligands in the treatment of obesity. Endocr Rev 2007; 28(6): 664-84.
[46] Calle EE, Thun MJ, Petrelli JM, Rodriguez C, Heath CW. Body-mass index and mortality in a prospective cohort of U.S. adults. N Engl J Med 1999; 341 (15): 1097-05.
[47] Björntorp P. Hazards in subgroups of human obesity. Eur J of Clin Invest 1984; 14: 239-41.
[48] Björntorp P. Obesity and the risk of cardiovascular disease. Ann Clin Res 1985; 17: 3-9.
[49] Kissebah AH, Evans DJ, Peiris A, Wilson CR. Endrocrine characteristics in regional obesities: role of sex steroids. In: Vague J, Björntorp P, Guy Grand B, Rebuffé-Scrive M, Vague P, Eds. Metabolic Complications of Human Obesities. Elsevier Science Publishers: Amsterdam 1985; pp.115-30.
[50] Guy-Grand B. Long-term pharmacoterapy in the management of obesity. In: Björntorp P, Rössner S, Eds. From Theory to Practice: Obesity in Europe: 88. London: John Libbey, 1989; pp. 311-8.
[51] Ioannides-Demos LL, Proietto J, McNeil JJ. Pharmacotherapy for obesity. Drugs 2005; 65(10): 1391-418.
[52] Kos K, Baker C, Kumar C. Current treatment strategies for obesity. Therapy 2005; 2(6): 955-67.
[53] Food and Drug Administration. Guidance for the clinical evaluation of weight-control drugs. Rockville (MD): FDA, 1996 Sep 24 [online]. Available from URL: http://www.fda.gov/ohrms/dockets/98fr/03d-0570-gdl0001.pdf [Accessed 2009 Jul 20]
[54] European Medicines Agency. Guideline on clinical investigation of medicine products used in weight control. CMP/EWP/281/96 Rev.1. London: The European Medicines Agency, 2007 Nov [online]. Available from URL: http://www.emea.europa.eu/pdfs/human/ewp/028196enfin.pdf [Accessed 2009 Jul 20]
[55] Brower V. Fighting fat. New drugs against obesity in the pipeline. EMBO Rep 2002; 3(7): 601-3.
[56] Rothman RB, Baumann MH, Dersch CM, *et al.* Amphetamine-type central nervous system stimulants release norepinephrine more potently than they release dopamine and serotonin. Synapse 2001; 39(1): 32-41.
[57] Greenway FL, Caruso MK. Safety of obesity drugs. Expert Opin Drug Saf 2005; 4(6): 1083-95
[58] Ryan DH, Kaiser P, Bray GA. Sibutramine: a novel new agent for obesity treatment. Obes Res 1995; 3(4): 553-9.
[59] Hansen DL, Toubro S, Stock MJ, Macdonald IA, Astrup A. Thermogenic effects of sibutramine in humans. Am J Clin Nutr 1998; 68(6): 1180-6.
[60] Padwal RS, Rucker D, Li SK, Curioni C, Lau DCW. Long term pharmacotherapy for obesity and overweight: updated meta-analysis. BMJ 2007; 335(7631): 1194-9.
[61] Chan JL, Mantzoros CS. Diagnosis, Evaluation, and Medical Management of Obesity and Diabetes. In: Mantzoros CS (org). Nutrition and Metabolism: Underlying Mechanisms and Clinical Consequences. Boston: Humana Press, 2009; pp.289-328.
[62] Halford JC. Obesity drugs in clinical development. Curr Opin Investig Drugs 2006; 7: 312-8.
[63] Grinspoon L, Bakalar JB. Marihuana. The forbidden medicine. London: Yale University Press 1997; pp.145-66.
[64] Abel EL. Cannabis: effects on hunger and thirst. Behav Biol 1975; 15: 255-81.
[65] Beal JE, Olson R, Lefkowitz L, *et al.* Long-term efficacy and safety of dronabinol for acquired immunodeficiency syndrome-associated anorexia. J Pain Symptom Manage 1997; 14: 7-14.
[66] Struwe M, Kaempfer SH, Geiger CJ, *et al.* Effect of dronabinol on nutritional status in HIV infection. Ann Pharmacother 1993; 27: 827-31
[67] Di Marzo V, Matias I. Endocannabinoid control of food intake and energy balance. Nat Neurosci 2005; 8: 585-9.
[68] Munro S, Thomas KL, Abu-Shaar M. Molecular characterization of a peripheral receptor for cannabinoids. Nature 1993; 365: 61-5
[69] Devane WA, Hanus L, Breuer A, *et al.* Isolation and structure of a brain constituent that binds to the cannabinoid receptor. Science 1992; 258: 1946-9.
[70] Sugiura T, Kondo S, Sukagawa A, *et al.* 2-Arachidonoylglycerol: a possible endogenous cannabinoid receptor ligand in brain. Biochem Biophys Res Commun 1995; 215: 89-97.
[71] Di Marzo V, Bifulco M, De Petrocellis L. The endocannabinoid system and its therapeutic exploitation. Nat Rev Drug Discov 2004; 3: 771-84.
[72] Begg M, Pacher P, Batkai S, *et al.* Evidence for novel cannabinoid receptors. Pharmacol Ther 2005; 106: 133-45.
[73] Mechoulam R, Ben-Shabat S, Hanus L, *et al.* Identification of an endogenous 2-monoglyceride, present in canine gut, that binds to cannabinoid receptors. Biochem Pharmacol 1995; 50: 83-90.
[74] Hanus L, Abu-Lafi S, Fride E, *et al.* 2-Arachidonoyl glycerol ether, endogenous agonist of the cannabinoid CB1 receptor. Proc Natl Acad Sci USA 2001; 98: 3662-5.
[75] De Petrocellis L, Cascio MG, Di Marzo V. The endocannabinoid system: a general view and latest additions. Br J Pharmacol 2004; 141: 765-74.

[76] Pagotto U, Marsicano G, Cota D, Lutz B, Pasquali R. The emerging role of the endocannabinoid system in endocrine regulation and energy balance. Endocr Rev 2006; 27: 73-100.
[77] Ameri A. The effects of cannabinoids on the brain. Prog Neurobiol 1999; 58: 315-48.
[78] Di Marzo V, Melck D, Bisogno T, De Petrocellis L. Endocannabinoids: endogenous cannabinoid receptor ligands with neuromodulatory action. Trends Neurosci 1998; 21: 521-8.
[79] Pacher P, Batkai S, Kunos G. The endocannabinoid system as an emerging target of pharmacotherapy. Pharmacol Rev 2006; 58: 389-462.
[80] Piomelli D. The molecular logic of endocannabinoid signalling. Nat Rev Neurosci 2003; 4: 873-84.
[81] Wilson RI, Nicoll RA. Endocannabinoid signaling in the brain. Science 2002; 296: 678-82.
[82] Giuffrida A, Beltramo M, Piomelli D. Mechanisms of endocannabinoid inactivation: biochemistry and pharmacology. J Pharmacol Exp Ther 2001; 298(1): 7-14.
[83] Cota D, Woods S. The role of the endocannabinoid system in the regulation of energy homeostasis. Curr Opin Endocrinol Diabetes 2005; 12: 338-51.
[84] Morton GJ, Cummings DE, Baskin DG, Barsh GS, Schwartz MW. Central nervous system control of food intake and body weight. Nature 2006; 443: 289-95.
[85] Bensaid M, Gary-Bobo M, Esclangon A, *et al.* The cannabinoid CB1 receptor antagonist SR141716 increases Acrp30 mRNA expression in adipose tissue of obese fa/fa rats and in cultured adipocyte cells. Mol Pharmacol 2003; 63: 908-14.
[86] Pagotto U, Valentina V, Pasquali R. The endocannabinoid system and the treatment of obesity. Ann Med 2005; 37: 270-5.
[87] Seeley RJ, Woods SC. Monitoring of stored and available fuel by the CNS: implications for obesity. Nat Rev Neurosci 2003; 4: 901-9.
[88] Schwartz MW, Woods SC, Porte D, Seeley RJ, Baskin DG. Central nervous system control of food intake. Nature 2000; 404: 661-71.
[89] Fride E. Cannabinoids and feeding: the role of the endogenous cannabinoid system as a trigger for newborn suckling. J Cannabis Ther 2002; 2: 51-62.
[90] Hollister LE. Hunger and appetite after single doses of marijuana, alcohol and dextroamphetamine. Clin Pharmacol Ther 1971; 12:45-9.
[91] Haney M, Ward AS, Comer SD, Foltin RW, Fischman MW. Abstinence symptoms following smoked marijuana in humans. Psychopharmacol 1999; 141: 395-404.
[92] Foltin RW, Brady JV, Fischman MW. Behavioral analysis of marijuana effects on food intake in humans. Pharmacol Biochem Behav 1986; 25: 577-82.
[93] Foltin RW, Fischman MW, Byrne MF. Effects of smoked marijuana on food intake and body weight of humans living in a residential laboratory. Appetite 1988; 11: 1-14.
[94] Williams CM, Kirkham TC. Anandamide induces overeating: mediation by central cannabinoid (CB1) receptors. Psychopharmacology 1999; 143: 315-7.
[95] Williams CM, Kirkham TC. Observational analysis of feeding induced by Delta9-THC and anandamide. Physiol Behav 2002; 76: 241-50.
[96] Jamshidi N, Taylor DA. Anandamide administration into the ventromedial hypothalamus stimulates appetite in rats. Br J Pharmacol 2001; 134: 1151-4.
[97] Kirkham TC, Williams CM, Fezza F, Di Marzo V. Endocannabinoid levels in rat limbic forebrain and hypothalamus in relation to fasting, feeding and satiation: stimulation of eating by 2-arachidonoyl glycerol. Br J Pharmacol 2002; 136: 550-7.
[98] Gomez R, Navarro M, Ferrer B, *et al.* A peripheral mechanism for CB1 cannabinoid receptor-dependent modulation of feeding. J Neurosci 2002; 22: 9612-7.
[99] Hao S, Avraham Y, Mechoulam R, Berry EM. Low dose anandamide affects food intake, cognitive function, neurotransmitter and corticosterone levels in diet-restricted mice. Eur J Pharmacol 2000; 392: 147-56.
[100] Kelley AE. Functional specificity of ventral striatal compartments in appetitive behaviors. Ann N Y Acad Sci 1999; 877: 71-90.
[101] Elmquist JK, Elias CF, Saper CB. From lesions to leptin: hypothalamic control of food intake and body weight. Neuron 1999; 22: 221-32.
[102] Cota D, Marsicano G, Lutz B, *et al.* Endogenous cannabinoid system as a modulator of food intake. Int J Obes Relat Metab Disord 2003; 27: 289-301.
[103] Hilairet S, Bouaboula M, Carriere D, Le Fur G, Casellas P. Hypersensitization of the Orexin 1 receptor by the CB1 receptor: evidence for cross-talk blocked by the specific CB1 antagonist, SR141716. J Biol Chem 2003; 278: 23731-7.
[104] Poncelet M, Maruani J, Calassi R, Soubrie P. Overeating, alcohol and sucrose consumption decrease in CB1 receptor deleted mice. Neurosci Lett 2003; 343: 216-8.
[105] Verty AN, McGregor IS, Mallet PE. The dopamine receptor antagonist SCH 23390 attenuates feeding induced by Delta9-tetrahydrocannabinol. Brain Res 2004; 1020(1-2): 188-95.
[106] Kirkham TC, Williams CM. Synergistic efects of opioid and cannabinoid antagonists on food intake. Psychopharmacology 2001; 153(2): 267-70.
[107] Verty AN, Singh ME, McGregor IS, Mallet PE. The cannabinoid receptor antagonist SR 141716 attenuates overfeeding induced by systemic or intracranial morphine. Psychopharmacol 2003; 168(3): 314-23.
[108] Burdyga G, Lal S, Varro A, Dimaline R, Thompson DG, Dockray GJ. Expression of cannabinoid CB1 receptors by vagal afferent neurons is inhibited by cholecystokinin. J Neurosci 2004; 24: 2708-15.
[109] Yan ZC, Liu DY, Zhang LL, *et al.* Exercise reduces adipose tissue via cannabinoid receptor type 1 which is regulated by peroxisome proliferator-activated receptor-delta. Biochem Biophys Res Commun 2007; 354: 427-33.
[110] Poirier B, Bidouard JP, Cadrouvele C, *et al.* The anti-obesity effect of rimonabant is associated with an improved serum lipid profile. Diabetes Obes Metab 2005; 7(1): 65-72.
[111] Kempf K, Hector J, Strare T, *et al.* Immune-mediated activation of the endocannabinoid system in visceral adipose tissue in obesity. Horm Metab Res 2007; 39: 596-600.
[112] Bluher M, Engeli S, Kloting N, *et al.* Dysregulation of the peripheral and adipose tissue endocannabinoid system in human abdominal obesity. Diabetes 2006; 55: 3053-60.
[113] Pagano C, Pilon C, Calcagno A, *et al.* The endogenous cannabinoid system stimulates glucose uptake in human fat cells via phosphatidylinositol 3-kinase and calcium-dependent mechanisms. J Clin Endocrinol Metab 2007; 92: 4810-9.

[114] Jesudason D, Wittert G. Endocannabinoid system in food intake and metabolic regulation. Curr Opin Lipidol 2008; 19: 344-8.
[115] Osei-Hyiaman D, DePetrillo M, Pacher P, *et al.* Endocannabinoid activation at hepatic CB1 receptors stimulates fatty acid synthesis and contributes to diet-induced obesity. J Clin Invest 2005; 115(5): 1298-305.
[116] Qi Y, Takahashi N, Hileman SM, *et al.* Adiponectin acts in the brain to decrease body weight Nat Med 2004; 10(5): 524-9.
[117] Ravinet Trillou C, Arnone M, Delgorge C, *et al.* Antiobesity effect of SR141716, a CB1 receptor antagonist, in diet-induced obese mice. Am J Physiol Regul Integr Comp Physiol 2003; 284: R345-53.
[118] Pischon T, Girman CJ, Hotamisligil GS, Rifai N, Hu FB, Rimm EB. Plasma adiponectin levels and risk of myocardial infarction in men. JAMA 2004; 291: 1730-7.
[119] Liu YL, Connoley JP, Wilson CA, Stock MJ. Effects of the cannabinoid CB1 receptor antagonist SR141716 on oxygen consumption and soleus muscle glucose uptake in Lep(ob)Lep(ob) mice. Int J Obes 2005; 29: 183-7.
[120] Rinaldi-Carmona M, Barth F, *et al.* SR141716A, a potent and selective antagonist of the brain cannabinoid receptor. FEBS Lett 1994; 350: 240-4.
[121] Barth, F. CB1 Cannabinoid Receptor Antagonists. In: Doherty A. (org) Annual Reports in Medicinal Chemistry 40th ed., Academic Press: EUA, 2005; pp. 103-8.
[122] Ducobu J, Sternon J. Rimonabant (Acomplia), specific inhibitor of the endocannabinoid system. Rev Med Brux 2005; 26: 165-8.
[123] Wierzbicki AS. Rimonabant: endocannabinoid inhibition for the metabolic syndrome. Int J Clin Pract 2006; 60: 1697-706.
[124] Boyd T, Fremming BA. Rimonabant - A selective CB1 antagonist. Ann Pharmacother 2005; 39: 684-90.
[125] Arnone M, Maruani J, Chaperon F, *et al.* Selective inhibition of sucrose and ethanol intake by SR 141716, an antagonist of central cannabinoid (CB1) receptors. Psychopharmacology 1997; 132(1): 104-6.
[126] Freedland CS, Poston JS, Porrino LJ. Effects of SR141716A, a central cannabinoid receptor antagonist, on food-maintained responding. Pharmacol Biochem Behav 2000; 67: 265-70.
[127] Colombo G, Agabio R, Diaz G, Lobina C, Reali R, Gessa GL. Appetite suppression and weight loss after the cannabinoid antagonist SR 141716. Life Sci 1998; 63: 113-7.
[128] Di Marzo V, Goparaju SK, Wang L, *et al.* Leptin-regulated endocannabinoids are involved in maintaining food intake. Nature 2001; 410: 822-5.
[129] Trillou CR, Arnone M, Delgorge C. Anti-obesity effect of SR141716, a CB1 receptor antagonist, in diet-induced obese mice. Am J Physiol Regul Integr Comp Physiol 2003; 284: 345-53.
[130] Herling AW, Kilp S, Elvert R, Haschke G, Kramer W. Increased energy expenditure contributes more to the body weight reducing effect of rimonabant than reduced food intake in candy-fed Wistar rats. Endocrinology 2008; 149: 2557-66.
[131] Gary-Bobo M, Elachouri G, Gallas JF, *et al.* Rimonabant reduces obesity-associated hepatic steatosis and features of metabolic syndrome in obese Zucker fa/fa rats. Hepatology 2007; 46: 122-9.
[132] Heshmati HM, Caplain H, Bellisle F. SR141716, a selective cannabinoid CB1 receptor antagonist, reduces hunger, caloric intake and body weight in overweight or obese men. Obes Res 2001; 9: 70.
[133] Pi-Sunyer FX, Marbury TC, Garland WT, *et al.* Rimonabant, a Selective CB1-Receptor Antagonist, Is a Valuable New Tool in the Treatment of Obesity. In: 86th Annual Meeting of the Endocrine Society 2004. New Orleans, USA 2004.
[134] Depres JP, Golay A, Sjostrom L. Effects of rimonabant on metabolic risk factors in overweight patients with dyslipidemia. N Engl J Med 2005; 353: 2121-34.
[135] Van Gaal LF, Rissanen AM, Scheen AJ, Ziegler O, Rossner S. Effect of the cannabinoid-1 receptor blocker rimonabant on weight reduction and cardiovascular risk factors in overweight patients: 1-year experience from the RIO-Europe study. Lancet 2005; 365: 1389-97.
[136] Van Gaal LF, Scheen AJ, Rissanen AM, Rössner S, Hanotin C, Ziegler O. RIO-Europe Study Group. Long-term effect of CB1 blockade with rimonabant on cardiometabolic risk factors: two year results from the RIO-Europe Study. Eur Heart J 2008; 29(14): 1761-71.
[137] Pi-Sunyer FX, Aronne LJ, Heshmati HM, Devin J, Rosenstock J. Effect of rimonabant, a cannabinoid-1 receptor blocker, on weight and cardiometabolic risk factors in overweight or obese patients. JAMA 2006; 295: 761-75.
[138] Scheen AJ, Finer N, Hollander P, Jensen MD, Van Gaal LF, RIO-Diabetes Study Group. Efficacy and tolerability of rimonabant in overweight or obese patients with type 2 diabetes: a randomized controlled study. Lancet 2006; 368(9548): 1660-72.
[139] Pagotto U, Vanuzzo D, Vicennati V, Pasquali R. Pharmacological therapy of obesity. G Ital Cardiol 2008; 9: 83S-93.
[140] Dixon JB, Dixon ME, O'Brien PE. Depression in association with severe obesity: changes with weight loss. Arch Intern Med 2003; 163(17): 2058-65.
[141] Onyike CU, Crum RM, Lee HB, Lyketsos CG, Eaton WW. Is obesity associated with major depression? Results from the Third National Health and Nutrition Examination Survey. Am J Epidemiol 2003; 158(12): 1139-47.
[142] Moreira FA, Crippa JAS. The psychiatric side-effects of rimonabant. Rev Bras Psiquiatr 2009; 31(2): 145-53.
[143] Rumsfeld JS, Nallamothu BK. The hope and fear of rimonabant. JAMA 2008; 299(13): 1601-2.
[144] Assessment report for Acomplia – London, 16 January EMEA/65105/2009.
[145] Assessment report for Zimulti - London, 16 January 2009 EMEA/65151/2009.
[146] FDA-Center for Drug Evaluation and Research Summary Minutes of the Endocrinologic and Metabolic Drugs Advisory Committee meeting on June 13, 2007. Available from: http://www.fda.gov/ohrms/ dockets/ac/07/minutes/2007-4306m1-final.pdf [Accessed 2009 Jul 10].

Phytochemicals as Potential Agents for Prevention and Treatment of Obesity and Metabolic Diseases

Taesun Park* and Yunjung Kim

Department of Food and Nutrition, Yonsei University, 262 Seongsanno, Seodaemun-gu, Seoul 120-749, Republic of Korea

Abstract: The high incidence of obesity and the lack of safe pharmaceutical agents have fuelled an increase in researches related to anti-obesity drugs. Although a number of pharmacological approaches have been investigated in recent years, few safe and therapeutically effective products have been developed. Phytochemicals are components of plants that convey healthful properties beyond their use as macronutrients or micronutrients. These compounds have biological properties such as antioxidant, modulation of detoxification enzymes, stimulation of the immune system, reduction of platelet aggregation, and modulation of hormone metabolism. Furthermore, the latest discoveries and studies on the cellular and molecular mechanisms of such phytochemicals suggest that they are potential agents in the treatment of obesity and associated diseases, and may be incorporated in food ingredients, dietary supplements, or drug components. The main focus of this chapter is to review the available information on various aspects of phytochemicals, with special reference to their effectiveness in reducing obesity and obesity-related diseases. The bioactives that have been derived from plants, including flavonoids, terpenoids, phenolic acids, and other categories of phytochemicals based on their structure, have shown interesting effects on adipose tissue such as the induction of apoptosis, the inhibition of adipocyte differentiation and lipid accumulation, and the induction of lipolysis. Besides the ample evidence of the anti-obesity effects of these phytochemicals in literature, the characterization of their properties and the accumulation of preclinical data could raise the possibility of a new application of these interesting phytochemicals as novel drug candidates or dietary supplements.

Keywords: Phytochemical, obesity, metabolic diseases, mechanism, drug candidate.

INTRODUCTION

Common obesity is a complex disease that results from the inappropriate control of the body's energy balance due to overfeeding and/or a sedentary way of life. In this context, both hypocaloric diets (decreased energy intake) and increased physical activity (increased energy output) result in loss of body weight and body fat. With these traditional approaches to weight loss, potential therapeutic agents could be important tools in preventing and/or treating obesity and associated metabolic diseases. Although a number of pharmacological approaches have been investigated in recent years, few therapeutically effective and safe products have been developed [1]. From ancient to modern times, some plants have been utilized as medicinal agents [2]. These medicinal agents initially took the form of crude drugs such as tinctures, teas, poultices, powders, and other herbal formulations [2, 3]. The specific plants to be used and the methods of application for particular ailments were passed down through oral history. Eventually information regarding medicinal plants was recorded in herbals. In more recent history, the use of plants as medicines has involved the isolation of bioactive compounds, beginning with the isolation of morphine from opium in the early 19th century [2, 4]. Many important bioactive compounds have been discovered from natural sources using bioactivity-directed fractionation and isolation [5]. These bioactive compounds are mostly secondary plant metabolites, and many naturally occurring pure compounds have become medicine, dietary supplements, and other useful commercial products.

Phytochemicals are the bioactive compounds of plants that do not deliver energy and are not yet classified as essential nutrients but possess healthful properties beyond their use as macronutrients or micronutrients. Plants usually produce such low-molecular-weight ingredients for their protection against pests and diseases, for the regulation of their growth, or as pigments, essence, or odor [6]. Scientists have identified thousands of phytochemicals, including flavonoids, glucosinolates (isothiocyanates and indoles),

*Corresponding author: Tel: 82 2 2123 3123; Fax: 82 2 365 3118; E-mail: tspark@yonsei.ac.kr

phenolic acids, phytates, and phytoestrogens (isoflavones and lignans), in vegetables, fruits, grains, legumes, and other plant sources. A vast variety of phytochemicals that are present in the daily human diet have been found to possess substantial antimutagenic and anticarcinogenic properties [7]. The chemopreventive effects of the majority of edible phytochemicals are often attributed to their antioxidative or anti-inflammatory activities [7-9]. Besides the edible chemopreventives in vegetables, fruits, herbs, and spices, some phytochemicals in diverse plants also have other beneficial health effects such as anti-obesity, lipid-lowering, and/or antidiabetic properties. Considering the above-mentioned facts, in this chapter, an overview of the present understanding of what and how phytochemicals prevent and treat obesity and associated metabolic diseases is provided. The bioactive compounds of plant origin that are discussed in this Chapter include flavonoids, phenolic acids, terpenes, and some other categories of phytochemicals. The biochemical and cellular events that are induced or modulated by these anti-obesity phytochemicals are summarized in Tables **1-4**.

FLAVONOIDS

Flavonoids are the most common phenolic compounds that are widely distributed in nature and are ubiquitous in plants, fruits, seeds, and vegetables. Flavonoids have the basic chemical structure of diphenylpropanes (C6–C3–C6), and are most often found attached to sugars (glycosides) or aglycones (e.g., quercetin or kaempferol) [10]. Flavonoids can be categorized into 13 classes that comprise more than 5,000 compounds. The most common flavonoids are flavones, flavonols, and their glycosides [11]. They possess anti-inflammatory, antiviral, antioxidant, hepatoprotective, antithrombotic, anticarcinogenic, and other biological effects [10]. A number of studies have been carried out to investigate the anti-obesity effects of flavonoids such as rutin, quercetin, kaempferol, myricetin, hesperidin, hesperetin, naringenin, naringin, green tea catechins (catechin, epigallocatechin gallate, and epicatechin gallate), theaflavins, cyanidins, and isoflavones (genistein, diadzein, and glycitien). The food sources, reported biological activities, and action mechanisms of these flavonoids are summarized in Table **1**.

Catechins: Catechin, Epigallocatechin Gallate and Epicatechin Gallate

Green tea, a beverage that is commonly consumed in Asian countries, is a significant source of a type of polyphenolic flavonoid known as (-)-catechin. Green tea catechins are mainly composed of catechin, epigallocatechin gallate (EGCG), epicatechin gallate (ECG), epigallocatechin, and epicatechin [12]. Among the numerous beneficial effects ascribed to tea consumption are anti-angiogenic, anticarcinogenic, antioxidant, anti-obesity, antihyperlipidemic, and antidiabetic effects [13-16]. For example, regular consumption of 5-6 or more cups of green tea or 200-300 mg of EGCG per day has demonstrated their usefulness in preventing cardiovascular and metabolic diseases [17]. Catechin-enriched tea has been found to reduce dietary lipid absorption in humans [18]. It has also been shown that green tea consumption increases energy expenditure and reduces the respiratory quotient in healthy humans [19]. Many of the aforementioned beneficial effects of green tea were recently attributed to its most abundant catechin, EGCG which accounts for up to 30% of the solids in green tea [20]. EGCG attenuated diet-induced obesity in animal models by reducing leptin levels and energy absorption, and by enhancing fat oxidation [20, 21]. A cross-over pilot study has indicated that diet supplementation with 300 mg of EGCG may also have beneficial effects on obese subjects, since it lowered the subjects' postprandial respiratory quotient [22]. Brown *et al.* investigated the effect of diet supplementation with EGCG among overweight or obese men aged 40-65 years [23]. Each tested participant was asked to take 400 mg capsules of EGCG twice daily for eight weeks. The study showed that EGCG has antihypertensive effects, which may be associated with the cardiovascular benefits of the consumption of green tea.

A recent report indicated that (-)-catechin may have some beneficial effects in the treatment of obesity-related diseases, especially type 2 diabetes [24]. (-)-Catechin enhanced the expression and secretion of adiponectin protein in a dose- and time-dependent manner. Furthermore, treatment with (-)-catechin increased insulin-dependent glucose uptake in differentiated adipocytes and augmented the expression of adipogenic marker genes, including peroxisome proliferator-activated receptor gamma (PPARγ), CCAAT-enhancer-binding protein alpha (C/EBPα), fatty acid synthase (FAS), and stearoyl-coenzymeA desaturase 1 (SCD1), when (-)-catechin was used in the treatment during the adipocyte differentiation. In a search for the molecular mechanism that is responsible for the inducible effect of (-)-catechin on adiponectin expression, it was found that (-)-catechin markedly suppresses the expression of Kruppel-like factor 7 (KLF7) protein, which has recently been reported as inhibiting the expression of adiponectin and other adipogenesis-related genes, including leptin, PPARγ, CEBPα, and aP2 in adipocytes [24]. Adiponectin is an adipocytokine that have anti-atherogenic, anti-inflammatory, and antidiabetic roles [25]. Thus, it represents a novel treatment target for insulin resistance and type-2 diabetes.

Bose *et al.* found that EGCG treatment attenuates hyperlipidemia and fatty liver in mice that were given a high-fat diet (HFD) [26]. In another study, EGCG and epicatechin gallate (ECG) attenuated hepatic lipid accumulation in human HepG2 cells [27]. EGCG is an *in vitro* and *in vivo* inhibitor of fatty acid synthase and acetyl-CoA carboxylase 1 (ACC1) [21, 28]. ACC1 is localized in the cytosol and inhibits the β-oxidation of fatty acids through malonyl-CoA formation, which results in the inhibition of fatty acid transport, mediated by carnitine palmitoyltransferase (CPT1), into the mitochondria [29]. EGCG also induced apoptosis in preadipocytes and inhibited adipogenesis in mature adipocytes. The apoptotic effects were dependent on cyclin-dependent kinase 2 (Cdk2) and caspase 3, and could be attributed to the inhibition of cell mitogenesis [30]. AMP-activated protein kinase (AMPK) is another target molecule for anti-obesity treatments, and it has been shown that EGCG inhibits adipocyte differentiation by activating AMPK [34]. EGCG has been known to stimulate the release of the intracellular reactive oxygen species (ROS), which rapidly activates AMPK and leads to apoptosis [31].

EGCG has also been shown to alleviate diabetes in genetically obese mice and rats [32]. EGCG reduced the glucose uptake in the rat intestine and significantly inhibited the sodium-dependent glucose transporter. In this experiment, ECG was even more potent than EGCG. Presently available *in vitro* data suggest that green tea catechins could reduce glucose absorption by inhibiting the gastro-intestinal enzymes that are involved in nutrient digestion. Furthermore, studies on animals have shown a significant increase in the glucose uptake in the skeletal muscle and a significant decrease in the glucose uptake in the adipose tissue following the ingestion of green tea catechins.

Theaflavins: Theaflavin, Theaflavin-3-Gallate, Theaflavin-3'-Gallate and Theaflavin-3, 3'-Digallate

Theaflavins are a group of natural polyphenol pigments found in black teas, which are among the world's most popular beverages. Theaflavins are categorized into theaflavin (TF), theaflavin-3-gallate (TF3G), theaflavin-3'-gallate (TF3'G), and theaflavin-3, 3'-digallate (TF3DG). Teas are classified into three major categories according to their manufacturing process: unfermented green tea, fully fermented black tea, and partially fermented oolong tea. Approximately 75% of teas consumed worldwide is black tea [33]. Theaflavins are formed from the polymerization of catechins at the fermentation stage during the manufacture of black tea. They contribute to the characteristic bright orange-red color of black tea, and account for 1-2% of the dried water extract from black tea [34]. In the production of black tea, EGCG is converted, together with epicatechin, during the enzymatic "fermentation" induced by polyphenol oxidase, into the most active TF3G. Teaflavins and catechins have recently received much attention as protective agents against cancer and cardiovascular disease [35, 36]. They are also believed to have a wide range of other pharmaceutical benefits, including antioxidative [37], hypolipidemic [38, 39], hypoglycemic [40], antihypertensive [41], anti-fatty liver, and anti-obesity [27] benefits.

A number of studies suggest that black tea consumption can lower total and low-density lipoprotein (LDL) cholesterol, as reviewed by Davies *et al.* [42]. The underlying mechanisms behind this beneficial effect might be the interference of black tea in the formation of dietary mixed micelles in the intestine [39] and its reduction of intestinal cholesterol absorption through the inhibition of pancreatic lipase activity [38]. Theaflavins, especially TF3G which is the most active theaflavin in terms of micelle formation, inhibit cholesterol incorporation in soluble micelles, [39]. Similar *in vitro* effects on decreased cholesterol incorporation in mixed micelles were reported by Ikeda *et al.* [43, 44], Raederstorff *et al.* [45], and others for green tea catechins, especially EGCG. In the study of Kobayashi *et al.*, the effect of theaflavins on postprandial hypertriacylglycerolemia was examined in rats, and the underlying mechanism of the action of the theaflavins was elucidated both *in vitro* and *in vivo* [38]. The administration of the theaflavins at 100 and 200 mg/kg of the body weight of the rats suppressed postprandial hypertriacylglycerolemia in a dose-dependent manner. Additionally, TF3G, TF3'G, and TF3DG, which have galloyl moieties, inhibited the activity of the pancreatic lipase in a dose-dependent manner, but TF did not, as it does not have a galloyl moiety [38]. Therefore, the presence of a gallate moiety in tea polyphenols seems to play a major inhibitory role in the formation of mixed micelles and in the inhibition of the pancreatic lipase activity.

In addition to the hypolipidemic effects of theaflavins, their hypoglycemic effect was revealed by Matsui *et al.* [40]. To clarify the postprandial glucose suppression effect of theaflavins, the researchers tested the inhibitory effects of theaflavins against α-glucosidase using an immobilized α-glucosidase assay system [46] which mimics the intestinal membrane-bound state of the sucrose-isomaltase complex [47]. The results indicated that theaflavins have a more potent antihyperglycemic effect than catechins by inhibiting α-glucosidase (maltase) activity, and subsequently inhibiting glucose production in the intestine [40]. To determine the maltase-inhibitory effects of theaflavins, the effects were observed in descending order of potency, as follows: TF3G, TF3DG, TF3′G, and TF. This suggests that the maltase inhibition induced by theaflavins is closely associated with the presence of a free hydroxyl group at the 3′-position of the TF as well as with the esterification of TF with a mono-gallate group [40].

Moreover, theaflavins may be active in the prevention of fatty liver and obesity. Rats that were treated with diets rich in theaflavins (TF, TF3G, or TF3DG, 50 mg/kg body weight) had more markedly reduced body weights than the HFD-fed controls [27]. Theaflavin-supplemented rats ate more but weighed less than the HFD controls, which suggests that theaflavins might increase energy expenditure. Similarly, the relative liver weight, epididymal fat mass, and plasma lipid levels were significantly reduced in the theaflavin-rich diet group than in the control rats. The researchers also provided evidence that theaflavins likely play a significant role in reducing cellular lipid accumulation by increasing AMPK phosphorylation in HepG2 cells, and that a ROS/serine-threonine kinase liver kinase B1/AMPK signaling module may be involved in this process [27].

Cyanidins

Cyanidins are considered the most widely spread anthocyanin in the plant kingdom. They are largely distributed in the human diet through crops, beans, fruits, vegetables, and red wines, which suggests that humans ingest daily significant amounts of these compounds from plant-based diets [48]. It has been reported that cyanidins have several pharmacological properties, including antioxidant, anticarcinogenic, anti-inflammatory, neuroprotective, skin-photoprotective, gastroprotective, anti-obesity, and antidiabetic effects [48].

Tsuda *et al.* investigated the potency of the therapeutic implications of cyanidin 3-glucoside in the prevention of obesity and diabetes. They assessed the potential role of purple corn color (PCC), which is rich in cyanidin 3-glucoside, in the prevention of obesity and in the amelioration of diabetes [49]. Cyanidin-3-glycoside, also known as kuromanin, is probably the most notorious and the most widely investigated among the cyanidin-glycosides [50]. Tsuda *et al.* found that dietary PCC significantly suppressed the HFD-induced increases in the body weight gain, the white and brown adipose tissue weights, and improved hyperglycemia, hyperinsulinemia, and hyperleptinemia, by suppressing the mRNA levels of the enzymes involved in fatty acid and triacylglycerol synthesis, lowering the mRNA level of the sterol regulatory element binding protein-1 (SREBP-1), and normalizing the increase in the mRNA level of the tumor necrosis factor (TNF)-α in the visceral adipose tissue [49]. In another study, the researchers found that rat and human adipocytes that were treated with cyanidin 3-glucoside [51] enhanced adipocytokine (adiponectin and leptin) secretion and upregulated the adipocyte-specific gene expression [52], and that the isolated rat adipocytes that were treated with cyanidin 3-glucoside and cyanidin demonstrated an up-regulation of hormone-sensitive lipase (HSL) and perilipin as well as enhancement of the lipolytic activity [53].

Cyanidin 3-glucoside stimulated *in vitro* insulin secretion from rodent pancreatic beta-cells (INS-1 832/13) at 4 and 10 mM glucose concentrations [54]. Among cyanidin glycosides, cyanidin 3-rutinoside has been proposed as a new non-competitive α-glucosidase inhibitor because of its ability to inhibit α-glucosidase from baker's yeast [55]. Another cyanidin glycoside, cyanidin 3-galactoside, has also been proposed as a new competitive α-glucosidase inhibitor due to its ability to inhibit α- glucosidase from rat intestinal acetone powder [56]. These outcomes suggest that cyanidins have a uniquely potent therapeutic advantage and important implications in the prevention of obesity and diabetes.

Isoflavones: Genistein, Daidzein, and Glycitein

Isoflavones are commonly found in soybeans and soy products. Isoflavones exist primarily in plants in an inactive form as β-D-glycosides (genistin, daidzin and glycitin). After ingested, isoflavone glycosides are hydrolyzed by interstinal glucosidases and are converted to corresponding bioactive aglycones (genistein, daidzein, and glycitein). The aglycones are then absorbed from the intestinal tract and conjugated mainly in the liver into glucuronides, which are either re-excreted through the bile and then reabsorbed through enterohepatic recycling, or excreted unchanged in the urine. The chemical structure of isoflavones is very similar to that of human estrogen. Because of this similarity in structure, they can interfere with the action of human estrogen [57]. Depending on the type of estrogen receptor in the cells, isoflavones may reduce or activate the activity of estrogen. The consumption of soy products has many health benefits, including protection against breast cancer, prostate cancer, menopausal symptoms, heart disease, and osteoporosis. Many of the health benefits of soy are derived from its isoflavones [57, 58].

A number of studies suggest that isoflavones (genistein, daidzein, and glycitein) may favorably affect adiposity, glucose homeostasis, insulin secretion, and lipid metabolism (Table **1**). Several epidemiological studies have reported that isoflavone consumption by postmenopausal women was correlated with lower body mass index and fasting insulin concentrations, and higher HDL levels [59-61]. Additionally, Japanese postmenopausal women who were treated with isoflavones for 24 weeks exhibited a lower body fat mass [62]. These results indicate the beneficial effects of isoflavones on excess body weight, hyperinsulinemia, and hyperlipidemia, which are the major cardiovascular risk factors commonly associated with obesity. Plasma triglycerides were more significantly reduced in Sprague-Dawley rats that were fed a mixture of synthetic daidzein and genistein (23.6 mg/kg body weight/day) than in those that were fed casein [63]. Hamsters that were fed pure synthetic daidzein (16 mg/kg body weight/day) had significantly lower plasma total cholesterol levels than those that were fed casein [64]. In another study, glycitein (13 mg/kg body weight/day) showed a more marked cholesterol-lowering effect than other isoflavones [65]. The researchers suggested that glycitein's greater cholesterol-lowering effect was due to its greater bioavailability, as reflected in its urinary recovery, than that of the other isoflavones [65].

In addition to the hypolipidemic effects of isoflavones, dietary supplementation with 500-1,500 ppm of genistein, with a serum equivalent of about 2 μM, decreases fat-pad weights by 50% in C57/BL6 mice [66]. Similarly, subcutaneous injections of genistein (8-200 mg/kg/day) in C57/BL6 ovariectomized mice for 21 days decreased the adipose tissue gain [66]. In contrast, in a study wherein male mice were exposed to daily oral doses of genistein of up to 50 mg/kg/day, the fat mass increased [67], whereas it decreased at doses of 200 mg/kg/day [67]. These results suggest that high pharmacological doses of isoflavones that yield serum levels in the micromolar range inhibit adipose tissue deposition. The mechanisms by which isoflavones reduce adiposity *in vivo* are still unclear. *In vitro* studies in which isolated rat adipocytes were used, however, showed that genistein and daidzein stimulate lipolysis by inhibiting cAMP phosphodiesterases [68, 69]. Furthermore, the exposure of cultured 3T3-L1 adipocytes to genistein has been reported to significantly activate AMPK and ACC [31]. AMPK is another target molecule for anti-obesity treatments, and genistein has been shown to inhibit adipocyte differentiation by activating AMPK. Genistein stimulated intracellular ROS release, which rapidly activated AMPK and led to apoptosis. The protein expressions of PPARs and C/EBP decreased in adipocytes that were treated with genistein [70]. Genistein also inhibited the mitotic clonal expansion of two-day post-confluent 3T3-L1 preadipocytes [70]. In an isolated perfused liver preparation, however, genistein reduced the incorporation of [^{14}C] glucose into lipids and increased the output of fatty acids into the medium [71]. These changes were accompanied by a decrease in the hepatic triacylglycerol content. Thus, genistein appears to have direct effects on lipid metabolism in the liver and the adipose tissue by affecting both lipogenesis and lipolysis.

Fewer studies have evaluated the effects of isoflavones on glucose homeostasis. In mice models of obesity and diabetes, treatment with genistein lowered glycemia [72]. Potential mechanisms by which isoflavones may improve glucose metabolism have been recently proposed. Recent reports indicate that genistein may itself have a direct beneficial effect on pancreatic β-cells. For example, genistein has been shown to stimulate insulin secretion in the insulin-secreting cell lines INS-1 and MIN6 and in mouse pancreatic islets, at nano- and micromolar concentrations [73]. Genistein and daidzein have been shown to prevent diabetes onset in non-obese diabetic mice by preserving the pancreatic β-cell function [74]. Similarly, Lee *et al.* (2006) recently reported that in rats that had streptozotocin-induced diabetes, diet supplementation with genistein (600 mg/kg of the diet) caused a twofold increase in the plasma insulin levels [75]. In additional studies, genistein was shown to inhibit islet tyrosine kinase activities and glucose- and sulfonylurea-stimulated insulin release without affecting the glucose metabolism [68]. Collectively, these data suggest that dietary soy and phytoestrogens may have therapeutic significance in reducing the severity of diabetes, and in improving β-cell survival and function. Further research is needed, however, first, to confirm, and then to analyze, in detail, how phytoestrogens exert antihyperglycemic actions through the pancreatic β-cells.

Kaempferol

Kaemferol is a natural flavonoid that has been isolated from tea, broccoli, strawberries, gooseberries, cranberries, *Euonymus alatus*, *Sauroupus androgynus*, *Delphinium*, witch hazel, grapefruit, brussel sprouts, apples, and other plant sources [76, 77]. A number of studies have been carried out to investigate the anti-obesity effects of kaempferol *in vitro* and *in vivo* (Table **1**). Yu *et al.* tested the toxicity and anti-obesity features of the compound 3-*O*-β-D-glucosyl-(1→6)-β-D-glucosyl-kaempferol (GGK), isolated from *Sauropus androgynus*, in rats fed an HFD. Sixty milligrams of GGK per kilogram of body weight, which was administered *via* gastric intubation, significantly reduced the food intake of rats, and the reduced food intake corresponded to decreases in the body weight gain [76].

The clinical relevance of PPARγ is highlighted by the currently marketed antidiabetic drugs, rosiglitazone and pioglitazone. As full PPARγ antagonists, they promote adipocyte differentiation and lipid storage. Kaempferol also significantly improved insulin-stimulated glucose uptake in mature 3T3-L1 adipocytes [77]. The potential mechanism by which kaempferol ameliorates hyperglycemia may partly be by serving as a ligand of PPARγ, and thus, improving insulin-stimulated glucose uptake in mature adipocytes, while lacking the capability to induce preadipocyte differentiation. Thus, kaempferol may potentially be developed as a safe and novel compound for anti-obesity and antidiabetes treatment.

Myricetin

Myricetin is a flavonol that is commonly found in teas, wines, berries, fruits, and medicinal plants (*Abelmoschus moschatus*). Its therapeutic potential is seen both in its anticarcinogenic, anti-inflammatory, antioxidative, antiviral, and antimicrobial properties and in its prevention of platelet aggregation [78-82]. The therapeutic benefits of myricetin in cardiovascular diseases associated with diabetes mellitus have also been reported [83-86]. Additionally, the insulinomimetic effect of myricetin on lipogenesis and glucose transport in the adipocytes of rats with non-insulin-dependent diabetes mellitus has been observed [87].

Liu *et al.* investigated the effects of myricetin on the healing of insulin resistance [83, 88]. Intravenous injection of myricetin (1 mg per kg of body weight) into genetically obese diabetic rats and rats that were fed high-fructose diets three times a day for one week and two weeks, respectively, reduced the value of the glucose-insulin index, an index of insulin resistance. In addition, myricetin treatment reversed the inability of insulin to increase the expression of the glucose transporter 4 (GLUT 4) and to increase the protein levels and phosphorylation of the insulin receptor substrate 1 (IRS1) in the soleus muscle of the obese rats. Myricetin treatment also increased the expression of the p85 regulatory subunit of phosphatidylinositol 3-kinase (PI3K) and promoted Akt serine phosphorylation in the soleus muscle of the diabetic rats [83, 88]. In another study, after two days of treatment with myricetin (3 mg per 12 h), hyperglycemia in diabetic rats was reduced by 50%, and the hypertriglyceridemia that is often associated with diabetes normalized [89]. Treatment with myricetin increased the hepatic glycogen synthase I activity and the glucose-6-phosphate content [89]. Myricein also stimulated glucose uptake in isolated rat adipocytes and enhanced insulin-stimulated lipogenesis in adipocytes at concentrations that ranged from 200 to 250 μM [87] and at low doses (10-100 μM), inhibited the transport of glucose in isolated rat adipocytes stimulated with insulin [90]. The increase in the lipogenesis might have been a consequence of increased glucose transport. Besides, myricetin prevented diabetic cataracts by inhibiting lens aldose reductase [91]. Taking all these together shows that myricetin may improve insulin sensitivity and reverse insulin resistance. Such effects may be mediated through enhanced insulin-mediated glucose transport signaling in the muscles and adipose tissues of obese diabetic rats.

Hesperetin and Hesperidin

Hesperetin belongs to the class of flavonoids called flavanones and is derived from the hydrolysis of its aglycone, hesperidin (hesperetin 7-rhammnoglucoside). Hesperetin, together with hesperidin, is abundant in citrus fruits, such as grapefruit and oranges. In Finland, the average daily intake of hesperetin has been estimated as 28.3 mg [92]. Hesperetin has been found to exhibit estrogenic, anticarcinogenic, antioxidative, anti-inflammatory and lipid-lowering properties [92-96].

With regard to the lipid-lowering propensity of hesperetin, Cha *et al.* [96] found that this compound, at a dietary level of 1%, attenuated the orotic-acid-dependent increase in the hepatic triacylglycerol level and activity of microsomal phosphatidate phosphohydrolase, an enzyme involved in the synthesis of triacylglyceride, in rat liver. Hesperetin, at a dietary level of 0.02%, lowered the plasma levels of cholesterol and triacylglyceride and the activity of 3-hydroxy-3-methylglutaryl-coenzyme (HMG-CoA) reductase, the rate-limiting enzyme in the cholesterol biosynthesis, and acyl CoA: cholesterol acyltransferase (ACAT), another key cholesterol-regulating enzyme involved in the esterification and absorption of cholesterol, in rats fed a high-cholesterol diet [96]. Studies of Wilcox *et al.* [94] have shown that hesperetin decreased the secretion of apolipoprotein B (apoB), an apolipoprotein that abounds in low-density and very-low-density lipoproteins, in human hepatoma cells (HepG2). Their study results also showed that hesperetin decreases the activities of ACAT2 and microsomal triacylglycerol transfer protein

(MTP), and increases the LDL receptor activity [94]. MTP plays a key role in apoB secretion by catalyzing the transfer of lipids to the nascent apoB molecule as it is cotranslationally translocated across the endoplasmic reticulum membrane [97, 98]. Furthermore, the increased LDL receptor activity contributed to the reduced accumulation of apoB in the media [94]. It has been seen that hesperetin's blockade of the cholesterol biosynthesis results in a lower intracellular supply of cholesterol, which triggers an over-expression of hepatic LDL receptors and enhances the clearance of circulating LDL particles [99]. Thus, hesperetin may affect various aspects of lipid metabolism and exert lipid-lowering activity *in vivo*.

Hesperidin is a flavanone glycoside that consists of the flavone hesperitin, which is bound to the disaccharide rutinose (Table **1**). The sugar causes hesperidin to be more soluble than hesperitin. Hesperidin is also mainly found in citrus fruits such as lemons and oranges. The highest concentration of hesperidin can be found in the white parts and pulps of the citrus peels. Hesperidin can also be found in green vegetables. Among naturally occurring flavonoids, hesperidin has been empirically proven to have no side-effects, as humans have been ingesting grapes and citrus fruits for a long time [100]. Hesperidin exhibits biological and pharmacological properties, such as anti-inflammatory, anticarcinogenic, antioxidant, lipid-lowering, and antidiabetic properties [101-104].

Hesperidin supplementation improves hyperglycemia in *db/db* mice by regulating the activities of the hepatic glucose metabolic enzymes involved in glycolysis and gluconeogenesis [102]. In another study, this compound was found to be beneficial in the lowering of the blood glucose level because it upregulates the hepatic glucokinase, PPARγ, and adipocyte GLUT4 [101]. Hesperidin was also found to be very effective in improving the lipid metabolism in *db/db* mice by suppressing the activities of hepatic lipid metabolizing enzymes, such as fatty acid synthase, glucose-6-phosphate dehydrogenase (G6PDH), and phosphatidate phosphohydrolase, and by increasing fecal triglyceride excretion [101]. Plasma cholesterol levels are regulated by cholesterol biosynthesis, the removal of cholesterol from the body's circulation, and the excretion of cholesterol *via* faecal sterols or bile acids. Numerous previous researches have reported the beneficial effects of hepatic HMG-CoA reductase and ACAT inhibitors on hypercholesterolaemia and atherosclerosis [105, 106]. In one study, hesperidin also led to a decrease in the plasma and hepatic cholesterol levels, which may have been partly due to the decreased activities of hepatic HMG-CoA reductase and ACAT and the increased fecal cholesterol excretion [101]. These coordinated responses of the hesperidin supplement seemed to play an important role in regulating the lipid and glucose metabolism in *db/db* mice [101].

Naringenin and Naringin

Naringenin is the predominat flavone in citrus fruits and grapefruit. It can also be absorbed from cooked tomato paste. This compound is considered to have a bioactive effect on human health as an antioxidant, a free radical scavenger, an anti-inflammatory agent, a carbohydrate metabolism promoter, and an immune system modulator. The average daily intake of naringenin in Finland has been estimated as 8.3 mg [92]. Harmon and Harp investigated the anti-obesity effects of naringenin [70] and found that it can reduce the adipose tissue mass by inhibiting preadipocyte proliferation. Naringenin at 50-100 μM inhibited the proliferation of preconfluent preadipocytes in a time- and dose-dependent manner [70], but the presence of naringenin during the induction of differentiation had no adverse effect on the subsequent adipogenesis [107].

Huong *et al.* demonstrated that naringenin has the physiologic effect of increasing hepatic fatty acid oxidation by up-regulating the gene expression of the enzymes involved in peroxisomal β-oxidation in mice [108]. The change may account for the propensity of this compound to lower serum lipid levels. This compound also caused significant increases in the activity levels of various enzymes involved in hepatic fatty acid oxidation, such as carnitine octanoyltransferase, acyl-coenzyme A oxidase, and 3-ketoacyl–coenzyme A thiolase [108]. Lee *et al.* also reported that naringenin at a 0.1% dietary level decreased the plasma cholesterol level and the hepatic levels of triacylglycerol and cholesterol in rats fed a high-cholesterol diet, which was accompanied by a decrease in the activity of HMG-CoA reductase and ACAT [109]. Naringenin decreased the secretion of apoB, an apolipoprotein that abounds in low-density and very-low-density lipoproteins, upregulated the mRNA expression of LDL receptors, and decreased the activities of ACAT and MTP, a key enzyme in apoB secretion, in HepG2 cells [94].

Harmon and Patel found that the grapefruit flavanone naringenin inhibited insulin-stimulated glucose uptake in 3T3-L1 adipocytes in a dose-dependent manner [107]. Naringenin inhibited the activity of PI3K, a key regulator of insulin-induced GLUT4 translocation. Although naringenin did not alter the phosphotyrosine status of the insulin receptor, insulin receptor substrate proteins, or PI3K, it inhibited the phosphorylation of the downstream signaling molecule, Akt. The physiologically attainable dose of 6 μM of naringenin reduced the insulin-stimulated glucose uptake by approximately 20%. This inhibitory effect remained 24 h after the removal of naringenin from the culture medium. Collectively, the findings suggest that regular consumption of naringenin may exacerbate insulin resistance in susceptible individuals *via* impaired glucose uptake in the adipose tissue. These adverse effects of naringenin on glucose homeostasis would depend on the ability of an individual to absorb and metabolize naringenin [107].

Naringin is the aglycone of naringenin (Table **1**). It is metabolized into the flavonone naringenin in humans. Naringin is the major flavonoid glycoside in citrus fruits and grapefruit, and which is what gives such fruits their bitter taste. Naringin exhibits biological and pharmacological properties, such as anti-inflammatory, anticarcinogenic, antioxidant, lipid-lowering, and antidiabetic properties [101-104]. Some studies have demonstrated that naringin may act as a regulator of plasma lipids in hypercholesterolemic animals, such as *db/db* mice or rats fed a HFD [101, 102, 110, 111]. Diet supplementation with 0.02% naringin for three weeks did not exhibit a hypolipidemic effect on rats fed a high-fat and high-cholesterol diet [113, 114]. Naringin improved the plasma and hepatic lipid metabolism in *db/db* mice by altering the hepatic-lipid-metabolizing enzyme activities and fecal lipids [101]. In addition, naringin improved hyperglycemia in type 2 diabetes mellitus mice by regulating the activities and expressions of the hepatic enzymes involved in glycolysis and gluconeogenesis and by up-regulating the hepatic and adipocyte PPARγ and GLUT4 [101, 102]. Naringin consumption (at 400 mg/day for eight weeks) lowered the plasma total and LDL-cholesterol concentrations in hypercholesterolemic subjects [111]. Naringin supplementation had no effect, however, on the plasma lipid levels in healthy control subjects [111]. These coordinated responses of the naringin supplement seemed to play an important role in regulating the lipid and glucose metabolism in hyperlipidemic or hyperglycemic subjects [101]. Naringin can, however, lower the hepatic cholesterol biosynthesis and levels of plasma lipids and glucose when supplemented for at least six weeks in these subjects [110, 111].

Quercetin

Quercetin, the most abundant of the flavonoids, forms the backbone for many other flavonoids including rutin (a glycosylated quercetin), hesperidin, and naringenin. Quercetin is found in various human foods such as red onions, grapes, apples, berries, cherries, broccoli, citrus fruits, and tea (*Camellia sinensis*), and in particularly high concentrations (180 mg per 100 g) in capers and lovage. The average daily human intake of quercetin ranges from 10 to 100 mg depending on eating habits [112]. Quercetin has a wide range of biological effects such as lowering of blood pressure [113, 114], reduction of body weight [113], and amelioration of hyperglycemia-related diseases [77, 115], as shown in animal models and, to some extent, in humans.

Edwards *et al.* recently published a randomized, double-blind, and placebo-controlled cross-over study that included patients with prehypertension (n = 19) and stage 1 hypertension (n = 22) [114]. The blood pressure of the prehypertensive patients did not change after their diet was supplemented with 730 mg of quercetin/day for 28 days. In contrast, significant reductions in systolic, diastolic, and mean arterial blood pressure were observed in the stage 1 hypertensive patients after quercetin treatment. Interestingly, quercetin did not affect the indices of oxidant stress that were measured in the plasma and urine, unlike in previous animal-based studies. Although many questions remain (on the optimal dosage, long-term-effects, efficacy compared with other antihypertensive agents, etc.), the study of Edwards *et al.* was the first to show that quercetin supplementation reduces blood pressure in hypertensive patients [114]. The increased nitric oxide (NO) availability caused by the elevated NO synthase (NOS) activity and the antioxidative activity in the DIO rats fed with quercetin is suggested as one of the causes of the suppressed elevation of the blood pressure [113].

Quercetin induces apoptosis in 3T3-L1 preadipocytes by decreasing the mitochondria membrane potential, down-regulating poly (ADP-ribose) polymerase (PARP) and Bcl-2, and activating caspase 3, Bax, and Bak [116]. In maturing preadipocytes, quercetin at 25 μM suppressed intracellular lipid accumulation by 15.9±2.5% and significantly decreased the expression of PPARγ, which acts as a key adipogenic transcription factor [117]. The breakdown of triglycerides in adipocytes and the release of glycerol and fatty acids are important in the regulation of energy homeostasis [118]. Quercetin caused a dose- and time-dependent increase in lipolysis in rat adipocytes, which was synergistic with epinephrine; and this effective lipolytic flavonoid was also reported to be a potent phosphodiesterase (PDE) inhibitor [119]. Taken together, these reports indicate that quercetin can have potential anti-obesity effects by inhibiting the differentiation of preadipocytes and inducing the apoptosis of mature adipocytes.

Table 1. Beneficial Effects of Flavonoids on Obesity and Associated Diseases

Bioactive Compound	Model (Treatment dosage and duration)	Beneficial effects	Mechanisms of action	Refs.
(-)-Catechin 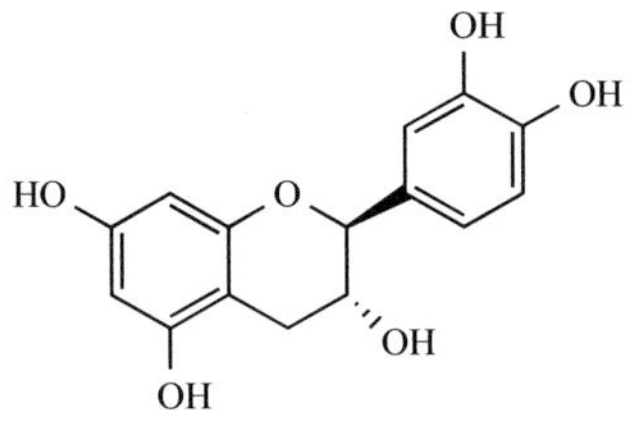	3T3-L1 adipocytes (50 μM)	Insulin-stimulated glucose uptake ↑	Adiponectin expression and secretion ↑ Adipogenic gene expression (PPARγ, C/EBPα, aP2) ↑	[24]
(-)-Epigallocatechin gallate	Obese men (300 mg/day, 3 days)	Postprandial RQ ↓		[22]
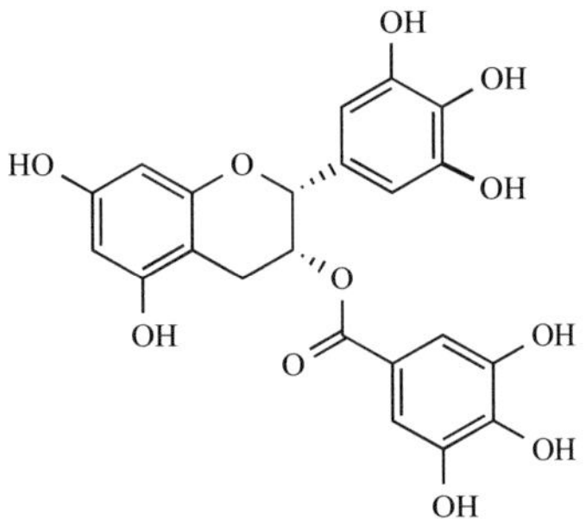	Obese men (800 mg/ day, 8wk)	Blood pressure ↓		[23]
	DIO mice and rats (0.32–1% wt/wt in diet, 16–20 wk)	Body weight ↓ Visceral fat weight ↓ Blood lipids ↓ Blood glucose ↓ Insulin resistance improved Fatty liver improved	Leptin secretion ↓ Fatty acid synthesis (FAS, G6PDH) ↓ Fatty acid oxidation (SCD1) ↑ Fecal lipids ↑	[21, 26]
	DIO mice (0.5–1% wt/wt in diet, 4 wk)	Body weight ↓ Visceral fat weight ↓ Blood lipids ↓ Blood glucose ↓	Hepatic fatty acid synthesis [malic enzyme, glucokinase (GK)] ↓ Hepatic fatty acid oxidation (SCD1) ↑ Epididymal leptin expression ↓ and fatty acid oxidation (SCD1) ↑	[28]
	db/db Mice and ZDF rats (0.5–1% wt/wt in diet, 7 wk)	Blood lipids ↓ Blood glucose ↓ Insulin resistance improved	Insulin secretion ↑ Fatty acid oxidation (ACO-1 and CPT-1) ↑ Hepatic glucose uptake (GK) ↑ Gluconeogenesis ↓	[32]
	3T3-L1 adipocytes (100 μM)	TG accumulation ↓	Apoptosis ↑ (apoptotic cell number ↑; Cdk2↓ and caspase-3 ↑) Adipogenic transcription factors (PPARγ1/2, C/EBPα and LXRα) expression ↓ Fatty acid oxidation (pACC/ACC and pAMPK/AMPK) ↑ GPDH activity ↓	[30, 31, 137, 138]
Epicatechin gallate 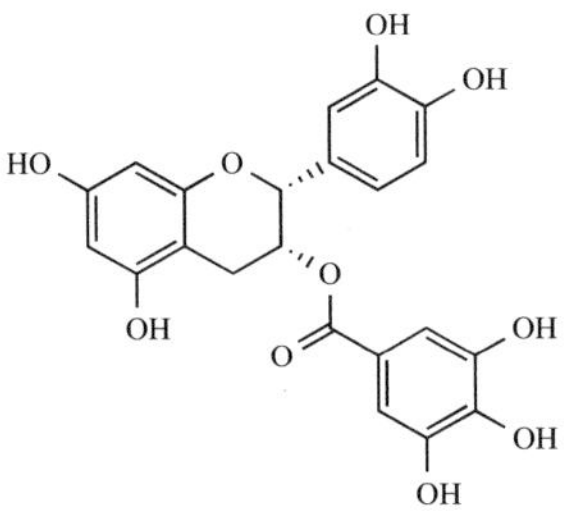	HepG2 cells (50 μM)	TG accumulation ↓	Adipogenic transcription factors (PPARγ2, C/EBPα) expression ↓	[27]
	Everted rat intestinal sacs and rabbit intestinal brush-border membrane vesicles (0.5–1 mM)	Glucose uptake ↓	Glucose transporter antagonist	[139]

(Table 1) Contd…..

Bioactive Compound	Model (Treatment dosage and duration)	Beneficial effects	Mechanisms of action	Refs.
Theaflavins: TF, TF3G, TF3´G, TF3DG 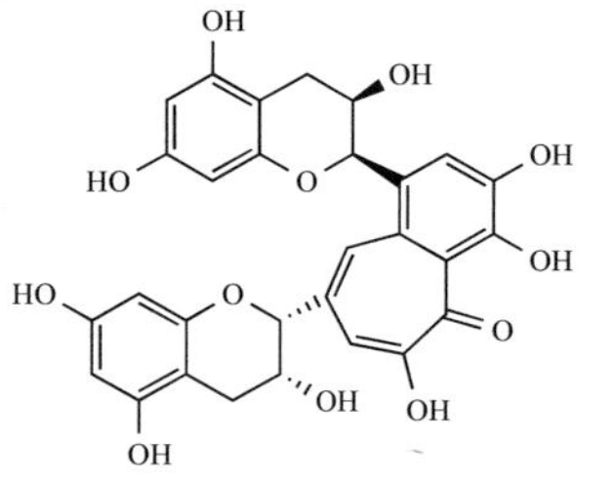 Teaflavin 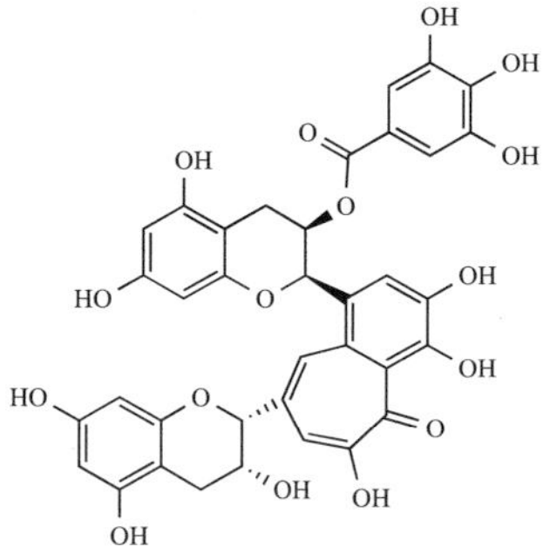 Teaflavin-3-gallate 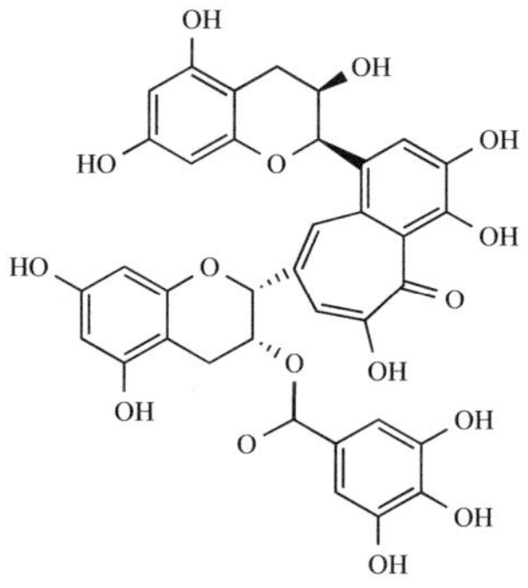 Teaflavin-3'-gallate	DIO rats (50 mg/kg BW)	Body weight ↓ Visceral fat weight ↓ Fatty liver ↓ Blood lipids ↓	Hepatic fatty acid oxidation (AMPK phosphorylation) ↑	[27]
	Rats (10 mg/ kg BW with maltose, 0–120 min) *In vitro* immobilized AGH assay system	Postprandial blood glucose ↓	α-Glucosidase (maltase) activity in the gut ↓	[40]
	Rats (100 or 200 mg/ kg BW with a lipid emulsion, 0–8 h) *In vitro* pancreatic lipase activity assay	Postprandial blood triglyceride ↓	Pancreatic lipase activity ↓ Intestinal triglyceride absorption ↓	[38]
	HepG2 cells (50μM)	TG accumulation ↓	Hepatic fatty acid oxidation (AMPK phosphorylation) ↑ and fatty acid synthesis (FAS) ↓	[27]
	In vitro micelle formation assay	Dietary mixed micelles formation ↓	Cholesterol incorporation into mixed micelles ↓	[39]
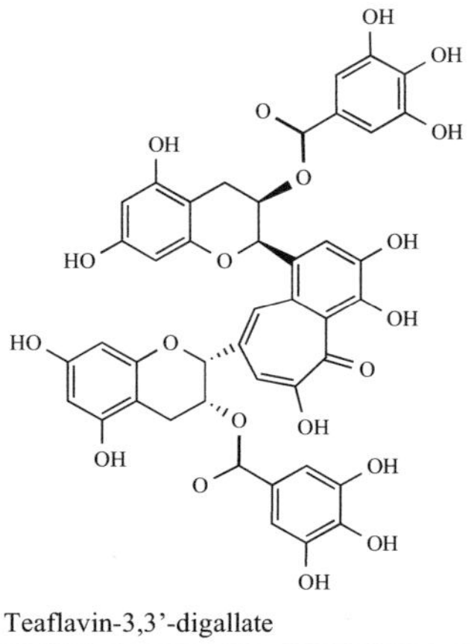 Teaflavin-3,3'-digallate				

(Table 1) Contd…..

Bioactive Compound	Model (Treatment dosage and duration)	Beneficial effects	Mechanisms of action	Refs.
Cyandin and Cyanidin 3-glucoside 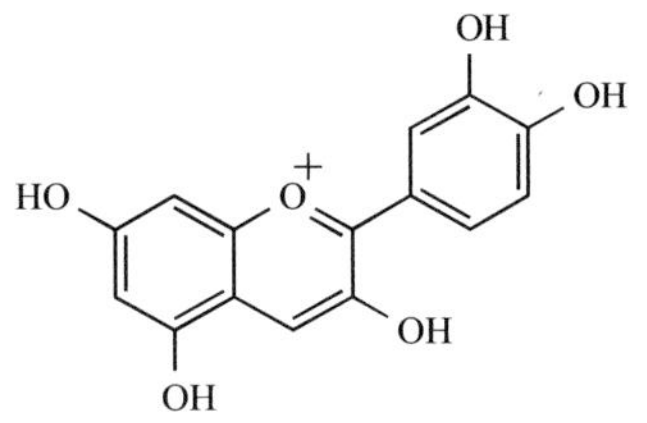 Cyanidin 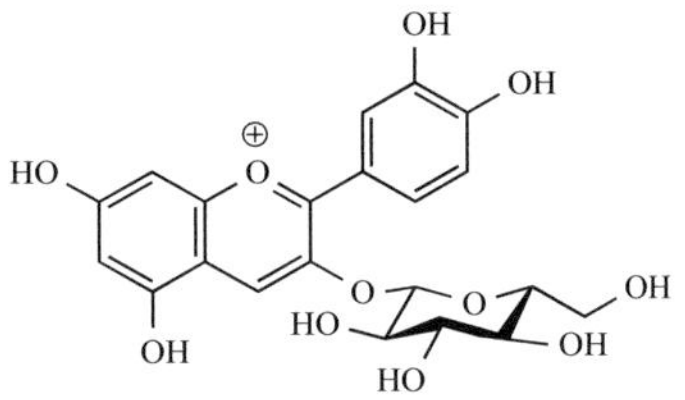 Cyanidin 3-glucoside	DIO mice (0.2% wt/wt in diet, 12 wk)	Body weight ↓ Visceral fat weight ↓ Blood lipids ↓ Fatty liver improved Insulin resistance improved	Adipogenic transcription factor (SREBP-1c) expression ↓, Adipogenic enzymes (FAS; ACS1; GPAT) ↓ Adipocytokines (leptin; TNF-α) ↓	[49]
	Isolated human adipocytes (100 μM)	TG accumulation ↓ Normalizing adipocytokine secretion Inflammation ↓	Adipogenic transcription factor (C/EBPα) mRNA↑ Adipocytokine expression change (adiponectin ↑; plasminogen activator inhibitor 1; IL-6 ↓) Lipolysis and fatty acid oxidation ↑ (UCP2, acylCoA oxidase 1, and perilipin ↑)	[52]
	Isolated rat adipocytes (100 μM)	TG accumulation ↓ Insulin resistance ↓	Adipogenic transcription factor (PPARγ and C/EBPα) ↑, Adipogenic genes (LPL, aP2, FAS, ME, GLUT 4) ↑ Adipocytokine (leptin and adiponectin) secretion ↑ Lipolysis and fatty acid oxidation ↑ (AMPK activation, UCP 2, HSL and perilipin) ↑	[51, 53]
	INS-1 832/13 cells (50μg/ml)	Insulin secretion ↑		[54]
Cyanidin-3-rutinoside 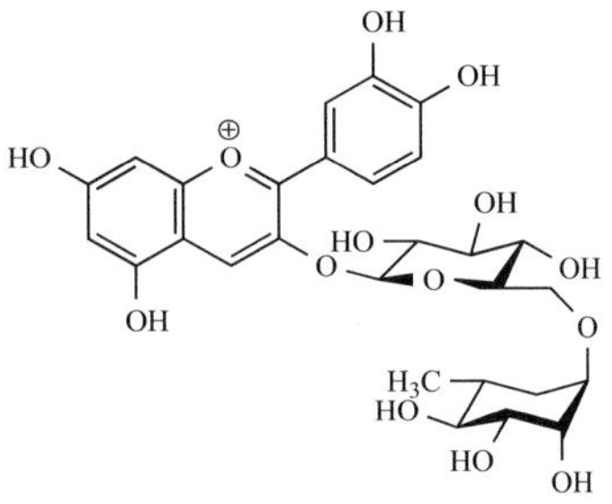	*In vitro* assay	α-Glucosidase activity↓	Competitive inhibitor of of α-glucosidase	[55]
Cyanidin-3-galactoside 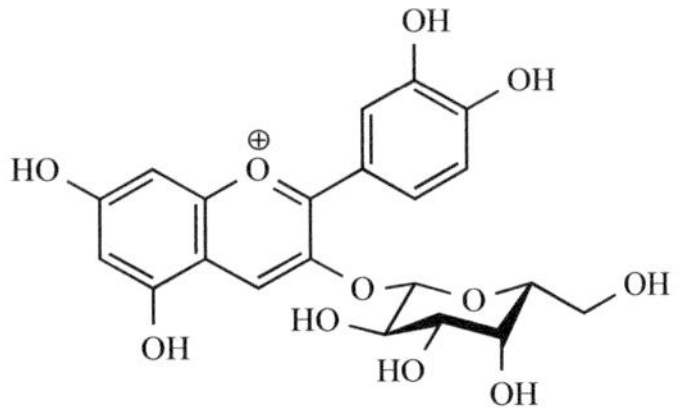	*In vitro* assay	α-Glucosidase activity↓	Competitive inhibitor of substrate of α-glucosidase	[56]
Soy isoflavones mixture	Postmenopausal women (75 mg/day, 6 mo)	BMI ↓ Body fat mass ↓ Blood HDL ↑		[62]
	Rats (0.038% wt/wt in diet, 3 wk)	Blood lipids (TG) ↓		[63]
	Hasmters (0.03% wt/wt in diet, 10 wk)	Blood TC ↓ Blood HDL ↓		[64]

(Table 1) Contd…..

Bioactive Compound	Model (Treatment dosage and duration)	Beneficial effects	Mechanisms of action	Refs.
Genistein 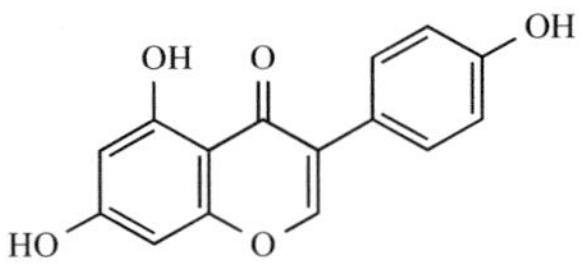	Postmenopausal women (≥ 1 mg/day)	BMI ↓ Body fat mass ↓ Waist size ↓ Blood HDL ↑		[59]
	Postmenopausal women (0.001-0.999 mg/day)	Blood HDL ↑ Fasting insulin ↓		[59]
	Mice (0.05-0.15% wt/wt in diet, 12 days)	Body fat mass ↓	LPL activity in adipose tissue ↓	[66]
	Mice (200 mg/kg, 15 days)	Body weight ↓ Body fat mass ↓		[67]
	Rats (0.01, 0.1% wt/wt in diet, 2 wk)	Blood lipids ↓ Fatty liver improved Lipogenesis ↓		[71, 140]
	db/db mice (0.02% wt/wt in diet, 5 wk)	Blood glucose ↓ Glucose tolerance ↑ Blood lipids ↓ Fatty liver improved	Hepatic gluconeogenesis (G6Pase and PEPCK activities) ↓ Hepatic glycolysis (GK activity) ↑ Hepatic fatty acid synthesis (FAS and G6PDH activity) ↓	[72]
	STZ-induced diabetic rats (0.06% wt/wt in diet, 3 wk)	Blood insulin ↑ Blood lipids ↓ Fatty liver improved	Hepatic gluconeogenesis (G-6-Pase activities) ↓ Hepatic glycolysis ↑ (GK activity) ↑	[75]
	Isolated rat adipocytes (0.1, 1 mM)	Lypolysis ↑ Insulin sensitivity ↑	cAMP phosphodiesterase ↓ Tyrosine kinase activity↓	[68]
	INS-1 and MIN6 cells (0.01-10 μM)	Insulin secretion ↑	cAMP/PKA activity ↑	[73]
Daidzein 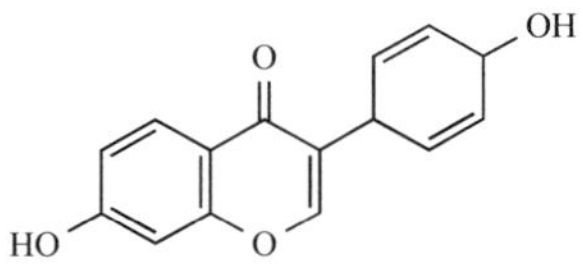	Non-obese diabetic mice (0.02% wt/wt in diet, 9 wk)	Blood glucose ↓ Blood insulin ↑ Blood lipids ↓ Fatty liver improved	Pancreatic β-cell function ↑ (C-peptide secretion↑, immune-histochemical insulin staining ↑) Hepatic gluconeogenesis (G6Pase and PEPCK activities) ↓ Hepatic fatty acid synthesis (malic enayme and G6PDH activity) ↓ Hepatic fatty acid oxidation (CPT activity) ↓	[74]
	Rat adipocytes (0.1, 1 mM)	Lypolysis ↑	PKA activity ↑	[69]
	3T3-L1 adipocytes (20-200 μM)	TG accumulation ↓ Adipocyte apoptosis ↑	Lypolysis (AMPK activity↑) ↑ ROS release ↑ PPARγ expression ↓	[31, 70]
Glycitein 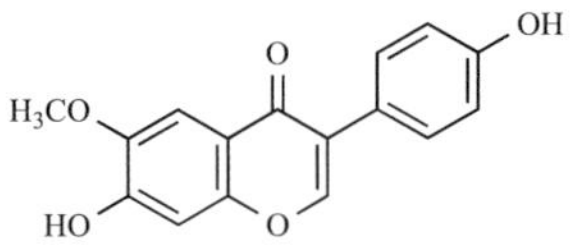	Ovariectomized rats (50 mg/kg BW)	Blood lipids ↓		[141]
	DIO Hamsters (0.025% wt/wt in diet, 4 wk)	Blood lipids (Cholesterol) ↓		[65]
Kaempferol 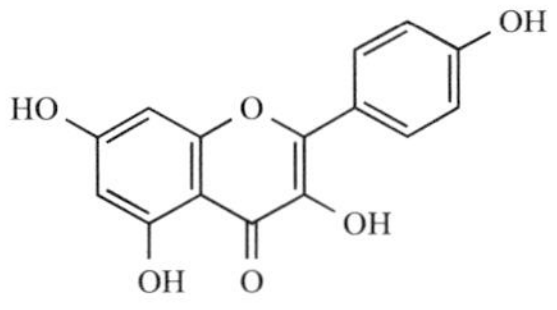	DIO rats (6−60 mg/kg BW, 4 wk)	Body weight gain ↓ Blood lipids ↓	Food intake ↓	[76]
	3T3-L1 adipocytes (20−50 μM)	Glucose uptake ↑ TG accumulation ↓	Adipogenesis ↓ Partial agonist of PPARγ	[77]

(Table 1) Contd…..

Bioactive Compound	Model (Treatment dosage and duration)	Beneficial effects	Mechanisms of action	Refs.
Myricetin 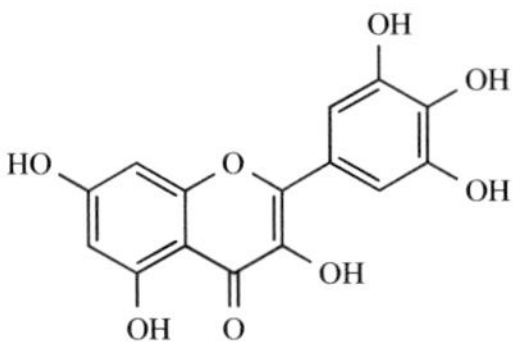	Obese Zucker rats (I.V. injection, 3 mg/kg BW/day, 1 wk)	Blood glucose ↓ Insulin resistance ↓	Post-receptor insulin signaling in muscle (GLUT 4, IRS-1, PI3-kinase, and Akt) ↑	[88]
	Diet-induced diabetic rats (I.V. injection, 3 mg/kg BW/day, 2 wk)	Blood glucose ↓ Insulin resistance ↓ Blood lipid (TG) ↓	Post-receptor insulin signalings in muscle (GLUT 4, IRS-1, PI3-kinase and Akt) ↑ Hepatic glycogen synthesis ↑	[83]
	Streptozotocin -induced diabetic rats (3 mg/12 h, 4 days)	Blood glucose ↓ Insulin resistance improved Blood lipid (TG) ↓	Hepatic glycogen synthesis and glucose-6-phosphate content ↑	[89]
	Isolated rat adipocytes (200–250 μM)	Glucose uptake ↑ TG accumulation ↓	GLUT 4' activity ↑	[87]
Hesperetin 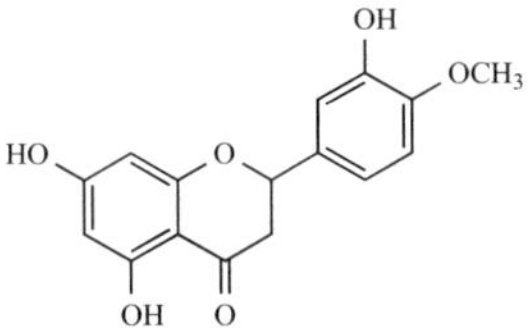	Hypercholesterolaemic rats (0.02% wt/wt in diet, 5 wk)	Blood lipids ↓ Atherogenic index ↓	HMG-CoA reductase and ACAT activities ↓ Fecal cholesterol excretion ↑	[95]
	Fatty liver rats (1% wt/wt in diet, 10 day)	Fatty liver improved	Hepatic triglyceride synthesis (phosphatidate phosphohydrolase, G6PDH, malic enzyme, DG acyltransferase activities)↓	[96]
	HepG2 cells (100–200 μM)	Lipids secretion ↓	ApoB-containing lipoprotein assembly (expression and activity of ACAT2 ↑ and MTP; LDL receptor expression ↑)	[94]
Hesperidin 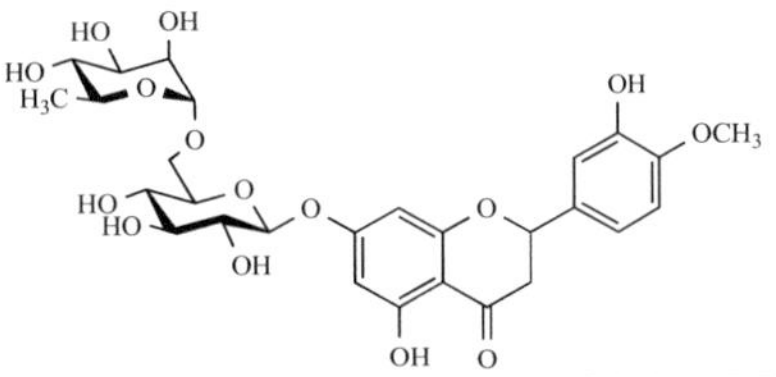	*db/db* Mice (0.02% wt/wt in diet, 5 wk)	Blood glucose ↓ Blood lipids ↓ Fatty liver improved Body weight ↑	Insulin and leptin secretion ↑ Hepatic glycolysis and ↓ glycogen synthesis ↑ HMG-CoA reductase and ACAT activities ↓ Fecal cholesterol excretion ↑	[101, 102]
Naringenin 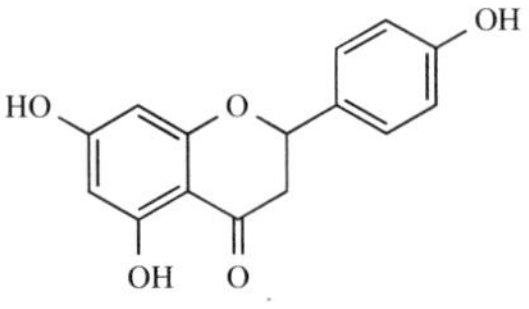	Mice fed normal diet (1% wt/wt in diet)	Blood lipids↓	Hepatic peroxisomal fatty acid oxidation ↑	[108]
	Hypercholesterolaemic rats (0.1% wt/wt in diet, 3 wk)	Blood lipids ↓ Fatty liver improved	HMG -CoA reductase and ACAT activities ↓	[109, 142]
	3T3-L1 adipocytes (50–100 μM)	Fat accumulation ↓	Adipocyte apoptosis ↑ (Preconfluent-preadipocytes growth ↓)	[70]
	HepG2 cells (100–200 μM)	Lipids secretion ↓	ApoB-containing lipoprotein assembly (expression and activity of ACAT2 and MTP; LDL receptor expression) ↓	[94]
	3T3-L1 adipocytes (6–100 μM)	Insulin-stimulated glucose uptake ↓	PI3K activity and Akt signaling ↓	[107]
Naringin 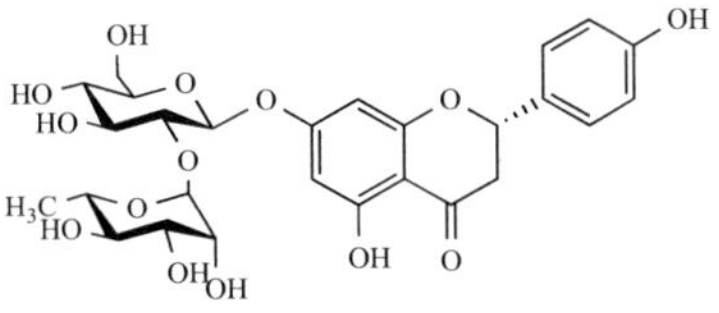	Hypercholesterolemic subjects (400 mg/ day, 8 wk)	Blood lipids ↓	Apolipoprotein B ↓	[111]
	db/db Mice (0.02% wt/wt in diet, 5wk)	Blood glucose ↓ Blood lipids ↓ Fatty liver ↓ Body weight	Insulin and leptin secretion ↑ Hepatic glycolysis and glycogen synthesis ↑ Gluconeogenesis ↓ HMG-CoA reductase and ACAT activities ↓ Fecal lipids excretion ↑	[101, 102]

(Table 1) Contd…..

Bioactive Compound	Model (Treatment dosage and duration)	Beneficial effects	Mechanisms of action	Refs.
	DIO rats (0.02 % wt/wt in diet, 6wk)	Blood lipids ↓	HMG-CoA reductase and ACAT activities ↓	[110]
Quercetin 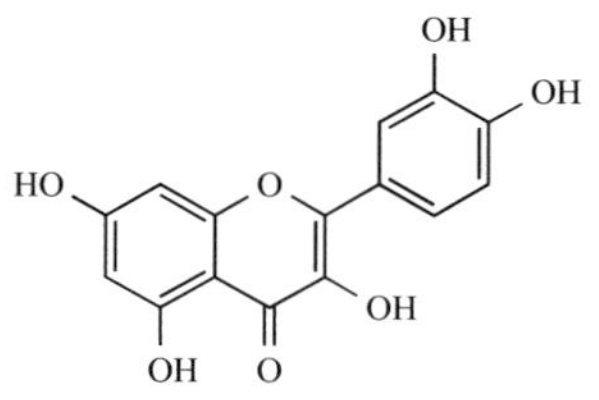	Men and women, stage 1 hypertension (730 mg/ day)	Blood pressure ↓		[114]
	DIO rats (0.5% wt/wt in diet, 4 wk)	Body weight gain ↓ Visceral fat weight ↓ Blood pressure ↓ Lipid peroxidation ↓	Nitric oxide synthase activity ↑ Antioxidative activity ↑	[113]
	Isolated rat adipocytes (10−100 μM)	Glucose uptake ↓	Direct interaction with GLUT4	[90]
	3T3-L1 cells (20−50 μM)	Glucose uptake ↑ Fat accumulation ↓	Partial agonist of PPARγ PPARγ1 expression ↓	[87, 117]
	3T3-L1 cells (50−250 μM)	Adipocyte apoptosis ↑	Caspase-3 dependent apoptotic cascade ↑	[116]
Rutin 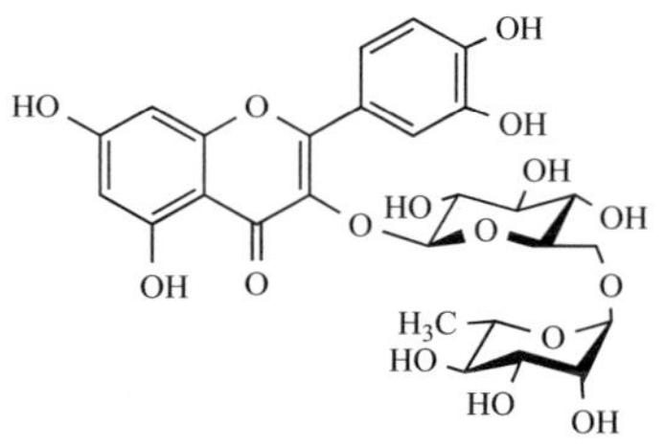	DIO mice (25−50 mg/kg BW, 4 wk)	Body weight ↓ Body weight gain ↓ Blood lipids ↓ Fatty liver ↓	Adipogenic transcription factors (PPARγ and C/EBPα) expression ↓	[134]
	DIO rats (50-100mg/kg BW, 8 wk)	Body weight ↓ Body weight gain ↓ Visceral fat weights ↓ Blood lipids ↓ Fatty liver ↓	Food efficiency ↓ GPDH activity ↓	[133]
	Hypercholesterolaemic rats (100 mg/kg BW, 4 wk)	Blood lipids ↓ Fatty liver ↓		[135]
	3T3-L1 cells (50−1, 650 μM)	Fat accumulation ↓	Adipogenic transcription factors expression (PPARγ and C/EBPα) ↓ GPDH activity ↓	[134, 136]

Strobel *et al.* [90] reported that quercetin interacts directly with GLUT4 to inhibit its uptake of glucose into the isolated rat adipocytes. In other *in vitro* studies, quercetin also directly worked on multiple targets within the insulin signaling pathway by inhibiting PI3K at relatively low concentrations [120-122] and modulating the activity of Akt/protein kinase B (PKB) and protein kinase C (PKC) [123-125]. In contrast, however, quercetin significantly improved insulin-stimulated glucose uptake in mature 3T3-L1 adipocytes [77]. Further experiments have proven that quercetin serves as a weak partial antagonist of PPARγ, and that unlike the traditional antagonist, quercetin cannot induce the differentiation of the preadipocyte 3T3-L1. Therefore, the potential mechanism by which quercetin ameliorates hyperglycemia may in part be by serving as a ligand of PPARγ, and thus, improving insulin-stimulated glucose uptake in mature adipocytes, while lacking the capability to induce preadipocyte differentiation, as shown in kaempferol [77].

Additionally, initial clinical data support the role of quercetin in the prevention of obesity and type 2 diabetes. A pilot study showed that QR-333, a topical compound that contains quercetin, safely induces relief from symptoms of diabetic neuropathy and improves quality of life [126]. The randomized, placebo-controlled, double-blind trial included 34 men and women with type 1 or 2 diabetes and diabetic neuropathy, who applied QR-333 or a placebo three times daily for four weeks to each foot wherein symptoms were experienced. QR-333 reduced the severity of the numbness, jolting pain, and irritation from the baseline values, was well tolerated, and improved quality-of-life measures.

Rutin

Rutin (3, 3′, 4′, 5, 7-pentahydrohyflavone-3-rhamnoglucoside) is a flavonol-type flavonoid that is found in many typical plants such as buckwheat, apples, teas, citrus fruits, parsley, mulberry, and tomatoes. It is also an important dietary constituent of other foods and plant-based beverages [127]. It has been reported that rutin has several pharmacological properties including antioxidant, anticarcinogenic, cytoprotective, neuroprotective, anti-platelet, antithrombic, vasoprotective and cardioprotective activities [128-132]. Besides, rutin was shown to prevent diet-induced obesity [133, 134], to reduce plasma leptin and insulin levels, and to alleviate dyslipidemia in obese mice and rats [133-135]. Choi *et al.* [134] and Hsu and Yen [136] reported that rutin efficiently suppresses adipogenesis in 3T3-L1 adipocytes. It appears to be mediated through the downregulated expression of adipo-genic transcription factors, such as PPARγ and C/EBPα, and adipocyte-specific proteins, such as leptin and then through the upregulated expression of adiponectin. Many studies have shown that rutin inhibits glycerol-3-phosphate dehydrogenase (GPDH), the cytosolic enzyme that plays an important role in the conversion of glycerol into triglyceride, in 3T3-L1 preadipocytes [134, 136] and in the fat and liver tissues of rats with HFD-induced obesity [133].

PHENOLIC ACIDS

Among plant materials, fruits, vegetables, grains, tea, coffee, and spices contain not only phenolic compounds that belong mainly to the flavonoids family, but also phenolic acids. The name "phenolic acids" generally describes phenols that possess only one carboxylic acid functionality [143]. Phenolic acids exhibit acidic properties due to the presence of the carboxylic acid group. Phenolic acids are aromatic secondary plant metabolites that are widely spread throughout the plant kingdom [144]. Hydroxybenzoic acids (C6–C1) and hydroxycinnamic acids (C6–C3) are phenolic acids that are predominantly found in plants [144]. The estimated daily consumption of phenolic acids ranges from 25 mg to 1 g, depending on the diet [143]. Most phenolic acids have shown excellent scavenging activity with respect to active oxygens such as superoxide anion radicals, hydroxyl radicals, and singlet oxygen. They have also been reported to exert anti-inflammatory, antimutagenic, and anticarcinogenic activities [143, 145]. Phenolic acids are currently being investigated for their potential anti-obesity activities. Some of them (gallic acid, capsaicin, curcumin, and coumaric acid) have anti-obesity properties (Table **2**).

Gallic Acid

Gallic acid (3,4,5-trihydroxybenzoic acid) is a phenolic compound that naturally abounds in tea leaves and vegetables, such as asparagus, broccoli, and aubergine [146]. It has been reported to have antioxidant, antimutagenic, anticarcinogenic, anti-allergic, and anti-inflammatory activities. It is expected to reduce the risk of disease and brings health benefits through daily intake [147]. In addition, gallic acid has shown antiproliferative activity in 3T3-L1 preadipocytes. Gallic acid increased the number of early and late apoptotic cells in a dose-dependent manner [148]. Hsu *et al.* investigated the effect of gallic acid on the apoptotic pathway in 3T3-L1 pre-adipocytes, and found that gallic acid triggers apoptosis by regulating Fas/FasL, p53, and Bcl-2 family members (Bad, Bak, Bax, Bcl-2, and Bcl-XL) and activating caspase cascade (caspase-3 and -9) [149]. Gallic acid's induction of cell apoptosis may prove to be a pivotal mechanism for decreased pre-adipocyte proliferation.

Gallic acid has a potential anti-obesity and hypolipidemic effect on HFD-fed mice. The addition of gallic acid to the HFD decreased the body weight gain the weights of the liver and the adipose tissue and the serum triglyceride, total cholesterol, insulin, and leptin levels and alleviated hepatic steatosis in rats. Gallic acid also reduced oxidative stress in rats with HFD-induced obesity [150]. More recently, Jang *et al.* found that the synthetic gallic acid - linoleic acid ester more effectively decreased the size of the adipocytes of mice with HFD-induced obesity relative to those of groups treated with gallic acid or linoleic acid [151]. Based on these observations, gallic acid may be useful in the treatment of obesity and raises the possibility of a new application as a dietary supplement.

Capsaicin

Capsaicin (8-methyl-*N*-vanillyl-*trans*-6-nonenamide) is a major pungent ingredient of red pepper, which is widely used as a spice [152]. Pepper is a potent analgesic and anti-inflammatory agent, and desensitizes different chemical irritants in long-term treatments [7]. Capsaicin has been reported to decrease energy intake [153], decrease the adipose tissue weight, and lower the serum triacylglycerol concentration by enhancing energy metabolism [154]. Capsaicin inhibits the growth of various immortalized and malignant cells [155] and induces apoptosis in transformed cells [156]. Capsaicin induces adipocyte apoptosis by collapsing the mitochondria membrane potential; activating caspase-3, Bax, and Bak; cleaving PARP and down-regulating Bcl-2. The researchers also suggested that capsaicin stimulated intracellular ROS release, which activated AMPK, and rapidly led to apoptosis [31].

Hsu and Yen demonstrated that capsaicin efficiently suppresses adipogenesis in 3T3-L1 preadipocytes, and adipocytes [157]. Capsaicin also inhibited lipid accumulation and the protein expression of PPARγ, C/EBPα, and leptin, but induced the up-regulation of adiponectin in 3T3-L1 adipocytes. In another study of

Hwang *et al.*, capsaicin was shown to inhibit the adipocyte differentiation process by activating AMPK [31], which is known to play a major role in energy homeostasis. It has been shown that dietary supplementation with capsaicin (0.014%) lowers the perirenal adipose tissue weight and the serum triglyceride level in obese rats [154]. These results indicate that the beneficial anti-adipogenesis activity of capsaicin that has been observed *in vitro* can be relevant *in vivo*.

Table 2. Beneficial Effects of Phenolic Acids on Obesity and Associated Diseases

Bioactive Compound	Model (Treatment dosage and duration)	Beneficial effects	Mechanisms of action	Ref.
Gallic acid 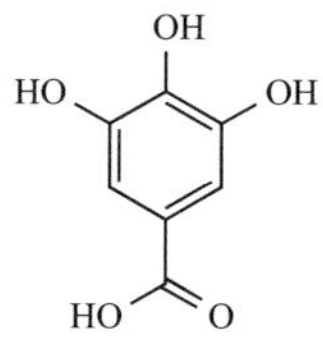 	DIO mice (0.1-0.2% wt/wt in diet, 10 wk)	Body weight ↓ Visceral fat weights ↓ Blood lipids ↓ Fatty liver improved	Antioxidant enzyme (GPx, GRd, GST) ↑ Blood insulin, leptin ↓	[150]
	DIO mice (1% wt/wt in diet, 7 wk)	Body weight ↓ Fatty liver improved Blood glucose ↓ Blood lipids ↓	Adipogenesis ↓	[151]
	3T3-L1 (50-250 μM)	Adipogenesis ↓ Adipocyte apoptosis ↑	Cell population and growth ↓ Antioxidant activity ↑	[148]
	3T3-L1 cells (10-250 μM)	Fat accumulation ↓	Cell growth ↓ Apotosis (FAS, FasL, p53, Bax, Bad, Bak, caspase-3, -9) ↑ Anti-Apotosis (Bcl-2, Bcl-X_L) ↓ HDAC activity ↓	[149]
Capsaicin 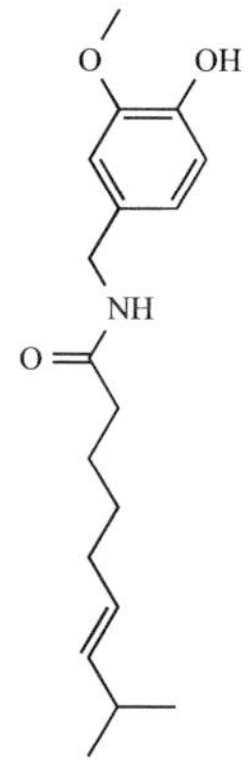 	DIO rats (0.014% wt/wt in diet, 10 day)	Visceral fat weights ↓ Blood lipids (TG) ↓	Hepatic G6PDH ↑ LPL activity in adipose tissue ↑	[154]
	DIO mice (0.015% wt/wt in diet, 10 wk)	Body weight gain ↓ Visceral fat weights ↓ Blood glucose, insulin ↓ Blood FFA, leptin ↓, adiponectin ↑ Fatty liver improved Adipocyte size ↓	Adipogenesis ↓ Glucose tolerance ↓ (GLUT4, IRS-1 ↑) Adipokine expression (adiponectin) ↓ Inflammation in adipose tissue and liver (TNFα, MCP1, IL-6, TRPV-1) ↓ Hepatic steatosis (PPARα, PGC-1α, CPT-1↑)↓	[158]
	DIO mice (I.P. injection: 2 mg/kg BW, 10 day) 3T3-L1 (100 μM)	Obesity-induced inflammation ↓	Adipokine expression (MCP1, COX-2, adiponectin) ↓ Inflammation (TNFα, IL-6, NF-κB) ↓	[163]
	DIO rats (I.P. injection: 6 mg/kg BW)	Blood glucose, insulin ↑ Blood FFA ↑	β-Adrenergic activator	[180]
	3T3-L1 cells (10-250 μM)	TG accumulation ↓	Apotosis (Bax, Bak, caspase-3, PARP) ↑ and Antiapotosis (Bcl-2) ↓ Adipogenic transcription factors (PPARγ and C/EBPα, leptin) expression ↓ AMPK activity ↑	[31, 157]

(Table 2) Contd…..

Bioactive Compound	Model (Treatment dosage and duration)	Beneficial effects	Mechanisms of action	Ref.
Curcumin 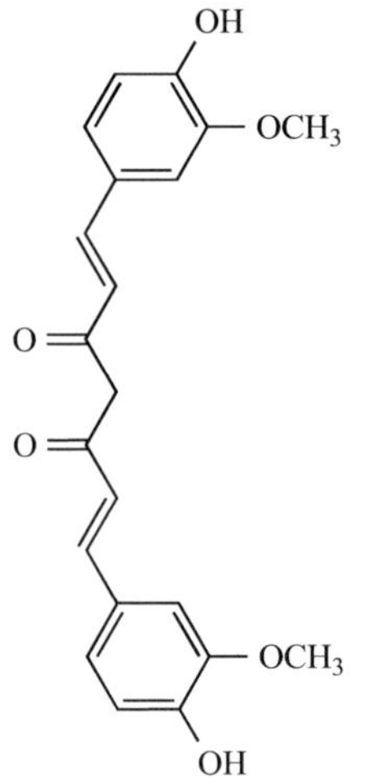	DIO mice, *ob/ob* mice (3% wt/wt in diet, 40-60 day)	Blood glucose ↓ Body weight ↓ Body fat ↓ Liver weight	Adipocyte size ↓ Adipokine expression (adiponectin ↑, F4-80 ↓) Stress response gene expression (Sirt1, HSP-70, 90, FoxO-1a) ↑ Hepatic NF-κB activity↓	[171]
	DIO mice (0.05% wt/wt in diet, 12 wk) 3T3-L1 cells (5-20 μmol/L)	Body weight ↓ Liver weight ↓ Blood cholesterol ↓	Cell growth ↓ Fatty acid oxidation (pACC and pAMPK) ↑ Adipokine-induced angiogenesis (VEGF-α, VEGFR-2) ↓ Adipogenic transcription factors (PPARγ and C/EBPα) expression ↓	[170]
	Hypercholesterolaemic rats (0.5% wt/wt in diet)	Blood lipids ↓ Fatty liver improved	Antioxidant activity ↑	[169]
	Streptozotocin -induced diabetic rats (0.5% wt/wt in diet, 8 wk)	Blood lipids ↓ Fatty liver improved	Cholesterol-7α-hydroxylase activity ↑ Hepatic HMG-CoA reductase acitivity ↓	[173]
	Hepatic stellate cells (10-30 μmol/L)	Fat accumulation ↓	TG, FFA, cholesterol accumulation ↓ LDL receptor ↓ SREBPs trans-activity ↓	[172]
	HepG2 cells (25-100 mM)	Fat accumulation ↓	LDL receptor ↑ Hepatic gene expression change (LXRα, SREBP2 ↑, FAT/CD36, FABP-1 ↓)	[175]
Coumaric aicd 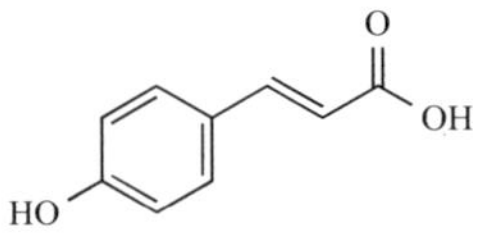	DIO mice (100 mg/kg BW, 8 wk)	Body weight ↓ Visceral fat weight ↓ Blood lipids ↓ Fatty liver ↓	Food intake and food efficiency ↓ Hepatic GPDH activity ↓ Oxidative stress ↓	[133]
	3T3-L1 cells (50-250 μM)	Fat accumulation ↓	Adipogenic transcription factor (PPARγ and C/EBPα) expression ↓ Adipocyte-specific protein (leptin) ↓ Adiponecton ↑	[136]

In addition to anti-obesity properties, dietary capsaicin (0.015%) lowered the fasting glucose and insulin levels, and markedly reduced the impairment of glucose tolerance in obese mice [158]. Obesity-induced inflammation plays a crucial role in the development of metabolic diseases such as insulin resistance, type 2 diabetes, hepatic steatosis, and cardiovascular diseases [159, 160]. Studies have shown that the dysregulation of proteins derived from adipose tissue, such as cytokines/chemokines and adipocytokines, results in impaired insulin signaling and lipid metabolism [161, 162]. Both the intraperitoneal injection of capsaicin (2 mg per kg of BW) and the dietary supplementation with capsaicin (0.015%) significantly decreased the expression levels of the TNFα, monocyte chemoattractant protein-1 (MCP-1), and interleukin (IL)-6 genes in the adipose tissue of obese mice, as did macrophage infiltration and transient receptor potential vanilloid (TRPV)1 expression in adipose tissue [158, 163]. At the same time, the mRNA/protein of adiponectin in the adipose tissue and the PPARα/ PPARγ-coactivator 1 α (PGC-1α) mRNA in the liver were increased. The levels of TNF α, MCP-1, and IL-6 mRNAs and of proteins in the liver were also markedly decreased by capsacin treatment. Taking all these together shows that dietary capsaicin appears to reduce obesity-induced glucose intolerance by not only suppressing inflammatory responses but also enhancing fatty acid oxidation in the adipose tissue and/or the liver, both of which are important peripheral tissues that affect insulin resistance. Hence, capsaicin may be useful as a dietary additive for reducing obesity-induced metabolic disorders.

Curcumin

Curcumin, a member of the curcuminoid family of compounds, is a yellow phenolic pigment that is obtained from the powdered rhizome of *Curcuma longa*. The dried ground rhizome of the perennial herb *Curcuma longa*, called turmeric in English, is a popular dietary spice in Asia that is used in curry. It is also an integral part of the ancient Hindu medicinal system called *Ayurveda*. In contrast to the maximum dietary consumption of 1.5 g per person per day in certain Southeast Asian communities, smaller quantities of turmeric tend to be used for medicinal purposes such as pain relief or wound healing [164]. Curcumin has no known dose-limiting toxicities and has been consumed by humans in dosages of up to 12 g/day without significant side-effects [165]. Curcumin has multiple pharmacological actions, such as antioxidant [166], anti-inflammatory [167], and anticancer [168] properties, which likely affect many of the interconnected pathological processes involved in apoptotic death.

A number of studies have been carried out to investigate the anti-obesity, antidiabetic, and lipid-lowering effects of curcumin [169-172]. The possible hypolipidemic effect of curcumin has been investigated in diet-induced hypercholesterolemic rats [169]. Curcumin mixed with the diet (0.5% wt/wt) decreased the serum total and LDL cholesterol levels, and increased the serum HDL cholesterol level. Curcumin also decreased the enzyme activities of serum aspartate aminotransferase (AST) and alanin aminotransferase (ALT), which increased in rats fed a high-cholesterol diet. Curcumin attenuated diet-induced hypercholesterolemia [169] by increasing the rate of cholesterol catabolism [173], increasing fecal excretion [174] and inducing changes in the expression of the genes involved in cholesterol homeostasis [175]. In addition, curcumin inhibited LDL oxidation in rabbits with experimental atherosclerosis [176].

Two independent dietary feeding studies indeed showed the beneficial effect of curcumin on body weight reduction and glucose metabolism [170, 171]. Ejaz *et al.* demonstrated that curcumin at cellular (3T3-L1 adipocytes) and whole organism levels (mice) displays remarkable potential health benefits in the prevention of obesity and associated metabolic disorders by suppressing angiogenesis in the adipose tissue, upregulating adipocyte energy metabolism and apoptosis, and downregulating preadipocyte differentiation [170]. In that study, curcumin at 5-20 μM suppressed 3T3-L1 differentiation, caused apoptosis, and inhibited adipokine-induced angiogenesis of human umbilical vein endothelial cells. The supplementation of the HFD with curcumin (0.05% wt/wt in the diet) did not affect food intake but reduced body weight gain, adiposity, and the microvessel density in the adipose tissue of mice. Curcumin increased AMPK phosphorylation, reduced glycerol-3-phosphate acyltransferase (GPAT)-1, and increased CPT-1 expression, which led to increased fatty acid oxidation and decreased fatty acid esterification. In addition, curcumin significantly lowered the serum cholesterol and the expression of PPARγ and C/EBP α, two key transcription factors in adipogenesis and lipogenesis. A relatively high dose of curcumin supplementation (3% wt/wt in the diet) resulted in a significant increase in the mice's food intake but to a small but significant decrease in their body weight and fat content [171]. Furthermore, compared with the control obese animals (both the DIO and *ob/ob* mice), the curcumin-treated obese mice had significantly decreased macrophage infiltration in their adipose tissue, increased forkhead box O-class (FoxO)-1 and adiponectin expression in their adipose tissue, and higher circulating adiponectin levels. Taking all these together shows that curcumin or related compounds warrant further investigation as novel adjunctive therapies for obesity and type 2 diabetes in humans.

Coumaric Acid

Coumaric acids are organic compounds that are hydroxy derivatives of cinnamic acid. They have three isomers: *o*-coumaric acid, *m*-coumaric acid, and *p*-coumaric acid, which differ in the position of the hydroxy substitution of the phenyl group. *p*-Coumaric acid is the most abundant isomer in nature. It can be found in a wide variety of edible plants such as peanuts, tomatoes, carrots, and garlic, and is an intermediate in the synthesis of many phenols. *p*-Coumaric acid has marked antioxidant and anti-inflammatory properties in rat colonic mucosa [177, 178] and inhibits platelet activity *in vitro* and *in vivo* [179].

The inhibitory effects of *o*-coumaric acid on 3T3-L1 adipocytes, as indicated by the decrease in the intracellular triglyceride content (61.3% decrease) and the GPDH activity (54.2% decrease), have been elucidated [136]. Anti-adipogenic effect of *o*-coumaric acid appears to be mediated through the downregulated expression of adipogenic transcription factors (PPARγ and C/EBPα) and adipocyte-specific proteins (leptin), and through the upregulated expression of adiponectin. The oil red O stained material showed, however, that the *o*-coumaric acid did not influence the cell number in the 3T3-L1 adipocytes. *o*-Coumaric acid has an anti-obesity effect and suppresses dyslipidemia, hepatosteatosis and oxidative stress in obese rats [133]. The feeding of the rats with *o*-coumaric acid (50 and 100 mg per kg of body weight) for eight weeks significantly deceased their body weight gain, the weights of their liver and adipose tissue, their serum parameters (triglyceride, phospholipid, total cholesterol, LDL-cholesterol, insulin, and leptin), and their hepatic steatosis.

TERPENES

Terpenes are widespread in nature, mainly in plants as constituents of essential oils that are used widely as natural flavor additives in food, as fragrance in perfumes, and in traditional and alternative medicine such as for aromatherapy. Many terpenes are hydrocarbons, but they also have oxygen-containing compounds such as alcohols, aldehydes, and ketones (terpenoids) [181]. Their building block is the hydrocarbon isoprene, $CH_2=C(CH_3)-CH=CH_2$. As chains of isoprene units are built up, the resulting terpenes are classified sequentially by size as hemiterpenes, monoterpenes, sesquiterpenes, diterpenes, sesterterpenes, triterpenes, and tetraterpenes [182]. The biological and ecochemical functions of terpenes have not yet been fully investigated. Some of them (astaxanthin, gamma linolenic acid, ginsenosides, oleanolic acid, and ursolic acid) have been known to have anti-obesity properties (Table **3**).

Astaxanthin

Astaxanthin belongs to the xanthophyll class of carotenoids and is closely related to β-carotene, lutein, and zeaxanthin, sharing with them many of the general metabolic and physiological functions attributed to carotenoids. Astaxanthin is contained in some seafoods, such as salmons (1.7-2.6 mg/100 g), crabs, and shrimps [183]. Several previous studies have demonstrated astaxanthin's wide variety of biological activities, including antioxidant [184, 185], antitumor [186], antidiabetic [187], and anti-inflammation activities [188]. Its antioxidant activity is greater than that of β-carotene or α-tocopherol [189]. Astaxanthin has inhibited LDL oxidation *in vitro* and *ex vivo* [190]. Ikeuchi *et al.* observed that astaxanthin alleviated HFD-induced increases in body weight and adipose tissue weight, and reversed the hepatic accumulation of triglyceride and hyperlipidemia in HFD-fed mice [191]. Furthermore, astaxanthin has beneficial effects on endurance exercise capacity by increasing the supply of free fatty acids in the blood in the early phase of exercise. The administration of astaxanthin decreases the utilization of glucose and increases the utilization of fatty acid as an energy source, which spares glycogen, during endurance exercise [191].

Gamma Linolenic Acid

Gamma linolenic acid (GLA, all *cis* 6, 9, 12-Octadecatrienoic acid, C18:3, n-6) is produced in the body from linoleic acid (all *cis* 6,9-octadecadienoic acid), an essential fatty acid in the omega-6 series, by the enzyme delta-6-desaturase [192]. Preformed GLA is present in trace amounts in green leafy vegetables and nuts. The most significant source of GLA for infants is breast milk. GLA is further metabolized into dihomogamma linlenic acid, which undergoes oxidative metabolism by cyclooxygenases and lipoxygenases to produce anti-inflammatory eicosanoids (series 1 prostaglandins and series 3 leukotrienes).

The availability of varying essential fatty acids (EFA) influences lipogenesis [193, 194], insulin sensitivity [195], and adipocyte differentiation [196]. These processes, in turn, provide credible links between the EFA status and the storage of dietary energy as fat. Schirmer *et al.* reported a distortion in the EFA distribution in obese humans, which is not resolved despite major weight loss [197]. There are many reports of similar distortions in the EFA metabolism in single-gene [198, 199] and multiple-gene [200] animal models of obesity. The consistent manifestation of this distorted EFA distribution in obese animals is a reduction in the proportion of arachidonate in the serum or membrane phospholipids and an increase in the proportion of arachidonate in the serum or liver cholesteryl esters. When the reduction in the phospholipid arachidonic acid in obese Zucker rats is corrected by administering dietary GLA to them to increase the arachidonic acid production in their liver, food intake and weight of the obese genotype were reduced. When the lean genotype of the Zucker rat was given the same dose of GLA, however, there was no effect on its food intake or body weight [199, 201]. It was further observed that GLA reduced weight regain in humans following major weight loss, which suggests the role of essential fatty acids in fuel partitioning in obesity-prone humans.

Ginsenosides (Rh_2, Rg_3 and Re)

Ginsenosides are triterpenoid glycosides of the dammarane series [202]. They are found exclusively in the plant genus *Panax*, such as in *Panax ginseng* (Asian ginseng) and *Panax quinquefolius* (American

Table 3. Beneficial Effects of Terpenes on Obesity and Associated Diseases

Bioactive Compound	Model (Treatment dosage and duration)	Beneficial effects	Mechanisms of action	Ref.
Astaxanthin 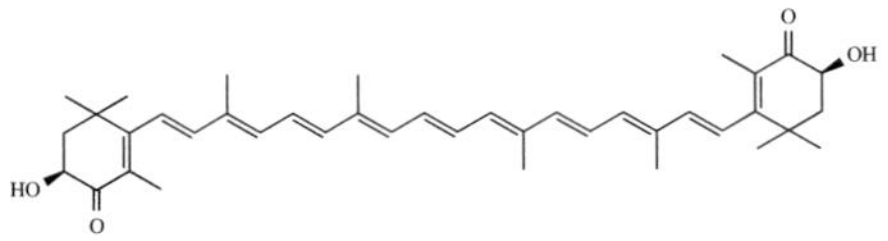	DIO mice (6 and 30 mg/kg BW, 60 day)	Body weight ↓ Visceral fat weight ↓ Blood lipids ↓ Fatty liver ↓	Respiratory quotient ↓	[191]
Gamma linoleic acid 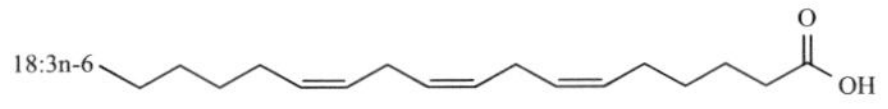	Obese humans (890 mg/d, 1 year)	Body weight regain ↓		[235]
	Obese Zucker rats (49 mg/ day)	Body weight ↓	Food intake ↓	[201]
Ginsenoside Rh2 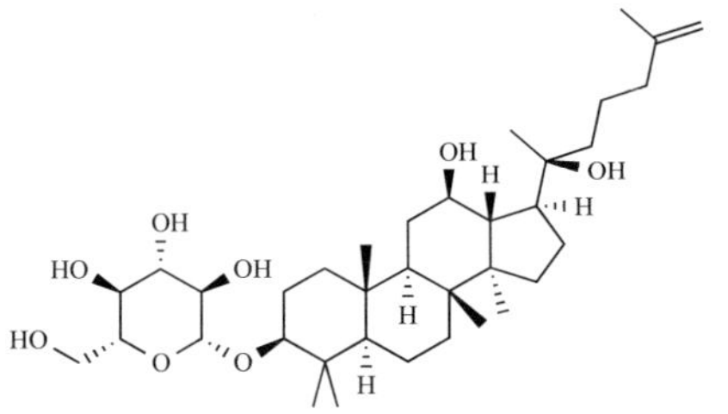	Streptozotocin -induced diabetic rats (1 mg/kg, 0-150 min)	Blood glucose ↓	β-Endorphin-like immunoreactivity ↑ GLUT4 translocation ↑	[212]
	3T3-L1 cells (20-40 μM)	Fat accumulation ↓	Adipogenesis ↓ (PPARγ activity ↓) AMPK signaling pathway (pAMPK, UCP2, CPT-1) ↑	[209]
	3T3-L1 cells (0.01-1 μM)	Fat accumulation ↓	Cell growth ↓ Glucocorticoid receptor activity ↑	[211]
Ginsenoside Rg3 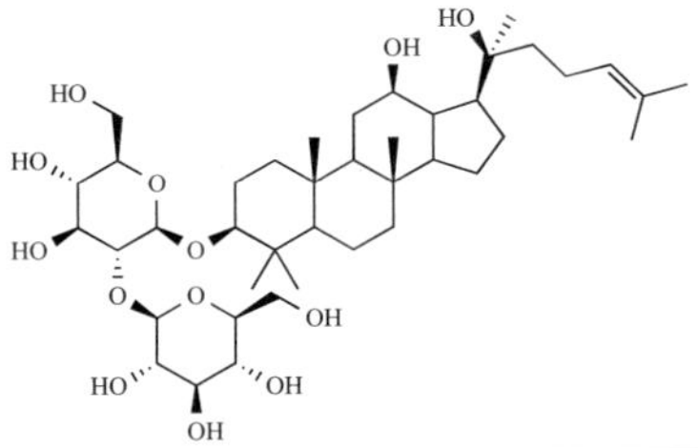	Hamster pancreatic β-cell line (HIT-T15) C2C12 myoblasts (10-100 μM)	Blood glucose ↓ Insulin secretion ↑	Fatty acid oxidation (pACC and pAMPK) ↑	[215]
	3T3-L1 cells (40-80 μM)	Fat accumulation ↓	Adipogenesis ↓ (PPARγ activity ↓) pAMPK ↑	[210]
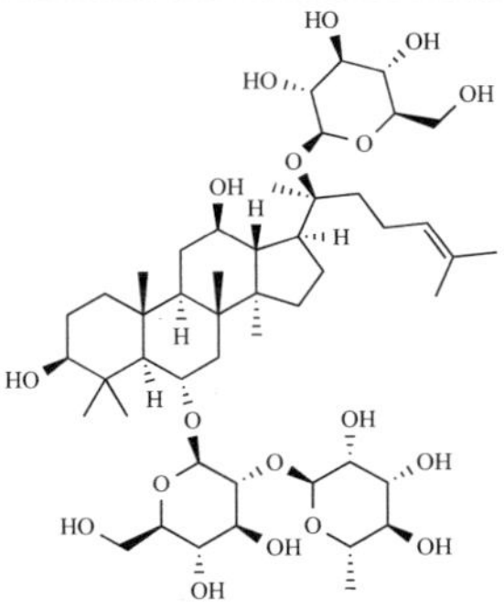 Ginsenoside Re	DIO rats (0.0.04% wt/wt in diet, 2 wk) 3T3-L1 (10 μM)	Glucose uptake ↑	GLUT4 translocation ↑ Insulin signaling molecules activities ↑ (tyr pIRS-1, PI3-kinase, Akt/PKCζ/λ ↑) NF-κB, JNK, MAPK, pERK, TNFα ↑	[213]
Oleanolic acid 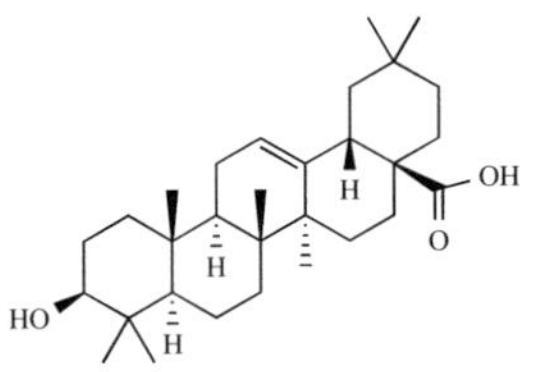	DIO mice (100 mg/kg BW, 14 day)	Body weight ↓ Visceral fat weight ↓ Blood glucose ↓ Blood insulin ↓	Anti-hyperglycemic gene (TGR5) ↑ Hepatic toxicity (ALT, AST, ALP) ↑	[222]
	DIO mice (50 mg/kg BW, 4 wk)	Body weight ↓ Blood lipids ↓ Fatty liver ↓	Lipid metabolism-related genes (Acacb, Gpd2, GPam, SREBP-1c) ↓ Inflammatory cytokine-related gene (IL-1β) ↓ Gluconeogenesis-related gene (G6pc) ↓ Insulin signaling-related genes (Irs2, Lep, Prkab2) ↑	[224]
	Hypercholesterolemic rats (100 mg/kg BW, 15 day)	Blood lipids ↓ Fatty liver ↓	Intestinal absorption, synthesis or storage of cholesterol (ACAT) ↓	[225]

(Table 3) Contd…..

Bioactive Compound	Model (Treatment dosage and duration)	Beneficial effects	Mechanisms of action	Ref.
Ursolic acid 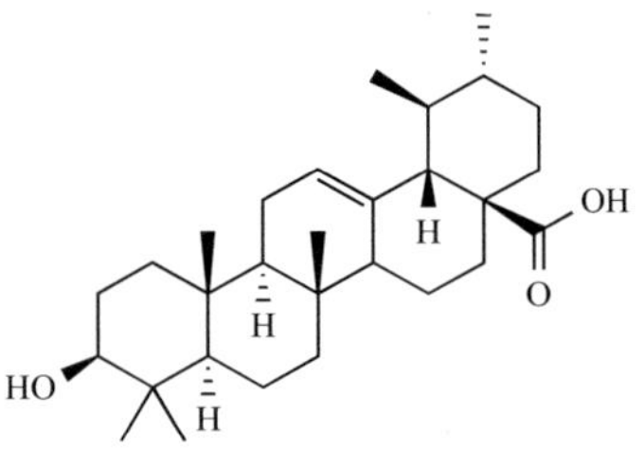	DIO mice (0.05% wt/wt in diet, 8 wk)	Fatty liver ↓ Blood glucose ↓ Blood insulin ↑	Lipid accumulation ↓	[228]
	STZ-induced mice fed a HFD (0.05% wt/wt in diet, 4 wk)	Blood glucose ↓ Blood insulin ↑ Blood C-peptide ↑	Splenic cytokine production (IL-2, IFN-γ ↑, TNF α) ↓	[234]
	Rats (50 and 100 mg/ kg BW with a lipid emulsion, 0–4 h) Isolated rat adipocytes (1–100 μM)	Blood lipids (TG) ↓	Pancreatic lipase activity ↓ cAMP/PDE activity ↓ Lipolysis ↑ (FFA release ↑) Phosphodiesterase (PDE) inhibition *(in vitro)* ↓	[226]
	Jurkat, 293, KBM-5, H1299, U937 cells (100 μM)	Tumorigenesis ↓	NF-κB, IKK, TNF α, PMA, TRAF2, COX-2, MMP-9, cyclin D1 activity ↓	[232]
	CHO/*h*IR cells, L6 myotubes (2 μM)	Glucose uptake ↑	Insulin signaling molecules ↑ (PTP1B ↓, pIR ↑)	[233]

ginseng), and the so-called ginseng saponins. Ginseng has been widely used as a tonic and a restorative remedy in oriental countries. Crude extracts of ginseng have also been traditionally used as remedies for lifestyle-related diseases such as arteriosclerosis, diabetes mellitus, hyperlipidemia, hypertension and obesity [203-206]. More than 30 ginsenosides have already been identified in *Panax ginseng* [202]. The adjuvanticity of saponins is assumed to be dependent on their amphipathic structure and on their functional groups such as aldehyde, carboxyl, acylate and glycoside [207, 208].

Hwang *et al.* recently examined the anti-obesity effects of ginsenoside Rh_2 [209] and Rg_3 [210], which are rich in ginseng *Radix rubra* (red ginseng), using cell culture systems, and investigated their anti-obesity molecular mechanisms. These two ginsenosides, at 20-40 μM, effectively inhibited adipocyte differentiation *via* PPAR-γ inhibition and AMPK activation [209, 210]. PPAR-γ is involved in adipogenesis, glucose and lipid homeostasis, and inflammatory responses. AMPK is a protein kinase that can be activated by stress, and its signaling plays an important role in the regulation of metabolic disorders. Ginsenoside Rh_2 can also regulate the expression of CPT-1 and UCP-2 in adipocytes [209], which are lipolysis molecules that are associated with obesity and diabetes. These study results indicated that ginsenoside Rh_2 and Rg_3 can be potent agents in the prevention of metabolic disorders, including obesity, through the AMPK signaling pathway. Another group obtained opposite results, however, using 3T3-L1 adipocytes. Niu *et al.* found that ginsenoside Rh_2, at markedly lower concentrations (0.01-1 μM) than in previous studies [209], can induce adipogenetic differentiation by activating the glucocorticoid receptor [211]. Glucocorticoids regulate lipid metabolism by promoting lipogenesis in the adipose tissue. The authors deemed it possible for ginsenoside Rh_2 to have multiple effects on adipocyte differentiation, but the detailed mechanisms for such need further investigation.

In relation to insulin sensitivity, Lai *et al.* reported increased gene expression in the mRNA and protein levels of GLUT4 in the soleus muscle of streptozotocin-induced diabetic rats when they were intravenously treated with ginsenoside Rh_2 [212]. Based on the cell culture system, ginsenoside Re was also found to enhance glucose uptake in 3T3-L1 adipocytes by enhancing insulin-induced GLUT4 translocation [213]. The inhibition of intracellular inflammatory molecules, including c-Jun N-terminal kinase (JNK) and the nuclear transcription factor κB (NF-κB), may be involved in this mechanism [213]. Serine phosphorylation of the insulin receptor substrate (IRS), which leads to the interruption of the signal transduction from the insulin receptor to the downstream molecules such as PI3K, is a major mechanism of insulin resistance. The phosphorylation is catalyzed by many serine kinases, such as JNK, IκB kinase (IKK), ribosomal protein S6 kinase (S6K), and PKC, in the inflammatory signaling pathways [214]. The inhibition of JNK and IKK will reduce the serine phosphorylation in the IRS proteins and prevent the inhibition of the IRS function. It is likely that ginseng extracts increase the insulin signaling activity by suppressing inflammatory responses. In another study, ginsenoside Rg_3 enhanced glucose-stimulated insulin secretion from pancreatic β-cells (HIT-T15) and activated AMPK and ACC in skeletal muscle cells (C2C12) [215]. All these show that ginsenoside Rg3 activation of AMPK inhibits ACC, decreases the malonyl-CoA levels, and stimulates fatty acid oxidation. The mechanisms of the antidiabetic and anti-obesity actions of ginsenosides appear to be related to insulin sensitization, insulin secretion, thermogenesis, and fatty acid oxidation.

Oleanolic Acid

3*β*-Hydroxyolean-12-en-28-oic acid, commonly called oleanolic acid, is one of the functional components of grape skin. Oleanolic acid belongs to the family of oleanane-type triterpenoids, which have been extensively studied in the oncology field. Triterpenoic acids, including oleanolic acid, together with its analogue and glycoside as well as free form, are widely distributed in plants [216, 217]. These triterpenoids have been known to exhibit multiple biological properties, such as hepatoprotection [218, 219], anti-inflammation [216, 220], and antitumor activities [221]. Oleanolic acid at 100 mg/kg/day showed some toxicity, however, since unlike in the non-treated HFD-fed mice, the transaminases (ALT and AST) and the alkaline phosphatase (ALP) activities were increased in the treated mice [222]. The increases in these liver enzymes probably indicate cholestasis, since the plasma total bilirubin levels were also increased [222]. Liu [223] reviewed all the pharmacological properties of oleanolic acid.

Oleanolic acid supplementation lowered the serum levels of total cholesterol and triglyceride and improved the fatty liver of rats that were fed a high-cholesterol diet [224]. The possible mechanism of this effect may be related to the lowering of the ACAT gene expression and the resulting decrease in the intestinal absorption, synthesis, or storage of exogenous and endogenous cholesterol [225]. The microarray analysis of the hepatic mRNA revealed reduced expression levels of lipogenic genes, including ACC and GPAT-1, probably due to the suppression of the transcription factor SREBP-1c expression [224].

Oleanolic acid lowers the serum glucose and insulin levels and enhances glucose tolerance in HFD-fed mice [222]. Oleanolic acid, a triterpenoid from olive leaves, is a highly specific and potent G protein-coupled receptor (TGR5) antagonist. TGR5 is a member of the G-protein coupled receptor group that is activated by bile acids and that mediates some of the various cellular and physiological effects of bile acids.

Ursolic Acid

Ursolic acid (3β-hydroxy-urs-12-en-28-oic acid), a natural pentacyclic triterpenoid carboxyl acid, is present in many fruits and herbs, including apples, bilberries, cranberries, *Actinidia arguta*, *Cornus mas*, basil, peppermint, rosemary, lavender, oregano, and thyme [226-228]. It is the major component of some traditional medicinal herbs and is well known to have a wide range of biological functions, including anticancer, antioxidative, anti-inflammatory, hepatoprotective, anti-allergic, gastroprotective, hypo-lipidemic, anti-atherosclerotic, and immunoregulatory functions [216, 223, 229-231]. Ursolic acid has been found to suppress NF-κB activation by inhibiting IKK, a kinase that is needed for NF-κB activation. This leads to the suppression of cyclin D1, cyclooxygenase-2, and matrix metalloproteinase-9 [232]. Thus, NF-κB has been linked to the above mentioned wide variety of diseases caused by dysregulated inflammation.

Several recent studies have investigated the promising effects of ursolic acid on the prevention and/or treatment of obesity and diabetes. Ursolic acid prevents lipid emulsion-induced increases in the plasma triacylglycerol by inhibiting the intestinal absorption of dietary fat through the inhibition of the pancreatic lipase activity [226]. Moreover, in one study, ursolic acid stimulated lipolysis in adipocytes by inhibiting cAMP-dependent phosphodiesterase. In another *in vivo* study, ursolic acid prevented HFD-induced glucose intolerance [228]. Zhang *et al.* reported that ursolic acid and its derivatives inhibit protein tyrosine phosphatase 1B (PTP1B), a key negative regulator of insulin signal transduction, which enhances insulin receptor phosphorylation and stimulates glucose uptake [233]. Compounds that inhibit PTP1B have potential use in therapeutic strategies for the treatment of diabetes and obesity. As competitive inhibitors of PTP1B, ursolic acid and its derivatives also inhibit T-cell protein tyrosine phosphatase and src homology phosphatase-2, but not leucocyte antigen-related phosphatase or protein tyrosine phosphatase α and ε, which are all possibly involved in the insulin pathway [233]. Furthermore, ursolic acid enhanced the pancreatic β-cell function in streptozotocin-induced diabetic mice that were fed an HFD [234]. Further studies could help to elucidate the potential role of this compound in weight loss and the treatment of diabetes.

OTHERS

In addition to the above-mentioned three classes of phytochemicals (flavonoids, phenolic acids and terpenes), other types of phytochemicals (*e.g.* alkaloid, stilbenoid, and lignan) also have been reported to possess anti-obesity properties. Alkaloids are naturally occurring chemical compounds containing basic nitrogen atoms. Many alkaloids are toxic to other organisms. They often have pharmacological effects and are used as medications, as recreational drugs, or in entheogenic rituals [236]. Examples are the local anesthetic and stimulant cocaine, caffeine, nicotine, the analgesic morphine, or the antimalarial drug quinine. Stilbenoids, hydroxylated derivatives of stilbene, are secondary products of heartwood formation in trees that can act as phytoalexins and antibiotics produced by plants that are under attack [237]. An example of stilbenoids is resveratrol which is found in grapes and which has been suggested to have many health benefits [238]. Lignans are one of the major classes of phytoestrogens, which are estrogen-like chemicals and also act as antioxidants. The principal lignan precursor found in flaxseed is secoisolariciresinol diglucoside, the first plant lignans identified in foods [239]. The biological effects and food sources of these compounds are summarized in Table **4**.

Berberine

Berberine is a botanical alkaloid found in the roots and barks of several plants, such as berberis, goldenseal (*Hydrastis canadensis)*, and *Coptis chinensis French*, an ancient Chinese herb that has been used for thousands of years in China to treat diabetes. Berberine is the main active compound of these herbs. Berberine has various pharmacological properties, including glucose-lowering [240, 241] and antimicrobial properties [242]. Many research groups [240, 243] have reported that berberine reduces body weight and significantly improves glucose tolerance and insulin action in obese and/or diabetic subjects. There is much evidence that berberine enhances insulin sensitivity, reduces hyperlipidemia [240, 243], and relieves fatty liver [244].

Berberine has been shown to reduce weight gain in both DIO rats and *db/db* mice [245]. It is well known that the inhibition of adipogenesis may contribute to the anti-obesity activity of berberine. A number of studies have shown that berberine suppresses adipocyte differentiation and reduces lipid accumulation in 3T3-L1 adipocytes [245-247]. In cells treated with berberine, the expressions of several lipogenic genes, including PPARγ, C/EBPα, SREBP-1c, fatty acid synthase (FAS), ACC, acyl-CoA synthase, lipoprotein lipase (LPL), aP2, and CD36, were suppressed. Since PPARγ and C/EBPα are master transcription regulators of adipogenesis, the inhibition of these two transcription factors may be the key mechanism in the inhibition of adipogenesis by berberine. Berberine has also been shown to markedly decrease the level of triglycerides, total cholesterol and LDL-cholesterol, and hepatic triglycerides in the blood of hamsters or diabetic rats fed with high-cholesterol diets [248, 249]. Two clinical trials demonstrated that berberine decreased the serum levels of triglycerides by 35%, of serum cholesterol by 29%, and of LDL-cholesterol by 25% in subjects with dyslipidemia [249]. One of the mechanisms by which berberine reduces cholesterol is related to the increased expression of the LDL receptor in both the mRNA and the protein in the liver [249]. Additionaly, Kim *et al.* suggested that berberine would relieve fatty liver and hyperlipidemia by modulating both the peripheral and central AMPK activities to increase the whole-body energy homeostasis [244].

The clinical study of Zhang *et al.* [250] indicated noteworthy reductions in the fasting and postprandial plasma glucose and hemoglobin A1c levels due to diet supplementation with 1.0 g of berberine daily for three months, compared with the placebo. Kim *et al.* [241] suggested that berberine's effects on cellular glucose metabolism may be indirect in that it may activate glucose transport in 3T3-L1 adipocytes by increasing the activity of GLUT1, with no appreciable effect on Akt/PKB or GLUT4 or response to PI3K inhibition. In contrast to the results of this study, Ko *et al.* [251] noted that berberine at 5 or 50 mM increased the tyrosine phosphorylation of IRS1 and the Akt/PKB phosphorylation to levels comparable to that produced with 10 nM insulin in 3T3-L1 adipocytes. Besides, many published studies consistently demonstrate that berberine is a strong inducer of Thr-172 phosphorylation in AMPK [240, 241, 243, 245, 248]. Phosphorylation of Thr-172 within the activation loop of the catalytic domain of the alpha sub-unit of AMPK is necessary for AMPK activity. Therefore, AMPK might be a target for berberine in the regulation of glucose metabolism.

Resveratrol

Resveratrol (*trans*-resveratrol, 3, 4', 5-trihydroxystilbene) is a polyphenol that is thought to be a phytoalexin, one of a group of compounds produced during times of environmental stress or pathogenic attack [238]. It is found principally in the skin of grapes, mulberry, *Polygonum cuspidatum*, and peanuts [252, 253]. Red wine is also a rich source of resveratrol and is thought to have cardioprotective effects associated with moderate consumption of wine. Besides resveratrol's cardioprotective property, it has been reported to have chemopreventive, antioxidant, antithrombotic, and anti-inflammatory properties [253-255].

Two independent dietary feeding studies with resveratrol indeed showed a beneficial effect on energy balance and health [256, 257]. Resveratrol increased the survival and longevity of mice that were fed a high-caloric diet and produced changes that mimicked caloric restriction, including improved insulin sensitivity and decreased fat accumulation and body weight. These changes were accompanied by an increased mitochondrial oxidative capacity [257] and increased mitochondrial density in the examined tissues [256, 257]. They were also associated with improved metabolic biomarkers (insulin, glucose, and the insulin-like growth factor 1) [256], reduced adiposity [256, 257], and improved endurance [257]. In another recent study on 3T3-L1 adipocytes, resveratrol down-regulated the expression of PPARγ, C/EBPα, SREBP-1c, FAS, HSL and LPL, and up-regulated the expression of the genes that regulate mitochondrial activity, such as sirtuin 3 (SIRT3), UCP1, and mitofusin 2 (Mfn2) [258]. The observation that resveratrol stimulated SIRT1 *in vitro* and in yeast [259] and the discovery of other members of this family with roles in energy metabolism [260] led to the speculation that sirtuins are potential targets for the treatment of the metabolic syndrome [261]. Activated SIRT1 further deacetylates the transcriptional coactivator PGC-1α at the promoter regions to induce the expression of the genes involved in mitochondrial biogenesis and fatty acid oxidation [262].

In addition to the anti-adipogenenic activity of resveratrol, it also decreased the severity of non-alcoholic fatty liver diseases (NAFLDs) in rats [263]. This effect was mediated, at least in part, by TNF-α inhibition and antioxidant activities. Resveratrol increased superoxide dismutase, glutathione peroxidase, and catalase, and decreased nitric oxide synthase in the liver of the rodents. There is evidence that resveratrol inhibits platelet aggregation and eicosanoid synthesis [264]. Resveratrol has also been shown to inhibit the expression of the tissue factor gene [265], the product of which initiates the coagulation cascade that results in thrombus formation. The perfusion of resveratrol prevents reperfusion-induced arrhythmias and mortality in rats, possibly due to its antioxidant and free-radical-scavenging activities as well as its ability to increase nitric oxide release [266]. Thus, the evidence to date suggests that resveratrol may alter the fat mass in maturing preadipocytes and may decrease the risk of cardiovascular disease *via* multiple mechanisms.

Secoisolariciresinol Diglucoside

Secoisolariciresinol is one of the most abundant dietary lignans in various foods, such as plant seeds, whole grains, legumes, vegetables, and fruits [58]. Secoisolariciresinol is the major lignin found in flaxseed and is present in a polymer that contains secoisolariciresinol diglucoside. Secoisolariciresinol and secoisolariciresinol diglucoside are known to have a number of health benefits, including reduction of the serum cholesterol levels, delaying of the onset of type 2 diabetes, and reduction of the formation of hormone-sensitive cancers such as breast, prostate, and colon cancers [267]. Following the consumption of secoisolariciresinol diglucoside, it is further converted by the bacteria in the colon of humans and other animals into aglycone secoisolariciresinol and the mammalian lignans, enterodiol and enterolactone [268]. The structures of enterodiol and enterolactone are similar to that of estradiol, an endogenous estrogen. This structural similarity accounts for the ability of these compounds to bind to estrogen receptors and to exert weak estrogenic or anti-estrogenic effects, depending on the presence of stronger estrogen [58]. It is well known that secoisolariciresinol has an estrogen-like activity and stimulates the cell growth of human breast cancer MCF-7 cells [269, 270].

Organic chemists are now studying the synthesis of secoisolariciresinol compounds. Stereoisomeric forms of secoisolariciresinol, such as (+)-, (-)-, and *meso*-secoisolariciresinol, have been synthesized, and several of their biological activities have been compared, to determine the relationship between the structure and activity of secoisolariciresinol. Tominaga *et al.* found that based on this relationship, all three stereoisomeric forms of secoisolariciresinol significantly suppressed triacylglycerol accumulation in 3T3-L1 adipocytes. Especially, (−)-secoisolariciresinol, the only isomer that accelerated adiponectin production among the socoisolariciresinol isomers, strongly inhibited triacylglycerol accumulation in 3T3-L1 adipocytes [271]. Furthermore, among the socoisolariciresionl isomers, only (−)-secoisolariciresinol had an estrogen-like activity [271].

Secoisolariciresinol diglucoside lowered the serum total and LDL cholesterol levels and reduced hypercholesterolemic atherosclerosis in rabbits by reducing their oxidative stress. Secoisolariciresinol diglucoside [272] and its mammalian metabolites, secoisolariciresinol, enterodiol, and enterolactone [273], have been shown to have antioxidant properties. The antioxidant activity of secoisolariciresinol and enterodiol is higher than that of vitamin E or the parent glucoside present in flaxseed [273]. Oxidative stress has been shown to be among the causes of both type 1 and type 2 diabetes. The administration of secoisolariciresinol diglucoside was reported to have effectively inhibited the development of diabetes in streptozotocin-induced diabetic rats [274]; diabetes-prone biobreeding rats, which are models of type 1 diabetes [275]; Zucker rats, which are models of type 2 diabetes [276].

Fukumitsu *et al.* recently examined the effects of the secoisolariciresinol diglucoside isolated from flaxseeds on HFD-induced obesity in C57BL/6 mice, and concluded that purified secoisolariciresinol diglucoside (0.5 and 1 % wt per wt in the diet) reduced HFD-induced visceral and liver fat accumulation, and improved hypercholesterolaemia, hyperinsulinaemia and hyperleptinaemia [277]. In the liver, the HFD that contained secoisolariciresinol diglucoside significantly reduced the mRNA level of the gene that is related to fatty acid synthesis, SREBP-1c. Secoisolariciresinol diglucoside administration reduces fatty acid synthesis by suppressing SREBP-1c expression in the liver, and promotes β-oxidation in the muscle by inducing adiponectin expression. The induction of adiponectin may also improve hyperinsulinaemia [277]. In another study of Felmlee *et al.*, secoisolariciresinol diglucoside and secoisolariciresinol decreased the rate of weight gain of female Wistar rats that were fed a standard diet and a diet with 1% cholesterol [278]. Taken together, these reports suggest that secoisolariciresinol and secoisolariciresinol diglucoside are potentially useful in preventing and improving obesity and its associated diseases.

Table 4. Beneficial Effects of Other Phytochemicals on Obesity and Associated Diseases

Bioactive Compound	Model (Treatment dosage and duration)	Beneficial effects	Mechanisms of action	Ref.
Berberine 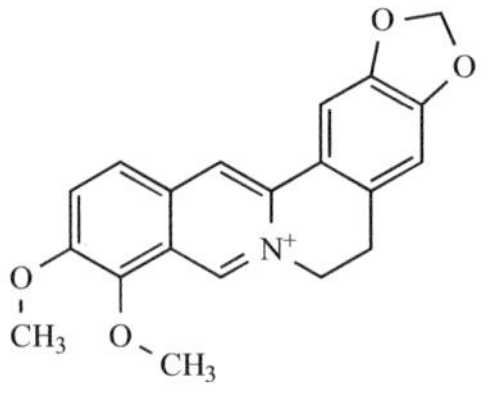	Hypercholesteromic patients (1 g/day, 3 month)	Blood lipids ↓		[249]
	DIO rats (250 mg/kg bw/day, 5 wk)	Fasting insulin ↓ Insulin sensitivity ↑		[243]
	DIO rats (380 mg/kg BW, 2 wk)	Body weight gain ↓ Blood lipids ↓		[245]
	DIO hamsters (50–100 mg/kg BW, 10 days)	Blood lipids ↓ Fatty liver improved	Hepatic LDL receptor expression ↓ Lipogenesis ↓	[248, 249]
	db/db Mice (5 mg/kg BW, 26 days)	Body weight ↓ Visceral fat weights ↓ Blood lipids ↓ TG accumulation ↓	Adipogenic transcription factors (PPARγ, C/EBPα, SREBP1c, aP2, FAS) ↓ Fatty acid oxidation ↑ (pACC and pAMPK ↑) Energy expenditure ↑ GLUT4 translocation ↑	[245]
	db/db Mice (5 mg/kg BW, 3 wk)	Body weight ↓ Liver weight ↓ Fatty liver improved Blood lipids ↓	Fatty acid oxidation (pACC, pAMPK, CPT-1, PGC-1α) ↑ Lipogenesis (PPARγ and FAS)↓ Inflammation (TNFα, IL-6, PAI-1, SAA3) ↓	[244]
	3T3-L1 adipocytes (1-20 μM)	Glucose uptake ↑ Insulin sensivity ↑	GLUT1 activity ↑ ERK and AMPK activity ↑ Fatty acid oxidation ↑ (pAMPK ↑) AMP/ATP ratio ↑ Anaerobic respiration ↑ (lactic acid release ↑)	[279, 241 243]
	3T3-L1 adipocytes (3-15 μM)	TG accumulation ↓	Adipogenic transcription factors (PPARγ, C/EBPα, SREBP1c, aP2, FAS) expression ↓ Fatty acid oxidation (pACC and pAMPK) ↑ GLUT4 translocation ↑	[245]

(Table 4) Contd…..

Bioactive Compound	Model (Treatment dosage and duration)	Beneficial effects	Mechanisms of action	Ref.
	3T3-L1 adipocytes (50 μM)	TG accumulation ↓ Glucose uptake ↑	TG accumulation ↓ GLUT4 transloca-tion pathway (pIRS-1, pAkt/PKB, GLUT4) ↑	[251]
	HepG2 cells (14-24 μg/ml)		Fatty acid oxidation (pAMPK) ↑	[248]
	- L6 myotubes, C2C12 myotubes, (3-20 μmol/L)	Insulin sensivity ↑ Glucose uptake ↑	Fatty acid oxida-tion (pAMPK) ↑ AMP/ATP ratio ↑ Anaerobic respira-tion (lactic acid release) ↑	[240, 243, 245]
Resveratrol 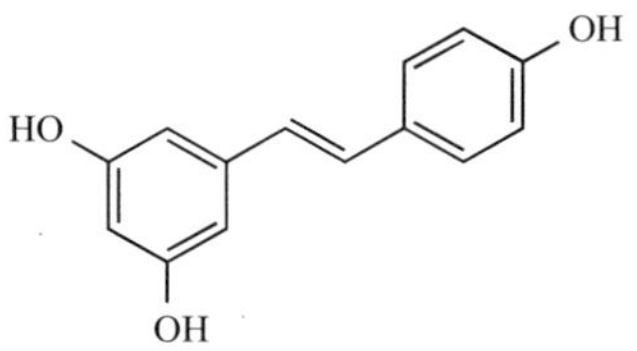	DIO Mice (0.002% wt/wt in diet, 110 wk)	Insulin sensitivity ↑	Glucose metabo-lism improved (insulin secretion, fasting blood glucose level, insulin-like growth factor-1 ↓) Mitochondria function (PGC1α) ↑ Fatty acid oxidation (AMPK) ↑	[256]
	DIO Mice (0.02-0.04% wt/wt in diet, 9 wk)	Body weight gain ↓ Visceral fat weights ↓ Insulin resistance ↓	Mitochondria function (PGC1α, NRF1, UCP3, myoglobin) ↑	[257]
	Human platelet (0-100 μM)	Platelet aggregation ↓		[264]
	HUVEC (100-200 μmol/L)	Inflammation ↓	LPS, TNFα, IL-1β, PMA activity ↓	[265]
	3T3-L1 (33.2 μM)	Adipogenesis ↓ Antioxidant activity ↑	Cell growth ↓	[116]
	3T3-L1 (25-100 μM)	Adipogenesis ↓ Mitochondrial activity↑	Adipogenic genes expression (PPARγ, C/EBPα, SREBP-1c, FAS, HSL, LPL) ↓ Energy expenditure (Sirt 3, UCP1, Mfn 2) ↑	[258]
	- Deacetylation assay (HeLa cells) - Cellular survival assay (HEK293 cells, 0.5 μM)	Cell survival ↑	Sirt1 activity ↑	[259]
	In vitro DPPH assay	Free radical scavenging activity ↑	Antioxidant activity ↑ NO release ↑	[265]
Secoisolariciresinol diglucoside 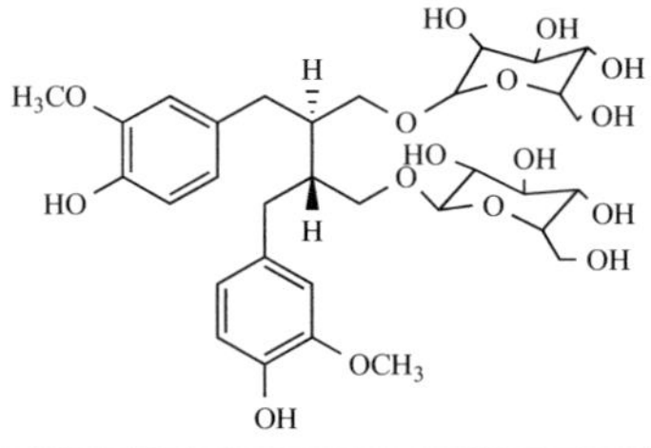	DIO mice (1% wt/wt in diet, 4 wk)	Blood lipids ↓ Fatty liver improved Visceral fat weights ↓	Adipogenic trans-cription factor expression (SREBP-1c) ↓ Fatty acid oxidation (CPT-1) ↑ Adipocytokine secre-tion (adiponectin) ↑ Blood insulin and leptin ↓	[277]
	ZDF rats (40 mg/kg BW, 10 wk)	Blood glucose ↓ Blood cholesterol ↓ Glycated hemoglobin ↓	Blood and pancreatic MDA ↓	[276]
	Streptozotocin induced diabetic rats (22 mg/kg BW, 24 days) Diabetic prone Bio-breeding rats (22 mg/kg BW)	Diabetes improved↓	Blood and pancreatic MDA ↓ Pancreatic antioxidant reserve ↑	[274, 275]

(Table 4) Contd…..

Bioactive Compound	Model (Treatment dosage and duration)	Beneficial effects	Mechanisms of action	Ref.
	Hypercholesterolaemic rats (3, 6 mg/kg BW, 4 wk)	Blood lipids ↓ Fatty liver improved	Hepatic ACAT2 expression ↓	[278]
	Hypercholesterolaemic rats (15 mg/kg BW, 8 wk)	Body weight ↓ Blood lipids ↓ Hypercholesterolemic atherosclerosis ↓		[280]
Secoisolariciresinols 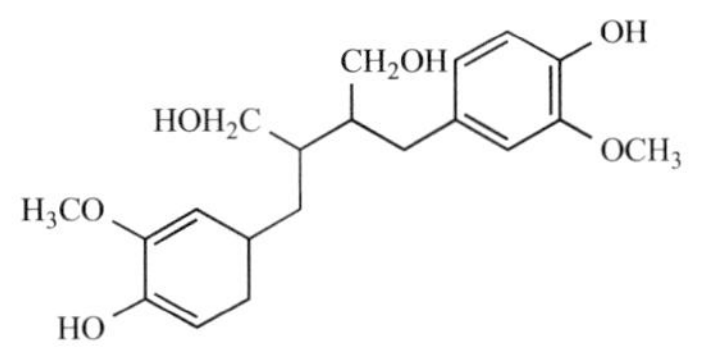	3T3-L1 cells (0.15 μM)	TG accumulation ↓		[271]

CONCLUSION AND FUTURE PROSPECTS

Although lifestyle change is accepted as the first-line treatment for obesity, the emphasis on reduced calorie intake and increased calorie expenditure to reduce weight has had disappointing results. The FDA has approved two products (orlistat and sibutramine) for long-term use in the treatment of obesity, and five other drugs (benzphetamine, diethylpropion, mazindol, phentermine, and phendimetrazine) for "short-term" use. All these drugs, except for orlistat, are sympathomimetrics or serotonin-norepinephrine reuptake inhibitors, and have been classified by the Drug Enforcement Agency as potentially abusive [281]. Orlistat is only minimally absorbed in the body, and its side-effects are those expected from its mechanism of action, which involves blocking the intestinal lipase. Orlistat acts on the gastrointestinal system and blocks the absorption of dietary fat, which results in an additional loss of 3-4% of the body weight over diet restriction alone in a two-year period [282]. Weight loss of 5-15% has been associated with improvements in obesity-related metabolic dysfunction [283, 284]. Therefore, medications that more effectively facilitate efforts to achieve both substantial and sustained weight loss over a long period of time are the ideal ways to combat the obesity epidemic.

The potential of natural products to treat obesity is still largely unexplored and might provide an excellent alternative strategy for the development of safe and effective anti-obesity drugs [285]. Interestingly, a growing body of published data indicates the promising role of phytochemicals in treating obesity and its associated metabolic diseases. Apart from the antioxidant and anti-inflammatory properties of phytochemicals, numerous *in vivo* studies have repeatedly indicated that the intake of some phytochemicals could inhibit HFD-induced obesity in mice, hamsters, rats, or even humans. The adipose tissue mass can be reduced by both inhibiting adipogenesis and inducing the apoptosis of adipocytes. Natural products that specifically target both pathways therefore have potential use in the treatment and prevention of obesity. *In vitro* studies have shown that some phytochemicals, such as quercetin, naringenin, EGCG, gallic acid, capsaicin and curcumin, efficiently induce apoptosis in 3T3-L1 pre-adipocytes and adipocytes. A possible molecular mechanism for the anti-obesity action of these phytochemicals in 3T3 preadipocytes was proposed to involve the mitochondria and mitogen-activated protein kinase (MAPK) pathway, with the subsequent induction of apoptosis. Apart from inducing apoptosis, several natural compounds such as rutin, quercetin, kaempferol, (−)-catechin, EGCG, theaflavins, cyanidin, daidzein, capsaicin, curcumin, coumaric acid, ginsenosides, secoisolariciresinol diglucoside and berberine inhibited adipogenesis by downregulating the adipogenic transcription factors in the 3T3-L1 adipocytes or in the adipose tissues of obese animals. Besides these two separate mechanisms of anti-obesity action, several phytochemicals stimulate lipolysis and increase fatty acid oxidation in adipocytes. For example, EGCG, cyanidin, cyaniding 3-glucoside, curcumin, ginsenosides, ursolic acid, resveratrol, secoisolariciresinol diglucoside and berberine stimulate a dose-dependent increase in lipolysis in the adipose tissue of rodents. Numerous phytochemicals discussed in this chapter have a potential benefit in preventing both obesity and metabolic disorder, such as hyperlipidemia, fatty liver, insulin resistance and hyperglycemia, and the actions for these compounds may involve multiple independent mechanisms, including decreased adipogenesis or lipogenesis, increased fatty acid oxidation, regulated hepatic glucose metabolism along with antioxidant activities.

The FDA mandates that an effective weight-management product should provide improvements in blood pressure, lipids, glycemia, or other beneficial outcomes that are commensurate with the degree of weight loss [286]. Drugs that act 'purely' on one end of the energy balance equation (that is, on energy intake or expenditure) may also fail to achieve significant long-term efficacy. Because body fat is likely to be regulated homeostatically, a change in either intake or expenditure alone will face resistance as compensatory adjustments are made. In the future, it is possible that phytochemicals having multiple mechanisms simultaneously may save this dilemma. Although there is much evidence of the anti-obesity effects of phytochemicals, characterizations of their properties as drug candidates or dietary supplements have been poorly explored. Further studies that focus on understanding their pharmacokinetics and identifying their target proteins, and the accumulation of preclinical data on these interesting phytochemicals, could raise the possibility of a new application of these natural compounds as novel drugs and/or dietary supplements.

ACKNOWLEDGEMENTS

This research was supported by the SRC program (Center for Food and Nutritional Genomics: grant number 2010-0001886) of the National Research Foundation (NRF) of Korea funded by Ministry of Education, Science and Technology. The authors thank Soomin Cho and Soyoung Park for their assistance in preparing the manuscript and illustrations.

REFERENCES

[1] Jandacek RJ, Woods SC. Pharmaceutical approaches to the treatment of obesity. Drug Discov Today 2004; 9: 874-80.

[2] Samuelsson G, Farah MH, Claeson P, *et al.* Inventory of plants used in traditional medicine in Somalia. I. Plants of the families Acanthaceae-Chenopodiaceae. J Ethnopharmacol 1991; 35: 25-63.

[3] Cox PA, Balick MJ. The ethnobotanical approach to drug discovery. Sci Am 1994; 270: 82-7.

[4] Pharmacognosy in the 21st century. J Pharm Pharmacol 2001; 53: 135-48.

[5] Itokawa H, Morris-Natschke SL, Akiyama T, Lee KH. Plant-derived natural product research aimed at new drug discovery. Nat Med (Tokyo) 2008; 62: 263-80.

[6] Perez-Vizcaino F, Duarte J, Andriantsitohaina R. Endothelial function and cardiovascular disease: effects of quercetin and wine polyphenols. Free Radic Res. 2006; 40: 1054-65.

[7] Surh YJ. Anti-tumor promoting potential of selected spice ingredients with antioxidative and anti-inflammatory activities: a short review. Food Chem Toxicol 2002; 40: 1091-7.

[8] Surh Y. Molecular mechanisms of chemopreventive effects of selected dietary and medicinal phenolic substances. Mutat Res. 1999; 428: 305-27.

[9] Surh YJ, Chun KS, Cha HH, *et al.* Molecular mechanisms underlying chemopreventive activities of anti-inflammatory phytochemicals: down-regulation of COX-2 and iNOS through suppression of NF-kappa B activation. Mutat Res 2001; 480: 243-68.

[10] Havsteen BH. The biochemistry and medical significance of the flavonoids. Pharmacol Ther 2002; 96: 167-202.

[11] Bravo L. Polyphenols: chemistry, dietary sources, metabolism, and nutritional significance. Nutr Rev 1998; 56: 317-33.

[12] Hu E, Liang P, Spiegelman BM. AdipoQ is a novel adipose-specific gene dysregulated in obesity. J Biol Chem 1996; 271: 10697-703.

[13] Sartippour MR, Shao ZM, Heber D, *et al.* Green tea inhibits vascular endothelial growth factor (VEGF) induction in human breast cancer cells. J Nutr 2002; 132: 2307-11.

[14] Kavanagh KT, Hafer LJ, Kim DW, *et al.* Green tea extracts decrease carcinogen-induced mammary tumor burden in rats and rate of breast cancer cell proliferation in culture. J Cell Biochem 2001; 82: 387-98.

[15] Osada K, Takahashi M, Hoshina S, Nakamura M, Nakamura S, Sugano M. Tea catechins inhibit cholesterol oxidation accompanying oxidation of low density lipoprotein *in vitro*. Comp Biochem Physiol C Toxicol Pharmacol 2001; 128: 153-64.

[16] Kao YH, Hiipakka RA, Liao S. Modulation of endocrine systems and food intake by green tea epigallocatechin gallate. Endocrinology 2000; 141: 980-7.

[17] Wolfram S. Effects of green tea and EGCG on cardiovascular and metabolic health. J Am Coll Nutr 2007; 26: 373S-88S.

[18] Hsu TF, Kusumoto A, Abe K, *et al.* Polyphenol-enriched oolong tea increases fecal lipid excretion. Eur J Clin Nutr 2006; 60: 1330-6.

[19] Dulloo AG, Duret C, Rohrer D, *et al.* Efficacy of a green tea extract rich in catechin polyphenols and caffeine in increasing 24-h energy expenditure and fat oxidation in humans. Am J Clin Nutr 1999; 70: 1040-5.

[20] Yang CS, Chen L, Lee MJ, Balentine D, Kuo MC, Schantz SP. Blood and urine levels of tea catechins after ingestion of different amounts of green tea by human volunteers. Cancer Epidemiol Biomarkers Prev 1998; 7: 351-4.

[21] Wolfram S, Raederstorff D, Wang Y, Teixeira SR, Elste V, Weber P. TEAVIGO (epigallocatechin gallate) supplementation prevents obesity in rodents by reducing adipose tissue mass. Ann Nutr Metab 2005; 49: 54-63.

[22] Boschmann M, Thielecke F. The effects of epigallocatechin-3-gallate on thermogenesis and fat oxidation in obese men: a pilot study. J Am Coll Nutr 2007; 26: 389S-95S.

[23] Brown AL, Lane J, Coverly J, *et al.* Effects of dietary supplementation with the green tea polyphenol epigallocatechin-3-gallate on insulin resistance and associated metabolic risk factors: randomized controlled trial. Br J Nutr 2009; 101: 886-94.

[24] Cho SY, Park PJ, Shin HJ, *et al.* (-)-Catechin suppresses expression of Kruppel-like factor 7 and increases expression and secretion of adiponectin protein in 3T3-L1 cells. Am J Physiol Endocrinol Metab 2007; 292: E1166-72.

[25] Pajvani UB, Du X, Combs TP, *et al.* Structure-function studies of the adipocyte-secreted hormone Acrp30/adiponectin. Implications fpr metabolic regulation and bioactivity. J Biol Chem 2003; 278: 9073-85.

[26] Bose M, Lambert JD, Ju J, Reuhl KR, Shapses SA, Yang CS. The major green tea polyphenol, (-)-epigallocatechin-3-gallate, inhibits obesity, metabolic syndrome, and fatty liver disease in high-fat-fed mice. J Nutr 2008; 138: 1677-83.

[27] Lin CL, Huang HC, Lin JK. Theaflavins attenuate hepatic lipid accumulation through activating AMPK in human HepG2 cells. J Lipid Res 2007; 48: 2334-43.

[28] Klaus S, Pultz S, Thone-Reineke C, Wolfram S. Epigallocatechin gallate attenuates diet-induced obesity in mice by decreasing energy absorption and increasing fat oxidation. Int J Obes (Lond) 2005; 29: 615-23.

[29] Tong L, Harwood HJ, Jr. Acetyl-coenzyme A carboxylases: versatile targets for drug discovery. J Cell Biochem 2006; 99: 1476-88.

[30] Wu BT, Hung PF, Chen HC, Huang RN, Chang HH, Kao YH. The apoptotic effect of green tea (-)-epigallocatechin gallate on 3T3-L1 preadipocytes depends on the Cdk2 pathway. J Agric Food Chem 2005; 53: 5695-701.

[31] Hwang JT, Park IJ, Shin JI, *et al.* Genistein, EGCG, and capsaicin inhibit adipocyte differentiation process via activating AMP-activated protein kinase. Biochem Biophys Res Commun 2005; 338: 694-9.

[32] Wolfram S, Raederstorff D, Preller M, *et al.* Epigallocatechin gallate supplementation alleviates diabetes in rodents. J Nutr 2006; 136: 2512-8.

[33] Graham HN. Green tea composition, consumption, and polyphenol chemistry. Prev Med 1992; 21: 334-50.

[34] Subramanian N, Venkatesh P, Ganguli S, Sinkar VP. Role of polyphenol oxidase and peroxidase in the generation of black tea theaflavins. J Agric Food Chem 1999; 47: 2571-8.

[35] Bushman JL. Green tea and cancer in humans: a review of the literature. Nutr Cancer 1998; 31: 151-9.

[36] Yang CS. Tea and health. Nutrition 1999; 15: 946-9.

[37] Leung LK, Su Y, Chen R, Zhang Z, Huang Y, Chen ZY. Theaflavins in black tea and catechins in green tea are equally effective antioxidants. J Nutr 2001; 131: 2248-51.

[38] Kobayashi M, Ichitani M, Suzuki Y, *et al.* Black-tea polyphenols suppress postprandial hypertriacylglycerolemia by suppressing lymphatic transport of dietary fat in rats. J Agric Food Chem 2009; 57: 7131-6.

[39] Vermeer MA, Mulder TP, Molhuizen HO. Theaflavins from black tea, especially theaflavin-3-gallate, reduce the incorporation of cholesterol into mixed micelles. J Agric Food Chem 2008; 56: 12031-6.

[40] Matsui T, Tanaka T, Tamura S, *et al.* alpha-Glucosidase inhibitory profile of catechins and theaflavins. J Agric Food Chem 2007; 55: 99-105.

[41] Lorenz M, Urban J, Engelhardt U, Baumann G, Stangl K, Stangl V. Green and black tea are equally potent stimuli of NO production and vasodilation: new insights into tea ingredients involved. Basic Res Cardiol 2009; 104: 100-10.

[42] Davies MJ, Judd JT, Baer DJ, *et al.* Black tea consumption reduces total and LDL cholesterol in mildly hypercholesterolemic adults. J Nutr 2003; 133: 3298S-302S.

[43] Ikeda I, Kobayashi M, Hamada T, *et al.* Heat-epimerized tea catechins rich in gallocatechin gallate and catechin gallate are more effective to inhibit cholesterol absorption than tea catechins rich in epigallocatechin gallate and epicatechin gallate. J Agric Food Chem 2003; 51: 7303-7.

[44] Ikeda I, Imasato Y, Sasaki E, *et al.* Tea catechins decrease micellar solubility and intestinal absorption of cholesterol in rats. Biochim Biophys Acta 1992; 1127: 141-6.

[45] Raederstorff DG, Schlachter MF, Elste V, Weber P. Effect of EGCG on lipid absorption and plasma lipid levels in rats. J Nutr Biochem 2003; 14: 326-32.

[46] Oki T, Matsui T, Matsumoto K. Evaluation of alpha-glucosidase inhibition by using an immobilized assay system. Biol Pharm Bull 2000; 23: 1084-7.

[47] Hauri HP, Wacker H, Rickli EE, Bigler-Meier B, Quaroni A, Semenza G. Biosynthesis of sucrase-isomaltase. Purification and NH2-terminal amino acid sequence of the rat sucrase-isomaltase precursor (pro-sucrase-isomaltase) from fetal intestinal transplants. J Biol Chem 1982; 257: 4522-8.

[48] Galvano F, La Fauci L, Vitaglione P, Fogliano V, Vanella L, Felgines C. Bioavailability, antioxidant and biological properties of the natural free-radical scavengers cyanidin and related glycosides. Ann Ist Super Sanita 2007; 43: 382-93.

[49] Tsuda T, Horio F, Uchida K, Aoki H, Osawa T. Dietary cyanidin 3-O-beta-D-glucoside-rich purple corn color prevents obesity and ameliorates hyperglycemia in mice. J Nutr 2003; 133: 2125-30.

[50] Galvano F, La Fauci L, Lazzarino G, *et al.* Cyanidins: metabolism and biological properties. J Nutr Biochem 2004; 15: 2-11.

[51] Tsuda T, Ueno Y, Aoki H, *et al.* Anthocyanin enhances adipocytokine secretion and adipocyte-specific gene expression in isolated rat adipocytes. Biochem Biophys Res Commun 2004; 16: 149-57.

[52] Tsuda T, Ueno Y, Yoshikawa T, Kojo H, Osawa T. Microarray profiling of gene expression in human adipocytes in response to anthocyanins. Biochem Pharmacol 2006; 71: 1184-97.

[53] Tsuda T, Ueno Y, Kojo H, Yoshikawa T, Osawa T. Gene expression profile of isolated rat adipocytes treated with anthocyanins. Biochim Biophys Acta 2005; 1733: 137-47.

[54] Jayaprakasam B, Vareed SK, Olson LK, Nair MG. Insulin secretion by bioactive anthocyanins and anthocyanidins present in fruits. J Agric Food Chem 2005; 53: 28-31.

[55] Adisakwattana S, Ngamrojanavanich N, Kalampakorn K, Tiravanit W, Roengsumran S, Yibchok-Anun S. Inhibitory activity of cyanidin-3-rutinoside on alpha-glucosidase. J Enzyme Inhib Med Chem 2004; 19: 313-6.

[56] Adisakwattana S, Charoenlertkul P, Yibchok-Anun S. alpha-Glucosidase inhibitory activity of cyanidin-3-galactoside and synergistic effect with acarbose. J Enzyme Inhib Med Chem 2009; 24: 65-9.

[57] Cederroth CR, Nef S. Soy, phytoestrogens and metabolism: A review. Mol Cell Endocrinol 2009; 304: 30-42.

[58] Bhathena SJ, Velasquez MT. Beneficial role of dietary phytoestrogens in obesity and diabetes. Am J Clin Nutr 2002; 76: 1191-201.

[59] Goodman-Gruen D, Kritz-Silverstein D. Usual dietary isoflavone intake is associated with cardiovascular disease risk factors in postmenopausal women. J Nutr 2001; 131: 1202-6.

[60] Goodman-Gruen D, Kritz-Silverstein D. Usual dietary isoflavone intake and body composition in postmenopausal women. Menopause 2003; 10: 427-32.
[61] Guthrie JR, Ball M, Murkies A, Dennerstein L. Dietary phytoestrogen intake in mid-life Australian-born women: relationship to health variables. Climacteric 2000; 3: 254-61.
[62] Wu J, Oka J, Higuchi M, *et al.* Cooperative effects of isoflavones and exercise on bone and lipid metabolism in postmenopausal Japanese women: a randomized placebo-controlled trial. Metabolism 2006; 55: 423-33.
[63] Demonty I, Lamarche B, Deshaies Y, Jacques H. Role of soy isoflavones in the hypotriglyceridemic effect of soy protein in the rat. J Nutr Biochem 2002; 13: 671-7.
[64] Song T, Lee SO, Murphy PA, Hendrich S. Soy protein with or without isoflavones, soy germ and soy germ extract, and daidzein lessen plasma cholesterol levels in golden Syrian hamsters. Exp Biol Med (Maywood) 2003; 228: 1063-8.
[65] Lee SO, Renouf M, Ye Z, Murphy PA, Hendrich S. Isoflavone glycitein diminished plasma cholesterol in female golden Syrian hamsters. J Agric Food Chem 2007; 55: 11063-7.
[66] Naaz A, Yellayi S, Zakroczymski MA, *et al.* The soy isoflavone genistein decreases adipose deposition in mice. Endocrinology 2003; 144: 3315-20.
[67] Penza M, Montani C, Romani A, *et al.* Genistein affects adipose tissue deposition in a dose-dependent and gender-specific manner. Endocrinology 2006; 147: 5740-51.
[68] Szkudelska K, Nogowski L, Szkudelski T. Genistein affects lipogenesis and lipolysis in isolated rat adipocytes. J Steroid Biochem Mol Biol 2000; 75: 265-71.
[69] Szkudelska K, Szkudelski T, Nogowski L. Daidzein, coumestrol and zearalenone affect lipogenesis and lipolysis in rat adipocytes. Phytomedicine 2002; 9: 338-45.
[70] Harmon AW, Harp JB. Differential effects of flavonoids on 3T3-L1 adipogenesis and lipolysis. Am J Physiol Cell Physiol 2001; 280: C807-13.
[71] Nogowski L, Mackowiak P, Kandulska K, Szkudelski T, Nowak KW. Genistein-induced changes in lipid metabolism of ovariectomized rats. Ann Nutr Metab 1998; 42: 360-6.
[72] Ae Park S, Choi MS, Cho SY, *et al.* Genistein and daidzein modulate hepatic glucose and lipid regulating enzyme activities in C57BL/KsJ-db/db mice. Life Sci 2006; 79: 1207-13.
[73] Liu D, Zhen W, Yang Z, Carter JD, Si H, Reynolds KA. Genistein acutely stimulates insulin secretion in pancreatic beta-cells through a cAMP-dependent protein kinase pathway. Diabetes 2006; 55: 1043-50.
[74] Choi MS, Jung UJ, Yeo J, Kim MJ, Lee MK. Genistein and daidzein prevent diabetes onset by elevating insulin level and altering hepatic gluconeogenic and lipogenic enzyme activities in non-obese diabetic (NOD) mice. Diabetes Metab Res Rev 2008; 24: 74-81.
[75] Lee JS. Effects of soy protein and genistein on blood glucose, antioxidant enzyme activities, and lipid profile in streptozotocin-induced diabetic rats. Life Sci 2006; 79: 1578-84.
[76] Yu SF, Shun CT, Chen TM, Chen YH. 3-O-beta-D-glucosyl-(1-->6)-beta-D-glucosyl-kaempferol isolated from Sauropus androgenus reduces body weight gain in Wistar rats. Biol Pharm Bull 2006; 29: 2510-3.
[77] Fang XK, Gao J, Zhu DN. Kaempferol and quercetin isolated from Euonymus alatus improve glucose uptake of 3T3-L1 cells without adipogenesis activity. Life Sci 2008; 82: 615-22.
[78] Hiermann A, Schramm HW, Laufer S. Anti-inflammatory activity of myricetin-3-O-beta-D-glucuronide and related compounds. Inflamm Res 1998; 47: 421-7.
[79] Hertog MG, Hollman PC, Katan MB, Kromhout D. Intake of potentially anticarcinogenic flavonoids and their determinants in adults in The Netherlands. Nutr Cancer 1993; 20: 21-9.
[80] Ono K, Nakane H, Fukushima M, Chermann JC, Barre-Sinoussi F. Differential inhibitory effects of various flavonoids on the activities of reverse transcriptase and cellular DNA and RNA polymerases. Eur J Biochem 1990; 190: 469-76.
[81] el-Gammal AA, Mansour RM. Antimicrobial activities of some flavonoid compounds. Zentralbl Mikrobiol 1986; 141: 561-5.
[82] Landolfi R, Mower RL, Steiner M. Modification of platelet function and arachidonic acid metabolism by bioflavonoids. Structure-activity relations. Biochem Pharmacol 1984; 33: 1525-30.
[83] Liu IM, Tzeng TF, Liou SS, Lan TW. Myricetin, a naturally occurring flavonol, ameliorates insulin resistance induced by a high-fructose diet in rats. Life Sci 2007; 81: 1479-88.
[84] Ong KC, Khoo HE. Biological effects of myricetin. Gen Pharmacol 1997; 29(2): 121-6.
[85] Liu IM, Liou SS, Lan TW, Hsu FL, Cheng JT. Myricetin as the active principle of Abelmoschus moschatus to lower plasma glucose in streptozotocin-induced diabetic rats. Planta Med 2005; 71: 617-21.
[86] Liu IM, Liou SS, Cheng JT. Mediation of beta-endorphin by myricetin to lower plasma glucose in streptozotocin-induced diabetic rats. J Ethnopharmacol 2006; 104: 199-206.
[87] Ong KC, Khoo HE. Insulinomimetic effects of myricetin on lipogenesis and glucose transport in rat adipocytes but not glucose transport translocation. Biochem Pharmacol 1996; 51: 423-9.
[88] Liu IM, Tzeng TF, Liou SS, Lan TW. Improvement of insulin sensitivity in obese Zucker rats by myricetin extracted from Abelmoschus moschatus. Planta Med 2007; 73: 1054-60.
[89] Ong KC, Khoo HE. Effects of myricetin on glycemia and glycogen metabolism in diabetic rats. Life Sci 2000; 67: 1695-705.
[90] Strobel P, Allard C, Perez-Acle T, Calderon R, Aldunate R, Leighton F. Myricetin, quercetin and catechin-gallate inhibit glucose uptake in isolated rat adipocytes. Biochem J 2005; 386: 471-8.
[91] Chaudhry PS, Cabrera J, Juliani HR, Varma SD. Inhibition of human lens aldose reductase by flavonoids, sulindac and indomethacin. Biochem Pharmacol 1983; 32: 1995-8.
[92] Erlund I, Meririnne E, Alfthan G, Aro A. Plasma kinetics and urinary excretion of the flavanones naringenin and hesperetin in humans after ingestion of orange juice and grapefruit juice. J Nutr 2001; 131: 235-41.
[93] Galati EM, Monforte MT, Kirjavainen S, Forestieri AM, Trovato A, Tripodo MM. Biological effects of hesperidin, a citrus flavonoid. (Note I): antiinflammatory and analgesic activity. Farmaco 1994; 40: 709-12.
[94] Wilcox LJ, Borradaile NM, de Dreu LE, Huff MW. Secretion of hepatocyte apoB is inhibited by the flavonoids, naringenin and hesperetin, via reduced activity and expression of ACAT2 and MTP. J Lipid Res 2001; 42: 725-34.
[95] Kim HK, Jeong TS, Lee MK, Park YB, Choi MS. Lipid-lowering efficacy of hesperetin metabolites in high-cholesterol fed rats. Clin Chim Acta 2003; 327: 129-37.

[96] Cha JY, Cho YS, Kim I, Anno T, Rahman SM, Yanagita T. Effect of hesperetin, a citrus flavonoid, on the liver triacylglycerol content and phosphatidate phosphohydrolase activity in orotic acid-fed rats. Plant Foods Hum Nutr 2001; 56: 349-58.

[97] Jamil H, Dickson JK, Jr., Chu CH, *et al.* Microsomal triglyceride transfer protein. Specificity of lipid binding and transport. J Biol Chem 1995; 270: 6549-54.

[98] Wetterau JR, Gregg RE, Harrity TW, *et al.* An MTP inhibitor that normalizes atherogenic lipoprotein levels in WHHL rabbits. Science 1998; 282: 751-4.

[99] Bilheimer DW, Grundy SM, Brown MS, Goldstein JL. Mevinolin and colestipol stimulate receptor-mediated clearance of low density lipoprotein from plasma in familial hypercholesterolemia heterozygotes. Proc Natl Acad Sci USA 1983; 80: 4124-8.

[100] Choe SC, Kim HS, Jeong TS, Bok SH, Park YB. Naringin has an antiatherogenic effect with the inhibition of intercellular adhesion molecule-1 in hypercholesterolemic rabbits. J Cardiovasc Pharmacol 2001; 38: 947-55.

[101] Jung UJ, Lee MK, Park YB, Kang MA, Choi MS. Effect of citrus flavonoids on lipid metabolism and glucose-regulating enzyme mRNA levels in type-2 diabetic mice. Int J Biochem Cell Biol 2006; 38: 1134-45.

[102] Jung UJ, Lee MK, Jeong KS, Choi MS. The hypoglycemic effects of hesperidin and naringin are partly mediated by hepatic glucose-regulating enzymes in C57BL/KsJ-db/db mice. J Nutr 2004; 134: 2499-503.

[103] Choi MS, Do KM, Park YS, *et al.* Effect of naringin supplementation on cholesterol metabolism and antioxidant status in rats fed high cholesterol with different levels of vitamin E. Ann Nutr Metab 2001; 45: 193-201.

[104] Bok SH, Lee SH, Park YB, *et al.* Plasma and hepatic cholesterol and hepatic activities of 3-hydroxy-3-methyl-glutaryl-CoA reductase and acyl CoA: cholesterol transferase are lower in rats fed citrus peel extract or a mixture of citrus bioflavonoids. J Nutr 1999; 129: 1182-5.

[105] Byington RP, Jukema JW, Salonen JT, *et al.* Reduction in cardiovascular events during pravastatin therapy. Pooled analysis of clinical events of the Pravastatin Atherosclerosis Intervention Program. Circulation 1995; 92: 2419-25.

[106] Delsing DJ, Offerman EH, van Duyvenvoorde W, *et al.* Acyl-CoA:cholesterol acyltransferase inhibitor avasimibe reduces atherosclerosis in addition to its cholesterol-lowering effect in ApoE*3-Leiden mice. Circulation 2001; 103: 1778-86.

[107] Harmon AW, Patel YM. Naringenin inhibits phosphoinositide 3-kinase activity and glucose uptake in 3T3-L1 adipocytes. Biochem Biophys Res Commun 2003; 305: 229-34.

[108] Huong DT, Takahashi Y, Ide T. Activity and mRNA levels of enzymes involved in hepatic fatty acid oxidation in mice fed citrus flavonoids. Nutrition 2006; 22: 546-52.

[109] Lee SH, Park YB, Bae KH, *et al.* Cholesterol-lowering activity of naringenin via inhibition of 3-hydroxy-3-methylglutaryl coenzyme A reductase and acyl coenzyme A:cholesterol acyltransferase in rats. Ann Nutr Metab 1999; 43: 173-80.

[110] Kim SY, Kim HJ, Lee MK, *et al.* Naringin time-dependently lowers hepatic cholesterol biosynthesis and plasma cholesterol in rats fed high-fat and high-cholesterol diet. J Med Food 2006; 9: 582-6.

[111] Jung UJ, Kim HJ, Lee JS, *et al.* Naringin supplementation lowers plasma lipids and enhances erythrocyte antioxidant enzyme activities in hypercholesterolemic subjects. Clin Nutr 2003; 22: 561-8.

[112] Bischoff SC. Quercetin: potentials in the prevention and therapy of disease. Curr Opin Clin Nutr Metab Care 2008; 11: 733-40.

[113] Yamamoto Y, Oue E. Antihypertensive effect of quercetin in rats fed with a high-fat high-sucrose diet. Biosci Biotechnol Biochem 2006; 70: 933-9.

[114] Edwards RL, Lyon T, Litwin SE, Rabovsky A, Symons JD, Jalili T. Quercetin reduces blood pressure in hypertensive subjects. J Nutr 2007; 137: 2405-11.

[115] Rivera L, Moron R, Sanchez M, Zarzuelo A, Galisteo M. Quercetin ameliorates metabolic syndrome and improves the inflammatory status in obese Zucker rats. Obesity (Silver Spring) 2008; 16: 2081-7.

[116] Hsu CL, Yen GC. Induction of cell apoptosis in 3T3-L1 pre-adipocytes by flavonoids is associated with their antioxidant activity. Mol Nutr Food Res 2006; 50: 1072-9.

[117] Yang JY, Della-Fera MA, Rayalam S, *et al.* Enhanced inhibition of adipogenesis and induction of apoptosis in 3T3-L1 adipocytes with combinations of resveratrol and quercetin. Life Sci 2008; 82: 1032-9.

[118] Frayn KN, Karpe F, Fielding BA, Macdonald IA, Coppack SW. Integrative physiology of human adipose tissue. Int J Obes Relat Metab Disord 2003; 27: 875-88.

[119] Kuppusamy UR, Das NP. Effects of flavonoids on cyclic AMP phosphodiesterase and lipid mobilization in rat adipocytes. Biochem Pharmacol 1992; 44: 1307-15.

[120] Matter WF, Brown RF, Vlahos CJ. The inhibition of phosphatidylinositol 3-kinase by quercetin and analogs. Biochem Biophys Res Commun 1992; 186: 624-31.

[121] Agullo G, Gamet-Payrastre L, Manenti S, *et al.* Relationship between flavonoid structure and inhibition of phosphatidylinositol 3-kinase: a comparison with tyrosine kinase and protein kinase C inhibition. Biochem Pharmacol 1997; 53: 1649-57.

[122] Walker EH, Pacold ME, Perisic O, *et al.* Structural determinants of phosphoinositide 3-kinase inhibition by wortmannin, LY294002, quercetin, myricetin, and staurosporine. Mol Cell 2000; 6: 909-19.

[123] Williams RJ, Spencer JP, Rice-Evans C. Flavonoids: antioxidants or signalling molecules? Free Radic Biol Med 2004; 36: 838-49.

[124] Gamet-Payrastre L, Manenti S, Gratacap MP, Tulliez J, Chap H, Payrastre B. Flavonoids and the inhibition of PKC and PI 3-kinase. Gen Pharmacol 1999; 32: 279-86.

[125] Gulati N, Laudet B, Zohrabian VM, Murali R, Jhanwar-Uniyal M. The antiproliferative effect of Quercetin in cancer cells is mediated via inhibition of the PI3K-Akt/PKB pathway. Anticancer Res 200; 26: 1177-81.

[126] Valensi P, Le Devehat C, Richard JL, *et al.* A multicenter, double-blind, safety study of QR-333 for the treatment of symptomatic diabetic peripheral neuropathy. A preliminary report. J Diabetes Complications 2005; 19: 247-53.

[127] Kuntic V, Pejic N, Ivkovic B, *et al.* Isocratic RP-HPLC method for rutin determination in solid oral dosage forms. J Pharm Biomed Anal 2007; 43: 718-21.

[128] Schwedhelm E, Maas R, Troost R, Boger RH. Clinical pharmacokinetics of antioxidants and their impact on systemic oxidative stress. Clin Pharmacokinet 2003; 42: 437-59.

[129] Sheu JR, Hsiao G, Chou PH, Shen MY, Chou DS. Mechanisms involved in the antiplatelet activity of rutin, a glycoside of the flavonol quercetin, in human platelets. J Agric Food Chem 2004; 52: 4414-8.

[130] Janbaz KH, Saeed SA, Gilani AH. Protective effect of rutin on paracetamol- and CCl4-induced hepatotoxicity in rodents. Fitoterapia 2002; 73: 557-63.

[131] La Casa C, Villegas I, Alarcon de la Lastra C, Motilva V, Martin Calero MJ. Evidence for protective and antioxidant properties of rutin, a natural flavone, against ethanol induced gastric lesions. J Ethnopharmacol 2000; 71: 45-53.

[132] Trumbeckaite S, Bernatoniene J, Majiene D, Jakstas V, Savickas A, Toleikis A. The effect of flavonoids on rat heart mitochondrial function. Biomed Pharmacother 2006; 60: 245-8.

[133] Hsu CL, Wu CH, Huang SL, Yen GC. Phenolic compounds rutin and o-coumaric acid ameliorate obesity induced by high-fat diet in rats. J Agric Food Chem 2009; 57: 425-31.

[134] Choi I, Park Y, Choi H, Lee EH. Anti-adipogenic activity of rutin in 3T3-L1 cells and mice fed with high-fat diet. Biofactors 2006; 26: 273-81.

[135] Ziaee A, Zamansoltani F, Nassiri-Asl M, Abbasi E. Effects of rutin on lipid profile in hypercholesterolaemic rats. Basic Clin Pharmacol Toxicol 2009; 104: 253-8.

[136] Hsu CL, Yen GC. Effects of flavonoids and phenolic acids on the inhibition of adipogenesis in 3T3-L1 adipocytes. J Agric Food Chem 2007; 55: 8404-10.

[137] Moon HS, Chung CS, Lee HG, Kim TG, Choi YJ, Cho CS. Inhibitory effect of (-)-epigallocatechin-3-gallate on lipid accumulation of 3T3-L1 cells. Obesity (Silver Spring) 2007; 15: 2571-82.

[138] Lin J, Della-Fera MA, Baile CA. Green tea polyphenol epigallocatechin gallate inhibits adipogenesis and induces apoptosis in 3T3-L1 adipocytes. Obes Res 2005; 13: 982-90.

[139] Kobayashi Y, Suzuki M, Satsu H, *et al.* Green tea polyphenols inhibit the sodium-dependent glucose transporter of intestinal epithelial cells by a competitive mechanism. J Agric Food Chem 2000; 48: 5618-23.

[140] Mackowiak P, Nogowski L, Nowak KW. Effect of isoflavone genistein on insulin receptors in perfused liver of ovariectomized rats. J Recept Signal Transduct Res 1999; 19: 283-92.

[141] Uesugi T, Toda T, Tsuji K, Ishida H. Comparative study on reduction of bone loss and lipid metabolism abnormality in ovariectomized rats by soy isoflavones, daidzin, genistin, and glycitin. Biol Pharm Bull 2001; 24: 368-72.

[142] Lee MK, Moon SS, Lee SE, *et al.* Naringenin 7-O-cetyl ether as inhibitor of HMG-CoA reductase and modulator of plasma and hepatic lipids in high cholesterol-fed rats. Bioorg Med Chem 2003; 11: 393-8.

[143] Stalikas CD. Extraction, separation, and detection methods for phenolic acids and flavonoids. J Sep Sci 2007; 30: 3268-95.

[144] Crozier A, Jaganath IB, Clifford MN. Dietary phenolics: chemistry, bioavailability and effects on health. Nat Prod Rep 2009; 26: 1001-43.

[145] Hsu CL, Yen GC. Phenolic compounds: evidence for inhibitory effects against obesity and their underlying molecular signaling mechanisms. Mol Nutr Food Res 2008; 52: 53-61.

[146] Yeh CT, Yen GC. Effect of vegetables on human phenolsulfotransferases in relation to their antioxidant activity and total phenolics. Free Radic Res 2005; 39: 893-904.

[147] Varin L, Marsolais F, Richard M, Rouleau M. Sulfation and sulfotransferases 6: Biochemistry and molecular biology of plant sulfotransferases. FASEB J 1997; 11: 517-25.

[148] Hsu CL, Huang SL, Yen GC. Inhibitory effect of phenolic acids on the proliferation of 3T3-L1 preadipocytes in relation to their antioxidant activity. J Agric Food Chem 2006 14; 54: 4191-7.

[149] Hsu CL, Lo WH, Yen GC. Gallic acid induces apoptosis in 3T3-L1 pre-adipocytes via a Fas- and mitochondrial-mediated pathway. J Agric Food Chem 2007; 55: 7359-65.

[150] Hsu CL, Yen GC. Effect of gallic acid on high fat diet-induced dyslipidaemia, hepatosteatosis and oxidative stress in rats. Br J Nutr 2007; 98: 727-35.

[151] Jang A, Srinivasan P, Lee NY, *et al.* Comparison of hypolipidemic activity of synthetic gallic acid-linoleic acid ester with mixture of gallic acid and linoleic acid, gallic acid, and linoleic acid on high-fat diet induced obesity in C57BL/6 Cr Slc mice. Chem Biol Interact 2008; 174: 109-17.

[152] Cordell GA, Araujo OE. Capsaicin: identification, nomenclature, and pharmacotherapy. Ann Pharmacother 1993; 27: 330-6.

[153] Yoshioka M, St-Pierre S, Drapeau V, *et al.* Effects of red pepper on appetite and energy intake. Br J Nutr 1999; 82: 115-23.

[154] Kawada T, Hagihara K, Iwai K. Effects of capsaicin on lipid metabolism in rats fed a high fat diet. J Nutr 1986; 116: 1272-8.

[155] Morre DJ, Chueh PJ, Morre DM. Capsaicin inhibits preferentially the NADH oxidase and growth of transformed cells in culture. Proc Natl Acad Sci USA 1995; 92: 1831-5.

[156] Macho A, Sancho R, Minassi A, Appendino G, Lawen A, Munoz E. Involvement of reactive oxygen species in capsaicinoid-induced apoptosis in transformed cells. Free Radic Res 2003; 37: 611-9.

[157] Hsu CL, Yen GC. Effects of capsaicin on induction of apoptosis and inhibition of adipogenesis in 3T3-L1 cells. J Agric Food Chem 2007; 55: 1730-6.

[158] Kang JH, Tsuyoshi G, Han IS, Kawada T, Kim YM, Yu R. Dietary capsaicin reduces obesity-induced insulin resistance and hepatic steatosis in obese mice fed a high-fat diet. Obesity (Silver Spring) 2010; 18: 780-7.

[159] Xu H, Barnes GT, Yang Q, *et al.* Chronic inflammation in fat plays a crucial role in the development of obesity-related insulin resistance. J Clin Invest 2003; 112: 1821-30.

[160] Weisberg SP, McCann D, Desai M, Rosenbaum M, Leibel RL, Ferrante AW, Jr. Obesity is associated with macrophage accumulation in adipose tissue. J Clin Invest 2003; 112: 1796-808.

[161] Matsuzawa Y, Funahashi T, Kihara S, Shimomura I. Adiponectin and metabolic syndrome. Arterioscler Thromb Vasc Biol 2004; 24: 29-33.

[162] Hausman DB, DiGirolamo M, Bartness TJ, Hausman GJ, Martin RJ. The biology of white adipocyte proliferation. Obes Rev 2001; 2: 239-54.

[163] Kang JH, Kim CS, Han IS, Kawada T, Yu R. Capsaicin, a spicy component of hot peppers, modulates adipokine gene expression and protein release from obese-mouse adipose tissues and isolated adipocytes, and suppresses the inflammatory responses of adipose tissue macrophages. FEBS Lett 2007; 581: 4389-96.

[164] Sharma RA, Gescher AJ, Steward WP. Curcumin: the story so far. Eur J Cancer 2005; 41: 1955-68.

[165] Lao CD, Ruffin MTt, Normolle D, *et al.* Dose escalation of a curcuminoid formulation. BMC Complement Altern Med 2006; 6:10.

[166] Dutta S, Padhye S, Priyadarsini KI, Newton C. Antioxidant and antiproliferative activity of curcumin semicarbazone. Bioorg Med Chem Lett 2005; 15: 2738-44.

[167] Lim CS, Jin DQ, Mok H, *et al.* Antioxidant and antiinflammatory activities of xanthorrhizol in hippocampal neurons and primary cultured microglia. J Neurosci Res 2005; 82: 831-8.
[168] Singh S, Khar A. Biological effects of curcumin and its role in cancer chemoprevention and therapy. Anticancer Agents Med Chem 2006 ; 6: 259-70.
[169] Arafa HM. Curcumin attenuates diet-induced hypercholesterolemia in rats. Med Sci Monit 2005; 11: BR228-34.
[170] Ejaz A, Wu D, Kwan P, Meydani M. Curcumin inhibits adipogenesis in 3T3-L1 adipocytes and angiogenesis and obesity in C57/BL mice. J Nutr 2009 ; 139: 919-25.
[171] Weisberg SP, Leibel R, Tortoriello DV. Dietary curcumin significantly improves obesity-associated inflammation and diabetes in mouse models of diabesity. Endocrinology 2008; 149: 3549-58.
[172] Kang Q, Chen A. Curcumin suppresses expression of low-density lipoprotein (LDL) receptor, leading to the inhibition of LDL-induced activation of hepatic stellate cells. Br J Pharmacol 2009; 157: 1354-67.
[173] Babu PS, Srinivasan K. Hypolipidemic action of curcumin, the active principle of turmeric (Curcuma longa) in streptozotocin induced diabetic rats. Mol Cell Biochem 1997; 166: 169-75.
[174] Rao DS, Sekhara NC, Satyanarayana MN, Srinivasan M. Effect of curcumin on serum and liver cholesterol levels in the rat. J Nutr 1970 ; 100: 1307-15.
[175] Peschel D, Koerting R, Nass N. Curcumin induces changes in expression of genes involved in cholesterol homeostasis. J Nutr Biochem 2007; 18: 113-9.
[176] Ramirez-Tortosa MC, Mesa MD, Aguilera MC, *et al.* Oral administration of a turmeric extract inhibits LDL oxidation and has hypocholesterolemic effects in rabbits with experimental atherosclerosis. Atherosclerosis 1999 ; 147: 371-8.
[177] Guglielmi F, Luceri C, Giovannelli L, Dolara P, Lodovici M. Effect of 4-coumaric and 3,4-dihydroxybenzoic acid on oxidative DNA damage in rat colonic mucosa. Br J Nutr 2003; 89: 581-7.
[178] Luceri C, Guglielmi F, Lodovici M, Giannini L, Messerini L, Dolara P. Plant phenolic 4-coumaric acid protects against intestinal inflammation in rats. Scand J Gastroenterol 2004 ; 39: 1128-33.
[179] Luceri C, Giannini L, Lodovici M, *et al.* p-Coumaric acid, a common dietary phenol, inhibits platelet activity *in vitro* and *in vivo*. Br J Nutr 2007; 97: 458-63.
[180] Kawada T, Watanabe T, Takaishi T, Tanaka T, Iwai K. Capsaicin-induced beta-adrenergic action on energy metabolism in rats: influence of capsaicin on oxygen consumption, the respiratory quotient, and substrate utilization. Proc Soc Exp Biol Med 1986; 183: 250-6.
[181] Paduch R, Kandefer-Szerszen M, Trytek M, Fiedurek J. Terpenes: substances useful in human healthcare. Arch Immunol Ther Exp (Warsz) 2007; 55: 315-27.
[182] Kohlert C, van Rensen I, Marz R, Schindler G, Graefe EU, Veit M. Bioavailability and pharmacokinetics of natural volatile terpenes in animals and humans. Planta Med 2000; 66: 495-505.
[183] Kishimoto Y, Tani M, Uto-Kondo H, *et al.* Astaxanthin suppresses scavenger receptor expression and matrix metalloproteinase activity in macrophages. Eur J Nutr 2010; 49: 119-26.
[184] Jacobsson LS, Yuan XM, Zieden B, Olsson AG. Effects of alpha-tocopherol and astaxanthin on LDL oxidation and atherosclerosis in WHHL rabbits. Atherosclerosis 2004; 173: 231-7.
[185] Jyonouchi H, Sun S, Iijima K, Gross MD. Antitumor activity of astaxanthin and its mode of action. Nutr Cancer 2000; 36: 59-65.
[186] Chew BP, Park JS, Wong MW, Wong TS. A comparison of the anticancer activities of dietary beta-carotene, canthaxanthin and astaxanthin in mice *in vivo*. Anticancer Res 1999; 19: 1849-53.
[187] Naito Y, Uchiyama K, Aoi W, *et al.* Prevention of diabetic nephropathy by treatment with astaxanthin in diabetic db/db mice. Biofactors 2004; 20: 49-59.
[188] Guerin M, Huntley ME, Olaizola M. Haematococcus astaxanthin: applications for human health and nutrition. Trends Biotechnol. 2003; 21: 210-216.
[189] Naguib YM. Antioxidant activities of astaxanthin and related carotenoids. J Agric Food Chem 2000; 48: 1150-4.
[190] Iwamoto T, Hosoda K, Hirano R, Kurata H, Matsumoto A, Miki W, *et al.* Inhibition of low-density lipoprotein oxidation by astaxanthin. J Atheroscler Thromb 2000; 7: 216-22.
[191] Ikeuchi M, Koyama T, Takahashi J, Yazawa K. Effects of astaxanthin in obese mice fed a high-fat diet. Biosci Biotechnol Biochem 2007; 71: 893-9.
[192] Kapoor R, Huang YS. Gamma linolenic acid: an antiinflammatory omega-6 fatty acid. Curr Pharm Biotechnol 2006; 7: 531-4.
[193] Strum-Odin R, Adkins-Finke B, Blake WL, Phinney SD, Clarke SD. Modification of fatty acid composition of membrane phospholipid in hepatocyte monolayer with n-3, n-6 and n-9 fatty acids and its relationship to triacylglycerol production. Biochim Biophys Acta 1987; 921: 378-91.
[194] Williams MA, Tinoco J, Yang YT, Bird MI, Hincenbergs I. Feeding pure docosahexaenoate or arachidonate decreases plasma triacylglycerol secretion in rats. Lipids 1989; 24: 753-8.
[195] Borkman M, Storlien LH, Pan DA, Jenkins AB, Chisholm DJ, Campbell LV. The relation between insulin sensitivity and the fatty-acid composition of skeletal-muscle phospholipids. N Engl J Med 1993; 328: 238-44.
[196] Serrero G, Lepak NM, Goodrich SP. Paracrine regulation of adipose differentiation by arachidonate metabolites: prostaglandin F2 alpha inhibits early and late markers of differentiation in the adipogenic cell line 1246. Endocrinology 1992 ; 131: 2545-51.
[197] Phinney SD, Davis PG, Johnson SB, Holman RT. Obesity and weight loss alter serum polyunsaturated lipids in humans. Am J Clin Nutr 1991; 53: 831-8.
[198] Blond JP, Henchiri C, Bezard J. Delta 6 and delta 5 desaturase activities in liver from obese Zucker rats at different ages. Lipids. 1989; 24: 389-395.
[199] Phinney SD, Tang AB, Thurmond DC, Nakamura MT, Stern JS. Abnormal polyunsaturated lipid metabolism in the obese Zucker rat, with partial metabolic correction by gamma-linolenic acid administration. Metabolism 1993; 42: 1127-40.
[200] Phinney SD, Fisler JS, Tang AB, Warden CH. Liver fatty acid composition correlates with body fat and sex in a multigenic mouse model of obesity. Am J Clin Nutr 1994; 60: 61-7.
[201] Thurmond DC, Tang AB, Nakamura MT, Stern JS, Phinney SD. Time-dependent effects of progressive gamma-linolenate feeding on hyperphagia, weight gain, and erythrocyte fatty acid composition during growth of Zucker obese rats. Obes Res 1993; 1: 118-25.

[202] Liu CX, Xiao PG. Recent advances on ginseng research in China. J Ethnopharmacol 1992; 36: 27-38.
[203] Han KH, Choe SC, Kim HS, *et al.* Effect of red ginseng on blood pressure in patients with essential hypertension and white coat hypertension. Am J Chin Med 1998; 26: 199-209.
[204] Inoue M, Wu CZ, Dou DQ, Chen YJ, Ogihara Y. Lipoprotein lipase activation by red ginseng saponins in hyperlipidemia model animals. Phytomedicine 1999; 6: 257-65.
[205] Kim JH, Hahm DH, Yang DC, Lee HJ, Shim I. Effect of crude saponin of Korean red ginseng on high-fat diet-induced obesity in the rat. J Pharmacol Sci 2005; 97: 124-31.
[206] Sotaniemi EA, Haapakoski E, Rautio A. Ginseng therapy in non-insulin-dependent diabetic patients. Diabetes Care 1995; 18: 1373-5.
[207] Soltysik S, Wu JY, Recchia J, *et al.* Structure/function studies of QS-21 adjuvant: assessment of triterpene aldehyde and glucuronic acid roles in adjuvant function. Vaccine 1995; 13: 1403-10.
[208] Kensil CR, Soltysik S, Wheeler DA, Wu JY. Structure/function studies on QS-21, a unique immunological adjuvant from Quillaja saponaria. Adv Exp Med Biol 1996; 404: 165-72.
[209] Hwang JT, Kim SH, Lee MS, *et al.* Anti-obesity effects of ginsenoside Rh2 are associated with the activation of AMPK signaling pathway in 3T3-L1 adipocyte. Biochem Biophys Res Commun 2007; 364: 1002-8.
[210] Hwang JT, Lee MS, Kim HJ, *et al.* Antiobesity effect of ginsenoside Rg3 involves the AMPK and PPAR-gamma signal pathways. Phytother Res 2009; 23: 262-6.
[211] Niu CS, Yeh CH, Yeh MF, Cheng JT. Increase of adipogenesis by ginsenoside (Rh2) in 3T3-L1 cell via an activation of glucocorticoid receptor. Horm Metab Res 2009; 41: 271-6.
[212] Lai DM, Tu YK, Liu IM, Chen PF, Cheng JT. Mediation of beta-endorphin by ginsenoside Rh2 to lower plasma glucose in streptozotocin-induced diabetic rats. Planta Med 2006; 72: 9-13.
[213] Zhang Z, Li X, Lv W, *et al.* Ginsenoside Re reduces insulin resistance through inhibition of c-Jun NH2-terminal kinase and nuclear factor-kappaB. Mol Endocrinol 2008; 22: 186-95.
[214] Ye J. Role of insulin in the pathogenesis of free fatty acid-induced insulin resistance in skeletal muscle. Endocr Metab Immune Disord Drug Targets. 2007; 7: 65-74.
[215] Park MW, Ha J, Chung SH. 20(S)-ginsenoside Rg3 enhances glucose-stimulated insulin secretion and activates AMPK. Biol Pharm Bull 2008; 31: 748-51.
[216] Banno N, Akihisa T, Tokuda H, *et al.* Triterpene acids from the leaves of Perilla frutescens and their anti-inflammatory and antitumor-promoting effects. Biosci Biotechnol Biochem 2004; 68: 85-90.
[217] Li JX, Hareyama T, Tezuka Y, Zhang Y, Miyahara T, Kadota S. Five new oleanolic acid glycosides from Achyranthes bidentata with inhibitory activity on osteoclast formation. Planta Med 2005; 71: 673-9.
[218] Liu Y, Kreppel H, Liu J, Choudhuri S, Klaassen CD. Oleanolic acid protects against cadmium hepatotoxicity by inducing metallothionein. J Pharmacol Exp Ther 1993; 266: 400-6.
[219] Kim JY, Lee KJ, Kim DH, *et al.* Cytokine-mediated induction of metallothionein in Hepa-1c1c7 cells by oleanolic acid. Biochem Biophys Res Commun 2004; 325: 792-7.
[220] Zhang Y, Jayaprakasam B, Seeram NP, Olson LK, DeWitt D, Nair MG. Insulin secretion and cyclooxygenase enzyme inhibition by cabernet sauvignon grape skin compounds. J Agric Food Chem 2004; 52: 228-33.
[221] Hsu HY, Yang JJ, Lin CC. Effects of oleanolic acid and ursolic acid on inhibiting tumor growth and enhancing the recovery of hematopoietic system postirradiation in mice. Cancer Lett 1997; 111: 7-13.
[222] Sato H, Genet C, Strehle A, *et al.* Anti-hyperglycemic activity of a TGR5 agonist isolated from Olea europaea. Biochem Biophys Res Commun 2007; 362: 793-8.
[223] Liu J. Pharmacology of oleanolic acid and ursolic acid. J Ethnopharmacol 1995; 49: 57-68.
[224] Yunoki K, Sasaki G, Tokuji Y, *et al.* Effect of dietary wine pomace extract and oleanolic acid on plasma lipids in rats fed high-fat diet and its DNA microarray analysis. J Agric Food Chem 2008; 56: 12052-8.
[225] Liu J. Oleanolic acid and ursolic acid: research perspectives. J Ethnopharmacol 2005; 100: 92-4.
[226] Kim J, Jang DS, Kim H, Kim JS. Anti-lipase and lipolytic activities of ursolic acid isolated from the roots of Actinidia arguta. Arch Pharm Res 2009; 32: 983-7.
[227] Aggarwal BB, Shishodia S. Suppression of the nuclear factor-kappaB activation pathway by spice-derived phytochemicals: reasoning for seasoning. Ann N Y Acad Sci 2004; 1030: 434-41.
[228] Jayaprakasam B, Olson LK, Schutzki RE, Tai MH, Nair MG. Amelioration of obesity and glucose intolerance in high-fat-fed C57BL/6 mice by anthocyanins and ursolic acid in Cornelian cherry (Cornus mas). J Agric Food Chem 2006; 54: 243-8.
[229] Sohn KH, Lee HY, Chung HY, Young HS, Yi SY, Kim KW. Anti-angiogenic activity of triterpene acids. Cancer Lett 1995; 94: 213-8.
[230] Balanehru S, Nagarajan B. Protective effect of oleanolic acid and ursolic acid against lipid peroxidation. Biochem Int 1991; 24: 981-90.
[231] Somova LO, Nadar A, Rammanan P, Shode FO. Cardiovascular, antihyperlipidemic and antioxidant effects of oleanolic and ursolic acids in experimental hypertension. Phytomedicine 2003; 10: 115-21.
[232] Shishodia S, Majumdar S, Banerjee S, Aggarwal BB. Ursolic acid inhibits nuclear factor-kappaB activation induced by carcinogenic agents through suppression of IkappaBalpha kinase and p65 phosphorylation: correlation with down-regulation of cyclooxygenase 2, matrix metalloproteinase 9, and cyclin D1. Cancer Res 2003; 63: 4375-83.
[233] Zhang W, Hong D, Zhou Y, *et al.* Ursolic acid and its derivative inhibit protein tyrosine phosphatase 1B, enhancing insulin receptor phosphorylation and stimulating glucose uptake. Biochim Biophys Acta 2006; 1760: 1505-12.
[234] Jang SM, Yee ST, Choi J, *et al.* Ursolic acid enhances the cellular immune system and pancreatic beta-cell function in streptozotocin-induced diabetic mice fed a high-fat diet. Int Immunopharmacol 2009; 9: 113-9.
[235] Schirmer MA, Phinney SD. Gamma-linolenate reduces weight regain in formerly obese humans. J Nutr 2007; 137: 1430-5.
[236] Ziegler J, Facchini PJ. Alkaloid biosynthesis: metabolism and trafficking. Annu Rev Plant Biol 2008; 59: 735-69.
[237] Joyce SA, Brachmann AO, Glazer I, *et al.* Bacterial biosynthesis of a multipotent stilbene. Angew Chem Int Ed Engl 2008; 47: 1942-5.
[238] Jang M, Cai L, Udeani GO, *et al.* Cancer chemopreventive activity of resveratrol, a natural product derived from grapes. Science 1997; 275: 218-20.
[239] Smeds AI, Eklund PC, Sjoholm RE, *et al.* Quantification of a broad spectrum of lignans in cereals, oilseeds, and nuts. J Agric Food Chem 2007; 55: 1337-46.

[240] Cheng Z, Pang T, Gu M, *et al.* Berberine-stimulated glucose uptake in L6 myotubes involves both AMPK and p38 MAPK. Biochim Biophys Acta 2006; 1760: 1682-9.
[241] Kim SH, Shin EJ, Kim ED, Bayaraa T, Frost SC, Hyun CK. Berberine activates GLUT1-mediated glucose uptake in 3T3-L1 adipocytes. Biol Pharm Bull 2007; 30: 2120-5.
[242] Lau CW, Yao XQ, Chen ZY, Ko WH, Huang Y. Cardiovascular actions of berberine. Cardiovasc Drug Rev 2001; 19: 234-44.
[243] Yin J, Gao Z, Liu D, Liu Z, Ye J. Berberine improves glucose metabolism through induction of glycolysis. Am J Physiol Endocrinol Metab 2008; 294: E148-56.
[244] Kim WS, Lee YS, Cha SH, *et al.* Berberine improves lipid dysregulation in obesity by controlling central and peripheral AMPK activity. Am J Physiol Endocrinol Metab 2009; 296: E812-9.
[245] Lee YS, Kim WS, Kim KH, *et al.* Berberine, a natural plant product, activates AMP-activated protein kinase with beneficial metabolic effects in diabetic and insulin-resistant states. Diabetes 2006; 55: 2256-64.
[246] Wang SH, Wang WJ, Wang XF, Chen W. Effect of Astragalus polysaccharides and berberine on carbohydrate metabolism and cell differentiation in 3T3-L1 adipocytes. Zhongguo Zhong Xi Yi Jie He Za Zhi 2004; 24: 926-8.
[247] Huang C, Zhang Y, Gong Z, *et al.* Berberine inhibits 3T3-L1 adipocyte differentiation through the PPARgamma pathway. Biochem Biophys Res Commun 2006; 348: 571-8.
[248] Brusq JM, Ancellin N, Grondin P, *et al.* Inhibition of lipid synthesis through activation of AMP kinase: an additional mechanism for the hypolipidemic effects of berberine. J Lipid Res 2006; 47: 1281-8.
[249] Kong W, Wei J, Abidi P, *et al.* Berberine is a novel cholesterol-lowering drug working through a unique mechanism distinct from statins. Nat Med 2004; 10: 1344-51.
[250] Zhang Y, Li X, Zou D, *et al.* Treatment of type 2 diabetes and dyslipidemia with the natural plant alkaloid berberine. J Clin Endocrinol Metab 2008; 93: 2559-65.
[251] Ko BS, Choi SB, Park SK, Jang JS, Kim YE, Park S. Insulin sensitizing and insulinotropic action of berberine from Cortidis rhizoma. Biol Pharm Bull 2005; 28: 1431-7.
[252] Chen L, Han Y, Yang F, Zhang T. High-speed counter-current chromatography separation and purification of resveratrol and piceid from *Polygonum cuspidatum*. J Chromatogr A 2001; 907: 343-6.
[253] Signorelli P, Ghidoni R. Resveratrol as an anticancer nutrient: molecular basis, open questions and promises. J Nutr Biochem 2005; 16: 449-66.
[254] Das S, Cordis GA, Maulik N, Das DK. Pharmacological preconditioning with resveratrol: role of CREB-dependent Bcl-2 signaling via adenosine A3 receptor activation. Am J Physiol Heart Circ Physiol 2005; 288: H328-35.
[255] Fremont L. Biological effects of resveratrol. Life Sci 2000; 66: 663-73.
[256] Baur JA, Pearson KJ, Price NL, *et al.* Resveratrol improves health and survival of mice on a high-calorie diet. Nature 2006; 444: 337-42.
[257] Lagouge M, Argmann C, Gerhart-Hines Z, *et al.* Resveratrol improves mitochondrial function and protects against metabolic disease by activating SIRT1 and PGC-1alpha. Cell 2006; 127: 1109-22.
[258] Rayalam S, Yang JY, Ambati S, Della-Fera MA, Baile CA. Resveratrol induces apoptosis and inhibits adipogenesis in 3T3-L1 adipocytes. Phytother Res 2008; 22: 1367-71.
[259] Howitz KT, Bitterman KJ, Cohen HY, *et al.* Small molecule activators of sirtuins extend Saccharomyces cerevisiae lifespan. Nature 2003; 425: 191-6.
[260] Michan S, Sinclair D. Sirtuins in mammals: insights into their biological function. Biochem J 2007; 404: 1-13.
[261] Guarente L. Sirtuins as potential targets for metabolic syndrome. Nature 2006; 444: 868-74.
[262] Gerhart-Hines Z, Rodgers JT, Bare O, *et al.* Metabolic control of muscle mitochondrial function and fatty acid oxidation through SIRT1/PGC-1alpha. EMBO J 2007; 26: 1913-23.
[263] Bujanda L, Hijona E, Larzabal M, *et al.* Resveratrol inhibits nonalcoholic fatty liver disease in rats. BMC Gastroenterol 2008; 8: 40.
[264] Pace-Asciak CR, Hahn S, Diamandis EP, Soleas G, Goldberg DM. The red wine phenolics trans-resveratrol and quercetin block human platelet aggregation and eicosanoid synthesis: implications for protection against coronary heart disease. Clin Chim Acta 1995; 235: 207-19.
[265] Pendurthi UR, Williams JT, Rao LV. Resveratrol, a polyphenolic compound found in wine, inhibits tissue factor expression in vascular cells : A possible mechanism for the cardiovascular benefits associated with moderate consumption of wine. Arterioscler Thromb Vasc Biol 1999; 19: 419-26.
[266] Hung LM, Chen JK, Huang SS, Lee RS, Su MJ. Cardioprotective effect of resveratrol, a natural antioxidant derived from grapes. Cardiovasc Res 2000; 47: 549-55.
[267] Thompson LU. Experimental studies on lignans and cancer. Baillieres Clin Endocrinol Metab 1998; 12: 691-705.
[268] Axelson M, Sjovall J, Gustafsson BE, Setchell KD. Origin of lignans in mammals and identification of a precursor from plants. Nature 1982; 298: 659-60.
[269] Falany JL, Macrina N, Falany CN. Regulation of MCF-7 breast cancer cell growth by beta-estradiol sulfation. Breast Cancer Res Treat 2002; 74: 167-76.
[270] Schafer TE, Lapp CA, Hanes CM, Lewis JB, Wataha JC, Schuster GS. Estrogenicity of bisphenol A and bisphenol A dimethacrylate *in vitro*. J Biomed Mater Res 1999; 45: 192-7.
[271] Tominaga S, Sugahara T, Nishimoto S, *et al.* The Effect of Secoisolariciresinol on 3T3-L1 adipocytes and the relationship between molecular structure and activity. Biosci Biotechnol Biochem 2009; 73: 35-9.
[272] Prasad K. Hydroxyl radical-scavenging property of secoisolariciresinol diglucoside (SDG) isolated from flax-seed. Mol Cell Biochem 1997; 168: 117-23.
[273] Prasad K. Antioxidant activity of secoisolariciresinol diglucoside-derived metabolites, secoisolariciresinol, enterodiol, and enterolactone. Int J Angiol 2000; 9: 220-5.
[274] Prasad K, Mantha SV, Muir AD, Westcott ND. Protective effect of secoisolariciresinol diglucoside against streptozotocin-induced diabetes and its mechanism. Mol Cell Biochem 2000; 206: 141-9.
[275] Prasad K. Oxidative stress as a mechanism of diabetes in diabetic BB prone rats: effect of secoisolariciresinol diglucoside (SDG). Mol Cell Biochem 2000; 209: 89-96.
[276] Prasad K. Secoisolariciresinol diglucoside from flaxseed delays the development of type 2 diabetes in Zucker rat. J Lab Clin Med 2001; 138: 32-9.

[277] Fukumitsu S, Aida K, Ueno N, Ozawa S, Takahashi Y, Kobori M. Flaxseed lignan attenuates high-fat diet-induced fat accumulation and induces adiponectin expression in mice. Br J Nutr 2008; 100: 669-76.

[278] Felmlee MA, Woo G, Simko E, Krol ES, Muir AD, Alcorn J. Effects of the flaxseed lignans secoisolariciresinol diglucoside and its aglycone on serum and hepatic lipids in hyperlipidaemic rats. Br J Nutr 2009;102: 361-9.

[279] Zhou L, Yang Y, Wang X, *et al.* Berberine stimulates glucose transport through a mechanism distinct from insulin. Metabolism. 2007; 56: 405-412.

[280] Prasad K. Reduction of serum cholesterol and hypercholesterolemic atherosclerosis in rabbits by secoisolariciresinol diglucoside isolated from flaxseed. Circulation 1999; 99: 1355-62.

[281] Bray GA. Are non-prescription medications needed for weight control? Obesity (Silver Spring) 2008; 16: 509-14.

[282] Foxcroft DR, Milne R. Orlistat for the treatment of obesity: rapid review and cost-effectiveness model. Obes Rev 2000; 1: 121-6.

[283] Douketis JD, Macie C, Thabane L, Williamson DF. Systematic review of long-term weight loss studies in obese adults: clinical significance and applicability to clinical practice. Int J Obes (Lond) 2005; 29: 1153-67.

[284] Avenell A, Broom J, Brown TJ, *et al.* Systematic review of the long-term effects and economic consequences of treatments for obesity and implications for health improvement. Health Technol Assess 2004; 8: 1-182.

[285] Birari RB, Bhutani KK. Pancreatic lipase inhibitors from natural sources: unexplored potential. Drug Discov Today 2007; 12: 879-89.

[286] Food and Drug Administration (FDA), Center for Drug Evaluation and Research (CDER). Draft. Guidance for industry. Developing products for weight management. 2007. Available at: http://www.fda.gov/cder/guidance/7544dft.pdf (last accessed January 2009).

Targeting the Opioid System: An Effective Treatment for Obesity?

Caroline Reid* and Caroline Davis

Department of Kinesiology and Health Science, York University 4700 Keele Street, Toronto, Ontario, Canada M3J 1P3, 503-10 Navy Wharf Court, Toronto, Ontario, M5V 3V2, Canada

Abstract: Because of the current obesity epidemic and its considerable effect on health, lifestyle, and longevity, there is a pressing need to further understand the neural pathways involved in the control of body weight, and the motivational states underlying ingestive behaviors. In a number of obese individuals, the homeostatic mechanisms that regulate energy consumption are overpowered by environmental influences, such as an abundance of highly palatable foods which are difficult to resist, and which can lead to their consumption beyond caloric need [1]. A strong liking for highly palatable foods has been linked to increased consumption [2, 3] and research has established that obese people show a greater liking and selection of sweet and fatty foods than their leaner counterparts [4-6]. Opioid peptides and opiate receptors are believed to mediate the affective response to highly palatable food [7-10]. Evidence suggests that the opioid system modulates one's perception of the hedonic properties of food and, consequently, food consumption [10, 11]. Therefore, the endogenous opioid system is likely to play an important role in food preferences and risk for obesity. Research suggests that targeting the opioid system may be an effective treatment option for certain individuals suffering from obesity. The following chapter will review the literature on the role of the opioid system in food consumption and examine the possibility that certain drugs, which target this system, are beneficial for weight loss and the treatment of obesity.

Keywords: Obesity, endogenous opioids, opioid antagonists, palatability, food intake.

INTRODUCTION

Eating is a behavior that is essential for survival; we all need to consume food in order to sustain life. Food supplies the body with a number of essential nutrients and is also an important part of energy homeostasis, the process by which body fuel stored in the form of adipose tissue remains relatively stable over long periods [12]. In order for this to occur, the amount of energy consumed must closely match the amount expended. However, for many individuals, the type and quantity of food ingested varies immensely from one meal to another, as well as from one day to the next. Body weight appears to be closely related to the amount of food consumed. Research has demonstrated that even a chronic mismatch of 100 calories per day in energy consumption and expenditure can lead to obesity over time [13]. Although many factors come into play to produce weight gain, evidence suggests that overeating is the main factor that has led to the population increase in body weigh over the past few years. The number of calories consumed daily has significantly increased during the same time period as the rise in obesity, and this increase in consumption is large enough to explain the population increase in body weight [14-16].

It was initially believed that a dysregulation in the body's homeostatic system was to blame for the consumption of food beyond caloric need. However, evidence now seems to suggest that hedonic drives tend to overpower satiety signals, leading to the overconsumption of food. A strong hedonic response to highly palatable foods has been linked to increased consumption [2, 3], and research has established that obese people show a greater liking and selection of sweet and fatty foods than their leaner counterparts [4-6]. For this reason, understanding how food interacts with brain-reward mechanisms is important in order to address overeating behaviors and help those suffering from obesity. One important group of neurotransmitters involved in the hedonics of food is the group called the endogenous opioids. Opioid peptides and their receptors are believed to mediate the affective response to highly palatable food [7-10]. Evidence suggests that the opioid system modulates one's perception of the hedonic properties of food (i.e. palatability) and, consequently, food consumption [10, 11]. Therefore, the endogenous opioid system is likely to play an important role in food preferences and the risk for obesity.

*Corresponding author: Tel: 416-623-0221; E-mail: creid@yorku.ca

Atta-ur-Rahman / M. Iqbal Choudhary (Eds.)

The following chapter will review the knowledge we have acquired thus far on the role of the endogenous opioids in food intake and will examine the potential effectiveness of opioid antagonists as anti-obesity drugs.

WHAT ARE ENDOGENOUS OPIOIDS?

Before discussing the role of the endogenous opioids in eating, it is important to first take a look at what these compounds are. The endogenous opioids are a group of neuro-transmitters which are part of the *neuropeptide* family. They are also referred to as *neuromodulators*, which are chemical transmitters that convey information to neighboring neurons by adjusting their level of sensitivity. In other words, they act either by enhancing or reducing the activities of neurons. Endogenous opioids bind to specific receptors which are widely distributed within the central nervous system (CNS), specifically in brain structures known to modulate food intake, reward, and pain [17]. Three main opioid receptors have been discovered and cloned, and given the names *mu, delta,* and *kappa* [18]. The opioid system plays a role in a wide range of functions, including nociception [19], memory [20], gastric motility [21, 22], immune status [23, 24], cell death [25, 26], renal excretion of sodium and water [27], hormone secretion [28], and, of course, food intake [29].

The opioid receptors are activated by endogenously produced opioid peptides as well as by exogenously administered opiates, such as morphine and heroin. The endogenous peptides for the *mu* opioid receptors include *endomorphin-1*, *endomorphin-2*, *β-endorphin*, *β-neoendorphin* and *dermorphin.* They show very high affinity and selectivity for the *mu* opioid receptors, whose activation results in a number of functions, such as the ones mentioned above [30]. Endogenous ligands for delta opioid receptors include *Leu5-enkephalin*, *Met5-enkephalin*, *Met5-enkephalin-Arg6-Phe7*, *Met5-enkephalin-Arg6-Gly7-Leu8*, *deltorphin*, *deltorphin I* and *deltorphin II.* Enkephalins and their analogs are also agonists at the *mu* opioid receptor. Ligands for the *kappa* opioid receptor include *dynorphin A* and *dynorphin B* [31]. The opioid receptor subtypes differ from each other regarding their contribution to specific actions [32]. Whereas *mu* opioid receptors have been shown to be involved in rewarding aspects of feeding, *kappa* ligands can lead to dysphoria [18, 33] and anhedonia [34]. Researchers believe that *dynorphin* is responsible for these depressive-like feelings. For example, microinjection studies have demonstrated that *dynorphin* decreases dopamine (DA) release in the basal ganglia of rats [35] and a study involving the "forced swim test" showed that cAMP response element binding protein (CREB), which activates a gene that makes *dynorphin*, increased immobility in the rats [33]. In other words, they gave up more easily (an illustration of learned helplessness).

Together, this system as a whole has been implicated in a wide range of addictions [36, 37], including alcoholism [38], heroin use and abuse [39, 40], and compulsive overeating [41, 42]. More and more, research suggests that the exact role of the endogenous opioid system in addictions and food intake is in what has been coined the 'liking' of these rewards.

OPIOIDS FOR 'LIKING'

The hedonic aspects of eating are processed in the mesocorticolimbic structures (see Fig. **1**), a series of synaptically interconnected circuits linking the prefrontal cortex, the amygdala, the ventral tegmental area (VTA), the nucleus accumbens (NAc) and the ventral pallidum (VP) with the medium forebrain bundle [18, 43]. Numerous studies have been performed to tease apart which areas of the brain are involved in the 'liking', 'wanting', or learning components of reward and how they interact to generate the experience of pleasure [44-51]. For many years, researchers have tried to shed light on which structures and neurotransmitters within the reward pathway are involved in the hedonics of food intake. Until a few years ago, the neurobiology of eating has largely emphasized the role of the DA system in food reward. It has been well established that DA in the NAc influences appetitive motivation for reward [48, 50, 52-54]. Researchers also believed that DA release directly caused the experience of pleasure [55]. More recently, however, evidence has suggested that the endogenous opioid system plays a prominent role in reward [11, 28, 29]. Research has demonstrated that opioids in the medial shell of the NAc contribute to the pleasurable feeling experienced from drugs, as well as from natural rewards such as food and sweetness [10, 53, 56-59]. In fact, evidence now points towards DA release not being able, in itself, to produce pleasurable reactions [60, 61]. The endogenous opioid system is also needed for this feeling to occur.

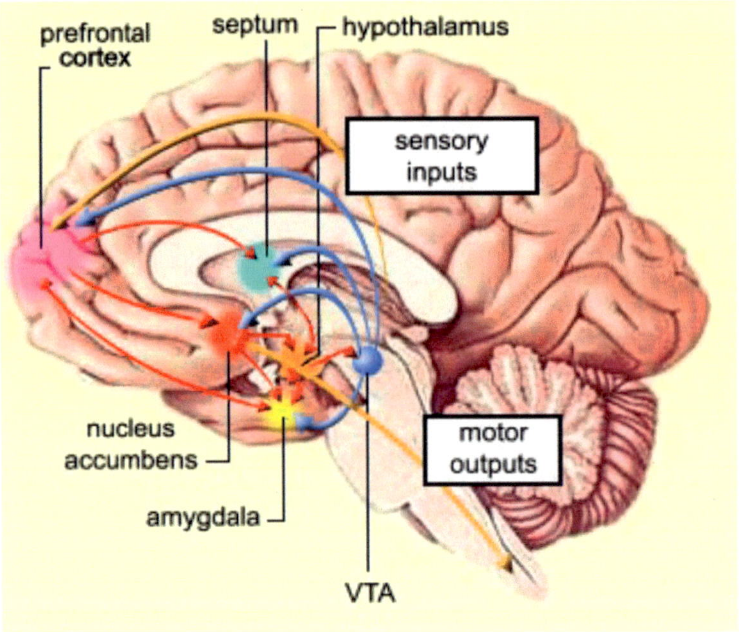

Fig. (1). Reward pathway of the brain.

In summary, and according to experts in the field of addiction, the endogenous opioids would be involved and needed in the 'liking' of rewards, whereas DA would be implicated in the 'wanting' of them [58, 62]. Liking and wanting are two distinct concepts, even though they may be hard to distinguish. Liking describes the actual pleasure (enjoyment) experienced from a reward, whereas wanting comprises the motivation to obtain the reward [62]. In other words, motivation can be seen as how hard one is willing to work to obtain the reward. Animal studies have been quite useful in helping us shed light on the difference between these two concepts. For instance, Smith and Berridge [63] activated a "hotspot" within the NAc of rats and examined the animals' behaviors after they were offered food. The authors observed two specific types of behaviors: the rats ate more food and exhibited greater liking responses, such as facial expressions.[1] The interesting finding was that, when they inhibited a part of the VP, the rats did not show any liking responses, but still ate increasing amounts of food. They seemed to be wanting something that did not give them pleasure. Their desire to consume was driven by something other than liking. These findings suggest that wanting is mediated by a pathway going from the NAc to the hypothalamus. By contrast, the liking circuit goes through the VP. The two impulses are thus independent and separable, even though the same brain centers are common to both. Nevertheless, in previous work [66], the same researchers found that directly stimulating the VP could modulate both liking and wanting food, or modulate wanting only, depending on what stimulus was used. Clearly, additional research is needed to further elucidate the regulatory mechanisms within specific areas of the reward pathway.

Patterns of liking and wanting have been extensively studied in drug addiction. Initially, when addicts start using a specific drug, they do so because they enjoy it (a representation of the liking concept); it produces a pleasurable feeling. However, as time goes on and they start using it more and more, something interesting happens. Drug addicts start wanting the drug more; however, they do not increase their liking of it [67]. Indeed, researchers have noticed that they will continue to seek the drug out even when they no longer experience pleasure from it. They appear to want the drug much more than they actually enjoy it. Researchers hypothesize that a neuropharmacological tolerance develops in the areas responsible for the pleasure response, whereas the neural systems that mediate wanting become sensitized [68]. Said differently, addiction results from an increased dissociation between wanting and liking. This same concept could be applied to certain types of compulsive overeating, such as Binge Eating Disorder (BED).[2] In BED, the reward system does not appear to be working optimally. The hunger drive, the pleasure experienced

---

[1] Changes caused by manipulating parts of the brain involved in the hedonics of food can be measured objectively by taste reactivity patterns, such as facial expressions, which are similar in a number of animals, such as human infants, apes, monkeys, and rats [64]. Sweet tastes tend to produce positive 'liking' expressions, such as tongue protrusions, whereas bitter tastes bring forth facial 'disliking' reactions such as gapes, etc. [65].

[2] BED is characterised by recurrent episodes of binge-eating, occurring at least twice a week for at least six months. Also, during most binge-eating episodes, three or more of the following behavioral indicators must be present: eating more quickly than normal, eating until feeling physically uncomfortable, eating large amounts of food when not feeling hungry, eating alone because one feels ashamed by the amount one is eating, and feeling disgusted with oneself, depressed, or extremely guilty after overeating. In addition, BED is not related to the regular use of inappropriate compensatory behaviors, such as purging or excessive exercise [69].

from food, as well as the desire to eat seem to have become separated. Binge eaters, who may start eating because of the immense pleasure they get from food, will eat until they feel extremely uncomfortable, an example of how people can end up wanting something they no longer enjoy.

Of the three types of reward component mentioned above, liking has been the least addressed in neuroscience studies. The studies that have been conducted thus far; however, suggest an important role of the endogenous opioid system in the pleasure experienced from food and manipulating this system can lead to changes in food intake.

ENDOGENOUS OPIOIDS AND FOOD INTAKE

Pleasure is an important part of life as it is essential for one to feel happy. Lacking pleasure can lead to a wide range of disorders, from depression to schizophrenia, to even addiction [62]. Not many experiences in life are more enjoyable than consuming a well-prepared meal. Because food is so rewarding, humans are strongly motivated to acquire it. Many individuals consume more food than is needed to survive, and there is compelling evidence to suggest that people's preference for energy-dense food may play a role in overeating. Our preference for highly palatable foods likely evolved because it had adaptive value, promoting the ingestion of foods that were good sources of needed nutrients. The high and increasing prevalence of overweight and obesity suggests, however, that the predispositions that were adaptive under circumstances where food was in short supply are no longer adaptive in today's environment where inexpensive foods high in sugar, fat, total energy, and salt are readily available. Some researchers believe that a biological predisposition to overeating may exist, which would lead certain individuals to engage in overconsumption [70]. In other words, overeating might be related to the 'sensitivity' or 'hedonic response' to particular qualities in foods.

Humans (and animals) have an innate liking for sweet and high fat foods [71, 72]. A number of studies (see [64] for a review) have examined the facial expressions of infants after the consumption of sweet tastes and found that sweet tastes elicited positive facial 'liking' expressions (tongue protrusions, smiling, etc.), whereas bitter tastes instead elicited facial 'disliking' expressions (see Fig. **2**). Food rewards like sugar seem to bring about typical 'liking' behaviors across mammal species [65]. For instance, a rat (or ape) chewing on sweets makes appreciative, lip-smacking facial expressions similar to that of a human baby. These indicators are an objective way to assess how much one likes a food, independent of how much one eats, or one's own subjective impressions of his/her enjoyment.

There is substantial evidence to suggest that the endogenous opioids help enhance the pleasure experienced from sweet and fatty food [41, 73]. Research has shown that stimulating opioid receptors can lead to an increase intake of palatable food [74]. In addition, opioid peptides are believed to mediate the affective response to highly palatable food [7-10]. For instance, the motivation to obtain food reinforcement was shown to decrease when *enkephalin* and *β-endorphin* were absent in the CNS and intake of palatable food increased when the *mu* opioid receptors within the ventral striatum were stimulated [75]. Several studies have shown that activation of opioid receptors leads to an increase in food intake [10, 76], and opioid peptides seem to play important roles in the control of ingestive behavior [77]. Researchers hold that stimulating opioid receptors leads animals to like the taste of food to a greater extent [7, 10, 57, 78-82].

As further evidence of the role of the endogenous opioids in food intake, administration of opioid antagonists have been found to lead to a decreased consumption of food, especially highly palatable food [83]. Opioid agonists[3], on the other hand, tend to increase consumption and pleasantness ratings of palatable food [11, 82]. For instance, microinjections of opioid agonist drugs, such as morphine and heroin, within the hedonic hotspots of the reward pathway, may increase by two or three times the normal number of 'liking' reactions to a sucrose taste [57, 63, 65, 66, 88]. Zhang and Kelley [89] found that microinjections of opioid agonists into the dorsal striatum of rats not only resulted in greater liking, but also led them to start eating. *Mu*-opioid agonists have also been found to increase food intake when injected into the entire NAc shell and related structures [56, 57, 90-92].

---

[3] Opioid agonists are drugs derived from (or related to) the opium poppy plant, *Papaver somniferum*. Opium contains more than 40 different alkaloids and the first one to be isolated was morphine [84]. Opiates bind to the mu, kappa, and delta receptors, however, most of them show a greater binding affinity to the mu receptors [85]. All opiates have an aromatic ring and a quaternary carbon atom linked to a tertiary amine group by two other carbon atoms [84]. The structure of morphine (which is the base of many of the opioid agnonists) consists of five rings forming a T-shaped molecule. More specifically, its structure is an ethanamine-bridged phenanthrene skeleton [86, 87]. Some of the well-know opiate agonists include heroin, codeine, oxymorphone, oxycodone, and hydromorphone [84].

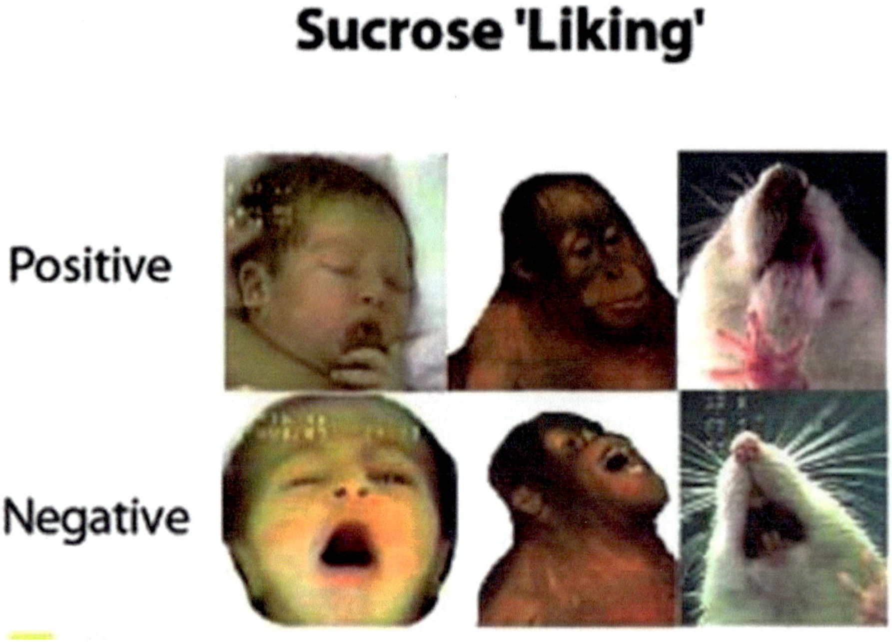

Fig. (2). Facial expressions of human infant, monkey, and rat in response to sweet and bitter tastes [67].

In addition, clinical studies and anecdotal reports suggest that opiate addiction is associated with heightened hedonic response to sweet taste [93] and that opiate withdrawal can sometimes be eased by sweets [29]. Studies have also shown that food cravings are reinforced by endogenous opiate release [73] and that consumption of a palatable food alters endogenous opioid levels in a number of areas in the brain [74]. Clinical studies suggest that plasma concentration levels of endorphin-1 may be higher in patients with eating disorders, such as bulimia nervosa, and in obese as opposed to normal-weight women [94-97]. Moreover, some researchers have found an increased preference for sweetened high-fat foods in obese individuals [2, 78]. Abnormalities in the secretion of endogenous opioid peptides could explain elevated sensory preference and overeating of sweet high-fat foods [78]. It is therefore probable that opioids modulate the development of food preferences and that the opioid system affects feeding in response to palatability rather than in response to metabolic needs, such as hunger. The above findings support the role of the endogenous opioid system in the hedonic impact of rewards.

GENETIC VARIABILITY INFLUENCES FOOD INTAKE

There is considerable variability in the degree to which individuals prefer certain types of food. While humans have a general and innate preference for sweet and fatty foods, there is a great deal of individual variability. In other words, some people like sweet foods more than others. Part of this variation can be explained by differences in our genetic make-up. For example, polymorphisms in the genes that regulate the reward pathways are known to play a role in how people differ in terms of their physiological, biochemical, and behavioral responses to natural rewards as well as drugs of abuse [98]. These variants help to explain why certain individuals prefer particular foods more than others – they find them more pleasurable and rewarding. Several genes have been linked to addictive behaviors and may also impact overeating, through their role in food preferences. Hedonic hyperphagia (overeating influenced by reward rather than the need for calories) often triggers excess caloric intake. Research has discovered that for many obese individuals, hedonic drives tend to overpower satiety signals, leading to food consumption beyond caloric need. Since the reward circuits that regulate drug and other forms of addiction are the same as those stimulated by highly palatable foods [67], it seems logical that genes that increase risk for addiction disorders may also increase the vulnerability to obesity. One such group of genes are those that code for the endogenous opioid system.

Numerous single nucleotide polymorphisms (SNPs) for the opioid receptors have been detected, but these SNPs are much more frequent in non-coding regions (i.e. introns[4]) of the gene than in translated

---

[4] An intron is a region within a gene that is not translated into protein.

sequences (i.e. exons[5]). Most of the coding polymorphisms are relatively rare, with allele frequencies around, or below, one percent [99]. The most prevalent polymorphic variant can be seen on the coding region variant of the mu-1 opioid receptor gene (*OPRM1*) known as the *A118G* SNP, located on exon 1 of chromosome 6 (*rs1799971*). This is a missense mutation where the nucleic acid *adenine* at base position 118 is replaced by *guanine* [99]. This SNP codes for a change in amino acids from *asparagine* (Asn) into *aspartic acid* (Asp) at position 40 [100-102]. Most people have two *adenine* alleles (A), while a few have either one or two *guanine* alleles (G). The frequency of this polymorphism (that is, having one or two G alleles) varies across populations, occurring in about two percent of individuals in some ethnic groups (e.g. African American) and up to fifty percent in others (e.g. Japanese) [98]. In terms of the rates for the *A118G* SNP in Caucasians, they have been found to vary between 10 to 14 percent [100, 103, 104]. However, it is still unknown whether these rates differ among individuals of various BMIs.

There are two main hypotheses in terms of the effects of the G allele. Some maintain that this mutation decreases binding to the receptors. For instance, some *in vitro* transfection studies have found that the G allele may be linked to lower mu opioid receptor protein expression compared to the A allele [105, 106] and could lead to a decreased binding of opioids on the mu receptors, which means one would need a lot more stimulation in order to activate them. This view holds that this allelic variation may therefore make the endogenous opioid system less reactive, causing vulnerability to addiction [107]. On the other hand, *in vivo* evidence indicates that the presence of the G allele increases opioid binding potential, making one more likely to experience pleasure from rewarding behaviors including feeding. The G allele is referred to as a *gain of function* mutation because of an enhanced responsiveness. In this case, the mutation results in an increase in the pleasure experienced from a reward. This view has received the most empirical support. For instance, *in vitro* studies have demonstrated that the *Asp40* variant (G allele) of the mu-opioid receptor binds β-endorphin three times more strongly than the more common *Asn40* variant (A allele) [101, 108]. Because food has a powerful stimulatory effect on the endogenous opioids, individuals carrying at least one copy of the G allele have been shown to exhibit a stronger sensitivity to highly palatable food [42, 109], and as a result might be at a higher risk of overeating and being overweight. In addition to food, several studies have demonstrated that the G allele of the *A118G* SNP relates to an increased risk of alcohol and heroin addiction [110-114]. Other studies have also linked this genotype with nicotine addiction [36, 37]. As with overeating, one reason why having at least one copy of the G allele might put some at risk of addiction is that they might find these substances more pleasure compared to those without the G allele. Regardless of the position one takes, the G allele has been associated with an increased risk of addictive behaviors and there is some research that supports the idea that it might play a role in overeating as well [42, 109].

A recent body of literature has examined the opioid receptors in food palatability (see Barbano *et al.* [28] for a review), however, there has only been one study to date linking genetic markers for these receptors to overeating and body weight. In this study, researchers examined the *A118G* SNP for the mu opioid receptors along with three genetic markers for DA [42] in two groups of obese individuals: one group of binge eaters and one group of non-binge eaters. Results indicated that the obese binge eating participants showed a significantly higher level of the G allele (the "at risk" allele) compared to their non-bingeing counterparts (see Fig. **3**). The findings suggest the binge eating group may engage in hedonic hyperphagia because of a greater liking of food. While further research is needed in order to replicate these findings, this study does offer preliminary evidence that targeting the opioid system in a subset of obese individuals may prove effective in helping them in their quest to lose weight and decrease their risk of a wide array of chronic diseases. One possible way of targeting the opioid system would be via administration of pharmacologic substances. Opioid antagonists inhibit the endogenous opioids and may be helpful in regulating people's eating behaviors, especially eating motivated by pleasure.

THE EFFECT OF OPIOID ANTAGONISTS ON FOOD INTAKE

Many opioid antagonists have been manufactured. The three most common opioid antagonists are naloxone, naltrexone, and nalmefene, and will therefore be the focus of the following section.[6] Antagonist

---

5 An exon is a region within a gene that codes for protein and affects gene expression, which in turn influences the phenotype.

6 Naloxone has been utilized widely in the treatment of opiate overdose [115]. When administered intravenously, its half-life is reported to be between one and two hours [116]. In contrast, the half-life of orally administered naltrexone is between 3.9 to 10.3 hours [117] and it is believed to be two to six times more potent than naloxone. Nalmefene has been reported to have roughly the same half-life as naltrexone when given orally [118], but has a considerably longer half-life than naloxone when administered intravenously [119].

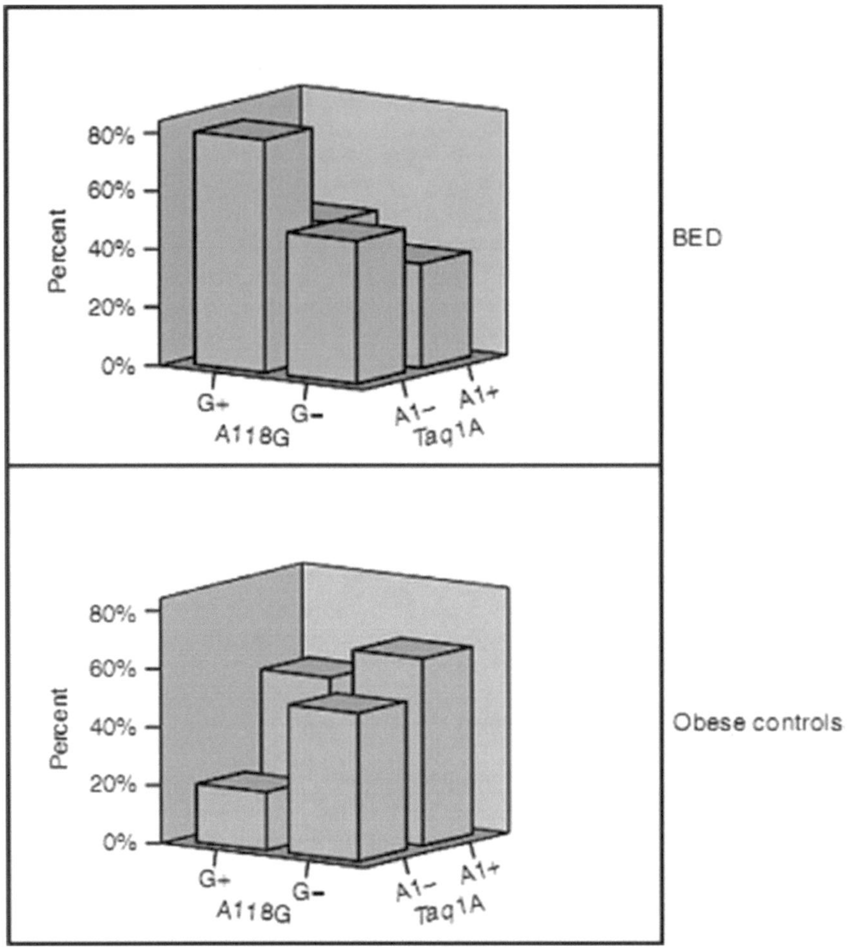

Fig. (3). Percentage of Obese participants with and without binge eating in each of the four gene-gene combination groups formed by the *Taq*1A ($A1^+$ *vs.* $A1^-$) and A118G (G^+ *vs.* G^-) SNPs.

drugs lead to a decrease in the target neurotransmitters' effects by either blocking the synthesis of the neurotransmitter molecule – causing the neurotransmitter molecules to leak from the vesicles and be destroyed by degrading enzymes – or by preventing the release of the neurotransmitter molecules from terminal buttons by blocking its receptors. Antagonists have been quite extensively examined in terms of their effects on ingestive behaviors, with quite interesting results [115].

The earliest evidence involving the endogenous opioids in the neurobiology of ingestive behavior comes from Holtzman [120] who found that the opioid antagonist naloxone led to a significant decrease in short-term food intake. Since then, a number of animal studies have demonstrated that antagonism of the endogenous opioids will reduce food intake [11, 82]. For instance, naloxone was found to decrease intake of a palatable food in a dose-dependent way in sated animals [28] and in those acutely (24 to 48 hours), versus chronically (80 percent of normal body weight), food deprived [81]. Similar results were observed in rats given unrestricted access to sucrose/saccharin solutions or sweet chow [121]. In addition, others have noticed a greater reduction in food intake after ingestion of an opioid antagonist, especially for very palatable food compared to normal chow [122, 123]. Furthermore, naloxone given peripherally and intracerebroventricularly was shown to decrease neuropeptide Y-induced food intake [124, 125]. However, a study by Kotz and colleagues [126] found that injecting either naloxone or naltrexone into the PVN of rats had a rather weak effect on PVN NPY-induced feeding, signifying that the PVN is not likely the site at which naloxone or naltrexone antagonize the effects of NPY. Marin-Bivens and Olster [127] also found that naltrexone administration reduced food intake over a period of 24 hours in obese Zucker rats.

The effects of opioid antagonists in humans were first noticed in detoxified male opiate addicts where about 10 percent of them experienced a significant reduction in appetite after being given a daily oral dose of 1500 mg of naltrexone [128]. Sternbach *et al.* [129] also reported that oral administration of naltrexone led to a reduction in body weight of two to five kilograms in detoxified opiate addicts after two to six weeks of treatment. Ever since then, experimental studies have confirmed the effect of opioid antagonists on food intake. Administration of naloxone has been found to reduce food intake in normal weight men [130] and normal-weight men and women [131, 132]. This change in consumption occurred even though subjective feelings of hunger and satiety remained unaltered. Similar results have been found in a number of studies of obese and normal weight individuals [133-136]. Furthermore, Yeomans and colleagues [137, 138] examined the effect of nalmefene and found that a single dose of 2.5 mg led to a 22 percent decrease in food intake in a buffet-style lunch. These researchers also noticed that this change occurred even though subjective ratings of hunger and satiety remained similar between the drug and placebo groups. Nalmefene had a greater effect on highly palatable foods, supporting the hypothesis that endogenous opioids are involved in reward-related aspects of feeding.

One possible explanation for the reduction in caloric intake, despite no apparent loss of appetite (or decrease in hunger) is that opioid antagonists lead individuals to dislike certain foods. For instance, naltrexone administration has been found to decrease the pleasantness of the food, without affecting appetite before mealtime [77, 80]. Research has also shown that a single-dose of naltrexone results in a significant reduction in preference for sweet tasting food [139], as well as sweet beverages and salty soups [140]. Naloxone was also found to decrease the pleasantness of sweet and fatty foods in female obese binge eaters and normal-weight controls [141]. These researchers also discovered that naloxone decreased total caloric intake in the binge eaters, but not in the controls. Another study involving humans showed that intake of nalmefene not only decreased caloric intake of a buffet-style meal but also reduced ratings of the pleasantness of the taste and smell of food [138]. Taken together, these findings support the notion that the endogenous opioid system plays an integral role in the liking of palatable food and in mediating taste responses. By blocking this system, people may eat less since they tend to not enjoy the taste of food as much.

OPIOID ANTAGONISTS AS A TREATMENT FOR OBESITY

Since studies have consistently shown that opioid antagonists can decrease short-term food consumption and influence food preferences in a number of species (including humans), researchers started directing their attention toward the effectiveness of these drugs in treating various forms of disordered eating. As a treatment approach, opioid antagonists were first used in patients with Prader-Willi, a genetic disorder characterized by hyperphagia, obesity, neonatal hypotonia, hypogonadism, stunted stature, and low intelligence [115, 142, 143]. Their effects on weight have since been studied in a number of experiments, both in animals and humans. For example, naltrexone was administered to both obese and lean mice for a period of five weeks [144]. Compared to the obese animals receiving the placebo, the naltrexone-injected obese mice gained weight more slowly, while the lean mice were unaffected by the drug. The authors concluded that this form of genetic obesity was characterized by high levels of endogenous opioids and a greater sensitivity to opioid antagonists. Naltrexone also decreased food intake over a 24-hour period, and led to a reduction in weight in obese Zucker rats [127]. One study of obese men [145] found a significant reduction in weight (4 kg +/- 3.97) in nine of 17 obese individuals who were given naltrexone (50 mg per day) for four months, compared to a placebo (0.96 kg +/- 4.95).

The remaining research on naltrexone has yielded very little, if any, support for this drug as an adequate weight-loss therapy. For instance, a double-blind study conducted by Atkinson and colleagues (1985) examined various doses of naltrexone (0, 50, and 100 mg) over an eight-week period. They did not find any significant differences in weight loss; however, women lost significantly more weight than men. The authors even noticed a slight increase in weight (+ 3.4 kg) in men taking 100 mg of naltrexone. Naltrexone was also studied over a period of ten weeks in a randomized parallel double-blind placebo controlled trial in both females (n=27) and males (n=14) who were considered to be between 30 and 100 percent over their ideal weight [146]. Participants who received naltrexone lost an average of 1.8 kg and those on the placebo lost 1.5 kg, which was not a significant difference between the groups. Later studies utilizing larger doses of naltrexone also did not find significant group differences. Malcolm *et al.* [147] examined the effects of 200 mg of naltrexone in 41 obese participants and found no significant effect of naltrexone on body weight compared to the placebo after eight weeks of treatment. Mitchell *et al.* [148] examined weight loss in 40 obese people who received 300 mg of naltrexone daily for eight weeks, while undergoing dietary counselling. They also failed to find any significant difference in the amount of weight loss between the groups. The weight loss experienced by those on the placebo was believed to be due to the dietary counselling program and this reduction was not improved by the addition of naltrexone. Maggio and colleagues [149], who also gave doses of up to 300 mg, did not find any significant effect of naltrexone either.

There appears to be an incongruity between the short-term effects of this drug on food intake and the more long-term effects on body weight. Research conducted on humans has largely failed to demonstrate a positive effect of naltrexone on long-term weight loss. It is possible that long-term administration of naltrexone may lead the body to engage in some type of compensatory mechanism or to build up a tolerance to the drug. One would therefore need to increase the dose to see any real results. However, the problem with doing this is that there are a number of side effects to this medication, especially when given over long periods of time and at high doses. Naltrexone can cause liver damage (hepatotoxicity [146, 148], nausea, vomiting [135, 136], and other gastrointestinal issues [149], as well as headaches, depression, and anxiety [150]. Consequently, this drug is not a recommended treatment for obesity, given that the side effects seem to outnumber the modest benefits it has on weight loss.

Studies of naloxone on body weight have been quite limited. Therefore, the use of naloxone and naltrexone is not recommended in the treatment of obesity due to their poor risk/benefit ratio. The use of naloxone is limited by the short action of the drug is contraindicated and the need for systematic administration, while naltrexone, especially at higher dosages, has potentially severe adverse effects, as outlined above. There is a growing need for development of long-acting, nontoxic, selective opiate antagonists with a strong and lasting effect on eating behavior.

Nalmefene, a newer long-acting opiate antagonist, may prove to be a better option since it does not appear to cause severe side effects. However, a study examining oral administration of this drug (up to 20 mg/kg) did not find any significant effect on food intake in mice [151]. In fact, on average, the mice taking nalmefene actually gained weight, which is contrary to the anticipated effects. Interestingly, when nalmefene was combined with subthreshold doses of AM251, an agonist for the CB1 cannabinoid receptor, there was a significant decrease in food intake in both lean and diet-induced obese mice [152]. Naloxone, combined with Rimonabant ®, another cannabinoid antagonist, led to a reduction in food intake and time spent eating in rats [153]. These findings suggest that a synergistic interaction may exist between opioid and cannabinoid systems in regulating eating behaviors.

Studies have also examined the effects of chronic administration of various lesser know opioid antagonists on body weight and food intake in rats. For example, Cole *et al.* [8] looked at the effects of selective long-acting opioid antagonists in rats given a palatable diet of pellets, fat, milk and water, compared to pellet-fed and diet-fed controls. They observed a significant decrease in weight after administration of beta-funaltrexamine (9%), naloxonazine (12%), [d-Ala^2, Leu5, Cys6]-enkephalin (7%) or naltrindole isothiocyanate (6%). The same group of researchers also noted a reduction in weight and food intake after chronic administration of various opioid antagonists in both lean and obese Zucker rats [154]. Another study examined the effects of opioid antagonists (trans-3,4-dimethyl-4-phenylpiperidines) on food intake in obese Zucker rats [155] and observed that long-term repeated administration of the antagonists LY88329 and LY117413 to these meal-fed animals led to a significant decrease in food consumption for as long as the drug was given. This decrease in food intake resulted in a significant reduction in body weight gain compared to obese rats having not received the drug. The authors also noted that the rats did not seem to build up a tolerance towards either drug [155].

Other opioid antagonists have been examined, such as the *phenylpiperidine* series, including the antagonist LY255582 [156, 157]. There is evidence of their effectiveness in producing weight loss in lean and meal-fed obese Zucker rats [156] and that LY255582 is a better appetite suppressant at lower doses compared to ephedrine, amphetamine, fenfluramine, naltrexone, and nalmefene [157]. The use of *nor-binaltorphimine* (NBNI), a specific and long-lasting *kappa* opioid antagonist, has demonstrated that some rats responded to the drugs – and those who did lost significantly more weight (three percent of initial body weight) than non responders and controls[7]. The authors concluded that a differential response to chronic opioid antagonism may exist in the obese Zucker rats [158]. Although research remains to be done on humans, these findings suggest that long-lasting *kappa* opioid antagonists may be effective treatments for obesity.

More recent findings suggest that combining an antidepressant with an opioid antagonist may also be an effective treatment for obesity. A press release by the pharmaceutical company Orexigen earlier this year [159] reported that their new drug Contrave®[8] – a mixture of the antidepressant bupropion and the opioid antagonist naltrexone – led to a mean decrease in body weight of 9.3 percent in a group of almost 800

7 Five rats were classified as responders, compared to six non-responders and five controls. The authors proposed that the differential response to the drug in these animals may be explained by the difference in overeating behavior. Those who exhibited binge eating-like behaviors were the ones who responded to the drug.

8 Contrave is undergoing Phase III clinical trials for obesity and is expected to have FDA approval in late 2009.

individuals. This was a significantly greater loss than in those taking the placebo. However, it fell short of the five percent placebo-corrected weight loss threshold for approval by the FDA. Drop-out rates at that point in the trial were 26 percent in the drug group and 13 percent in those taking the placebo. The main side effects reported were nausea, hives, anxiety, headache, constipation and dizziness. On the other hand, participants taking Contrave® reported significant improvement in their quality of life, markers of cardiovascular risk, and decreases in food cravings. The most recent findings from three of the Phase III trials have demonstrated that between 48 and 56 percent of people on Contrave® lost at least five percent of their body weight after 56 weeks, compared to 16-17 percent of those on the placebo [159].

A group of researchers [160] have also reported that combining bupropion with naltrexone helps prevent the classic weight plateau observed in so many studies that examine opioid antagonists on their own. It will be interesting to see if there are certain subsets of obese individuals who will respond better to this drug than to existing treatments (potentially those with an enhanced opioid system due to genetic differences). It has been hypothesized that Contrave® may have the most benefit in those who struggle with emotional eating, hedonic hyperphagia, as well as food addictions and mood disorders [161]. Both bupropion and naltrexone have well-established side effects, therefore, a cautious assessment of risk-benefit ratios will be necessary. Nonetheless, for individuals who will respond well to, and tolerate the combination of bupropion and naltrexone, Contrave®, when utilized alongside behavioral modification, may be an important tool in weight management and the prevention of many of the complications associated with obesity.

CONCLUSION

Substantial evidence supports the role of the endogenous opioid system in the regulation of food intake and feeding behavior. In particular, endogenous opioids and their receptors have been implicated in the hedonic aspects of food intake. Because they regulate the experienced palatability of food, their genetic variants are likely to influence the risk of overeating in some people. In light of the current obesity epidemic, individual differences in endogenous opioid availability and/or their receptor densities may help us understand why so many people seem to be eating beyond caloric need. Targeting the opioid system (in certain individuals) may be an effective treatment option for those looking to reduce their consumption of palatable food and lose weight. Selective opiate antagonists, including naloxone, naltrexone, and nalmefene, have proven to have a robust short-term effect on food intake and eating behavior in animal as well as in humans. However, their long-term effectiveness in reducing weight in obese individuals has proven to be quite limited. These drugs also come at a potentially very serious cost to one's health. With current advances in pharmacology, however, there may be some better drug choices for obese persons. For example, the newly developed drug Contrave® may have some effectiveness in treating obesity. It is also likely that developing effective drugs will require targeting more than one system in the CNS, as evidence points to the fact that the endogenous opioid system works closely with the cannabinoid system in the control of ingestive behaviors. Even if these newly developed drugs only help prevent future weight gain, without leading to significant weight loss, they may still be worth exploring. Stopping the progression of weight gain could be an important first step in the fight against obesity. Also, given our current inability to effectively manage obesity by behavioral modification alone, any safe and effective drug developed to help treat obesity should be welcomed by the medical community. The single biggest challenge in developing anti-obesity drugs will be, however, to match the right patients with the right medications.

REFERENCES

[1] French SA, Story M, Jeffery RW. Environmental influences on eating and physical activity. Annu Rev Public Health 2001; 22: 309-35.

[2] Geiselman PJ, Anderson AM, Dowdy ML, West DB, Redmann SM, Smith SR. Reliability and validity of a macronutrient self-selection paradigm and a food preference questionnaire. Physiol Behav 1998; 63: 919-28.

[3] Weaver MR, Brittin HC. Food preferences of men and women by sensory evaluation versus questionnaire. Fam Con Sci Res J 2001; 29: 288-301.

[4] Drewnoswki A. Why do we like fat? J Am Diet Assoc 1997; 97: S58-S62.

[5] Drewnowski A. Taste preferences and food intake. Ann Rev Nutr 1997; 17: 237-53.

[6] Mela DJ. Determinants of food choice: relationships with obesity and weight control. Obes Res 2001; 9 (Suppl 4): 249S-55S.

[7] Cooper SJ, Kirkham TC. Opioid mechanisms in the control of food consumption and taste preferences. Exp Pharmacol 1993; 104: 239-62.

[8] Cole JL, Leventhal L, Pasternak GW, Bowen WD, Bodnar RJ. Reductions in body weight following chronic central opioid receptor subtype antagonists during development of dietary obesity in rats. Brain Res 1995; 678: 168-76.

[9] Giraudo SQ, Grace MK, Billington CJ. Levine AS.Differential effects of neuropeptide Y and the mu-agonist DAMGO on 'palatability' vs. 'energy'. Brain Res 1999; 834: 160-3.
[10] Kelley AE, Bakshi VP, Haber SN, Steininger TL, Will MJ, Zhang M. Opioid modulation of taste hedonics within the ventral striatum. Physiol Behav 2002; 76: 365-77.
[11] Glass MJ, Billington CJ, Levine AS. Opioids and food intake: distributed functional neural pathways? Neuropeptides 1999; 33: 360-8.
[12] Woods SC, Seeley RJ, Porte D Jr, Schwartz MW. Signals that regulate food intake and energy homeostasis. Science 1998; 280: 1378-83.
[13] Wynne W, Stanley S, Bloom S. The gut and regulation of body weight. J Clin Endocrinol Metab 2004; 89: 2576-82.
[14] Putnam JJ, Allshouse JE. Food consumption, prices, and expenditures, 1970–97. Economic Research Services, USDA, Stat.Bulletin, Washington, DC 1999.
[15] Centres for Disease Control and Prevention, Prevalence of overweight and obesity among adults with diagnosed diabetes – US, 1988-1994 and 1999-2002. J Am Med Assoc 2004; 293: 546-7.
[16] Nielsen SJ, Popkin BM. Patterns and trends in food portion sizes, 1977-1998. JAMA 2003; 289: 450-3
[17] Pert CB, Kuhar MJ, Snyder SH. Opiate receptor: autoradiographic localization in rat brain. Proc Natl Acad Sci USA 1976; 73: 3729-33.
[18] Cota D, Tschöp MH, Horvath TL, Levin AS. Cannabinoids, opioids and eating behavior: The molecular face of hedonism? Brain Res Rev 2005; 51: 85-107.
[19] Gradin M, Schollin J. The role of endogenous opioids in mediating pain reduction by orally administered glucose among newborns. Pediatrics 2005; 115: 1004-7.
[20] Vaccarino AL, Kastin AJ. Endogenous opiates: 2000. Peptides 2001; 22: 2257-328.
[21] Dubois A. Endogenous opioids, gastric motility, and gastric emptying. Gastroenterol Clin Biol 1987; 11: 56B-61.
[22] Tsuchida D, Fukuda H, Koda K, Miyazaki M, Pappas TN, Takahashi T. Central effect of mu-opioid agonists on antral motility in conscious rats. Brain Res 2004; 1024: 244-50.
[23] Lysle DT, Luecken LJ, Maslonek KA. Modulation of immune status by a conditioned aversive stimulus: evidence for the involvement of endogenous opioids. Brain Behav Immun 1992; 6: 179-88.
[24] Nelson CJ, Schneider GM, Lysle DT. Involvement of central mu- but not delta- or kappa-opioid receptors in immunomodulation. Brain Behav Immun 2000; 14: 170-84.
[25] Tegeder I, Geisslinger G. Opioids as modulators of cell death and survival--unraveling mechanisms and revealing new indications. Pharmacol Rev 2004; 56: 351-69.
[26] Yin D, Mufson RA, Wang R, Shi Y. Fas-mediated cell death promoted by opioids. Nature 1999; 397: 218.
[27] Kapusta DR, Obih JC. Central kappa opioids blunt the renal excretory responses to volume expansion by a renal nerve-dependent mechanism. J Pharmacol Exp Ther 1995; 273: 199-205.
[28] Barbano MF, Cador M. Differential regulation of the consummatory, motivational, and anticipatory aspects of feeding behavior by dopaminergic and opioidergic drugs. Neuropsychopharmacology 2006; 31: 1371-81.
[29] Bodnar RJ, Klein GE. Endogenous opiates and behavior: 2003. Peptides 2004; 25: 2205-56.
[30] Okada Y, Tsuda Y, Bryant SD, Lazarus LH. Endomorphins and related opioid peptides. Vitam Horm 2002; 65: 257-79.
[31] Waldhoer M, Bartlett SE, Whistler JL. Opioid receptors. Annu Rev Biochem 2004; 73: 953-90.
[32] Law PY, Loh HH. Regulation of opioid receptor activities. J Pharmacol Exp Ther 1999; 289: 607-24.
[33] Todtenkopf MS, Marcus JF, Portoghese PS, Carlezon WA, Jr. Effects of kappa-opioid receptor ligands on intracranial self-stimulation in rats. Psychopharmacology (Berl) 2004; 172: 463-70.
[34] Carlezon WA, Béguin C, DiNieri JA, *et al.* Depressive-like effects of the κ-opioid receptor agonist salvinorin a on behavior and neurochemistry in rats. J Pharmacol Exper Ther 2006; 316: 440-7.
[35] You ZB, Herrera-Marschitz M, Terenius L. Modulation of neurotransmitter release in the basal ganglia of the rat brain by dynorphin peptides. J Pharmacol Exp Ther 1999; 290: 1307-15.
[36] Berrendero F, Kieffer BL, Maldonado R. Attenuation of nicotine-induced antinociception, rewarding effects, and dependence in mu-opioid receptor knock-out mice. J Neurosci 2002; 22: 10935-40.
[37] Kreek MJ. Cocaine, dopamine and the endogenous opioid system. J Addict Dis 1996; 15: 73-96.
[38] Herz A. Endogenous opioid systems and alcohol addiction. Psychopharmacology (Berl) 1997; 129: 99-111.
[39] Tanda G, Pontieri FE, Di Chiara G. Cannabinoid and heroin activation of mesolimbic dopamine transmission by a common mu1 opioid receptor mechanism. Science 1997; 276: 2048-50.
[40] Van Ree JM, Niesink RJ, Van Wolfswinkel L, *et al.* Endogenous opioids and reward. Eur J Pharmacol 2000; 405: 89-101.
[41] Mercer ME, Holder MD. Food cravings, endogenous opioid peptides, and food intake: a review. Appetite 1997; 29: 325-52.
[42] Davis CA, Levitan RD, Reid C, *et al.* Dopamine for "wanting" and opioids for "liking": a comparison of obese adults with and without binge eating. Obesity (Silver Spring) 2009; 17: 1220-5.
[43] Koob GF. Drugs of abuse: anatomy, pharmacology and function of reward pathways. Trends Pharmacol Sci 1992; 13: 177-84.
[44] Baldo BA, Kelley AE. Discrete neurochemical coding of distinguishable motivational processes: insights from nucleus accumbens control of feeding. Psychopharmacology (Berl) 2007; 191: 439-59.
[45] Balleine BW, Killcross S. Parallel incentive processing: an integrated view of amygdala function. Trends Neurosci 2006; 29: 272-9.
[46] Beaver JD, Lawrence AD, van Ditzhuijzen J, Davis MH, Woods A, Calder AJ. Individual differences in reward drive predict neural responses to images of food. J Neurosci 2006; 26: 5160-6.
[47] Di Chiara G, Bassareo V. Reward system and addiction: what dopamine does and doesn't do. Curr Opin Pharmacol 2007; 7: 69-76.
[48] Wise RA. Role of brain dopamine in food reward and reinforcement. Philos Trans R Soc Lond B Biol Sci 2006; 361: 1149-58.
[49] Kringelbach ML. Food for thought: hedonic experience beyond homeostasis in the human brain. Neuroscience 2004; 26: 807-19.
[50] Schultz W. Behavioral theories and the neurophysiology of reward. Annu Rev Psychol 2006; 57: 87-115.
[51] Everitt BJ, Robbins TW. Neural systems of reinforcement for drug addiction: from actions to habits to compulsion. Nat Neurosci 2005; 8: 1481-9.

[52] Berridge KC, Robinson TE. What is the role of dopamine in reward: hedonic impact, reward learning, or incentive salience? Brain Res Brain Res Rev 1998; 28: 309-69.
[53] Kalivas PW, Volkow ND, The neural basis of addiction: pathology of motivation and choice. Am J Psychiatry 2005; 162: 1403-13.
[54] Palmiter RD. Is dopamine a physiologically relevant mediator of feeding behavior? Trends Neurosci 2007; 30: 375-81.
[55] Wise RA, Rompre PP. Brain dopamine and reward. Annu Rev Psychol 1989; 40: 191-225.
[56] Zhang M, Gosnell BA, Kelley AE. Intake of high-fat food is selectively enhanced by mu opioid receptor stimulation within the nucleus accumbens. J Pharmacol Exp Ther 1998; 285: 908-14.
[57] Pecina S, Berridge KC. Opioid site in nucleus accumbens shell mediates eating and hedonic 'liking' for food: map based on microinjection Fos plumes. Brain Res 2000; 863: 71-86.
[58] Berridge KC. Pleasures of the brain. Brain Cogn 2003; 52: 106-28.
[59] Bodnar RJ, Lamonte N, Israel Y, Kandov Y, Ackerman TF, Khaimova E. Reciprocal opioid-opioid interactions between the ventral tegmental area and nucleus accumbens regions in mediating mu agonist-induced feeding in rats. Peptides 2005; 26: 621-9.
[60] Pecina S, Berridge KC, Parker LA. Pimozide does not shift palatability: separation of anhedonia from sensorimotor suppression by taste reactivity. Pharmacol Biochem Behav 1997; 58: 801-11.
[61] Wyvell CL, Berridge KC. Intra-accumbens amphetamine increases the conditioned incentive salience of sucrose reward: enhancement of reward "wanting" without enhanced "liking" or response reinforcement. J Neurosci 2000; 20: 8122-30.
[62] Berridge KC, Kringelbach ML. Affective neuroscience of pleasure: reward in humans and animals. Psychopharmacology (Berl) 2008; 199: 457-80.
[63] Smith KS, Berridge KC. Opioid limbic circuit for reward: interaction between hedonic hotspots of nucleus accumbens and ventral pallidum. J Neurosci 2007; 27: 1594-605.
[64] Berridge KC. Measuring hedonic impact in animals and infants: microstructure of affective taste reactivity patterns. Neurosci Biobehav Rev 2000; 24: 173-98.
[65] Pecina S, Berridge KC. Hedonic hot spot in nucleus accumbens shell: where do mu-opioids cause increased hedonic impact of sweetness? J Neurosci 2005; 25: 11777-86.
[66] Smith KS, Berridge KC. The ventral pallidum and hedonic reward: neurochemical maps of sucrose "liking" and food intake. J Neurosci 2005; 25: 8637-49.
[67] Kelley AE, Berridge KC. The neuroscience of natural rewards: relevance to addictive drugs. J Neurosci 2002; 22: 3306-11.
[68] Robinson TE, Berridge KC. Addiction. Annu Rev Psychol 2003; 54: 25-53.
[69] American Psychiatric Association. Diagnostic and Statistical Manual. 4th ed (Text Revision). American Psychiatric Association Press: Washington, DC 2000.
[70] Mela DJ, Rogers PJ. Food, eating and obesity: The psychobiological basis of food control, Chapman and Hall: London 1998.
[71] Drewnowski A, Greenwood MR. Cream and sugar: human preferences for high-fat foods. Physiol Behav 1983; 30: 629-33.
[72] Mela DJ. Why do we like what we like? J Sci Food Agric 2000; 81: 10-16.
[73] Pelchat ML. Of human bondage: food craving, obsession, compulsion, and addiction. Physiol Behav 2002; 76: 347-52.
[74] Kelley AE, Will MJ, Steininger TL, Zhang M, Haber SN. Restricted daily consumption of a highly palatable food (chocolate Ensure(R)) alters striatal enkephalin gene expression. Eur J Neurosci 2003; 18: 2592-8.
[75] Hayward MD, Pintar JE, Low MJ. Selective reward deficit in mice lacking beta-endorphin and enkephalin. J Neurosci 2002; 22: 8251-8.
[76] Will MJ, Franzblau EB, Kelley AE. Nucleus accumbens mu-opioids regulate intake of a high-fat diet via activation of a distributed brain network. J Neurosci 2003; 23: 2882-8.
[77] Yeomans MR, Gray RW. Opioid peptides and the control of human ingestive behaviour. Neurosci Biobehav Rev 2002; 26: 713-28.
[78] Drewnowski A, Krahn DD, Demitrack MA, Nairn K, Gosnell BA. Naloxone, an opiate blocker, reduces the consumption of sweet high-fat foods in obese and lean female binge eaters. Am J Clin Nutr 1995; 61: 1206-12.
[79] Bodnar RJ, Glass MJ, Ragnauth A, Cooper ML. General, mu and kappa opioid antagonists in the nucleus accumbens alter food intake under deprivation, glucoprivic and palatable conditions. Brain Res 1995; 700: 205-12.
[80] Yeomans MR, Gray RW. Effects of naltrexone on food intake and changes in subjective appetite during eating: evidence for opioid involvement in the appetizer effect. Physiol Behav 1997; 62: 15-21.
[81] Levine AS, Weldon DT, Grace M, Cleary JP, Billington CJ. Naloxone blocks that portion of feeding driven by sweet taste in food-restricted rats. Am J Physiol 1995; 268: R248-52.
[82] Soderpalm AH, Berridge KC. Food intake after diazepam, morphine or muscimol: microinjections In the nucleus accumbens shell. Pharmacol Biochem Behav 2000; 66: 429-34.
[83] Lamonte N, Echo JA, Ackerman TF, Christian G, Bodnar RJ. Analysis of opioid receptor subtype antagonist effects upon mu opioid agonist-induced feeding elicited from the ventral tegmental area of rats. Brain Res 2002; 929: 96-100.
[84] Schiff PLJ. Opium and its alkaloids. Am J Pharm Educ 2002; 66.
[85] Bailey CP, Connor M. Opioids: cellular mechanisms of tolerance and physical dependence. Curr Opin Pharmacol 2005; 5: 60-8.
[86] Thorpe DH. Opiate structure and activity--a guide to understanding the receptor. Anesth Analg1984; 63: 143-51.
[87] Furst S, Hosztafi S. The chemical and pharmacological importance of morphine analogues. Acta Physiol Hung 2008; 95: 3-44.
[88] Mahler SV, Smith KS, Berridge KC. Endocannabinoid hedonic hotspot for sensory pleasure: anandamide in nucleus accumbens shell enhances 'liking' of a sweet reward. Neuropsychopharmacology 2007; 32: 2267-78.
[89] Zhang M, Kelley AE. Enhanced intake of high-fat food following striatal mu-opioid stimulation: microinjection mapping and fos expression. Neuroscience 2000; 99: 267-77.
[90] Evans KR, Vaccarino FJ. Amphetamine- and morphine-induced feeding: evidence for involvement of reward mechanisms. Neurosci Biobehav Rev 1990; 14: 9-22.
[91] Will MJ, Franzblau EB, Kelley AE. The amygdala is critical for opioid-mediated binge eating of fat. Neuroreport 2004; 15: 1857-60.
[92] Echo JA, Lamonte N, Ackerman TF, Bodnar RJ. Alterations in food intake elicited by GABA and opioid agonists and antagonists administered into the ventral tegmental area region of rats. Physiol Behav 2002; 76: 107-16.

[93] Willenbring ML, Morley JE, Krahn DD, Carlson GA, Levine AS, Shafer RB. Psychoneuroendocrine effects of methadone maintenance. Psychoneuroendocrinology 1989; 14: 371-91.

[94] Givens JR, Wiedemann E, Andersen RN, Kitabchi AE. beta-Endorphin and beta-lipotropin plasma levels in hirsute women: correlation with body weight. J Clin Endocrinol Metab 1980; 50: 975-6.

[95] Olson GA, Olson RD, Kastin AJ. Endogenous opiates: 1991. Peptides 1992; 13: 1247-87.

[96] Waller DA, Kiser RS, Hardy BW, Fuchs I, Feigenbaum LP, Uauy R. Eating behavior and plasma beta-endorphin in bulimia. Am J Clin Nutr 1986; 44: 20-3.

[97] Zelissen PM, Koppeschaar HP, Erkelens DW, Thijssen JH. Beta-Endorphin and adrenocortical function in obesity. Clin Endocrinol (Oxf) 1991; 35: 369-72.

[98] Kreek MJ, Bart G, Lilly C, LaForge KS, Nielsen DA. Pharmacogenetics and human molecular genetics of opiate and cocaine addictions and their treatments. Pharmacol Rev 2005; 57: 1-26.

[99] Mayer P, Hollt V. Allelic and somatic variations in the endogenous opioid system of humans. Pharmacol Ther 2001; 91: 167-77.

[100] Bergen AW, Kokoszka J, Peterson R, *et al.* Mu-opioid receptor gene variants: Lack of association with alcohol dependence. Molecular Psychiatry 1997; 2: 490-494.

[101] Van den Wildenberg E, Wiers RW, Dessers J, *et al.* A functional polymorphism of the mu-opioid receptor gene (OPRM1) influences cue-induced craving for alcohol in male heavy drinkers. Alcohol Clin Exp Res 2007; 31: 1-10.

[102] Wendel B, Hoehe MR. The human mu opioid receptor gene: 5' regulatory and intronic sequences. J Mol Med 1998; 76: 525-32.

[103] Bond C, LaForge KS, Mingting T, *et al.* Single-nucleotide polymorphism in the human mu opioid receptor gene alters b-endorphin binding and activity: possible implications for opiate addiction. Proc Natl Acad Sci USA 1998; 95: 9608-13.

[104] Gelernter J, Kranzler H, Cubells J. Genetics of two mu-opioid receptor gene (OPRM1) exon 1 polymorphisms: Population studies, and allele frequencies in alcohol- and drug-dependent subjects. Mol Psychiatry 1999; 4: 476-83.

[105] Beyer A, Koch T, Schroder H, Schulz S, Höllt V. Effect of the A118G polymorphism on binding affinity, potency, and agonist-mediated endocytosis, desensitization, and resensitization of the human mu-opioid receptor. J Neurochem 2004; 89: 553-60.

[106] Kroslak T, Gianotti RG, LaForge KS, Ho AA, Kreek MJ. Signaling properties of the human opioid receptor hMOR and the polymorphic variant hMOR(A118G), International Narcotic Research Conference, Perpignon, France 2003.

[107] Zhang Y, Wang D, Johnson AD, Papp AC, Sadee W. Allelic expression imbalance of human mu opioid receptor (OPRM1) caused by variant A118G. J Biol Chem 2005; 280: 32618-24.

[108] Wand GS, McCaul M, Yang X, *et al.* The mu-opioid receptor gene polymorphism (A118G) alters HPA axis activation induced by opioid receptor blockade. Neuropsychopharmacology 2002; 26: 106-14.

[109] Nathan PJ, Bullmore ET. From taste hedonics to motivational drive: central mu-opioid receptors and binge-eating behaviour. Int J Neuropsychopharmacol 2009: 1-14.

[110] Bart G, Heilig M, LaForge KS, *et al.*Substantial attributable risk related to functional mu-opioid receptor gene polymorphism in association with heroin addiction in central Sweden. Mol Psychiatry 2004; 9: 547-49.

[111] Bencherif B, Wand GS, McCaul ME, *et al.* Mu-opioid receptor binding measured by [11C]Carfentanil postiron emission tomography is related to craving and mood in alcohol dependence. Biological Psychiatry 2004; 55: 255-62.

[112] Bergen G, Kreek MJ, Ott J, *et al.* Increased attributable risk related to a functional mu-opoid receptor gene polymorphism in association with alcohol dependence in central Sweden. Neuropsychopharmacology 2005; 30: 417-22.

[113] Bray GA. Medical consequences of obesity. J Clin Endocrinol Metab 2004; 89: 2583-9.

[114] Schinka JA, Town T, Abdullah L, *et al.* A functional polymorphism within the mu-opioid receptor gene and risk for abuse of alcohol and other substances. Mol Psychiatry 2002; 7: 224-8.

[115] de Zwaan M, Mitchell JE. Opiate antagonists and eating behavior in humans: A review. J Clin Pharmacol 1992; 32: 1060-72.

[116] Aitkenhead AR, Derbyshire DR, Pinnock CA, Achola K, Smith G. Pharmacokinetics of intravenous naloxone in healthy volunteers. Anesthesiology 1984; 61: A381.

[117] Crabtree BL. Review of naltrexone, a long-acting opiate antagonist. Clin Pharmacol 1984; 3: 273-80.

[118] Dixon R, Gentile J, Hsiao J, Howes J, Garg D, Weidler D. Safety and kinetics after single and multiple oral doses of a new opioid antagonist. J Clin Pharmacol 1987; 27: 233-9.

[119] Dixon R, Howes J, Gentile J, *et al.* Nalmefene: Intravenous safety and kinetics of a new opioid antagonist. Clin Pharmacol Ther 1986; 39: 49-53.

[120] Holtzman SG. Suppression of appetitive behavior in the rat by naloxone: lack of effect of prior morphine dependence. Life Sci 1979; 24: 219-26.

[121] Cleary J, Weldon DT, O'Hare E, Billington C, Levine AS. Naloxone effects on sucrose-motivated behavior. Psychopharmacology 1996; 126: 110-14.

[122] Hutchinson AC, Simpson GR, Randall JF, *et al.* Assessment of SNC 80 and naltrindole within a conditioned taste aversion design. Pharmacol Biochem Behav 2000; 66: 779-87.

[123] Giraudo SQ, Grace MK, Welch CC, Billington CJ, Levine AS. Naloxone's anorectic effect is dependent upon the relative palatability of food. Pharmacol Biochem Behav 1993; 46: 917-21.

[124] Levine AS, Morley JE, Gosnell BA, Billington CG, Bartness TJ. Opioids and consumatory behavior. Brain Res Bull 1985; 14: 663-72.

[125] Schick RR, Schusdziarra V, Nussbaumer C, Classen M. Neuropeptide Y and food intake in fasted rats: effect of naloxone and site of action. Brain Res 1991; 552: 232-9.

[126] Kotz CM, Grace MK, Briggs J, Levine AS, Billington CJ. Effects of opioid antagonists naloxone and naltrexone on neuropeptide Y-induced feeding and brown fat thermogenesis in the rat. Neural site of action. J Clin Invest 1995; 96: 163-70.

[127] Marin-Bivens CL, Olster DH. Opioid receptor blockade promotes weight loss and improves the display of sexual behaviors in obese Zucker female rats. Pharmacol Biochem Behav 1999; 63: 515-20.

[128] Zaks A, Jones T, Fink M, Freedman AM. Naloxone treatment of opiate dependence. J Am Med Assoc 1971; 215: 2108-10.

[129] Sternbach HA, Annitto W, Pottash ALC, Gold MS. Anorexic effects of naltrexone in man. Lancet 1982; 1: 388-9.

[130] Thompson DA, Welle SL, Lilavivat U, Pinecaud L, Campbell RG. Opiate receptor blockade in man reduces 2-deoxy-D-glucose-induced food intake but not hunger, thirst, and hypothermia. Life Sci 1982; 31: 847-52.

[131] Cohen MR, Cohen RM, Pickar D, Murphy DL. Naloxone reduces food intake in humans. Psychosom Med 1985; 2: 132-8.

[132] Trenchard E, Silverstone T. Naloxone reduces the food intake of normal human volunteers. Appetite 1983; 4: 43-50.
[133] Atkinson RL. Naloxone decreases food intake in obese humans. J Clin Endocrinol Metab 1982; 55: 196-8.
[134] Wolkowitz OM, Doran OR, Cohen MR, Cohen RM, Wise TN, Pickar D. Effect of naloxone on food consumption in obesity. N Engl J Med 1985; 313: 327.
[135] Spiegel TA, Stunkard AJ, Shrager EE, O'Brien CP, Morrison MF, Stellar E. Effect of naltrexone on food intake, hunger, and satiety in obese men. Physiol Behav 1987; 40: 135-41.
[136] Hollister LE, Johnson K, Boukhabza D, Gillepsie HK. Aversive effects of naltrexone in subjects not dependent on opiates. Drug Alcohol Depend 1981; 8: 37-41.
[137] Yeomans MR, Wright P, Macleod HA, Critchley JA. Effects of nalmefene on feeding in humans. Dissociation of hunger and palatability. Psychopharmacology (Berl) 1990; 100: 426-32.
[138] Yeomans MR, Wright P. Lower pleasantness of palatable foods in nalmefene-treated human volunteers. Appetite 1991; 16: 249-59.
[139] Fantino M, Hosotte J, Apfelbaum M. An opioid antagonist, naltrexone, reduces preference for sucrose in humans. Am J Physiol 1986; 251: R91-R96.
[140] Bertino M, Beauchamp GK, Engelman K. Naltrexone, an opioid blocker, alters taste perception and nutrient intake in humans. Am J Physiol 1991; 261: R59-63.
[141] Drewnowski A, Krahn DD, Demitrack MA, Nairn K, Gosnell BA. Taste responses and preferences for sweet high-fat foods: evidence for opioid involvement. Physiol Behav 1992; 51: 371-9.
[142] Zlotkin SH, Fettes IM, Stallings VA. The effects of naltrexone, an oral beta-endorphin antagonist, in children with the Prader-Willi syndrome. J Clin Endocrinol Metab 1986; 63: 1229-32.
[143] Johnson RD. Opioid involvement in feeding behaviour and the pathogenesis of certain eating disorders. Med Hypotheses 1995; 45: 491-7.
[144] Recant L, Voyles NR, Luciano M, Pert CB. Naltrexone reduces weight gain, alters "beta-endorphin", and reduces insulin output from pancreatic islets of genetically obese mice. Peptides 1980; 1: 309-13.
[145] Novi RF, Lamberto M, Visconti P, *et al.* [The role of opioid antagonists in the treatment of obesity. Results of a clinical trial with naltrexone]. Minerva Endocrinol 1990; 15: 121-3.
[146] Malcolm R, O'Neil PM, Sexauer JD, Riddle FE, Currey HS, Counts C. A controlled trial of naltrexone in obese humans. Int J Obes 1985; 9: 347-53.
[147] Malcolm R, O'Neil PM, Von JM, Dickerson PC. Naltrexone and dysphoria: a double-blind placebo controlled trial. Biol Psychiatry 1987; 22: 710-6.
[148] Mitchell JE, Morley JE, Levine AS, Hatsukami D, Gannon M, Pfohl D. High-dose naltrexone therapy and dietary counseling for obesity. Biol Psychiatry 1987; 22: 35-42.
[149] Maggio CA, Presta E, Bracco EF, *et al,* Naltrexone and human eating behavior: a dose-ranging inpatient trial in moderately obese men. Brain Res Bull 1985; 14: 657-61.
[150] Atkinson RL, Berke LK, Drake CR, Bibbs ML, Williams FL, Kaiser DL. Effects of long-term therapy with naltrexone on body weight in obesity. Clin Pharmacol Ther 1985; 38: 419-22.
[151] Chen RZ, Huang RR, Shen CP, MacNeil DJ, Fong TM. Chronic administration of nalmefene leads to increased food intake and body weight gain in mice. Eur J Pharmacol 2004; 495: 63-6.
[152] Chen RZ, Huang RR, Shen CP, MacNeil DJ, Fong TM. Synergistic effects of cannabinoid inverse agonist AM251 and opioid antagonist nalmefene on food intake in mice. Brain Res 2004; 999: 227-30.
[153] Tallett AJ, Blundell JE, Rodgers RJ. Endogenous opioids and cannabinoids: system interactions in the regulation of appetite, grooming and scratching. Physiol Behav 2008; 94: 422-31.
[154] Cole JL, Berman N, Bodnar RJ. Evaluation of chronic opioid receptor antagonist effects upon weight and intake measures in lean and obese Zucker rats. Peptides 1997; 18: 1201-7.
[155] Shaw WN, Mitch CH, Leander JD, Zimmerman DM. Effect of phenylpiperidine opioid antagonists on food consumption and weight gain of the obese Zucker rat. J Pharmacol Exp Ther 1990; 253: 85-9.
[156] Rothman RB, Xu H, Char GU, *et al.* Phenylpiperidine opioid antagonists that promote weight loss in rats has high affinity for the kappa 2B (enkephalin-sensitive) binding site. Peptides 1993; 14: 17-20.
[157] Shaw WN, Mitch CH, Leander JD, Mendelsohn LG, Zimmerman DM. The effect of the opioid antagonist LY255582 on body weight of the obese Zucker rat. Int J Obes 1991; 15: 387-95.
[158] Jarosz PA, Metzger BL. The effect of opioid antagonism on food intake behavior and body weight in a biobehavioral model of obese binge eating. Biol Res Nurs 2002; 3: 198-209.
[159] Orexigen Pharmaceuticals, Contrave Obesity Research Phase 3 Program Meets Co-Primary and Key Secondary Endpoints; Exceeds FDA Efficacy Benchmark for Obesity Treatments, 2009.
[160] Greenway FL, Whitehouse MJ, Guttadauria M, *et al.* Rational design of a combination medication for the treatment of obesity. Obesity (Silver Spring) 2009; 17: 30-9.
[161] Sharma AM. Orexigen's Obesity Drug Contrave Meets FDA Benchmark, 2009.

Development of Melanin Concentrating Hormone Receptor R1 Antagonists for the Pharmacological Treatment of Obesity

Gildardo Rivera[*,1], Antonio Monge[2] and Virgilio Bocanegra-Garcia[1]

[1]*Departamento de Farmacia y Química Medicinal, Unidad Académica Multidisciplinaria Reynosa Aztlán, Universidad Autónoma de Tamaulipas, Calle 16 y Lago de Chápala, s/n, 88740, Reynosa, México*

[2]*Unidad de Investigación y Desarrollo de Medicamentos, Centro de Investigación en Farmacobiología Aplicada (CIFA), Universidad de Navarra, Calle Irunlarrea, s/n, 31008, Pamplona, España*

Abstract: In this chapter we review the development of melanin concentrating hormone receptor 1 (MCH-R1) antagonists as a new perspective for the pharmacological treatment of obesity. We will initially focus on melanin concentrating hormone (MCH): structure, localization and function in the regulation of feeding behavior and energy balance and two receptors for MCH in humans. We will then review the discovery of the first MCH-R1 antagonists, the drug-design strategies used to obtained new series of MCH-R1 antagonists and an analysis of their structure-activity relationship. Finally, we will evaluate the absorption, distribution, metabolism and excretion, efficacy, safety and toxicity in preclinical and clinical trials.

Keywords: Development, Melanin concentrating hormone (MCH), Melanin concentrating hormone receptor 1 (MCH-R1), Structure-activity relationship (SAR), Obesity.

MELANIN CONCENTRATING HORMONE

Melanin-concentrating hormone (MCH) was initially characterized as a factor mediating color change in teleost fish as a cyclic heptadecapeptide that regulates adaptive changes in pigmentation [1]. MCH has the opposite effect of the hormone, alpha melanocyte stimulating hormone (alpha-MSH) which causes darkening of fish pigmentation, since MCH causes concentration of pigment in melanophores, producing a lightening of pigmentation. This phenomenon helps the fish to camouflage themselves from predators in different environments.

In mammals, MCH is expressed in the lateral hypothalamus (LH), which has been shown to finely regulate the balance between energy intake and expenditure in rodents [2-4], displaying high sequence conservation in the ring structure with the salmon counterpart from which it was originally isolated [1, 5]. MCH is the natural ligand for the seven-transmembrane G-protein-coupled receptors known as melanin concentrating hormone receptor 1(MCH-R1) and melanin concentrating hormone receptor 2 (MCH-R2) [6]. MCH in mammals was discovered because several studies reported the presence of neurons, which coincidentally crossreacted with antibodies to alpha-MSH but did not stains with antibodies to other products of the preproopiomelanocortin gene (POMC) [7]. In mammals, MCH is identical between rat, rabbit, mouse and human and highly homologous to the fish peptide. Unlike fish, in mice there does not seem to be a direct role for MCH in regulating skin or hair color since MCH and MCH-R1 knock-out (KO) animals both have normal brown coat color [8].

Rat, mouse and human mRNA sequences have a high degree of homology, with 90% overall nucleotide identity. The preprohormone encoded comprises 165 residues. MCH is generated *via* a posttranslation proteolytic cleavage at arginines 145 and 146 by proconvertases in the hypothalamic neurons. In mammalian brains, MCH is expressed primarily in the LH and zona incerta (ZI) with projections to numerous areas in the brain that suggest its involvement in feeding, arousal and sensorimotor integration. No association between MCH and mammalian pigmentation has been found [9, 10].

Analysis of the mRNA of MCH of rodent indicated that the prohormone precursor of MCH (Pmch) encodes a preprohormone with two other potential neuropeptide products, designated neuropeptide E-I

*Corresponding author: Tel: (+52) 899 921 33 40, Ext. 124; Fax: (+52) 899 923 06 22; E-mail: gildardors@hotmail.com

Atta-ur-Rahman / M. Iqbal Choudhary (Eds.)

(NEI) and neuropeptide G-E (NGE) [11]. In the mammalian brain, MCH is predominantly expressed in the perikarya of the LH area, and the ZI and projects widely throughout the central nervous system (CNS) [5, 9].

Despite that originally MCH was described as a hormone that affected fish pigmentation, and that even it is expressed in human melanocytes, it has been shown to function as a neuropeptide involved in several homeostatic processes such as energy, sleep/arousal, and emotionality [12-16]. The distribution of MCH in mammalian brains suggested that it might be involved in mediating "motivated behaviors". However, the role of the peptide remained obscure until 1996 when, with the use of reverse transcription polymerase chain reaction (RT-PCR) differential display, the expression of Pmch mRNA was found to be increased in leptin-deficient ob/ob (lep $^{ob/ob}$) mice [17]. MCH is also expressed at low levels in some peripheral tissues, and may play a role in mediating gut inflammation, vaginal artery contraction, and beta-cell islet function [18-20].

Pmch expression increase was similar to that seen with the known orexigenic neuro-peptide Y (NPY), suggesting that MCH might play a role in appetite. This was confirmed when it was found that intracerebroventricular (ICV) administration of 5 ug of MCH to rats led to a rapid increase in chow consumption. Compared with vehicle, MCH treated animals eat two- to threefold more over a six hour period. Feeding can also be induced by injection of MCH directly into the paraventricular nucleus [21].

As an orexigenic peptide, MCH interacts with other neuropeptides that influence feeding behavior. For example, MCH is a mutual functional antagonist of the anorectic peptide alpha-MSH, which inhibits appetite. Further evidence regarding the role of MCH in energy homeostasis comes from mice in which the Pmch gene is either ablated or over-expressed. Mice lacking MCH are about 25% leaner that their wild-type littermates [22]. Additional effects of MCH *in vivo* in mice include an increase in water consumption, which is independent of feeding [23, 24]. As MCH-containing neurons innervate many different brain regions, the exact mechanisms in which MCH mediates effects on food intake are quite complex and have not been completely worked out.

Early studies with MCH suggested an interaction between MCH and the hypothalamic-pituitary-adrenal (HPA) axis. A role for MCH in the regulation of emotion and stress responses is also supported by anatomical and neurochemical studies. MCH-R1 receptors are densely expressed in the nucleus accumbes (Nac) shell and also distributed in monoaminergic nuclei such as the locus coeruleus and dorsal raphe nucleus, in which MCH-containing fibers are also detected. These brain areas are implicated in the regulation of emotion and stress [25, 26]. A major role for MCH in energy homeostasis has been established based on physiological, genetic and pharmacologic studies in animal models. Initial data supporting a role for MCH in energy homeostasis came from a RT-PCR differential display experiment, in which the expression of pro-MCH mRNA was found to be increased in lep $^{ob/ob}$ mice [17], suggesting that MCH might have orexigenic action. MCH genetic models lend further support for a major role of MCH in energy homeostasis; KO mice lacking MCH are lean and hypophagic, while MCH over-expression transgenic mice are hyperphagic and develop obesity [22, 27]. Also, central administration of MCH has been shown to promote feeding [17], while MCH-R1 mRNA levels rise as a result of starvation and leptin deficiency [28] and MCH circulatory levels are high in obese Zucker rats [29]. MCH also stimulates insulin and leptin release in insulinoma cell lines and 3T3- L1 adipose cells, respectively [30, 31] and regulates pituitary hormones [32-35].

MCH exerts its physiological action through binding to its cognate receptors. Rodents display a single receptor (MCH-R1) while humans also possess a second receptor (MCH-R2) of yet unknown function [6, 36, 37].

MCH ANIMAL MODELS

The importance of MCH system in energy metabolism was also confirmed by genetic interventions in animal models [38]. Mice devoid of MCH are lean and hypophagic [22], while mice over-expressing MCH are obese and hyperphagic [27].

The genetic ablation of the MCH locus produces animals that are hypophagic and lean. The first report was one in which MCH gene expression was knocked-out in C57Bl/6 mice (MCH -/-) and it was found that MCH -/- mice were hypophagic and lean with respect to their normal littermates. Also, the resting energy expenditure in MCH-/- mice was elevated, which accounted in part for their leanness [22]. In addition, the MCH KO mice also show an osteoporotic phenotype due to a high bone turnover [39].

Although extensive work in rodents has implicated this gene in obesity, to date, linkage of genetic defect causing severe human obesity still needs to be established [40, 41]. Transgenic over-expression of MCH in the lateral hypothalamus results in transgenic FVB or C57B1/6 mice resulted in mice being obese, hyperlipidemic, and hyperinsulinemic with islet hyperplasia [27].

The most compelling evidence supporting these functions derives from the manipulation of ligand levels in rodents. For instance, artificially enhancing MCH levels in the brain induces a hyperphagic state [27, 42]. In another study it was proved that mice chronically exposed to MCH gained more weight than vehicle treated controls. Chronic ICV infusion of MCH (14 days, 10 ug/day) in normal C57BL/6J mice caused a slight, but significant increase in body weight on a normal fat diet; on moderate high-fat diet (about 33% fat), mice infused with MCH became hyperphagic and had elevated plasma glucose, leptin and insulin levels and gained 22% of the initial body weight compared to about 4.5% body weight gain in vehicle-treated mice after a 14 day treatment with MCH. ICV infusion of MCH in mice on a moderately high fat diet results in increased body weight accompanied by hyperphagia and significant increases in fat and liver weights. Expression levels of key modulators of energy expenditure in brown adipose tissue such as acyl-Coa oxidase, carnitine palmitoyltransferase, and uncoupling protein-1 were also down regulated. In addition, plasma glucose, insulin and leptin levels were increased [43, 44].

Decreased energy expenditure has also been explained by the reduction of plasma thyroid stimulating hormone (TSH) after ICV administration of MCH in rats [33]. Exogenous administration of MCH to hypothalamic explants has been shown to increase the release of orexigenic neurotransmitter such as NPY and Agouti-related protein (AGRP) and decrease the release of anorectic neurotransmitters as alpha-MSH and cocaine-and-amphetamine-regulated transcript (CART) [45]. Central ICV administration of MCH elicits increased food intake and body weight gain in rodents and in sheep [46]. Further support for the notion that MCH can regulate food intake was provided by a number of studies that demonstrated that injection of MCH directly into rat brain ventricles promoted food and water intake [17, 24].

Abbot *et al.* dissected this effect on food intake by MCH further by injecting the peptide into discrete brain regions and found that MCH administered directly into arcuate and paraventricular nucleus, but not LH area, supraoptic nucleus, medial preoptic area, anterior hypothalamic area, or ventromedial nucleus produced sustained food intake responses in satiated rats [45]. It was found that MCH also increased the release of orexigenic peptides, NPY and AGRP, and MCH also decreased the release of anorexic peptides, alpha-MSH and CART from hypothalamic explants, suggesting that at least part of the MCH-induced food intake effect might be due to regulating release of these other orexigenic or anorexic peptides from various hypothalamic regions. A role for the ability of MCH to affect energy expenditure and thermogenesis was provide by a study in which Wistar rats were exposed to cold, in that study, hypothalamic mRNA analysis by RT-PCR of cold-exposed rats indicated that mRNA for MCH, in addition to many other genes, was elevated by cold exposure [47]. Jeon *et al.* reported that aging-related reductions in insulin sensitivity and elevated body weight were reduced in age-matched MCH KO mice, suggesting that the lean body mass in young MCH KO mice is maintained throughout the adulthood [48].

MCH deficiency in ob/ob mice results in dramatic reduction in body fat. These mice show increased basal metabolic temperature, lower plasma glucocorticoid levels, improved glucose tolerance, and reduced expression of stearoyl-Coa desaturase [49]. Apart from genetic modifications to the receptor or the MCH gene itself, obese phenotypic models such as obese Zucker rats and ob/ob mice exhibit high hypothalamic levels of MCH [29, 50]. With the demonstration that MCH neuron cell bodies were localized primarily to the LH area and ZI it strongly supported a role for MHC in food intake [9]. This notion was further supported by studies that showed that MCH mRNA expression levels in hypothalamus were over-expressed in $lep^{ob/ob}$ mice and were increased even more by fasting in both $lep^{ob/ob}$ mice and in lean controls [17]. Similarly, hypothalamic fa/fa Zucker rats [29], in diet-induced obese rats and mice and in obese A^y mice that ectopically-express the endogenous alpha-MSH antagonist, agouti, supporting roles of MCH in these diverse rodent models of obesity [51].

MCH RECEPTORS

MCH-R1

The first high-affinity receptor for MCH was identified simultaneously be several groups using different pharmacological approaches [36, 52-54]. MCH-R1 is expressed primarily in the CNS with highest levels in Nac, hippocampus, olfactory bulb, pyriforms cortex and the amygdala. There is also significant expression in the ventromedial and arcuate nucleus of the hypothalamus [8]. MCH-R1 was found to be identical to the previously cloned orphan receptor SLC-1 and it belongs to the superfamily of G protein-coupled receptors (GPCRs) [55]. MCH-R1 is a 353 aminoacids long, with all the hallmark features of the superfamily, including seven transmembrane helice, a DRY motif and the end the third intracellular loop and three potential glycosylation sites at the N-terminus with about 32% amino acid homology with somatostatin receptor family members and the gene has been localized to chromosome 22q13.3. MCH-R1 is highly homologous between species, has similar affinity for MCH peptide analogs and has similar distribution between species [56-58]. Comparison of the human and the rodent receptors shows a high degree of conservation between species. Isolation of MCH spurred efforts resulting in identification of its receptor MCH-R1 (SLC-1/GPR24) using reverse pharmacology techniques. MCH-R1 was originally cloned and named SLC-1 (or GPR24), an orphan receptor without a known ligand [55]. Three years later in 1999, three independent groups find the ligand by a reverse-pharmacology approach in which peptide libraries or brain extracts were screened in functional assays in stable cell lines that over-expressed the receptor in an attempt to find the ligand. Reverse genetic approaches were used to deorphanize SLC-1 as a high affinity receptor for MCH [36]. MCH-R1, GPCRs previously known as orphan receptor SLC-1, was identified by several groups using different pharmacological approaches [36, 52]. All three groups found that MCH activated a transient increase in intracellular Ca^{2+} concentration and inhibited adenylyl cyclase activity and one group showed that it was through interaction with pertussis-toxin sensitive Galpha $_{i/o}$ GTP binding proteins [54].

MCH-R1 has been shown to modulate cellular function via coupling to at least three distinct heterotrimeric G-proteins, Gi, Go and Gq. Signals propagated through Gq lead to the accumulation of inositol phosphates, and the release of intracellular calcium stores. Signaling through G_i and G_o inhibits adenylate cyclase activity, and activates mitogen-activated protein (MAP) kinase. The impact of these various G-protein mediated signaling events on the biological activities attributed to MCH *in vivo*, has yet to be resolved. MCH-R1 has been found to couple to Gi, Go and Gq proteins, activating diverse signaling pathways, whereas MCH-R2 is exclusively coupled to Gq proteins. Both receptors have a similar distribution in the CNS [6, 59-61]. The high expression of MCH-R1 in hypothalamic ventromedial and dorsomedial regions was of particular interest as these regions regulate feeding behavior and energy expenditure [9, 53]. Based on those observations several reports suggest that MCH plays an important role in energy homeostasis. Genetic manipulations have shed light on the role of MCH in energy homeostasis. MCH-deficient mice have reduced body weight and leanness due to hypophagia and increased metabolic rate when compared to their wild-type littermates [22].

MCH-R1 has received most of the attention probably because of the fact that MCH-R1 is expressed in rodents, which has allowed for suitable animal models to probe its neurobiological functions. Many published studies indicate that MCH-R1 is involved in biological processes related to mammalian feeding behavior and energy expenditure [4, 62] because is expressed in the brain regions where MCH fibers were identified, in particular in centers modulating feeding behavior [9, 26, 36,], and in some peripheral tissues [3, 8, 30, 31, 63]. In addition, it has been suggested that MCH-R1 plays a key role in anxiety and mood disorders since MCH-R1 antagonist have been found to have anxiolytic and antidepressant effects in various animal models [64-66]. It has also been suggested the possibility that MCH-R1 in involved in modulating cardiovascular activity in addition to regulating energy homeostasis and the MCH-R1 may be crucial for the coordination of normal responses to weight loss [67].

MCH-R1 is highly expressed in the brain, with moderate to weak expression in other tissues, including muscle, eye, tongue and adipose tissue [36]. The distribution of MCH-R1 in the brain has been investigated in detail in the rat [25] and the expression pattern was found to be very broad throughout the CNS. Expression is seen in the cortex, basal ganglia, hypothalamus and brainstem. The presence of MCH-R1 in the arcuate and ventromedial nucleus of the hypothalamus is consistent with MCH regulating food intake and energy balance. However, the highest level of expression is seen in extrahypothalamic areas that process olfactory information, like the anterior olfactory nucleus, the pyriform cortex and the olfactory tubercle. Very high levels of MCH-R1 are also found in the shell of the Nac, an area involved in rewarding aspects of motivated behaviors, such as food intake. Significant amounts are also present in the amygdale and hippocampus, potentially implicating MCH in regulating emotions, such as fear and anxiety, and also as potential regulator of memory. Therefore, MCH is probably involved in many other behaviors, some of which might be important in food intake, such as olfaction and reward, in addition to regulating general mood and arousal levels. The mechanism underlying the effects of MCH on energy homeostasis are no clear, although food intake, locomotor activity and resting energy expenditure probably play a major role. Differences exist between mice lacking the MCH prohormone and mice lacking MCH-R1. Those lacking MCH-R1 are hyperphagic, hypermetabolic and have higher locomotor activity, whereas those lacking the

MCH prohormone have slightly decreases feeding and slightly increased energy expenditure. MCH-R2 does not exist in rodent species, hence its potential role in feeding and energy balance remains uncertain.

Among orexigenic peptides in the hypothalamus MCH is the only known peptide whose ablation results in leanness [29]. In contrast to the MCH KO model, none of the KO models of these peptides changed the feeding pattern and body weight. Therefore, it may be possible that specific MCH receptor antagonists like compounds would be more effective that the other orexigenic peptide receptor antagonists in inhibiting food intake and the treatment of obesity. Interestingly, recent studies that evaluated the role of MCH in the presence of MCH-R1 in rhesus monkeys indicate that there was no compensation by MCH-R2 on antagonist of MCH-R1[68].

MCH-R1 Animal Models

MCH-R1 has been inactivated in mice by homologous recombination [69-71]. Mice lacking functional MCH-R1 maintained on regular chow diet exhibited decreased fat mass, increased activity and, surprisingly, were found to be hyperphagic compared with their wild-type littermates. When placed on a high-fat diet, MCH-R1 deficient mice gained significantly less weight, suggesting that inactivation of MCH-R1 protected them from diet-induced obesity. Also, pharmacological blockade of MCH-R1 using specific antagonist produced similar effects [64]. These results indicate that the MCH system is effective in reducing body weight under conditions in which leptin is ineffective and make the MCH receptor a viable target for the treatment of obesity. After the MCH receptors were cloned, several groups reported within five months of each other the effect of MCH-R1 KO on phenotype in obesity-prone C57B1/6 mice. In contrast to MCH peptide KO mice, MCH-R1 KO mice were hyperphagic, but remained lean on a regular chow diet. On a high-fat diet, MCH-R1 KO mice gained less weight than wild type mice. Energy expenditure and activity levels were significantly elevated in MCH-R1 KO mice, suggesting that the resistance to high fat diet was primarily mediate by an increase in metabolic activity not food intake.

Rodents only express MCH-R1, and genetic elimination of this locus results in animals that have a decreased fat content relative to their littermates. Genetic disruption of MCH-R1 on the other hand results in mice that are surprisingly hyperphagic, but also hypermetabolic, and obesity-resistant. The reasons for this discrepancy are unknown. Paradoxically, unlike the ligand deficient animals, these animals are hyperphagic and have no change in body weight relative to their littermates. This phenotype is the result of an increase in lean body mass, which is at least partially attributable to increased locomotor activity. However, the loss of the MCH-R1 locus also disrupts the basal metabolic rate, such that receptor deficient animals have an increased metabolic rate relative to control animals. MCH-R1 (-/-) mice are resistant to high-fat, diet-induced obesity. These mice are hyperphagic and hypermetabolic with lower levels of insulin and leptin. MCH-R1 KO mice are lean and hypophagic [69, 70]. Although there are no reports of the effects of MCH antagonist in humans, increased MCH receptor levels were observed in the infundibular nucleus levels in human post-mortem brain tissue from cachectic patients [72]. Although MCH-R1 (-/-) mice has desirable body weight loss, adverse physiological changes that may limit the use of an MCH antagonist as an antiobesity drug need to be addressed. For example, the KO mice seem to have increased sympathetic tone resulting in an increased heart rate [73].

The differences in feeding behavior, between MCH-deficient and receptor KO mice probably results from deletion of peptides that are generated from preprohormone MCH processing by proconvertases [74, 75]. Additionally, mice overexpression the MCH gene demonstrated obesity traits, hyperphagia, hyperglycemia and insulin resistance [76], whilst transgenic MCH-R1 KO mice displayed hyperactivity, a lean phenotype and were resistant to diet-induced obesity [77, 78]. Consequently, MCH-R1 antagonists are currently being pursued by several laboratories as means to reduce food intake and body weight, hopefully serving as effective pharmacological treatments for obesity.

MCH-R1 receptor antagonists have been shown to be effective at modulating feeding and diet induced obesity [79, 80]. Consistent with the wide distribution of MCH-R1 in the brain, the MCH system is expected to be involved in various physiological functions and indeed a MCH-R1 antagonist has been shown to have antidepressant and anxiolytic activity [64, 81, 82]. MCH-R1 antagonists have also been reported to improve social memory in a social recognition test [83]. On the other hand, MCH-R1 KO mice exhibit cognitive deficits in inhibitory passive avoidance test [84].

MCH-R2

Higher mammals express at least two receptors for the MCH ligand. Two years after the cloning of MCH-R1, database scanning revealed a second high-affinity receptor for MCH, with significant homology to the core region of MCH-R1. The human MCH-R2 receptor is 340 amino acids long and its gene resides on the long arm of chromosome 6 [60, 85]. The overall homology between the two MCH receptors is quite low. They share only 38% identical amino acids and 44% amino acid identity, with the highest homology in the transmembrane domains that form part of the putative MCH-binding pocket. MCH-R2, is species specific, most notably it is absent in rodents, a fact that has impaired study of its function [6, 56, 60, 85]. It has similar distribution to MCH-R1 with the notable exceptions that in the hypothalamus, MCH-R2 receptors are abundant in LH area and anterior hypothalamus, but not in dorsomedial hypothalamus, whereas MCH-R1 is abundant in dorsomedial, but not anterior or LH area. MCH-R2 is also primarily expressed in the CNS, with highest expression in cortex, amygdale and Nac [8]. Uniquely, MCH-R2 is not functional expressed in mice, rats, rabbits or guinea pigs, making it more difficult to target for drug discovery efforts. Most groups reported that MCH-R2 functionally coupled to Ca^{2+} mobilization solely, not to inhibition of adenylyl cyclase [6, 60, 86-88]. Like MCH-R1, MCH-R2 also belongs to the rhodopsin family of GPCRs. Key elements of both receptors include a 7-transmembrane (7TM) motif, N-linked glycosylation sites in the N-terminal region that are important for full activity, an aspartic acid-arginine-tyrosine motif located in the cytosolic region of helix 3 (TM3) region and Asp123 and Asp113 in the TM3 regions of MCH-R1 and MCH-R2, respectively, that may be involved in ligand binding.

MCH-R1 is expressed in all mammals, in contrast to MCH-R2, which is present in dogs, ferrets, primates and humans but absent in rodents [56]. In higher species, the expression pattern of MCH-R2 mRNA is similar to MCH-R1 with the highest expression observed in the brain, notably in the frontal cortex, amygdale and Nac. Both MCH receptors are also expressed in areas associated with energy homeostasis such as the arcuate nucleus and the ventral medial hypothalamus [6, 87]. The distribution of MCH-R2 in the CNS suggests that it may mediate physiology similar to MCH-R1, however the physiological importance of MCH-R2 is difficult to assess because of its absence in rodent models [89].

HUMAN GENETICS

Several single nucleotide polymorphism haven been identified in the two MCH receptors within different ethnic groups. Two studies identified the same polymorphisms in the MCH-R1 gene that resulted in a nonconservative single amino acid change, R248Q that cosegregated with obesity across more than one generation. Mutations in the control groups at very rare frequencies have also been reported. Another mutation (rs133068) found by Bell *et al.* was within the promoter region of the MCH-R1 gene and seemed to convey protection against obesity [40, 90]. Hawes *et al.* reported single nucleotide polymorphisms (SNPs) in MCH-R2 genes. In their study, four SNPs of the MCH-R2 gene were identified in the coding region, two of these produced amino acid substitutions in the protein [41].

MCH AS ANTI-OBESITY DRUG TARGET

The MCH/MCH-R1 system is considerate as a promising therapeutic target for the treatment of the obesity because, is a peptide that stimulates food intake produced by neurons in the lateral hypothalamic area. These neurons are hypothesized to be downstream of POMC and NPY/AGRP neurons in the energy homeostasis pathway [87]. Other research has been suggested the orexigenic action of MCH is mediated via the NPY Y81 receptor and be independent of galanin and melanocortin receptor [91, 92]. Leptin and insulin are hormones that circulate in proportion to body adiposity and activate POMC neurons while inhibiting NPY/AGRP neurons, thus promoting weight loss. In contrast, the gastric hormone ghrelin stimulates NPY/AGRP neurons and promotes weight gain. MCH neurons are inhibited by input from POMC cells, whereas NPY/AGRP neurons are proposed to have the opposite effect. Because voluntary weight loss lowers insulin and leptin levels while raising ghrelin levels, a set of arcuate nucleus responses (activation of NPY/AGRP neurons and inhibition of POMC neurons) is engaged that activates MCH neurons. This pathway can be disrupted by pharmacological antagonism of MCH-R1 receptor. Takekawa *et al.* mentioned to several lines of evidence suggest that MCH plays an important function in feeding behavior and energy balance and those MCH receptor antagonists could be major potential targets for the treatment of obesity [68].

MELANIN CONCENTRATING HORMONE RECEPTOR 1 ANTAGONISTS

Discovery of the First MCH-R1 Antagonists

Peptide Derivatives

Schering-Plough was the first to discover a functional and competitive peptide antagonist on the human MCH-R1, which was the analogue of human MCH D-Ala^{11} with a K_B of 15.8 μM, with this type of peptide antagonist being very important in the development of MCH antagonists, since they initially permitted the identification of key interactions with its two receptors, MCH-R1 and MCH-R2. The analysis of the interaction of the cloned human hormone and peptide analogues substituted in Alanine helped determine that the chains of Arginine^{6} and Methionine^{8} moderately contribute to a reorganization of both receptors; this being important for Arginine^{6} chirality since this causes a significant decrease in the selectivity of the MCH-R2 [93]. In addition, by analyzing various MCH analogues with a 5-aminovaleric acid substituent at positions 9, 10 and/or 14, 15, it was determined that the segments of Leucine^{9}-Glycine^{10} and Arginine^{14}-Proline^{15} of the disulfide ring are the main structural elements that determine the ability and selectivity for MCH derived peptide analogues to act as antagonists [94, 95]. Despite these advances, peptide compounds have not been reported as potential antagonists of MCH-R1 in clinical trials for the treatment of obesity.

Small Molecules

Initially, Takeda Pharmaceutical Company discovered the first small molecule selective MCH antagonist called T-226296 (**1**), which is orally active, with an inhibitory concentration 50 (IC_{50}) value of 5.5 nM. On the other hand, through a series of assays on MCH receptor affinity, Synaptic discovered SNAP-7941(**2**) (Fig. **1**), with a K_b value of 0.3 nM.

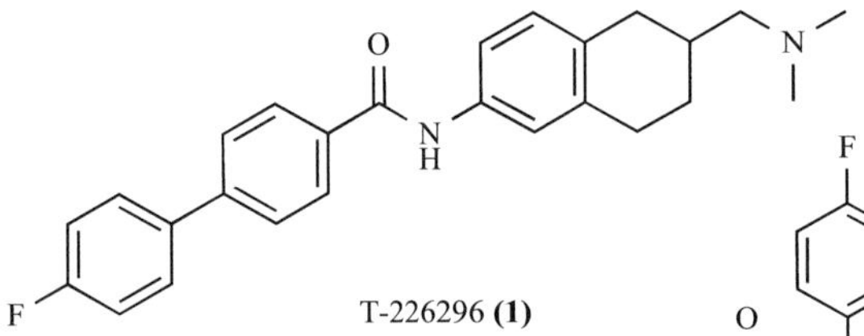
T-226296 (**1**)

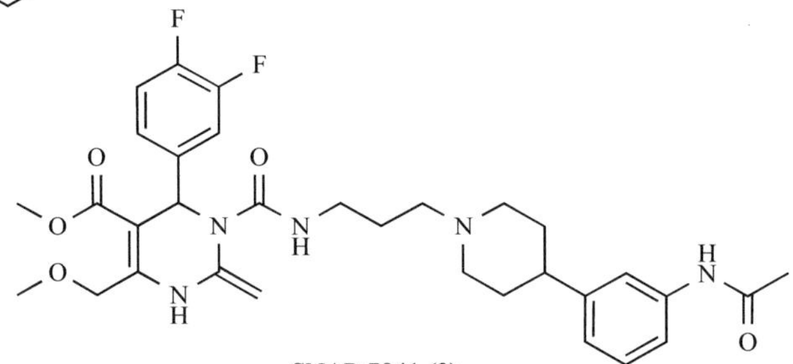
SNAP-7941 (**2**)

Fig. (1). Structures of compounds T-226296 (**1**) and SNAP-7941 (**2**).

Thus, in the development of MCH-R1 antagonists, T-226296 and SNAP-7941 were two of the first small molecules that helped to establish and develop a series of strategies, mostly from research groups of various pharmaceutical companies, to obtain new and more selective MCH-R1 antagonists in recent years for the pharmacologic treatment of obesity and which are described below.

Drug-Design Strategies to MCH-R1 Antagonists

Carboxamide Derivatives

One of the initial strategies in the development of MCH-R1 antagonists was the synthesis of analogues of T-226296; the compound SB-568849 (**3**) (Fig. **2**), which presented a K_i value of 7.7 nM, was discovered in this way, as well as DABA-821 (**4**) (Fig. **2**), which presented a K_i value of 39.3 nM and an IC_{50} value of 14.0 nM [96].

Afterwards, the design of more potent MCH-R1 antagonists was based on limiting the conformation of the three regions of SB-568849. First, they focused on the basic side chain; second, on the hydrophobic part represented by the biphenyl moiety; and third, on the amide group. Thus, the above changes led to the determination that cyclization of the basic side chain literally reduces affinity for MCH receptors. Also, restricting the conformation of the biphenyl fraction to a planar conformation led to a significant loss of affinity for the MCH-R1, this trend being independent of the basic side chain and the methylation of the

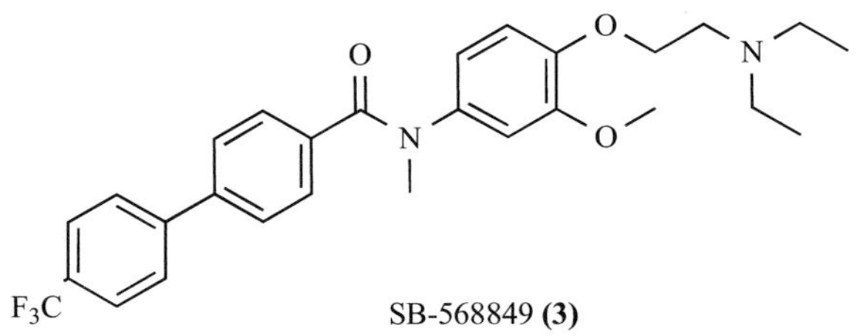

SB-568849 **(3)**

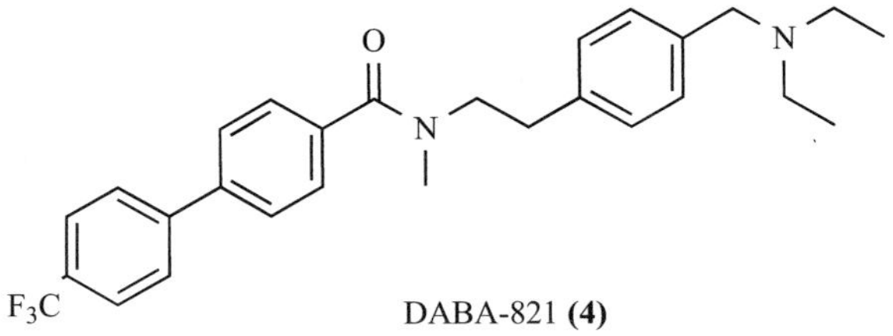

DABA-821 **(4)**

Fig. (2). Structures of compounds SB-568849 **(3)** and DABA-821 **(4)**.

nitrogen of the amide group. Surprisingly, the limitation of conformation of the amide group relatively increased receptor affinity. However, the results of aqueous stability studies of these compounds were poor because the ring of these derivatives opens at a pH 7. Years later, optimization of analogue molecules of SB-568849 was achieved using quinozaline, benzotriazole and thienopyrimidinone rings instead of the classic biphenyl fraction, providing rigidity to the amide group. These new molecules showed good water stability and a low *in vitro* sensitivity by human liver microsome (HLM) metabolism. This strategy turned out to be one of the best used for the design of carboxamide derived MCH-R1 antagonists, since the incorporation of a thienopyrimidinone ring (considered an isoster of the biphenyl group) served to reduce the conformation of the amide group and led to the discovery of GW3430 (**5**) (Fig. **3**), which presented an IC_{50} value of 9.3 nM [97, 98].

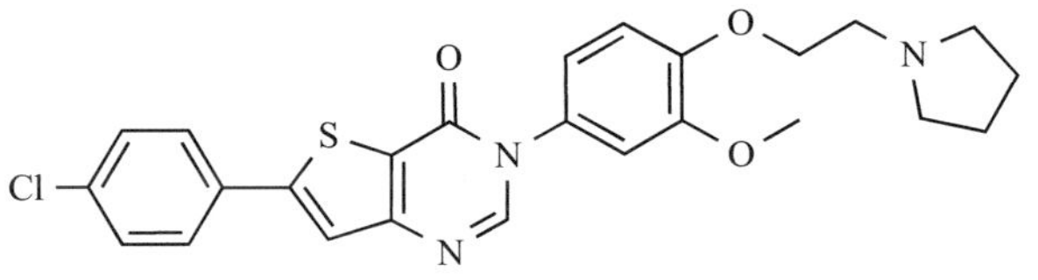

GW3430 **(5)**

Fig. (3). Structure of compound GW3430 **(5).**

The study of the structure-activity relationship (SAR) shows that potency increases when the biphenyl group is substituted by 4-chlorophenylthienopyrimidinone, which determines a preference for small lypophilic substituents in the *para* position of the aromatic ring on the left side of the molecule, suggesting that the aryl ring may be located in a tight hydrophobic pocket of the receptor; in addition, the carbonyl group of the pyrimidinone ring appears to be crucial for the antagonist activity of these compounds, speculating that carbonyl oxygen is acting as a hydrogen acceptor [99-101]. Also, from the analysis of various analogs of GW3430 on MCH-R1 and MCH-R2 receptors, key elements has been determined for both receptors, which include a 7-transmembrane (7TM) motif, N-linked glycosylation sites in the N-terminal region that are important for full activity, an aspartic acid-arginine-tyrosine motif located in the cytosolic region of the helix 3 (3TM) region and Asp123 and Asp113 in the 3TM regions of MCH-R1 and MCH-R2, respectively. It was also established that substituents at position 4 and 6 of the basic thieno[3.2.d] pyrimidinone ring increases the potency of the compounds and it is suggested that analogues that present a steric demand for basic substituents and a hydroxyl group on the right side allow better interaction with the receptor. Additionally, the results of coupling these compounds showed that the carbonyl group of the pyrimidinone ring forms hydrogen bonds with the amino acid Tyr273. In contrast, on the right side of the molecule, compounds with large substituents in the basic amine chain can cause unfavorable steric interactions that result in a loss of potency, suggesting that interactions must be present through hydrogen or ionic bonding and indicating the importance of Asp123 as a key protein element that helps provide more potency to the compounds [102]. Other substitutions have been carried out such as the incorporation of a naphthalene or benzothiophene group that have proven to be a good addition because of an increase in affinity, but this requires the presence of a hydroxyl group or a basic nitrogen. Both options appear to be good because since they increase the possibility of forming hydrogen bonds with Asp123 residues of the receptor. Thus, one of the best MCH-R1 antagonists developed is compound (**6**) (Fig. **4**), which has an aromatic benzothiophene substituent on the right side of the molecule and a 4-chlorothienopyrimidinone fraction on the left side [103].

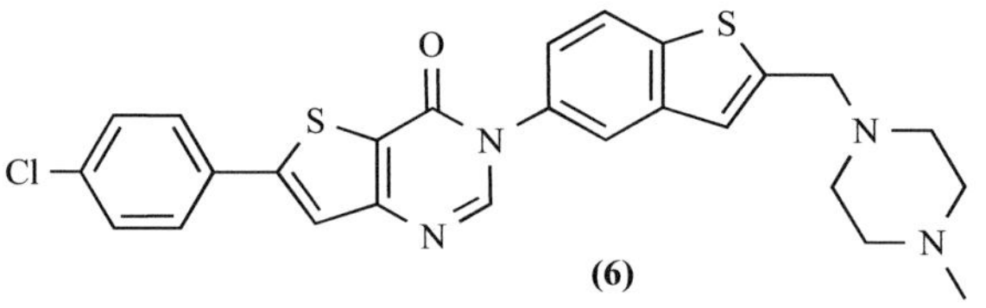

(6)

Fig. (4). Structure of compound (**6**).

A new class of MCH inhibitors was subsequently identified, such as compound (**7**) (Fig. **5**) that includes isosteric benzimidazole on the right side of the molecule, maintaining the 4-chlorothienopyrimidinone fraction. SAR studies established that regioselective substitutions on the benzimidazole ring can affect bioavailability and potency [99].

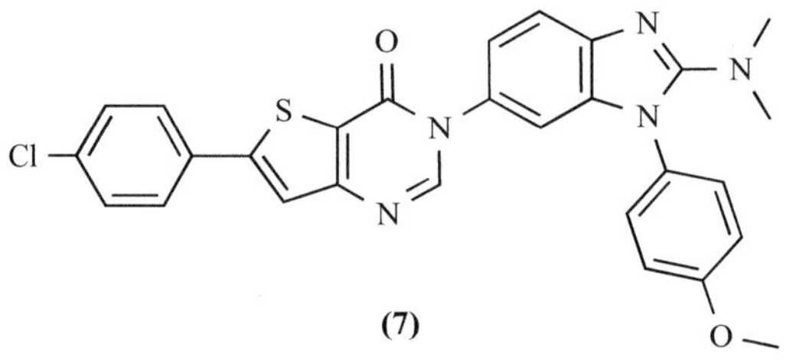

(7)

Fig. (5). Structure of compound (**7**).

Another strategy in the development of MCH-R1 antagonists was to design new benzamides derived ligands with a hydrophobic fraction based on the similarity of the MCH-R1 receptor binding site and of several dopaminergic receptors, such as dopamine D2 and D3, introducing the 2-methoxybenzamide system in the central part of the molecule as a potential hydrogen donor and acceptor site, like compound (**8**) (Fig. **6**). Using a SAR study, it was determined that the elimination of the 2-methoxy group from carboxamide derived biphenyl results in a complete loss of affinity. Furthermore, it was determined that the hydrophilic properties at the *para* position were unfavorable in benzamide derivatives and that the substituents that disrupt the planarity of the system around the central benzamide are not adequate. Urea group also exhibit a high affinity in comparison with amides. This may be due to the involvement of urea in the interaction with the receptor by hydrogen bonds [104].

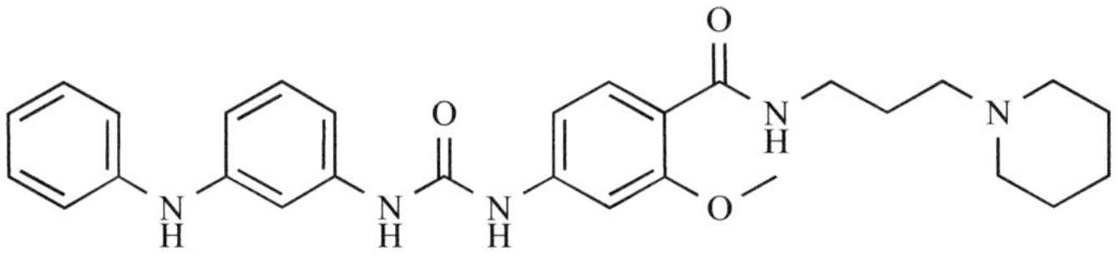

(8)

Fig. (6). Structure of compound (**8**).

Aminoaryl derived substituents have also been reported having a 3-aminopyrrolidine fraction as the central part of the molecule and on the left side the classic biphenyl fragment is maintained, with compound (**9**) (Fig. **7**), which has a K_i value of 2.3 nM, being one of the best derivatives. However, these compounds undergo rapid metabolic clearance when administered to rats; [105] therefore, a possible effective strategy suggested for reducing the elimination of compounds and optimizing half-life was to carry out modifications of the benzamide group in bicyclic compounds, maintaining a carbonyl group, possibly to promote the interaction of this group with Gln212 from transmembrane 5 of the MCH-R1 [106, 107].

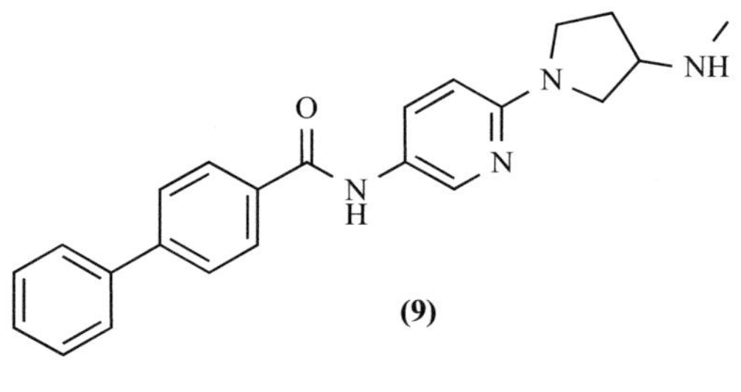

(9)

Fig. (7). Structure of compound **(9)**.

3-aminopyrrolidine derivatives have been designed incorporating on the left side of the molecule the substituted biphenyl substituent and limiting the conformation of carbonyl with the formation of a chromone derived ring, like compound (**10**) (Fig. **8**), which has subnanomolar affinity values and a 66% oral bioavailability in rats. However, it was determined that the incorporation of a methoxy group in the phenyl ring is apparently responsible for the rapid elimination of these compounds by HLM [108].

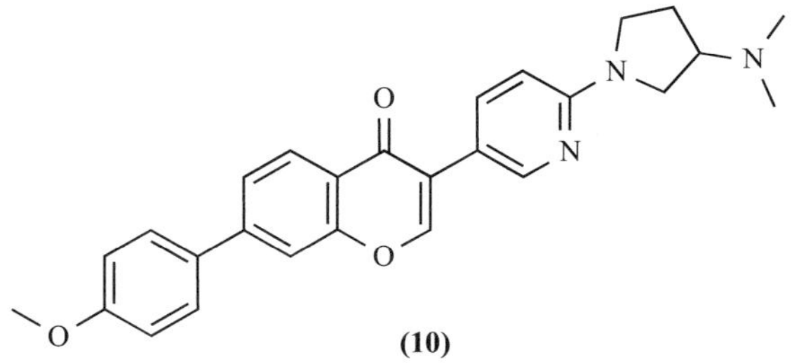

(10)

Fig. (8). Structure of compound **(10)** derived from chromones.

Moreover, and continuing with the design of 3-aminopyrrolidine derived compounds, structural analogues of compound (**11**) (Fig. **9**) that differ only in substitutions at the *para* position of the phenyl ring incorporating a chlorine atom or a trifluoromethyl group, presented an affinity of 7.3 and 1.1 nM, respectively. Although the affinity of compounds is similar, the ability to inhibit calcium flow as a function of time was markedly influenced by substitutions on the left side of the molecule. Therefore, it is likely that the presence of chlorine or trifluoromethyl substituents is responsible for a steric effect as well as a redistribution of electron density. This shows that steric interferences between the receptor and the substituted compounds are key factors that influence the inhibitory potency of this type of compounds [109].

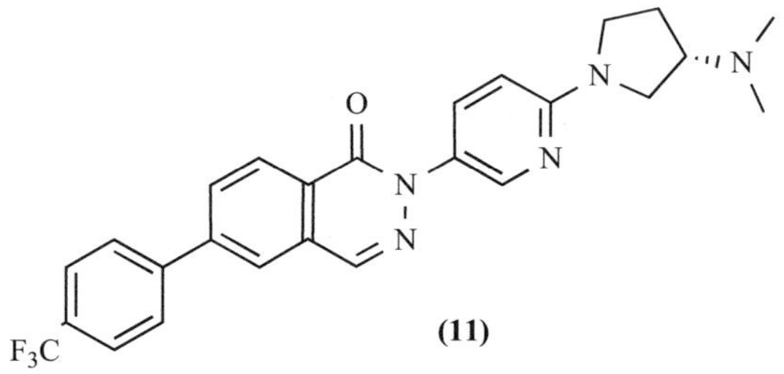

(11)

Fig. (9). Structure of compound **(11).**

Several molecular modeling studies have led to the establishment of key pharmacophore points for biological activity on the MCH receptors. For example, the design of a new class of potent MCH-R1 antagonists was based on a replacement of the carboxamide group of the structure, identifying as part of a pharmacophore to a tertiary amide, an amine and a terminal aromatic ring. Although other studies suggest a pharmacophore with the following characteristics: a positive nitrogen, a hydrogen acceptor group and the presence of two hydrophobic fragments, parts of this pharmacophore have been validated by a similar study conducted by the Argenta research group that helped to identify some of the same features [110]. Docking studies suggest that carboxamide derived compounds are integrated into the transmembrane region between helices 3, 6 and 7. The docking model suggests that basic amines interact inside the receptor with Asp123, while the biaryl system is involved in π-stacking and π-cationic interactions near the receptor surface. Also, amide appears to be involved in the interaction by forming hydrogen bonds with Gln79 and Arg197 with the oxygen atom of the carbonyl group, which acts as a hydrogen donor [106, 110].

An alternative in the design of new MCH-R1 antagonist derivatives was the incorporation of systems such as benzoyl, 4-aminopiperidine and naphthalene. This led to the identification of compound (R)-isomer **(12)** (Fig. **10**), which presents excellent MCH-R1 antagonist activity with a K_i value of 7 nM. The SAR study of this type of derivatives led to the determination that a hydroxyl group rich in electrons or a fluorine atom at *meta* position in the phenyl ring enhance interaction with the receptor in comparison with non-substituted compounds. It was also observed that large substituents in the nitrogen atom reduce *in vitro* activity, suggesting that the basic nitrogen may play an important role in affinity as well as in the conformational orientation of the benzamide group [111].

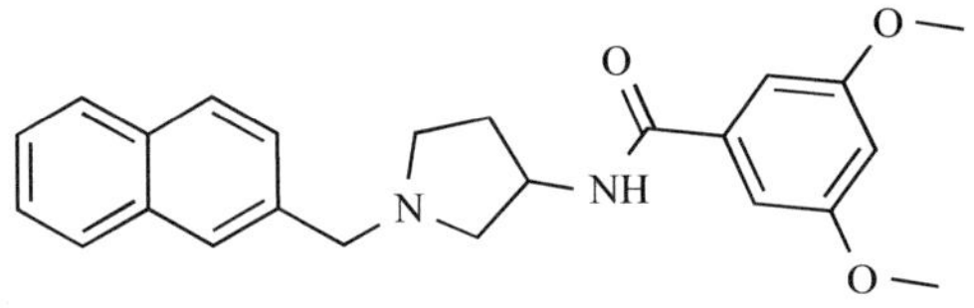

(12)

Fig. (10). Structure of compound **(12)**.

One drawback that has occurred in the development of MCH-R1 antagonist compounds is the effect that they have on human ether-a-go-go related gene (hERG). For example, ketopiperazine derived compound **(13)** (Fig. **11**) shows potency as an orally effective MCH-R1 antagonist; however, compound **(13)** presented hERG-blocking activity [112].

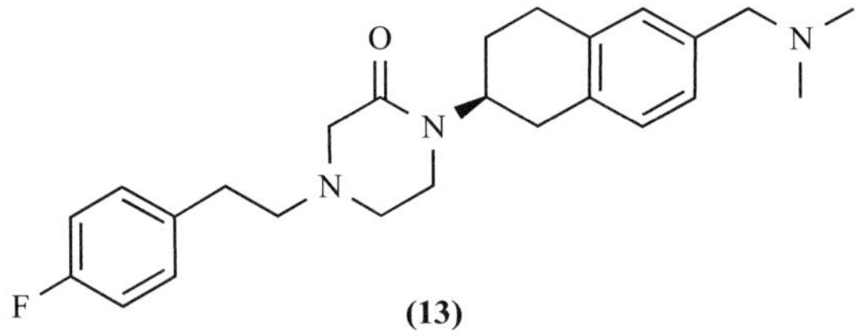

(13)

Fig. (11). Structure of compound **(13)**.

Continuing with the strategy of incorporating ketopiperazine as a central part, compound **(14)** (Fig. **12**) was discovered, which in a study in diet-induced obesity (DIO) rats did not promote weight loss hypothesizing that this compound has no *in vivo* activity due to its lack of exposure to MCH receptors in the brain and the hydrophilic nature of the compound, which may contribute to its inability to cross the blood-brain barrier (BBB): this is why the synthesis of compounds with increased lipophilicity to address the difficulty of crossing the BBB associated with the presence of phenylethyl ketopiperazine of compound **(14)** was considered. Thus, compound **(15)** derived from pyrazolopiperazinones was synthesized (Fig. **12**).

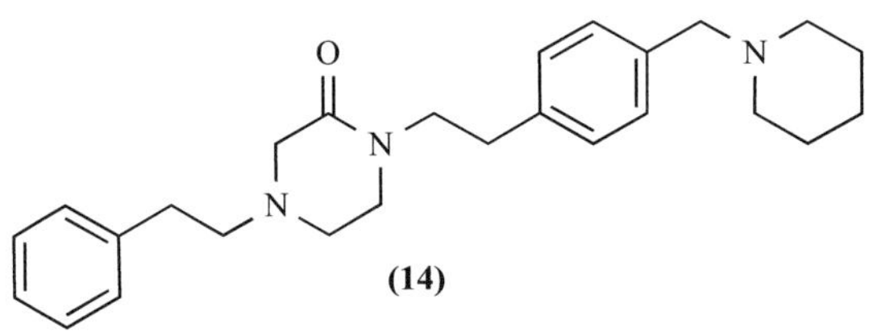

(14)

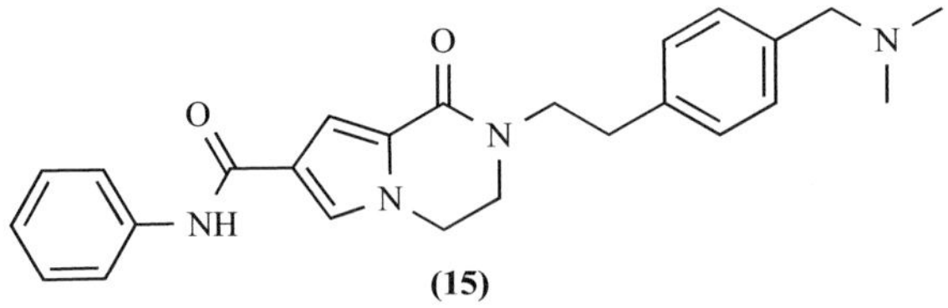

(15)

Fig. (12). Structures of compounds **(14)** and **(15)**.

However, results show that derivatives of this type are not active *in vivo*, probably because of little BBB penetration. It is suggested that the general orientation of the structure of the compound plays a more important role than the polar character of the spacer for receptor interaction and that the amide is not necessary to show high interaction affinity with the MCH-R1. Eliminating the amide group of the compound, results in a complete loss of affinity for the MCH-R1 and the selectivity for 5-HT_{2C} receptors [113].

As part of the research process of new MCH-R1 antagonists, compounds that determine key interactions with hERG channels have been developed. It has been proposed that compound (**16**) (Fig. **13**) can interact through the tertiary amine in a cation-π interaction with the Tyr-652 residue of the hERG channel. In addition, the lipophilic fractions of the molecule, like biphenyls and tetrahydronaphthalenes, can interact with hydrophobic residues of the hERG channel such as Phe-656. This has allowed the design of new compounds that have the introduction of nitrogen in the terminal aromatic ring of the right fragment of the molecule that considerably decreases the activity on hERG.

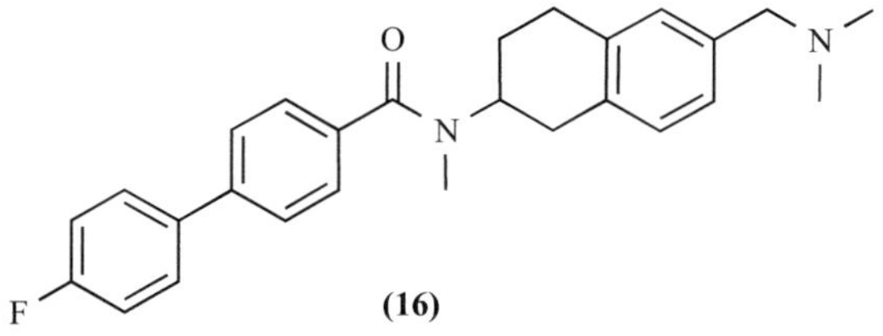

(16)

Fig. (13). Structure of compound (**16**).

Another strategy that has been carried out to reduce the effects on hERG is the incorporation of polar groups next to the tertiary amine. Unfortunately, the effects were not adequate, even though it decreased the selectivity on 5-HT_{2C} receptors. Subsequently, aminomethyl tetrahydronaphthalene ketopiperazine derivatives were developed in order to make the compounds more selective for hERG through substitutions of the benzylic tertiary amine and 4-fluorophenyl sites, suggesting that hydrophobic volume and non aromaticity are required for high affinity on hERG receptors. In short, the importance of the relationship between the basicity of amines and the activity on hERG was determined; establishing that an imidazole analog is a more potent hERG blocker, even if it is a less basic tertiary amine, possibly due to the fact that the imidazole ring can participate in π - π interactions as well as cationic interactions with hERG ion channels [114-118].

One of the strategies more currently used by pharmaceutical companies is high throughput screening (HTS). With this tool aminopiperidin coumarin derived MCH-R1 antagonists have been identified with moderate affinity with an IC_{50} value of 191 nM. SAR studies rapidly showed that substitutions in C6 are essential for improving antagonist function and affinity. An example is the incorporation of chlorine at the C6 position that allowed efficient penetration of the BBB at a dose of 10 mg/kg [119]. Compound **(17)** (Fig. **14**) showed moderate cross-reactivity against three GPC receptors that also bind amino ligands and it

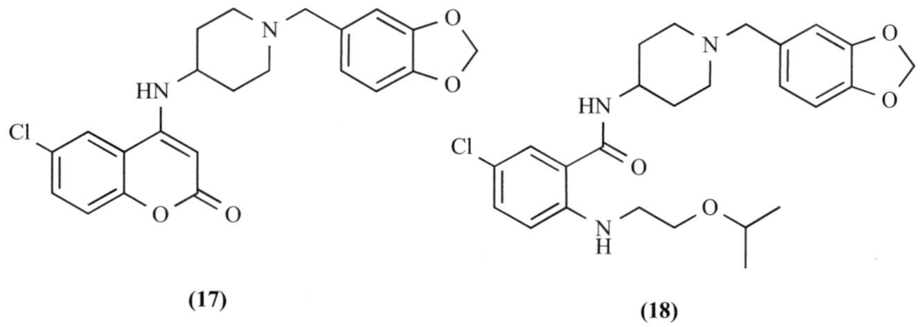

(17) **(18)**

Fig. (14). Structures of compounds **(17)** and **(18)**.

did not show appreciable affinity for the MCH-R2 receptor or to other receptors that have been implicated in weight loss such as galanin, cannabinoids, serotonin, or ion transport receptors, among others. However, adverse cardiovascular effects of this type of compounds led to the optimization of existing lead compounds, obtaining new MCH-R1 antagonists such as those derived from *ortho*-aminobenzamides and nicotinamides. An example is compound (**18**) (Fig. **14**). The introduction of hydrophobic substituents at the *ortho* position of the phenyl ring led to a significant reduction in MCH-R1 inhibition, although this suggests that the introduction of an *ortho*-amino group on the benzamide should allow conformational restriction via an intramolecular hydrogen bond between the amine and the carbonyl groups [120].

On the other hand, 4-amino-2-(3, 4-dichlorophenyl)butyl benzamide derived compounds were developed as MCH-R1 antagonists with a K_i value of 4.1 μM. The SAR study determined that there is a dramatic reduction in potency when the 3,5-dichlorobenzamide group is replaced with a substituted dihalophenyl urea. However, the introduction of an aryl group in the *para* position can strongly increase potency, obtaining compounds with nanomolar activity, such as compound (**19**) (Fig. **15**), which has a K_i value of 0.84 nM [121]. Subsequently, using a computer model of passive absorption, piperidine derivatives like compound (**20**) were designed (Fig. **15**); these were predicted to have compatible features such as good oral absorption and this later resulted in the discovery of MCH-R1 antagonists based on biaryl piperidines with nanomolar activity [122, 123].

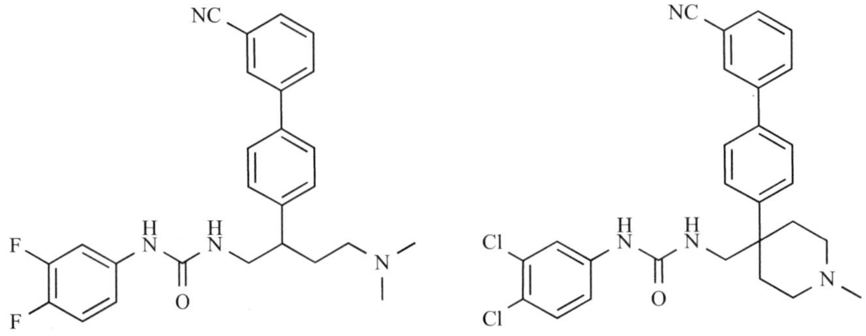

(19) **(20)**

Fig. (15). Structures of compounds **(19)** and **(20)**.

Another strategy common in medicinal chemistry and employed in the design of MCH-R1 antagonists was the hybridization between SNAP-7941 and chlorohaloperidol. This resulted in the discovery of an antagonist compound also known as SNAP-94847 (**21**) (Fig. **16**) with a high affinity and selectivity for MCH-R1 with a K_i of 2.2 nM [124].

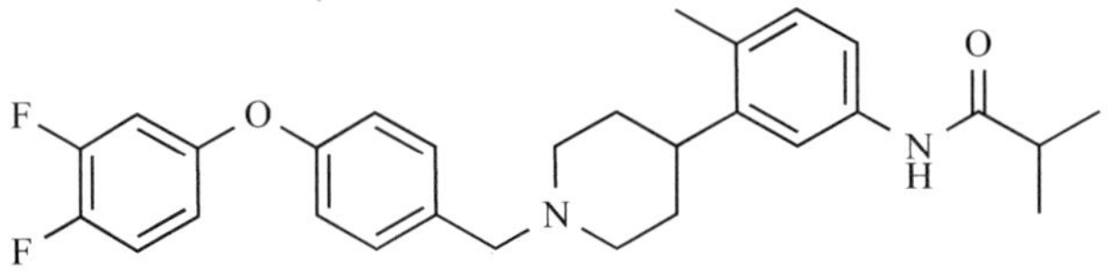

(21)

Fig. (16). Structure of compound SNAP-94847 **(21).**

Urea Derivatives

The development of urea derived MCH-R1 antagonist compounds arose from a series of antagonist compounds related to bis (aminopyrrolidines) ureas (APUs) based on a γ-aminobutyramide (GABA) core. However, the flexible nature of the GABA molecules were a concern because of the multitude of possible conformations available for a possible selectivity, as well as the negative impact of a large number of rotatable bonds on pharmacokinetic parameters [125].

Previously and consistently, several observations determined that the stereochemistry influences the potency of the compounds, this being consistent with experimental data. For example, it was confirmed that the stereochemistry of the pyrrolidine ring near the carboxamide group is more critical for high affinity than the analogous centers on the right side of the molecule. In this way compound (**22**) (Fig. **17**), which has a functional activity with an IC_{50} value of 14 nM, was discovered. Using a SAR study it was determined that the electron donating/withdrawing capacity of the substituent at the *para* position does not seem important in the terminal aryl of the biarylcarboxamide. However, the incorporation of more lipophilic substituents at this position results in a dramatic reduction in potency, which suggests that the same steric factor may play a role; it has also been determined that moving a secondary amine to a tertiary amine results in reduced affinity, but the presence of a basic core in this region of the molecule is important for functional activity. It was later determined in this type of compounds that the stereochemical preference is slightly different from the original compounds of the APU series, the most potent isomer being the diastereomer (S, R), represented by compound (**22**) (Fig. **17**). These data suggest that a conformational change in the amide group allows the adoption of a slightly different conformation in the interaction of the compound on the receptor pocket, which led to the substitution of the biphenyl group by the 4-chlorophenyl-thienopyrimidinone fraction, allowing the discovery of compound (**23**) (Fig. **17**) [126]. However, APU derived compounds have low metabolic stability in *in vitro* studies with HLM and have only moderate oral exposure in rats, which probably occurs via oxidative deamination of the pyrrolidine ring on the right side producing in the process 3-pyrrolidinone. These results suggest that the receptor region surrounding this part of the molecule is relatively open, of lipophilic nature, and prefers relatively non-polar groups [127].

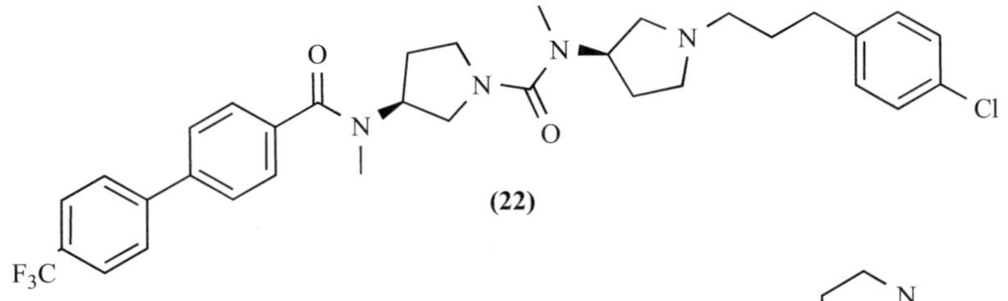

(22)

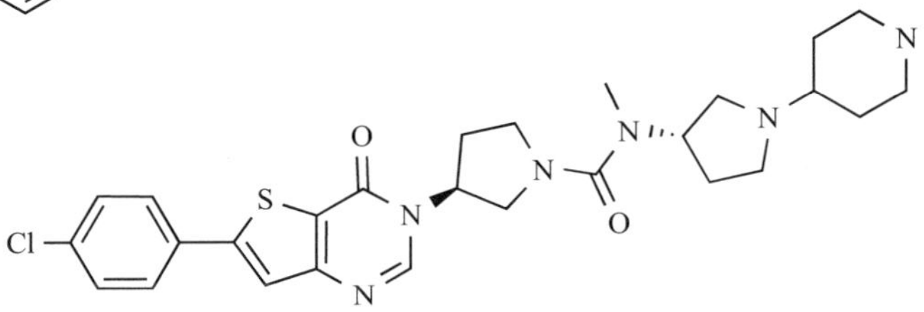

(23)

Fig. (17). Structures of compounds **(22)** and **(23)**.

Significant inhibition of CYP2D6 and low BBB penetration were identified as two problems of analogs of compounds (**22**) and (**23**), so the left and right side of the molecule were modified. On the left side electron donor substituent that could favor affinity were incorporated. These results confirm the hypothesis that the receptor binding pocket around the biaryl group is sensitive to certain steric changes, as well as the addition of only tertiary amines where the presence of a hydrogen donor on the ligand is crucial for binding and inhibiting the potency of the CYP2D6 enzyme. Likewise, it was determined that reducing the basicity of the amine by the introduction of a trifluoromethyl substituent resulted in a reduction in CYP2D6 activity [128]. Certain changes around the biaryl fraction were explored based on the structure of bis-amino-pyrrolidines ureas, incorporating the 5-phenyl-2-thiophenylcarboxamide, which allowed the discovery of compound (**24**) (Fig. **18**) [129].

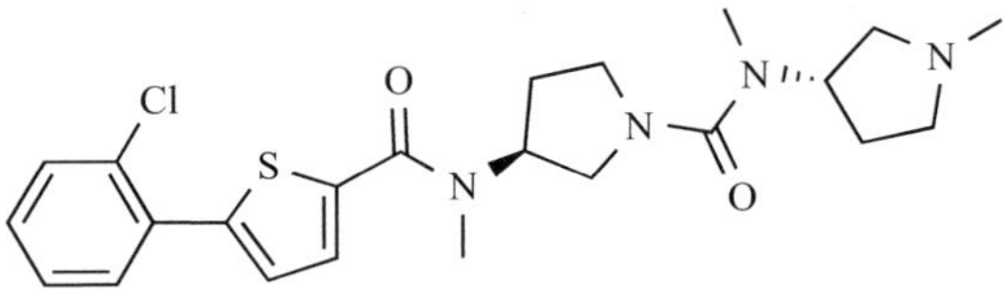

(24)

Fig. (18). Structure of compound **(24)**.

Shering-Plough Pharmaceutical, in the design of new MCH-R1 antagonists, revealed a number of urea derived compounds with the general structure (**25**) (Fig. **19**). These derivatives showed a K_i value of less than 100 nM. Additionally, the optimization of benzylpiperidine derived compounds allowed the development of a series of MCH antagonists with general structure (**26**) (Fig. **19**) with a K_i value of 5 nM [130].

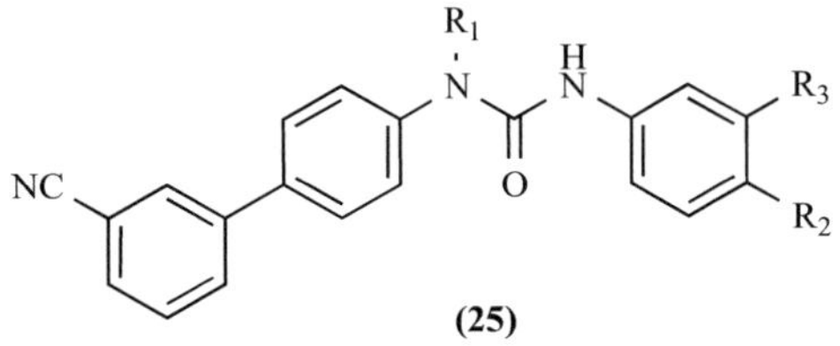

(25)

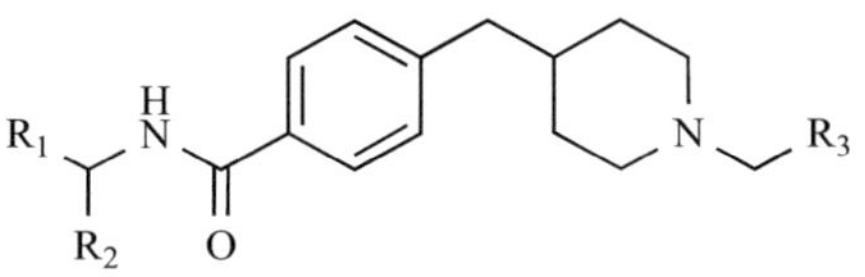

(26)

Fig. (19). Structures of compounds **(25)** and **(26)**.

Following a HTS strategy, Shering-Plough identified a series of biarylurea derived compounds as potent antagonists for the treatment of obesity. One of these compounds is a potent but non selective MCH-R1 antagonist with a K_i of 3.9 nM, which also has an antagonistic effect on M2 muscarinic receptors with a K_i of 532 nM. The SAR study of compounds derived from general structure (**25**) determined that methylation of urea results in decreased affinity, which confirms the importance of the hydrogen N-H of the urea group and its possible link in the interaction with the receptor. It was shown for these compounds that the *meta* substitution is preferred in the terminal ring of the biaryl fragment over *ortho* and *para* substitutions, with the cyano group being the best substituent at the *meta* position. However, some analogues have potent reuptake inhibition of 5-HT transporters with a K_i of 27 nM. SAR studies of pyrrolidine analogues helped in the identification of compound (**27**) (Fig. **20**), which shows an excellent profile in terms of MCH-R1 affinity and selectivity over other receptors such as NPY, 5-HT, M2 and MCH-R2 [131].

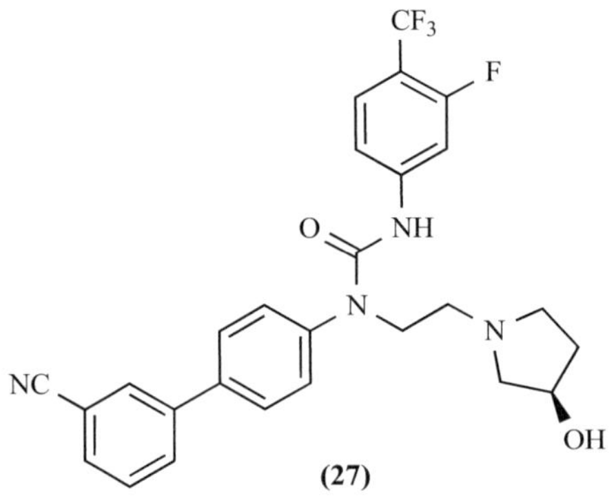

(27)

Fig. (20). Structure of compound (**27**).

Modifications of the central phenyl were later studied and the bicycloalkyl urea ring was discovered as a viable option, which is present in compound (**28**) (Fig. **21**) as an MCH-R1 antagonist. It was determined that the *trans* isomer is much more active than the *cis* isomer and cyclohexane was proposed as a substitute for the central phenyl ring [132]. A different modification of biaryl aniline was carried out, which resulted

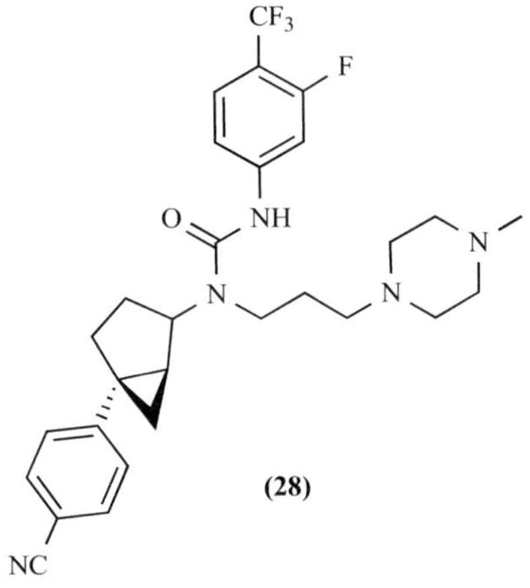

(28)

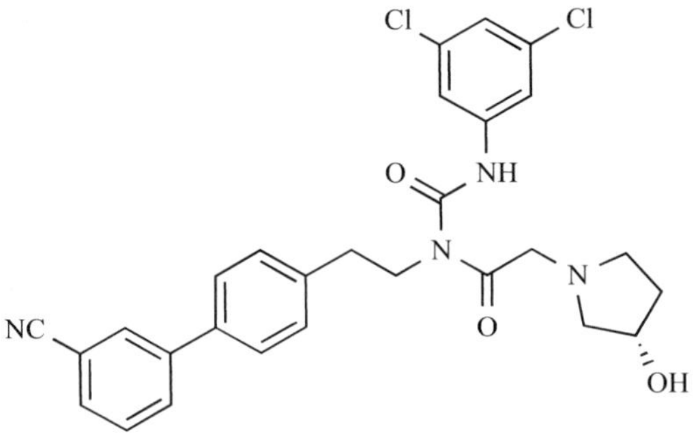

(29)

Fig. (21). Structures of compounds (**28**) and (**29**).

in the discovery of biaryl diamides as potent MCH-R1 antagonists, compound (**29**) is an example (Fig. **21**), possibly determining that considerable loss of activity in a series of biaryl methylenes derived compounds could be due to a number of changes in the orientation of the biaryl fraction as well as the interaction with the receptor provided by the hydrogen of urea [133].

In the design of APU derived MCH-R1 antagonists, urea isosteres were used, such as aminobenzimidazole, which occurs in compound (**30**) (Fig. **22**). Biological activity results show that all new aminobenzimidazole derived compounds were inactive in interaction assays with MCH-R2, which indicates MCH-R1 receptor selectivity. Additionally, it was determined that alkylation of the benzimidazole nitrogen causes active compounds to substantially lose their activity, indicating that the benzimidazole hydrogen plays a key role in the interaction with MCH-R1 [134].

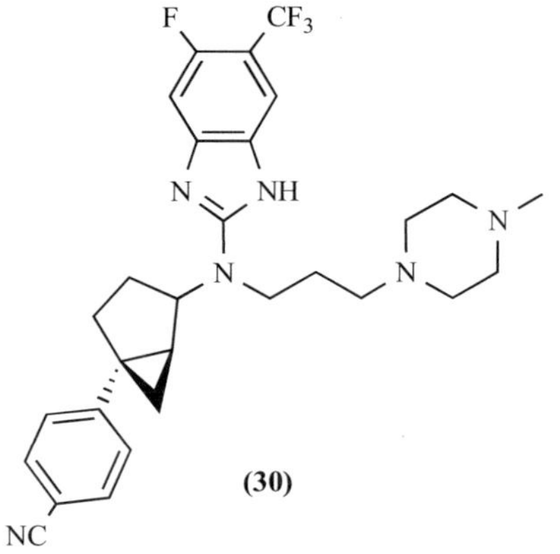

(30)

Fig. (22). Structure of compound **(30)**.

Pyrazine and pyrimidine analogues of biarylamines were synthesized mainly because of their close resemblance to the biarylamine derived MCH-R1 antagonist (**27**). However, these simple changes drastically decreased affinity for MCH-R1. Bicyclo (4.1.0) heptane derived compounds were subsequently discovered as compound (**31**) (Fig. **23**); with this it was determined that the urea phenyl ring requires one or two electron withdrawing groups at the *para* or *meta* position and that the basicity of the nitrogen side chain is also very important because if basicity decreases, the activity against MCH-R1 decreases as a result [135]. An alternative to biaryl aniline and bicyclo (4.1.0) heptane rings was the incorporation of the cyclopentyl core that would further benefit molecular weight reduction, a property that has been shown to favorably impact bioavailability. With this type of compounds, saturation of the cyclopentyl substructure provides *cis* and *trans* derivatives, of which the *trans* isomer is the most powerful. In particular, substitutions with electron withdrawing groups in position 3, 4 or 3, 5 are required on the aryl urea, such as those in compound (**32**) (Fig. **23**) [136].

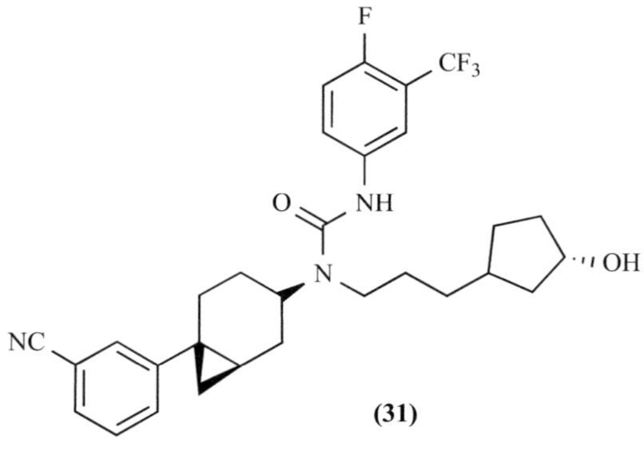

(31)

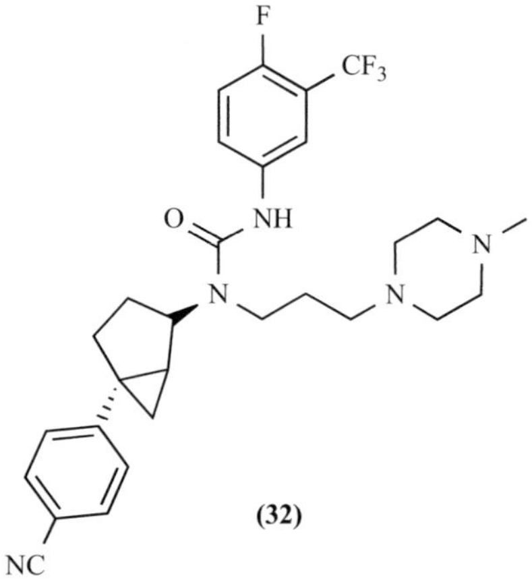

(32)

Fig. (23). Structures of compounds **(31)** and **(32)**.

SAR studies have determined that halogen atoms or a trifluomethyl group on aryl urea improve the pharmacokinetic properties of analogues of compound (**32**). The incorporation of cyclic amines on the terminal side chain is important in order to provide better selectivity of MCH-R1 than on muscarinic receptors and serotonin transport and reuptake. It was observed in this type of compounds that the basicity of the nitrogen atom is essential for MCH-R1 activity. These findings support previous observations in SAR studies of the side-chain of the biaryl series [131]. Also, a difference in *meta* substitution of the terminal aryl ring results in a significant decrease in activity, while the cyano substituent offers significant pharmacokinetic advantages such as an increase in the area under the curve (AUC) and in half-life. Strong evidence indicates that the substituents at position *para* provide receptor occupancy above 90% at 6 hours post-dose and the bicyclo fragment has been established as an effective substitute for biaryl anilines [137]. The discoveries of bicyclo (3.1.0) hexyl ureas derived antagonists were subsequently reported. In this type of compounds sulfone, amide and amine substituents in the aryl and amide urea and small alkyl amides in the bicyclo at the *meta* or *para* position showed a significant reduction of hERG inhibition, although the pharmacokinetic properties are altered and present a decrease in the AUC, suggesting that cyclic amides can provide greater stability of the compounds *in vivo* [138].

Biarylether derivatives have been synthesized. Based on these compounds several observations have been determined: a tertiary amine is preferred over a primary amine; The presence of a tertiary amine is common in MCH-R1 antagonists and represent a key point in the interaction with the receptor suggesting that the NH of the urea group is involved in a key interaction through hydrogen bonds with the receptor, a fact mentioned by other authors. This led to the discovery of the compound known as AMGN-608450 (**33**) (Fig. **24**), which has an IC_{50} value of 1.0 nM [139, 140].

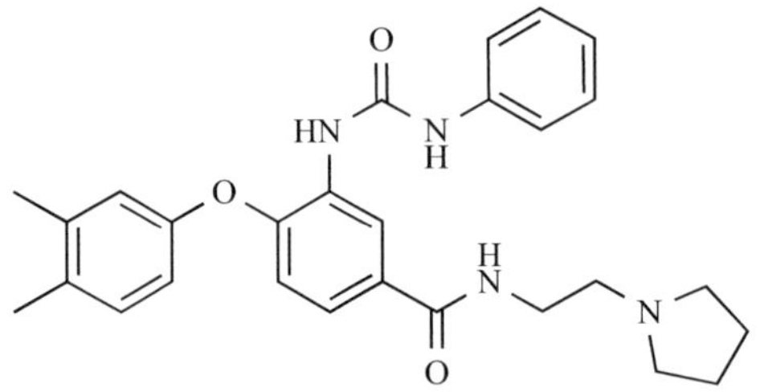

AMGN-608450 (**33**)

Fig. (24). Structure of compound AMGN-608450 (**33**).

In the program to discover new MCH-R1 antagonists, new potential spacers and substituents with different structural requirements have also explored, for example an amide group for the urea fraction or a methyl, or a nitrogen or oxygen atom, determining the following order of importance, O > NH, NME $\geq$ CH_2. This indicates that the amide fraction serves as a hydrogen donor in the interaction with the MCH-R1 receptor. In contrast, the 3-cyano group is the best substituent in the biaryl fraction in piperidine derivatives as in compound (**34**) (Fig. **25**), although interestingly some analogues that have a non-basic piperidine fraction are also very potent MCH-R1 antagonists with fractions such as benzimidazole and imidazole,

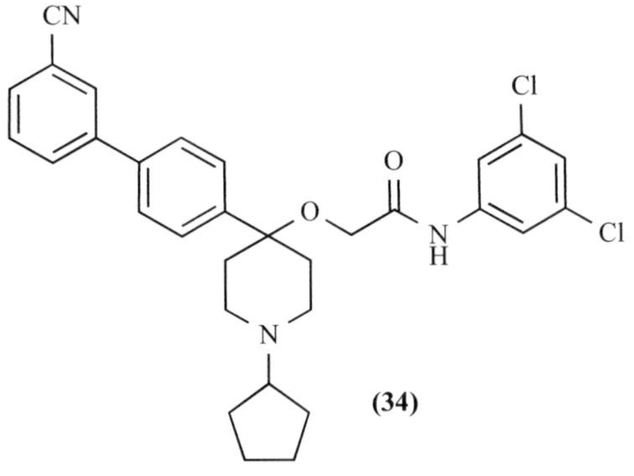

(**34**)

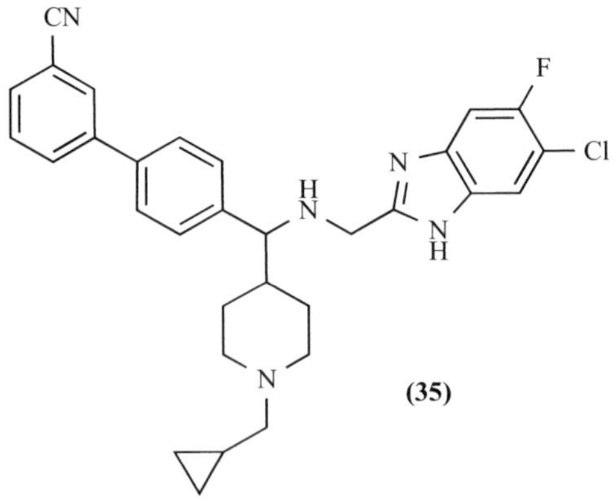

(**35**)

Fig. (25). Structures of compounds (**34**) and (**35**).

which have been used as isosteric replacements of the amide fraction to reduce the instability caused by the amide bond [141]. Changing the nitrogen of the biarylaniline fragment because of its mutagenic effect for a carbon atom of a vinyl group has also been suggested. Thus, the phenylamide fragment is replaced by an isosteric such as benzimidazole as in compound (**35**) (Fig. **25**). The SAR study of this type of compound shows that the fluor atom in position 5 and the trifluoromethyl group in position 6 are the best substituents. Furthermore, it was determined that the 3-cyano group in the terminal aryl is optimal for MCH-R1 affinity. Polar substituents such as N-piperidine are also tolerated, although these have less potency. Synthesized alkene analogues also have good exposure in rats, indicating that the substituted tetra olefins are metabolically more stable [142].

Diverse leading structures were identified using HTS, as in compound (**36**) (Fig. **26**), which presented a K_i value of 5 nM. Using SAR studies modifications of the amide substituents on the left and the substituent of the nitrogen of piperidine on the right side of the molecule were explored in order to determine the effect of changes in the basicity of the nitrogen atom on biological activity, determining that on the left side of the molecule, the benzyl amines were more active than other alkyl amines, suggesting that a *para* substitution is much better than a halogen atom substitution at the *meta* or *ortho* position. However, biological evaluation revealed that the biphenyl unit does not favor affinity [130]. Furthermore, using functional tests with MCH HEK293 cell lines compound (**37**), which presented an IC_{50} value of 0.13 nM, was found (Fig. **26**) [143].

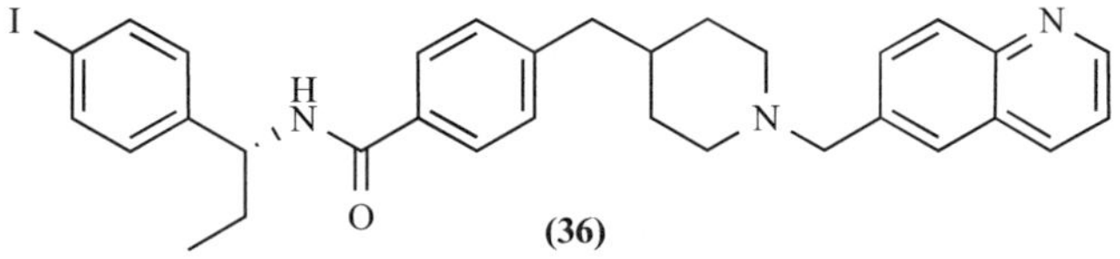

(36)

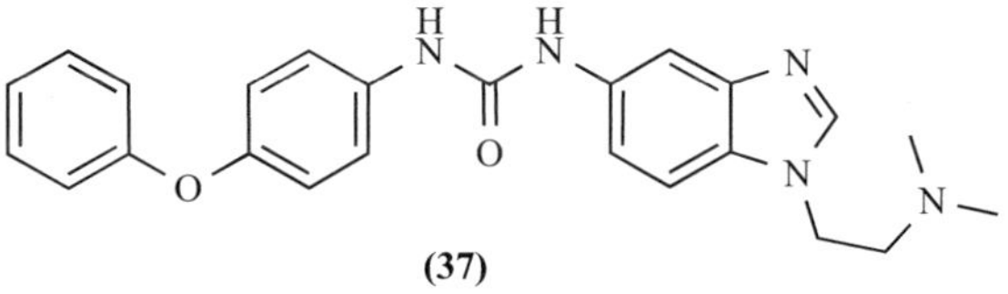

(37)

Fig. (26). Structures of compounds **(36)** and **(37)**.

Quinoline and Quinazoline Derivatives

The development of quinoline and quinazoline derived compounds as MCH-R1 antagonists was based on general structure (**38**) (Fig. **27**). SAR studies indicated that unicycle, bicyclic or tricyclic systems must be aromatic in origin with a substituent at R1 to increase charge density. At R2 the presence of a hydrogen atom is preferred since it favors MCH-R1 affinity and R3 and R4 should preferably present aliphatic substituents [144]. Following this strategy compound A-224940 (**39**) with an IC_{50} value of 91 nM was later discovered (Fig. **27**). The SAR study of this compound determined that the retention of basic nitrogen in the side chain is indicated to improve BBB passage and half-life, while large hydrophobic aliphatic substituents reduce affinity for MCH-R1 [145].

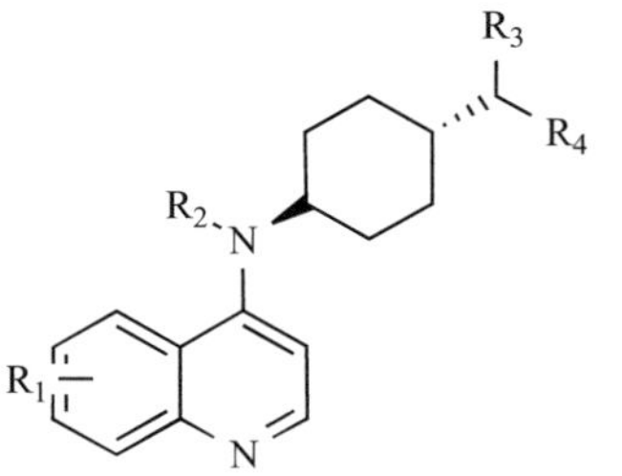

(38)

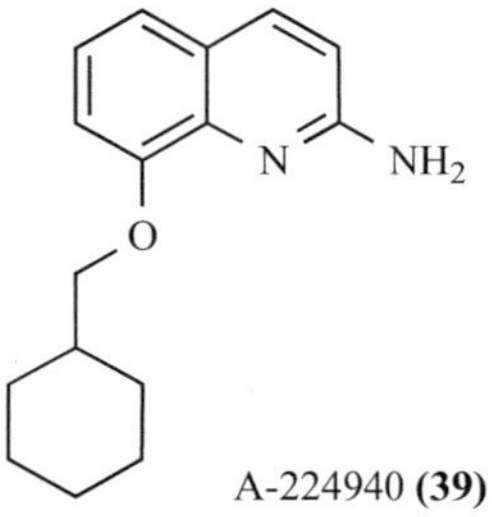

A-224940 **(39)**

Fig. (27). Structures of compounds **(38)** and A-224940 **(39)**.

Moreover, coupling studies confirmed the need for potential ligands for the western hydrophobic side of the receptor as was observed with compound T-226296. Studies suggest that Asp123 interacts preferentially with the nitrogen of the central quinoline. Thus, in compound (**40**) (Fig. **28**), which presents an IC_{50} value of 1.9 nM, it was suggested that the western side aromatic ring is coplanar with the quinoline system and high volume *para* substituents are optimal for MCH-R1 affinity. The importance of the basicity of amines was also observed, although it was found that piperidine analogues were less potent, corroborating the idea that electron donor properties of the 2-amino group are more important than any direct interaction with the binding site [106, 146]. Additionally, a series of new analogues of quinolines, which contain a basic amino group and two aromatic groups linked by an appropriate spacer, was designed. Thus, biaryl derivatives such as compound (**41**) (Fig. **28**) have potent binding to MCH-R1. However, placing a heteroatom at the benzene junction is harmful for activity. Another strategy for obtaining potent MCH-R1 antagonists was the placement of polar groups. Hydrogen bond acceptor substituents on the tertiary amine region and hydrogen methylation of the amide nitrogen allow conformational restriction around the amide group, which allows compounds to interact with the receptor in a favorable way [147]. Several authors have hypothesized that constriction of this amide bond within a cycle, forming a rigid system can improve activity [148, 149].

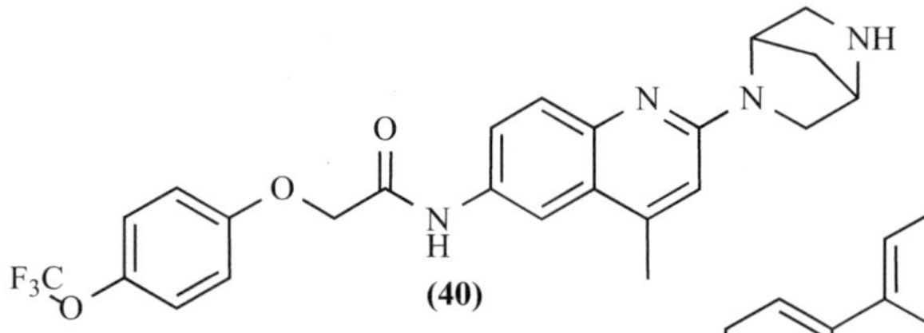

(**40**)

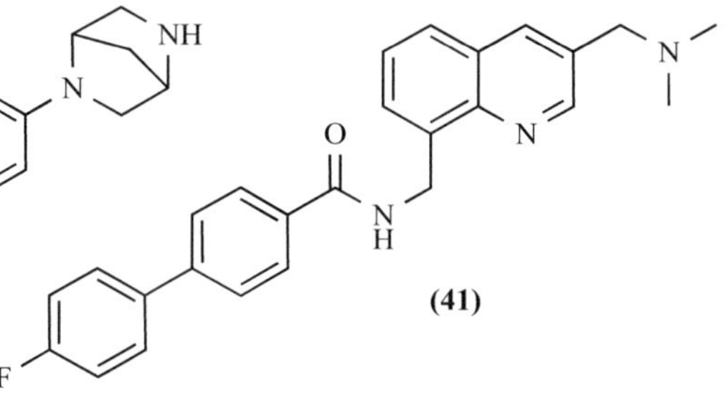
(**41**)

Fig. (28). Structures of compounds (**40**) and (**41**).

Argenta also developed 2-aminoquinoline derived compounds like compound (**42**) (Fig. **29**) with an IC_{50} value of 55 nM and good physicochemical properties. SAR studies indicated that ethyl or methyl substituents on the basic nitrogen did not significantly affect activity; the methyl substituent on the amide spacer has a detrimental effect; an aromatic group on the right side seems to be essential for proper activity, where changes in an aliphatic group produce poor activity and substitutions at *para* in terminal aromatic group seem to be necessary for potency. Additionally, lipophilic substituents such as chlorine seem to provide better potency than the methoxy group with a more polar nature.

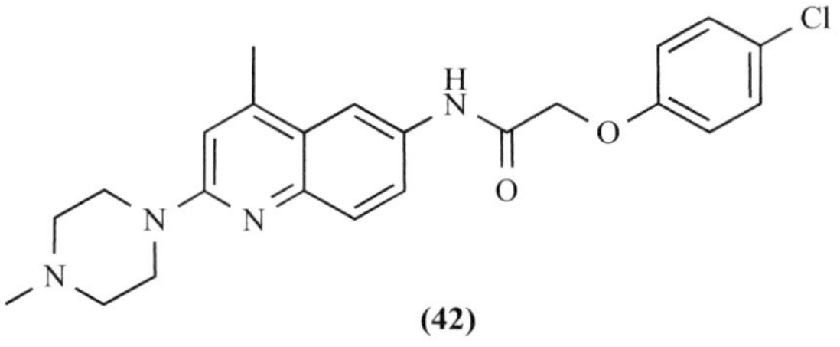

(**42**)

Fig. (29). Structure of compound (**42**).

Using the bovine rhodopsin model [150] analogue coupling studies of compound (**42**) have been conducted, postulating the following three interactions; first, a salt bridge formed between the tertiary amine of the piperazine moiety and Asp172, which is located at the extracellular end of helix 3. Second, in mutagenesis studies, the mutation D172A completely abolished MCH (agonists) binding, showing this residue to be critically important in the formation of the MCH peptide/receptor complex. Interestingly, Asp172 is in a position identical to that of the critical Asp residue found in biogenic amine receptors. Third, the amide carbonyl forms a hydrogen bond with the side chain of Gln325 located on helix 6, and the terminal chlorophenyl moiety is situated in an aromatic binding region comprising a number of phenylalanine residues from helices 5 and 6 [139].

It was also found that the removal of electron withdrawing substituents in these compounds, such as chlorine, methoxy, or trifluoromethyl provide more potent compounds. Furthermore, a steric requirement is needed in the *para* position and the basic nitrogen is not essential for MCH-R1 receptor affinity. However, these compounds showed affinity for other receptors in particular 5-HT_{2B} and 5-HT_{2C}; this is of great importance because 5-HT receptor activation has been implicated in the mechanism associated with cardiac valve disease and is the reason why D-fenfluramine was removed from the market [151]. Amino-piperidin quinoline derived compounds have been identified and characterized where SAR studies determined that small hydrophobic groups at position 6 on the quinoline-2(1H) ring confer high potency and substitutions on the quinazoline-2(1H) ring system do not adversely affect this class of compounds. Thus, compound **(43)** (Fig. **30**) provided derived anti-obesity agents with a better efficacy and safety window compared with benzamide and coumarin derivatives that have been previously described [152]. A series of potent and selective MCH-R1 inhibitors have been developed based on piperidine glycinamide derivatives [153]. However, these compounds have problems with moderate pharmacological properties mainly due to amide hydrolysis. These problems were minimized by designing structurally rigid compounds like compound **(44)** (Fig. **30**) of which tetrahydroisoquinoline showed better pharmacological properties. It was determined that the acylation and sulfonation of the piperidine nitrogen completely eliminates MCH-R1 receptor affinity, but groups such as hydroxipentyl, tetrahydropyranyl, and tetrahydrothienyl cyclopropyl urea helped to discover the most active compounds. These results determined that basic nitrogens are important for MCH-R1 affinity and show that the biaryl fraction of the molecule is less tolerant of substitutions, with the 3-cyanophenyl group substituent being the best in the biaryl region and heterocyclic substitutions such as 2-pyrrolyl and quinoline decreasing MCH-R1 affinity [134].

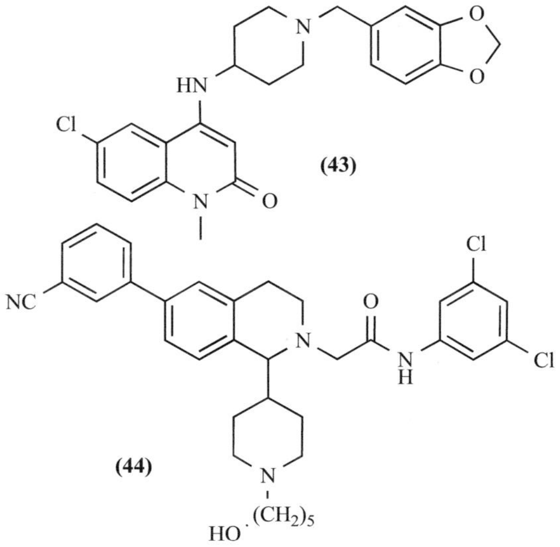

(43)

(44)

Fig. (30). Structures of compounds **(43)** and **(44)**.

Taisho Pharmaceuticals designed a series of quinazoline derived compounds as potent and selective MCH-R1 antagonists. Some compounds had an IC_{50} value of approximately 100 nM. The design of this type of derivatives allowed the identification of compound AR129330 **(45)** by HTS (Fig. **31**). SAR studies indicated that substitutions of the 4-amino and the terminal phenyl group of quinazoline are crucial for activity on the MCH-R1 receptor and form two key points in the pharmacophore together with *trans*-1,4-cyclohexane-dimethylenamine serving as a spacer of the two groups in a three dimensional space. Changing the relative orientation of the substituents around the cyclohexyl ring of AR29330 from *trans* to *cis* allows the creation of a compound with reduced activity. It is suggested that the stereochemistry of the spacer between the aromatic ring and the quinoxaline group are decisive factors for MCH-R1 affinity [154]. Subsequently, through a system optimization strategy of the space of the linker and the aromatic ring of the right portion of compound AR129330, ATCO175 was identified **(46)** (Fig. **31**) with a more potent antagonist activity for MCH-R1 with an IC_{50} value of 3.4 nM. It is important to point out the selectivity of the compound on MCH-R1 receptors rather than on α_{2A} receptors representing an improvement over compound AR129330. It was also shown that sulfonamide derivatives in general have a tendency to be metabolically less stable than those derived from amides and amines in rats and HLM assays [154]. Later efforts focused on finding the optimal distance between the two regions of the pharmacophore in *cis*-4-amine aminomethylcyclohexil derivatives, determining that the distance of three atoms is the optimum length for the cyclohexane and benzene ring. However, improving metabolic stability by maintaining good activity on MCH-R1 is only possible by modifying the position of the nitrogen atom. This optimization allowed the discovery of ATC0065 (**47**) (Fig. **31**) as a metabolically more stable MCH antagonist [100].

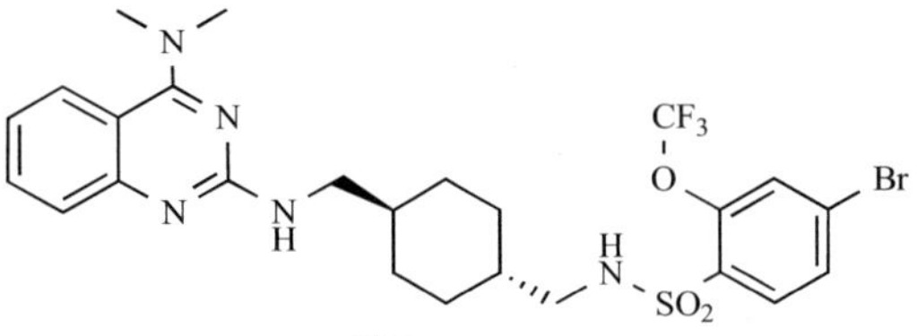

(45)

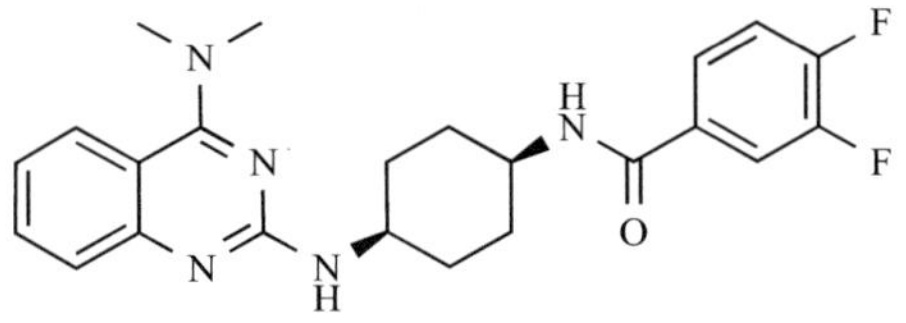

(46)

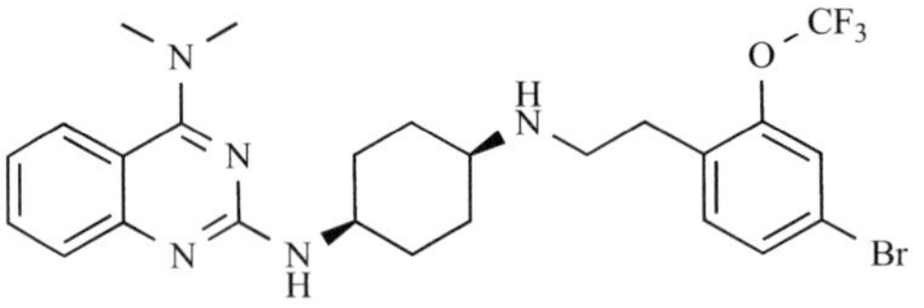

(47)

Fig. (31). Structures of compounds **(45)**, **(46)** and **(47)**.

Others Derivatives

Interestingly, other compounds without carboxamide, sulfonamide or urea fractions have been reported as MCH-R1antagonists. For example, piperazine and piperidine derived antagonists, such as compounds (**48**) and (**49**) (Fig. **32**) from the Neurogen group, are known for not using an amide or urea group in their structure [155]. Tularik synthesized a series of MCH-R1 antagonists, one of the best is compound (**50**) (Fig. **32**) [156].

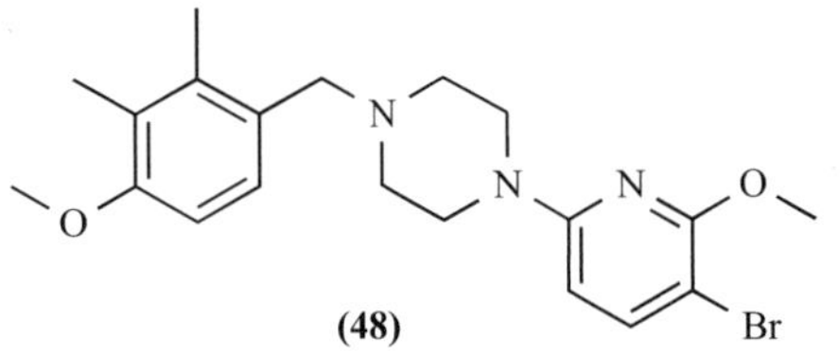

(48)

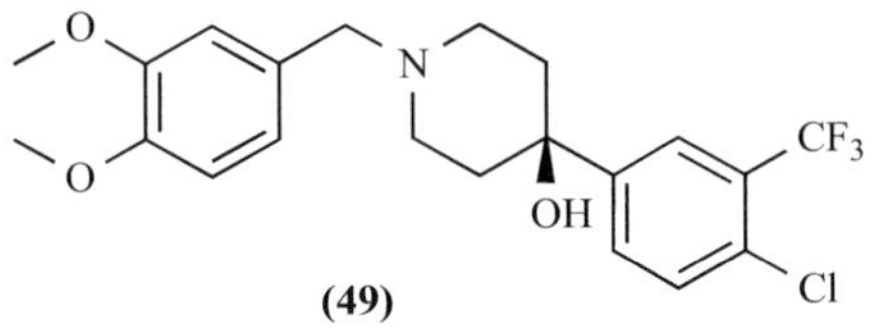

(49)

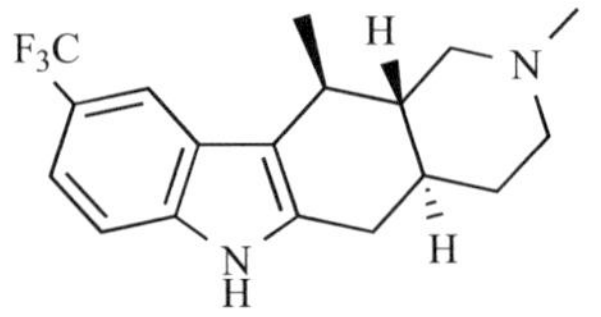

(50)

Fig. (32). Structures of compounds **(48)**, **(49)** and **(50)**.

Pharmacokinetic and Pharmacodynamic Properties

Carboxamides

Several carboxamide derived MCH-R1 antagonist compounds have presented interesting results of biological activity. In this section we mention the most relevant data regarding the most important antagonist compounds discovered so far by different research groups. The *in vivo* study of compound T-226296, after oral administration in rats at a dose of 30 mg/kg produced total suppression of food intake induced by the administration of MCH, which indicates that this compound has oral activity for the MCH-R1 receptor through passage of the BBB. However, one disadvantage was that this compound also showed affinity for the MCH-R2 receptor and receptors related with ion transport [68]. Later studies showed that T-226296 has an antagonistic effect because it reduces feeding by reducing meal size in obese rodents. Additionally, DABA-821, an analogue of T-226296, caused a dose-dependent weight loss in mice at a dose of 3 mg/kg compared with the vehicle. An autopsy at the end of treatment determined that body weight reduction was due solely to a reduction of adipose tissue mass and not to a reduction in other tissues such as skeletal muscle [157].

On the other hand, SNAP-7941, one of the first small molecule MCH antagonists, presented affinity for both the MCH-R1 receptor and 5-HT, NPY and galanin (GAL) receptors [158]. *In vivo* studies have determined that acute treatment with SNAP-7941 reduces appetite in rats and chronic treatment produces a significant sustained weight reduction in rats. Additionally, it has been shown that systemic administration of SNAP-7941 is capable of inhibiting the effects of central administration of MCH, presenting a moderate effect on food intake in comparison with fenfluramine; however, in DIO rats, SNAP-7941 produces a greater reduction in maintained body weight than with fenfluramine, suggesting that fenfluramine and SNAP-7941 have different mechanisms of action, and that SNAP-7941 causes a chronic blockade of MCH and low reduction in body weight that continues until the end of treatment [159]. Two other carboxamide derivatives that have shown interesting biological data are SB-568846, which exhibits good water solubility, a good pharmacokinetic profile and an oral bioavailability of 80% in rats and GW3430, which is active orally and causes a significant and dose-dependent weight loss of 13.3% in obese AKE mice over a period of 12 days at a dose of 3 mg/kg [160]. Additionally, the analogue of GW3430, compound (**8**), presents interesting data because during 21 days of oral treatment once daily at a dose of 1, 3 and 1 mg/kg, it produced a dose-dependent weight loss of 1.1, 3.2 and 11.8%, respectively. In the same study, rimonabant, a cannabinoid receptor antagonist approved by the FDA, caused a weight loss of 8.4% [103]. In addition, several analogs of compound GW3430 have shown excellent pharmacokinetic results, for example, compound (**51**) (Fig. **32**) exhibits a good oral bioavailability of 19% with a low clearance rate of 11 mL/min/kg and a good half-life of 8 hours; however, substitution with a fluor atom or a trifluoromethyl group at position 4 of the phenylpiperazine can block the potential metabolism of these compounds and significantly increase half-life to 16 hours. Furthermore, piperazine methylation can produce a compound with a bioavailability of 98%, a suitable half-life of 7.7 hours and a clearance of 39.7 mL/min/kg with this being the best compound of this type of derivatives since it also does not have activity on ion and hERG channels receptors [102]. With regard to the pharmacodynamic properties of compound (**51**) (Fig. **33**), it induces weight loss in a model of DIO AKR/J rats and after oral administration for 26 days at 1, 3 and 10 mg/kg daily, produced a dose-dependent weight loss of 4.8, 9.4 and 16.9%, respectively. An analysis of the concentration of the compound in serum and brain determined that the compound is absorbed in the circulation. Additionally, the carboxamide derivative, compound (**11**) exhibits a good oral bioavailability of 32% and good efficacy *in vivo* in rats suggests that in addition to its anorectic effects, MCH-R1 antagonists may lead to metabolic changes [105].

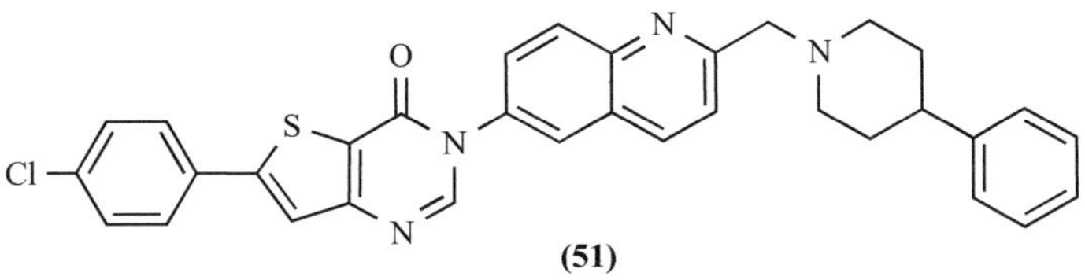

(51)

Fig. (33). Structure of compound **(51)**.

Moreover, it has been postulated that the non-relationship between *in vitro* and *in vivo* activity of the compounds may be due to poor penetration of the BBB, an essential requirement for MCH-R1 antagonists, since these receptors are mainly in the central nervous system [113]. Based on the above, several compounds that do not present the classic biphenyl or phenylthienopyrimidinone fraction of MCH-R1 antagonists in their structure have presented biological activity results of great interest. Thus, compound (**51**) (Fig. **33**) derived from piperonyl produced the best combination of a potent functional antagonist with metabolic stability and an exposure value in the brain with an AUC of 4.17 µg.h/g and in plasma of 6.35 µg.h/mL at an oral dose of 10 mg/kg in DIO mice [119]. Moreover, compound **(51)** presented prolonged exposure in the brain at an oral dose of 30 mg/kg with a dose-dependent weight loss that led to normalization of body weight in 13 days of dosing. However, this compound did not present an acceptable therapeutic index with regard to multiple adverse hemodynamic cardiovascular parameters after administration of an intravenous dose in dogs. In addition, vascular toxicity has been observed at low micromolar concentrations in anesthetized dog trials [119]. Unfortunately, although oral doses appeared to be well tolerated in chronic studies of efficacy, these compounds cause hemodynamic effects at low concentrations, which limit their development. Interestingly, a structural analogue showed a similar profile in the pentobarbital anesthetized dog cardiovascular model, suggesting that the effect of cardiotoxicity is linked to the special conformation of the structure of the compound and not to the activity on the MCH-R1 receptor [111, 119]. The need to screen the compounds against cardiovascular adverse effects at an early stage in an optimization program of leading compounds, incorporating cardiovascular tests in an inaction-anesthetized rat model was also identified. This method of early detection reflects a high priority on cardiovascular safety and represents a new quick strategy to find lead compounds in a drug discovery program [111]. Additionally, aminopiperidine derived MCH-R1 antagonist compounds (**52**) and (**53**) (Fig. **34**) showed a high plasma concentration and sustained efficacy in dose-dependent weight loss in an obese mouse model. The optimization of these compounds led to the discovery of compound (**54**) (Fig. **34**) that is effective orally in a DIO mouse model, maintaining a favorable cardiovascular profile in rats and showing a marked improvement on blood pressure effects in a dog cardiovascular model in comparison with other series. With regard to cardiovascular safety, this compound became the best heterocycle from a series of aminopiperidine derivatives. However, this analog showed QT interval prolongation in dogs, which was associated with an affinity for hERG channels with an unexpected functional potency for blocking these channels [159].

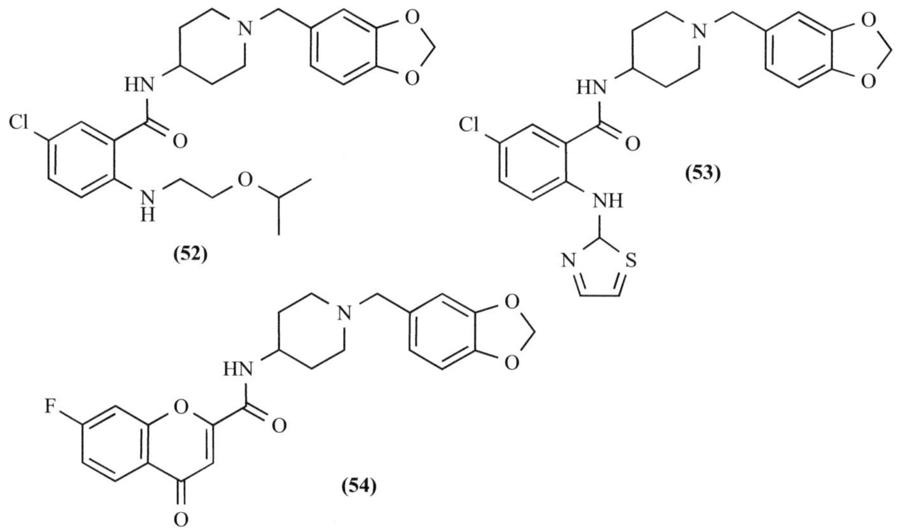

Fig. (34). Structures of compounds **(52)**, **(53)** and **(54)**.

The optimization of pyrrolidinethylindol derivatives as MCH-R1 antagonists led to the discovery of compound (**55**) (Fig. **35**). This compound has a high affinity for the MCH-R1 receptor and proved to be a potent inhibitor of MCH measured by the release of Ca^{2+}, showing good exposure in the CNS and plasma at an oral dose in DIO mice, being the first MCH-R1 antagonist that is effective at an oral dose in a model of chronic weight loss [160].

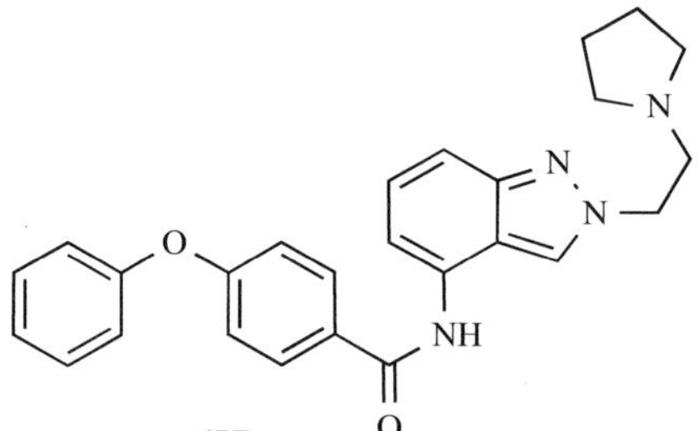

(55)

Fig. (35). Structure of compound **(55)**.

SNAP-94847 exhibits a bioavailability of 59%, a low blood and plasma clearance of 4.2 L/hr/kg and 3.3 L/hr/kg, respectively, and a half-life of 5.2 h in rats. Interestingly, brain levels in rats at 4 h were 2.3 times higher than plasma levels at an oral dose of 10 mg/kg. It has also been reported that MCH stimulates water intake independent of food intake, so the effect of SNAP-94847 on water intake was evaluated, determining that the compound inhibits water intake induced by MCH administration at doses of 1, 2.5 and 10 mg/kg.

Urease

In urea derived MCH-R1 antagonists, there have also been problems with the pharmacokinetic and pharmacodynamic properties of compounds. For example, compound (**22**) is rapidly metabolized *in vitro* with HLM with an intrinsic clearance of 50 mL/min/kg. These data predict that the compound will also be rapidly eliminated *in vivo* [125]. In contrast, compound (**24**) has a promising stability in *in vitro* metabolic profiles and exhibits good stability in HLM trials with no significant inhibition of major CYP450 metabolizing enzymes [127]. In addition, MCH-R1 antagonist compounds derived from spyrohydantoin with a K_i value of 50 nM have been discovered. However, these compounds showed potent inhibition of CYP3A4 with an IC_{50} value of 35 nM, which hinders their metabolism. It was determined that the imidazole ring is involved in a potent inhibition of CYP3A4, although the imidazole can be replaced by a 3 or 4-pyridyl fraction with no loss of activity on MCH-R1 receptors. Finally, compound (**25**) was discovered, which has better pharmacokinetic properties with a clearance of 25 mL/kg and an IC_{50} greater than 10 000 nM on CYP3A4. Additionally, compound (**27**), a urea derivative, presents good plasma levels after oral administration in rats, including good levels in the brain, 579 ng/n at 6 hours, with excellent *in vitro* activity and moderate *in vivo* activity. These compounds stopped being developed because of the presence of high mutagenicity of the biarylaniline subunit [131]. Compound (**27**) was orally effective in an obese rodent model of 28 days, showing a decrease in food intake and a selective decrease in fat mass in relation to lean body mass. It has been mentioned that there is no evidence from preliminary studies that the same biarylamine is formed *in vivo* from MCH-R1 antagonist compounds that contain this fragment in its molecule. These compounds are considered inappropriate for development because of the potential risk of exposure to this highly mutagenic precursor, suggesting that substitutions in the distal aryl ring may have little or no effect in relation to the effects of mutagenicity of biarylamines and that the changes of the aniline part of the molecule could have a major impact on the mutagenic effects [135]. Another urea derivative with interesting biological data is compound (**33**) with a half-life of 1.5 hours and a maximum concentration in the brain of 31.5 ng/g [140]. Two analogues of compound (**35**) have presented a robust reduction in food intake after an oral dose of 30 mg/kg in a fasted DIO mouse model and compound 46 showed good anorexigenic activity *in vivo*, producing a 38% reduction in milk consumption when administered orally to mice at a dose of 10 mg/kg [144, 145]. Subsequently, structural changes in compound (**39**) produced two potent MCH-R1 antagonists with IC_{50} values of 3.0 and 5.0 nM and an AUC in the brain of 11 ng.hr/mL and 9521 ng.hr/mL. However, it must be considered that several studies have shown that an *ex vivo* affinity of 60% correlates with activity in the DIO rat model. These results have established *ex vivo* affinity as one of the primary indicators of *in vivo* efficacy [135]. Finally, GlaxoSmithKline reported in 2004 a phase I clinical evaluation of the first MCH antagonist compound, an analogue of compound GW3430, for the pharmacological treatment of obesity [99, 155]. In the same year Amgen also reported that its compound AMG-076 was ready to enter Phase I clinical evaluation. However, to date, the status of these compounds has not been reported and in recent years only NGD-4715 from the company Neurogen has been included in a phase I clinical evaluation study [112]. Several companies have dedicated great efforts to develop new small molecule derivatives as potential MCH-R1 receptor antagonists for the pharmacological treatment of obesity. However, a limited number of these compounds have progressed to clinical trials. This is possibly due to the absorption, distribution, metabolism and excretion properties that these drugs must have and the safety profile necessary because of the cardiovascular risk that they can cause because of their activity on hERG and the induction of prolonged QTc.

CONCLUSION

There have been several approaches to obtain active compounds suitable to be used as MCH-R1 antagonist and help to reduce weight, such as the peptidic, carboxamide, urea and quinoline derivatives reviewed in this chapter. However there have been several degrees of success in reaching this goal, especially in achieving good pharmacodynamic and pharmacokinetic properties and this along with safety concerns of the use of such compounds on humans, further investigations is still necessary in order to validate MCH-R1 as a drug target or discard it in order to study other more promising drug targets.

REFERENCES

[1] Kawauchi H, Kawazoe I, Tsubokawa M, Kishida M, Baker BI. Characterization of melanin-concentrating hormone in chum salmon pituitaries. Nature 1983; 30: 321-3.

[2] Mouri T, Takahashi K, Kawauchi H, *et al*. Melanin-concentrating hormone in the human brain. Peptides 1993; 14: 643-6.

[3] Saito Y, Nothacker HP, Civelli O. Melanin-concentrating hormone receptor: an orphan receptor fits the key. Trends Endocrinol Metab 2000; 11: 299-303.
[4] Schwartz MW, Woods SC, Porte D Jr, Seeley RJ, Baskin DG. Central nervous system control of food intake. Nature 2000; 404: 661-71.
[5] Vaughan JM, Fischer WH, Hoeger C, Rivier J, Vale W. Characterization of melanin-concentrating hormone from rat hypothalamus. Endocrinology 1989; 125: 1660-5.
[6] Sailer AW, Sano H, Zeng Z, McDonald TP, *et al.* Identification and characterization of a second melanin-concentrating hormone receptor, MCH-2R. Proc Natl Acad Sci USA 2001; 98: 7564-9.
[7] Köhler C, Haglund L, Swanson LW. A diffuse alpha MSH-immunoreactive projection to the hippocampus and spinal cord from individual neurons in the lateral hypothalamic area and zona incerta. J Comp Neurol 1984; 223: 501-14.
[8] Pissios P, Bradley RL, Maratos-Flier E. Expanding the scales: The multiple roles of MCH in regulating energy balance and other biological functions. Endocr Rev 2006; 27: 606-20.
[9] Bittencourt JC, Presse F, Arias C, *et al.* The melanin-concentrating hormone system of the rat brain: an immune and hybridization histochemical characterization. J Comp Neurol 1992; 319: 218-45.
[10] Saper CB, Chou TC, Elmquist JK. The need to feed: homeostatic and hedonic control of eating. Neuron 2002; 36: 199-211.
[11] Nahon JL. The melanocortins and melanin-concentrating hormone in the central regulation of feeding behavior and energy homeostasis. C R Biol 2006; 329: 623-38.
[12] Adamantidis A, de Lecea L. Physiological arousal: a role for hypothalamic systems. Cell Mol Life Sci 2008; 65: 1475-88.
[13] Borowsky B, Durkin MM, Ogozalek K, *et al.* Antidepressant, anxiolytic and anorectic effects of a melanin-concentrating hormone-1 receptor antagonist. Nat Med 2002; 8: 825-30.
[14] Gehlert DR, Rasmussen K, Shaw J, *et al.* Preclinical evaluation of melanin-concentrating hormone receptor 1 antagonism for the treatment of obesity and depression. J Pharmacol Exp Ther 2009; 329: 429-38.
[15] Adamantidis A, de Lecea L. A role for Melanin-Concentrating Hormone in learning and memory. Peptides 2009; 30: 2066-70.
[16] Lakaye B, Coumans B, Harray S, Grisar T. Melanin-concentrating hormone and immune function. Peptides 2009; 30: 2076-80.
[17] Qu D, Ludwig DS, Gammeltoft S, *et al.* A role for melanin-concentrating hormone in the central regulation of feeding behavior. Nature 1996; 380: 243-7.
[18] Aughton KL, Hamilton-Smith K, Gupta J, Morton JS, Wayman CP, Jackson VM. Pharmacological profiling of neuropeptides on rabbit vaginal wall and vaginal artery smooth muscle *in vitro*. Br J Pharmacol 2008; 155: 236-43.
[19] Kokkotou E, Mastaitis JW, Qu D, *et al.* Characterization of [Phe(13), Tyr(19)]-MCH analog binding activity to the MCH receptor. Neuropeptides 2000; 34: 240-7.
[20] Pissios P, Ozcan U, Kokkotou E, *et al.* Melanin concentrating hormone is a novel regulator of islet function and growth. Diabetes 2007; 56: 311-9.
[21] Rossi M, Choi SJ, O'Shea D, Miyoshi T, Ghatei MA, Bloom SR. Melanin-concentrating hormone acutely stimulates feeding, but chronic administration has no effect on body weight. Endocrinology 1997; 138: 351-5.
[22] Shimada M, Tritos NA, Lowell BB, Flier JS, Maratos-Flier E. Mice lacking melanin-concentrating hormone are hypophagic and lean. Nature 1998; 396: 670-4.
[23] Clegg DJ, Air EL, Benoit SC, Sakai RS, Seeley RJ, Woods SC. Intraventricular melanin-concentrating hormone stimulates water intake independent of food intake. Am J Physiol Regul Integr Comp Physiol 2003; 284: R494-9.
[24] Morens C, Nørregaard P, Receveur JM, Van Dijk G, Scheurink AJ. Effects of MCH and a MCH1-receptor antagonist on (palatable) food and water intake. Brain Res 2005; 1062: 32-8.
[25] Hervieu GJ, Cluderay JE, Harrison D, *et al.* The distribution of the mRNA and protein products of the melanin- concentrating hormone (MCH) receptor gene, slc-1, in the central nervous system of the rat. Eur J Neurosci 2000; 12: 1194-216.
[26] Saito Y, Cheng M, Leslie FM, Civelli O. Expression of the melanin-concentrating hormone (MCH) receptor mRNA in the rat brain. J Comp Neurol 2001; 435: 26-40.
[27] Ludwig DS, Tritos NA, Mastaitis JW, *et al.* Melanin-concentrating hormone overexpression in transgenic mice leads to obesity and insulin resistance. J Clin Invest 2001; 107: 379-86.
[28] Kokkotou E, Jeon JY, Wang X, *et al.* Mice with MCH ablation resist diet-induced obesity through strain-specific mechanisms. Am J Physiol Regul Integr Comp Physiol 2005; 289: R117-24.
[29] Stricker-Krongrad A, Dimitrov T, Beck B. Central and peripheral dysregulation of melanin-concentrating hormone in obese Zucker rats. Brain Res Mol Brain Res 2001; 92: 43-8.
[30] Bradley RL, Kokkotou EG, Maratos-Flier E, Cheatham B. Melanin-concentrating hormone regulates leptin synthesis and secretion in rat adipocytes. Diabetes 2000; 49: 1073-7.
[31] Tadayyon M, Welters HJ, Haynes AC, Cluderay JE, Hervieu G. Expression of melanin-concentrating hormone receptors in insulin-producing cells: MCH stimulates insulin release in RINm5F and CRI-G1 cell-lines. Biochem Biophys Res Commun 2000; 275: 709-12.
[32] Kennedy AR, Todd JF, Dhillo WS, *et al.* Effect of direct injection of melanin-concentrating hormone into the paraventricular nucleus: further evidence for a stimulatory role in the adrenal axis via SLC-1. J Neuroendocrinol 2003; 15: 268-72.
[33] Kennedy AR, Todd JF, Stanley SA, *et al.* Melanin-concentrating hormone (MCH) suppresses thyroid stimulating hormone (TSH) release, *in vivo* and *in vitro*, via the hypothalamus and the pituitary. Endocrinology 2001; 142: 3265-8.
[34] Murray JF, Mercer JG, Adan RA, *et al.* The effect of leptin on luteinizing hormone release is exerted in the zona incerta and mediated by melanin-concentrating hormone. J Neuroendocrinol 2000; 12: 1133-9.
[35] Tsukamura H, Thompson RC, Tsukahara S, *et al.* Intracerebroventricular administration of melanin-concentrating hormone suppresses pulsatile luteinizing hormone release in the female rat. J Neuroendocrinol 2000; 12: 529-34.
[36] Saito Y, Nothacker HP, Wang Z, Lin SH, Leslie F, Civelli O. Molecular characterization of the melanin-concentrating-hormone receptor. Nature 1999; 400: 265-9.
[37] Mori M, Harada M, Terao Y, *et al.* Cloning of a novel G protein-coupled receptor, SLT, a subtype of the melanin-concentrating hormone receptor. Biochem Biophys Res Commun 2001; 283: 1013-8.
[38] Pissios P. Animals models of MCH function and what they can tell us about its role in energy balance. Peptides 2009; 30: 2040-4.

[39] Bohlooly-Y M, Mahlapuu M, Andersén H, *et al.* Osteoporosis in MCHR1-deficient mice. Biochem Biophys Res Commun 2004; 318: 964-9.

[40] Gibson WT, Pissios P, Trombly DJ, *et al.* Melanin-concentrating hormone receptor mutations and human obesity: functional analysis. Obes Res 2004; 12: 743-9.

[41] Hawes BE, Green B, O'Neill K, *et al.* Identification and characterization of single-nucleotide polymorphisms in MCH-R1 and MCH-R2. Obes Res 2004; 12: 1327-34.

[42] Rossi M, Choi SJ, O'Shea D, Miyoshi T, Ghatei MA, Bloom SR. Melanin-concentrating hormone acutely stimulates feeding, but chronic administration has no effect on body weight. Endocrinology 1997; 138: 351-5.

[43] Gomori A, Ishihara A, Ito M, *et al.* Chronic intracerebroventricular infusion of MCH causes obesity in mice. Melanin-concentrating hormone. Am J Physiol Endocrinol Metab 2003; 284: E583-8.

[44] Ito M, Gomori A, Ishihara A, *et al.* Characterization of MCH-mediated obesity in mice. Am J Physiol Endocrinol Metab 2003; 284: E940-5.

[45] Abbott CR, Kennedy AR, Wren AM, *et al.* Identification of hypothalamic nuclei involved in the orexigenic effect of melanin-concentrating hormone. Endocrinology 2003; 144: 3943-9.

[46] Whitlock BK, Daniel JA, McMahon CD, *et al.* Intracerebroventricular melanin-concentrating hormone stimulates food intake in sheep. Domest Anim Endocrinol 2005; 28: 224-32.

[47] Pereira-da-Silva M, Torsoni MA, Nourani HV, *et al.* Hypothalamic melanin-concentrating hormone is induced by cold exposure and participates in the control of energy expenditure in rats. Endocrinology 2003; 144: 4831-40.

[48] Jeon JY, Bradley RL, Kokkotou EG, *et al.* MCH-/- mice are resistant to aging-associated increases in body weight and insulin resistance. Diabetes 2006; 55: 428-34.

[49] Segal-Lieberman G, Bradley RL, Kokkotou E, *et al.* Melanin-concentrating hormone is a critical mediator of the leptin-deficient phenotype. Proc Natl Acad Sci USA 2003; 100: 10085-90.

[50] Sahu A. Leptin decreases food intake induced by melanin-concentrating hormone (MCH), galanin (GAL) and neuropeptide Y (NPY) in the rat. Endocrinology 1998; 139: 4739-42.

[51] Morton GJ, Mystkowski P, Matsumoto AM, Schwartz MW. Increased hypothalamic melanin concentrating hormone gene expression during energy restriction involves a melanocortin-independent, estrogen-sensitive mechanism. Peptides 2004; 25: 667-74.

[52] Bächner D, Kreienkamp H, Weise C, Buck F, Richter D. Identification of melanin concentrating hormone (MCH) as the natural ligand for the orphan somatostatin-like receptor 1 (SLC-1). FEBS Lett 1999; 457: 522-4.

[53] Chambers J, Ames RS, Bergsma D, *et al.* Melanin-concentrating hormone is the cognate ligand for the orphan G-protein-coupled receptor SLC-1. Nature 1999; 400: 261-5.

[54] Lembo PM, Grazzini E, Cao J, *et al.* The receptor for the orexigenic peptide melanin-concentrating hormone is a G-protein-coupled receptor. Nat Cell Biol 1999; 1: 267-71.

[55] Kolakowski LF Jr, Jung BP, Nguyen T, *et al.* Characterization of a human gene related to genes encoding somatostatin receptors. FEBS Lett 1996; 398: 253-8.

[56] Tan CP, Sano H, Iwaasa H, *et al.* Melanin-concentrating hormone receptor subtypes 1 and 2: species-specific gene expression. Genomics 2002; 79: 785-92.

[57] Berman JR, Skariah G, Maro GS, Mignot E, Mourrain P. Characterization of two melanin-concentrating hormone genes in zebrafish reveals evolutionary and physiological links with the mammalian MCH system. J Comp Neurol 2009; 517: 695-710.

[58] Mizusawa K, Saito Y, Wang Z, Kobayashi Y, Matsuda K, Takahashi A. Molecular cloning and expression of two melanin-concentrating hormone receptors in goldfish. Peptides 2009; 30: 1990-6.

[59] Hawes BE, Kil E, Green B, O'Neill K, Fried S, Graziano MP. The melanin-concentrating hormone receptor couples to multiple G proteins to activate diverse intracellular signaling pathways. Endocrinology 2000; 141: 4524-32.

[60] An S, Cutler G, Zhao JJ, *et al.* Identification and characterization of a melanin-concentrating hormone receptor. Proc Natl Acad Sci USA 2001; 98: 7576-81.

[61] Saito Y, Nothacker HP, Wang Z, Lin SH, Leslie F, Civelli O. Molecular characterization of the melanin-concentrating-hormone receptor. Nature 1999; 400: 265-9.

[62] Shearman LP, Camacho RE, Sloan Stribling D, *et al.* Chronic MCH-1 receptor modulation alters appetite, body weight and adiposity in rats. Eur J Pharmacol 2003; 475: 37-47.

[63] Verlaet M, Adamantidis A, Coumans B, *et al.* Human immune cells express ppMCH mRNA and functional MCHR1 receptor. FEBS Lett 2002; 527: 205-10.

[64] Borowsky B, Durkin MM, Ogozalek K, *et al.* Antidepressant, anxiolytic and anorectic effects of a melanin-concentrating hormone-1 receptor antagonist. Nat Med 2002; 8: 825-30.

[65] Chaki S, Funakoshi T, Hirota-Okuno S, *et al.* Anxiolytic- and antidepressant-like profile of ATC0065 and ATC0175: nonpeptidic and orally active melanin-concentrating hormone receptor 1 antagonists. J Pharmacol Exp Ther 2005; 313: 831-9.

[66] Chaki S, Yamaguchi J, Yamada H, *et al.* ATC0175: an orally active melanin-concentrating hormone receptor 1 antagonist for the potential treatment of depression and anxiety. CNS Drug Rev 2005; 11: 341-52.

[67] Messina MM, Overton JM. Cardiovascular effects of melanin-concentrating hormone. Regul Pept 2007; 139: 23-30.

[68] Takekawa S, Asami A, Ishihara Y, *et al.* T-226296: a novel, orally active and selective melanin-concentrating hormone receptor antagonist. Eur J Pharmacol 2002; 438: 129-35.

[69] Marsh DJ, Weingarth DT, Novi DE, *et al.* Melanin-concentrating hormone 1 receptor-deficient mice are lean, hyperactive, and hyperphagic and have altered metabolism. Proc Natl Acad Sci USA 2002; 99: 3240-5.

[70] Chen Y, Hu C, Hsu CK, *et al.* Targeted disruption of the melanin-concentrating hormone receptor-1 results in hyperphagia and resistance to diet-induced obesity. Endocrinology 2002; 143: 2469-77.

[71] Chung S, Saito Y, Civelli O. MCH receptors/gene structure-*in vivo* expression. Peptides 2009; 30: 1985-9.

[72] Unmehopa UA, Van Heerikhuize JJ, Spijkstra W, *et al.* Increased melanin concentrating hormone receptor type I in the human hypothalamic infundibular nucleus in cachexia. J Clin Endocrinol Metab 2005; 90: 2412-9.

[73] Astrand A, Bohlooly-Y M, Larsdotter S, *et al.* Mice lacking melanin-concentrating hormone receptor 1 demonstrate increased heart rate associated with altered autonomic activity. Am J Physiol Regul Integr Comp Physiol 2004; 287: R749-58.

[74] Viale A, Ortola C, Hervieu G, *et al.* Cellular localization and role of prohormone convertases in the processing of pro-melanin concentrating hormone in mammals. J Biol Chem 1999; 274: 6536-45.

[75] Gonzalez MI, Vaziri S, Wilson CA. Behavioral effects of alpha-MSH and MCH after central administration in the female rat. Peptides 1996; 17: 171-7.

[76] Neary NM, Goldstone AP, Bloom SR. Appetite regulation: from the gut to the hypothalamus. Clin Endocrinol (Oxf) 2004; 60: 153-60.

[77] Jebb SA, Siervo M, Murgatroyd PR, Evans S, Frühbeck G, Prentice AM. Validity of the leg-to-leg bioimpedance to estimate changes in body fat during weight loss and regain in overweight women: a comparison with multi-compartment models. Int J Obes (Lond) 2007; 31: 756-62.

[78] Seeley RJ, Woods SC. Monitoring of stored and available fuel by the CNS: implications for obesity. Nat Rev Neurosci 2003; 4: 901-9.

[79] Handlon AL, Zhou H. Melanin-concentrating hormone-1 receptor antagonists for the treatment of obesity. J Med Chem 2006; 49: 4017-22.

[80] Mashiko S, Ishihara A, Gomori A, *et al.* Antiobesity effect of a melanin-concentrating hormone 1 receptor antagonist in diet-induced obese mice. Endocrinology 2005; 146: 3080-6.

[81] David DJ, Klemenhagen KC, Holick KA, *et al.* Efficacy of the MCHR1 antagonist N-[3-(1-{[4-(3,4-difluorophenoxy)phenyl]methyl}(4-piperidyl))-4-methylphenyl]-2-m ethylpropanamide (SNAP 94847) in mouse models of anxiety and depression following acute and chronic administration is independent of hippocampal neurogenesis. J Pharmacol Exp Ther 2007; 321: 237-48.

[82] Smith DG, Davis RJ, Rorick-Kehn L, *et al.* Melanin-concentrating hormone-1 receptor modulates neuroendocrine, behavioral, and corticolimbic neurochemical stress responses in mice. Neuropsychopharmacology 2006; 31: 1135-45.

[83] Millan MJ, Gobert A, Panayi F, *et al.* The melanin-concentrating hormonel receptor antagonists, SNAP-7941 and GW3430, enhance social recognition and dialysate levels of acetylcholine in the frontal cortex of rats. Int J Neuropsychopharmacol 2008; 11: 1105-22.

[84] Adamantidis A, Thomas E, Foidart A, *et al.* Disrupting the melanin-concentrating hormone receptor 1 in mice leads to cognitive deficits and alterations of NMDA receptor function. Eur J Neurosci 2005; 21: 2837-44.

[85] Hill J, Duckworth M, Murdock P, *et al.* Molecular cloning and functional characterization of MCH2, a novel human MCH receptor. J Biol Chem 2001; 276: 20125-97.

[86] Rodriguez M, Beauverger P, Naime I, *et al.* Cloning and molecular characterization of the novel human melanin-concentrating hormone receptor MCH2. Mol Pharmacol 2001; 60: 632-9.

[87] Wang S, Behan J, O'Neill K, *et al.* Identification and pharmacological characterization of a novel human melanin-concentrating hormone receptor, mch-r2. J Biol Chem 2001; 276: 34664-70.

[88] Schwarz DA, Allen MM, Petroski RE, *et al.* Manipulation of small-molecule inhibitory kinetics modulates MCH-R1 function. Mol Cell Endocrinol 2006; 259: 1-9.

[89] Yang J, Yuan C, Wei L, Yi F, Song F. Melanin-concentrating hormone receptor 2 affects 3T3-L1 preadipocyte differentiation. Mol Cell Endocrinol 2009; 311: 11-7.

[90] Bell CG, Meyre D, Samson C, *et al.* Association of melanin-concentrating hormone receptor 1 5' polymorphism with early-onset extreme obesity. Diabetes 2005; 54: 3049-55.

[91] Chaffer CL, Morris MJ. The feeding response to melanin-concentrating hormone is attenuated by antagonism of the NPY Y(1)-receptor in the rat. Endocrinology 2002; 143: 191-7.

[92] Rossi M, Beak SA, Choi SJ, *et al.* Investigation of the feeding effects of melanin concentrating hormone on food intake-action independent of galanin and the melanocortin receptors. Brain Res 1999; 846: 164-70.

[93] Bednarek MA, Feighner SD, Hreniuk DL, *et al.* Short segment of human melanin-concentrating hormone that is sufficient for full activation of human melanin-concentrating hormone receptors 1 and 2. Biochemistry 2001; 40: 9379-86.

[94] Audinot V, Lahaye C, Suply T, *et al.* [125I]-S36057: a new and highly potent radioligand for the melanin-concentrating hormone receptor. Br J Pharmacol 2001; 133: 371-8.

[95] Bednarek MA, Hreniuk DL, Tan C, *et al.* Synthesis and biological evaluation *in vitro* of selective, high affinity peptide antagonists of human melanin-concentrating hormone action at human melanin-concentrating hormone receptor 1. Biochemistry 2002; 41: 6383-90.

[96] Witty DR, Bateson J, Hervieu GJ, *et al.* Discovery of potent and stable conformationally constrained analogues of the MCH R1 antagonist SB-568849. Bioorg Med Chem Lett 2006; 16: 4872-8.

[97] Kennedy AR, Todd JF, Dhillo WS, *et al.* Effect of direct injection of melanin-concentrating hormone into the paraventricular nucleus: further evidence for a stimulatory role in the adrenal axis via SLC-1. J Neuroendocrinol 2003; 15: 268-72.

[98] Witty DR, Bateson JH, Hervieu GJ, *et al.* SAR of biphenyl carboxamide ligands of the human melanin-concentrating hormone receptor 1 (MCH R1): discovery of antagonist SB-568849. Bioorg Med Chem Lett 2006; 16: 4865-71.

[99] Carpenter AJ, Al-Barazanji KA, Barvian KK, *et al.* Novel benzimidazole-based MCH R1 antagonists. Bioorg Med Chem Lett 2006; 16: 4994-5000.

[100] Kanuma K, Omodera K, Nishiguchi M, *et al.* Identification of 4-amino-2-cyclohexylaminoquinazolines as metabolically stable melanin-concentrating hormone receptor 1 antagonists. Bioorg Med Chem 2006; 14: 3307-19.

[101] Hertzog DL, Al-Barazanji KA, Bigham EC, *et al.* The discovery and optimization of pyrimidinone-containing MCH R1 antagonists. Bioorg Med Chem Lett 2006; 16: 4723-7.

[102] Tavares FX, Al-Barazanji KA, Bishop MJ, *et al.* 6-(4-chlorophenyl)-3-substituted-thieno[3,2-d]pyrimidin-4(3H)-one-based melanin-concentrating hormone receptor 1 antagonist. J Med Chem 2006; 49: 7108-18.

[103] Tavares FX, Al-Barazanji KA, Bigham EC, *et al.* Potent, selective, and orally efficacious antagonists of melanin-concentrating hormone receptor 1. J Med Chem 2006; 49: 7095-107.

[104] Receveur JM, Bjurling E, Ulven T, Little PB, Nørregaard PK, Högberg T. 4-Acylamino-and 4-ureidobenzamides as melanin-concentrating hormone (MCH) receptor 1 antagonists. Bioorg Med Chem Lett 2004; 14: 5075-80.

[105] Huang CQ, Baker T, Schwarz D, *et al.* 1-(4-Amino-phenyl)-pyrrolidin-3-yl-amine and 6-(3-amino-pyrrolidin-1-yl)-pyridin-3-yl-amine derivatives as melanin-concentrating hormone receptor-1 antagonists. Bioorg Med Chem Lett 2005; 15: 3701-6.

[106] Ulven T, Frimurer TM, Receveur JM, *et al.* 6-Acylamino-2-aminoquinolines as potent melanin-concentrating hormone 1 receptor antagonists. Identification, structure-activity relationship, and investigation of binding mode. J Med Chem 2005; 48: 5684-97.

[107] Dyck B, Markison S, Zhao L, *et al.* A thienopyridazinone-based melanin-concentrating hormone receptor 1 antagonist with potent *in vivo* anorectic properties. J Med Chem 2006; 49: 3753-6.
[108] Dyck B, Zhao L, Tamiya J, *et al.* Substituted chromones and quinolones as potent melanin-concentrating hormone receptor 1 antagonists. Bioorg Med Chem Lett 2006; 16: 4237-42.
[109] Schwarz DA, Allen MM, Petroski RE, *et al.* Manipulation of small-molecule inhibitory kinetics modulates MCH-R1 function. Mol Cell Endocrinol 2006; 259: 1-9.
[110] Rivera G, Bocanegra-García V, Galiano S, *et al.* Melanin-concentrating hormone receptor 1 antagonists: a new perspective for the pharmacologic treatment of obesity. Curr Med Chem 2008; 15: 1025-43.
[111] Kym PR, Souers AJ, Campbell TJ, *et al.* Screening for cardiovascular safety: a structure-activity approach for guiding lead selection of melanin concentrating hormone receptor 1 antagonists. J Med Chem 2006; 49: 2339-52.
[112] Méndez-Andino JL, Colson AO, Meyers KM, *et al.* The efficacy and cardiac evaluation of aminomethyl tetrahydronaphthalene ketopiperazines: a novel class of potent MCH-R1 antagonists. Bioorg Med Chem 2007; 15: 2092-105.
[113] Meyers KM, Méndez-Andino J, Colson AO, *et al.* Novel pyrazolopiperazinone- and pyrrolopiperazinone-based MCH-R1 antagonists. Bioorg Med Chem Lett 2007; 17: 657-61.
[114] Fernandez D, Ghanta A, Kauffman GW, Sanguinetti MC. Physicochemical features of the HERG channel drug binding site. J Biol Chem 2004; 279: 10120-7.
[115] Cavalli A, Poluzzi E, De Ponti F, Recanatini M. Toward a pharmacophore for drugs inducing the long QT syndrome: insights from a CoMFA study of HERG K(+) channel blockers. J Med Chem 2002; 45: 3844-53.
[116] Sanguinetti MC, Mitcheson JS. Predicting drug-hERG channel interactions that cause acquired long QT syndrome. Trends Pharmacol Sci 2005; 26: 119-24.
[117] Meyers KM, Kim N, Méndez-Andino JL, *et al.* Aminomethyl tetrahydronaphthalene biphenyl carboxamide MCH-R1 antagonists--Increasing selectivity over hERG. Bioorg Med Chem Lett 2007; 17: 814-8.
[118] Bilodeau MT, Balitza AE, Koester TJ, *et al.* Potent N-(1,3-thiazol-2-yl)pyridin-2-amine vascular endothelial growth factor receptor tyrosine kinase inhibitors with excellent pharmacokinetics and low affinity for the hERG ion channel. J Med Chem 2004; 47: 6363-72.
[119] Kym PR, Iyengar R, Souers AJ, *et al.* Discovery and characterization of aminopiperidinecoumarin melanin concentrating hormone receptor 1 antagonists. J Med Chem 2005; 48: 5888-91.
[120] Vasudevan A, LaMarche MJ, Blackburn C, *et al.* Identification of ortho-amino benzamides and nicotinamides as MCHr1 antagonists. Bioorg Med Chem Lett 2005; 15: 4174-9.
[121] Guo T, Shao Y, Qian G, *et al.* Discovery and SAR of biaryl piperidine MCH1 receptor antagonists through solid-phase encoded combinatorial synthesis. Bioorg Med Chem Lett 2005; 15: 3696-700.
[122] Egan WJ, Merz KM Jr, Baldwin JJ. Prediction of drug absorption using multivariate statistics. J Med Chem 2000; 43: 3867-77.
[123] Guo T, Hunter RC, Gu H, Rokosz LL, Stauffer TM, Hobbs DW. Discovery and SAR of 4-amino-2-biarylbutylurea MCH 1 receptor antagonists through solid-phase parallel synthesis. Bioorg Med Chem Lett 2005; 15: 3691-5.
[124] Smith DG, Hegde LG, Wolinsky TD, *et al.* The effects of stressful stimuli and hypothalamic-pituitary-adrenal axis activation are reversed by the melanin-concentrating hormone 1 receptor antagonist SNAP 94847 in rodents. Behav Brain Res 2009; 197: 284-91.
[125] Grey J, Dyck B, Rowbottom MW, *et al.* Bis(aminopyrrolidine)-derived ureas (APUs) as potent MCH1 receptor antagonists. Bioorg Med Chem Lett 2005; 15: 999-1004.
[126] Zhang M, Tamiya J, Nguyen L, *et al.* Thienopyrimidinone bis-aminopyrrolidine ureas as potent melanin-concentrating hormone receptor-1 (MCH-R1) antagonists. Bioorg Med Chem Lett 2007; 17: 2535-9.
[127] Rowbottom MW, Vickers TD, Dyck B, *et al.* Synthesis and structure-activity relationships of retro bis-aminopyrrolidine urea (rAPU) derived small-molecule antagonists of the melanin-concentrating hormone receptor-1 (MCH-R1). Part 1. Bioorg Med Chem Lett 2006; 16: 4450-7.
[128] Hudson S, Kiankarimi M, Rowbottom MW, *et al.* Synthesis and structure-activity relationships of retro bis-aminopyrrolidine urea (rAPU) derived small-molecule antagonists of the melanin-concentrating hormone receptor-1 (MCH-R1). Part 2. Bioorg Med Chem Lett 2006; 16: 4922-30.
[129] Rowbottom MW, Vickers TD, Dyck B, *et al.* Synthesis and structure-activity relationships of biarylcarboxamide bis-aminopyrrolidine urea derived small-molecule antagonists of the melanin-concentrating hormone receptor-1 (MCH-R1). Bioorg Med Chem Lett 2005; 15: 3439-45.
[130] Su J, McKittrick BA, Tang H, *et al.* Discovery of melanin-concentrating hormone receptor R1 antagonists using high-throughput synthesis. Bioorg Med Chem 2005; 13: 1829-36.
[131] Palani A, Shapiro S, McBriar MD, *et al.* Biaryl ureas as potent and orally efficacious melanin concentrating hormone receptor 1 antagonists for the treatment of obesity. J Med Chem 2005; 48: 4746-9.
[132] McBriar MD, Guzik H, Xu R, *et al.* Discovery of bicycloalkyl urea melanin concentrating hormone receptor antagonists: orally efficacious antiobesity therapeutics. J Med Chem 2005; 48: 2274-7.
[133] Palani A, Shapiro S, McBriar MD, *et al.* Biaryl diamides as potent melanin concentrating hormone receptor 1 antagonists. Bioorg Med Chem Lett 2005; 15: 5234-6.
[134] Sasikumar TK, Qiang L, Burnett DA, *et al.* Novel aminobenzimidazoles as selective MCH-R1 antagonists for the treatment of metabolic diseases. Bioorg Med Chem Lett 2006; 16: 5427-31.
[135] Xu R, Li S, Paruchova J, *et al.* Bicyclic[4.1.0]heptanes as phenyl replacements for melanin concentrating hormone receptor antagonists. Bioorg Med Chem 2006; 14: 3285-99.
[136] Vieth M, Siegel MG, Higgs RE, *et al.* Characteristic physical properties and structural fragments of marketed oral drugs. J Med Chem 2004; 47: 224-32.
[137] McBriar MD, Guzik H, Shapiro S, *et al.* Discovery of orally efficacious melanin-concentrating hormone receptor-1 antagonists as antiobesity agents. Synthesis, SAR, and biological evaluation of bicyclo[3.1.0]hexyl ureas. J Med Chem 2006; 49: 2294-310.
[138] McBriar MD, Guzik H, Shapiro S, *et al.* Bicyclo[3.1.0]hexyl urea melanin concentrating hormone (MCH) receptor-1 antagonists: impacting hERG liability via aryl modifications. Bioorg Med Chem Lett 2006; 16: 4262-5.

[139] Clark DE, Higgs C, Wren SP, *et al.* A virtual screening approach to finding novel and potent antagonists at the melanin-concentrating hormone 1 receptor. J Med Chem 2004; 47: 3962-71.

[140] Ma V, Bannon AW, Baumgartner J, *et al.* Solid-phase synthesis and structure-activity relationships of novel biarylethers as melanin-concentrating hormone receptor-1 antagonists. Bioorg Med Chem Lett 2006; 16: 5066-72.

[141] Wu WL, Burnett DA, Caplen MA, *et al.* Design and synthesis of orally efficacious benzimidazoles as melanin-concentrating hormone receptor 1 antagonists. Bioorg Med Chem Lett 2006; 16: 3674-8.

[142] Wu WL, Burnett DA, Spring R, *et al.* Synthesis and structure-activity relationships of piperidine-based melanin-concentrating hormone receptor 1 antagonists. Bioorg Med Chem Lett 2006; 16: 3668-73.

[143] Keil S, Falk E, Frick W, Glombik H, Schwink L, Schaefer HL, Wendler W. New (oxazolylalkyl)-cycloalkyl)-alkyl)-benzoic acid derivatives, are peroxisome proliferator activated receptor agonists or antagonists used e.g. for treating lipid metabolism disorders, type II diabetes, syndrome X and obesity. DE10223273 (2003).

[144] Collins CA, Phelan KM, Verzal MK, Gao J, Hartandi K, Kym PR, Vasudevan A, Akritopoulou-Zanze I. Antagonist of melanin concentrating hormone and their uses. WO03070244 (2003).

[145] Vasudevan A, Wodka D, Verzal MK, *et al.* Synthesis and evaluation of 2-amino-8-alkoxy quinolines as MCHr1 antagonists. Part 2. Bioorg Med Chem Lett 2004; 14: 4879-82.

[146] Arienzo R, Clark DE, Cramp S, *et al.* Structure-activity relationships of a novel series of melanin-concentrating hormone (MCH) receptor antagonists. Bioorg Med Chem Lett 2004; 14: 4099-102.

[147] Warshakoon NC, Sheville J, Bhatt RT, *et al.* Design and synthesis of substituted quinolines as novel and selective melanin concentrating hormone antagonists as anti-obesity agents. Bioorg Med Chem Lett 2006; 16: 5207-11.

[148] Goodfellow V, Zhang M, Tamiya J. Melanin-cocnentrating hormone receptor antagonists and compositions and methods related thereto. WO2005047293 (2005).

[149] Barvian KK, Handlon AL, Hertzog DL, Hyman CE. 3-(4-aminophenyl)thienopyrimid-4-one derivatives as MCH R1 antagonists for the treatment of obesity, diabetes, depression and anxiety. WO2005042541 (2005).

[150] Palczewski K, Kumasaka T, Hori T, *et al.* Crystal structure of rhodopsin: A G protein-coupled receptor. Science 2000; 289: 739-45.

[151] Luthin DR. Anti-obesity effects of small molecule melanin-concentrating hormone receptor 1 (MCHR1) antagonists. Life Sci 2007; 81: 423-40.

[152] Blackburn C, LaMarche MJ, Brown J, *et al.* Identification and characterization of amino-piperidinequinolones and quinazolinones as MCHr1 antagonists. Bioorg Med Chem Lett 2006; 16: 2621-7.

[153] Wu WL, Burnett DA, Spring R, *et al.* Synthesis and structure-activity relationships of piperidine-based melanin-concentrating hormone receptor 1 antagonists. Bioorg Med Chem Lett 2006; 16: 3668-73.

[154] Kanuma K, Omodera K, Nishiguchi M, *et al.* Lead optimization of 4-(dimethylamino)quinazolines, potent and selective antagonists for the melanin-concentrating hormone receptor 1. Bioorg Med Chem Lett 2005; 15: 3853-6.

[155] Bakthavatchalam R, Hutchison A, Thurkauf A. Melanin concentrating hormone receptor ligands. WO0204433 (2002).

[156] Jeffrey TM, Xi C, Xiaoqi C, Juan J, Leping L, Pingchen T. Fused heterocyclic compounds. WO02004043958 (2004).

[157] Eric Hu X, Wos JA, Dowty ME, *et al.* Small-molecule melanin-concentrating hormone-1 receptor antagonists require brain penetration for inhibition of food intake and reduction in body weight. J Pharmacol Exp Ther 2008; 324: 206-13.

[158] Chiu G, DeLeon JE, Lagu B, Noble S, Wetzel J, Gluchowski C, Marzabadi MR, Nagarathnam D. Selective melanin concentrating hormone-1 (MCH1) receptor antagonists and uses thereof. WO0206245 (2002).

[159] Lynch JK, Freeman JC, Judd AS, *et al.* Optimization of chromone-2-carboxamide melanin concentrating hormone receptor 1 antagonists: assessment of potency, efficacy, and cardiovascular safety. J Med Chem 2006; 49: 6569-84.

[160] Souers AJ, Gao J, Brune M, *et al.* Identification of 2-(4-benzyloxyphenyl)-N-[1-(2-pyrrolidin-1-yl-ethyl)-1H-indazol-6-yl]acetamide, an orally efficacious melanin-concentrating hormone receptor 1 antagonist for the treatment of obesity. J Med Chem 2005; 48: 1318-21.

CBR1 Blockade and New Anti-Obesity Drugs Development: Targeting the Adipose Tissue

Laurence Hoareau, Karima Bencharif and Régis Roche*

Groupe d'Etude sur l'Inflammation Chronique et l'Obésité (GEICO), Plateforme CYROI - Université de La Réunion, 2 rue Maxime Rivière, 97490 Sainte Clotilde, France

Abstract: The discovery and the characterization of the cannabinoid receptor 1 (CBR1) as well as the finding of its involvement in the regulation of satiety, has initiated the race for the development of antagonist molecules with the admitted purpose to counteract obesity. The first one which reach the clinical trials, was the SR141716, or Rimonabant, and a large number of studies were conducted with this molecule. The RIO, STRADIVARIUS, SERENADE and ADAGIO studies clearly showed that Rimonabant led to a loss of weight, an increase of HDL-C levels, a decrease of triglycerides and blood pressure, an improvement of the insulin response and glucose uptake, as well as an increase of adiponectin levels. Surprisingly, numerous effects of this molecule seem to be linked to a peripheral action. In particular, Rimonabant has a strong anti-inflammatory action on liver and on fat cells, which could explain its beneficial effects on the insulino-resistance. However, the molecule possesses major side effects, limitating its commercial development. These effects are inherent to the central action of the CBR1 antagonists. To eliminate these problems, it will be necessary to develop molecules which have only peripheral effects. Beside this, other molecules with a more important fat specificity could be of a strong interest, such as Cholesteryl Ester Transfert Protein (CETP) inhibitors. Indeed, this type of molecules gives good clinical results with no central effect. So, despite the commercial failure of Torcetrapib, it is likely that we will see the development of several molecules targeting CETP and yet with limited side effects.

Keywords: Endocannabinoid, SR141716, obesity, adipocyte, adipose tissue.

INTRODUCTION: THE ENDOCANNABINOID SYSTEM

In recent years a great deal of attention has been paid to the central and peripheral components of energy metabolism in order to develop pharmacological modulators of appetite and energy expenditure, with the ultimate aim of fighting the obesity epidemic. One of the biggest and most surprising discoveries of the last ten years was the description of the endocannabinoid system (endoCB) as well as its influence on appetite and metabolism [1-6]. The endocannabinoid system is composed of receptors, endoCB, and endoCB synthesis, transport and degradation systems [7]. An endoCB is an endogenous molecule able to bind to a cannabinoid receptor and to activate the transduction pathways of the signal to which the receptor is coupled. Three endoCBs have been identified (Fig. **1**): arachidonoyl ethanolamide (AEA or anandamide), 2-arachidonoyl glycerol (2-AG) and 2-AG ether (noladin ether).

Studies, which have mainly concentrated on anandamide and 2-AG, show that these molecules possess all of the characteristics of the neuro-transmitters, except for their mode of storage and release. Indeed, the endoCB are synthesized (in the neurons and the astrocytes) "upon demand", following stimulation of the various receptors, and bring about the hydrolysis of membrane lipid precursors. Due to their lipid nature, the endoCB are not stored in synaptic vesicles and freely diffuse after their production [8]. Two principal receptors have been described as belonging to the cannabinoid system: CB1, present primarily in the brain [2, 4] and to a lesser extent at the peripheral level, and CB2, localized mainly on the cells of the immune system [5].

The cannabinoid receptors belong to the 7-transmembrane domain family of receptors and are coupled with Gi/o proteins. In 1990, the first receptor, CB1, was cloned from the central nervous system (CNS) [4], opening the way for research into the endocannabinoid system. Rapidly, a second receptor, CB2, was cloned from the spleen of rats [5, 9], followed by the identification of other endogenous molecules, able to bind to CB receptors. CB2 receptors display 44% homology with CB1. If the expression profile of CB1 is

*Corresponding author: Tel: +262 262 93 88 40; E-mail: regis.roche@adipsculpt.com

Atta-ur-Rahman / M. Iqbal Choudhary (Eds.)

extremely broad (central nervous system, peripheral tissues), that of CB2 would seem to be restricted to the peripheral cells. However, this assertion has recently been disproved [10]. It should be noted, and this is important for what follows, that CB1 is strongly expressed in many different area of the CNS, in particular within the hypothalamus.

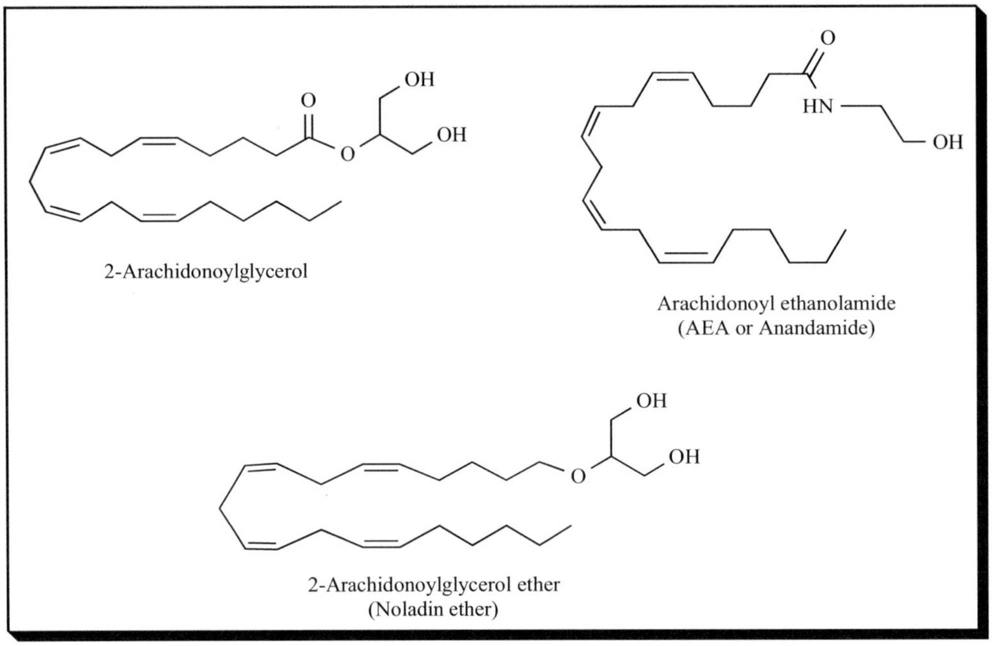

Fig. (1). Structures of the three different identified endocannabinoids.

CANNABINOIDS, ANTAGONISTS AND APPETITE

The appetite stimulating effect of marijuana in humans has been known for several centuries [11] and numerous studies have shown that the administration of cannabinoids stimulates feeding in animal models [12, 13]. Based upon observations that the cannabinoids were present in the areas of the brain that control food behaviour [14], the endogenous cannabinoid system was proposed as one of the modulators of this process [15, 16]. Moreover, CB1 receptor deficient mice are thin and resistant to the effect of a high-fat diet [15, 17].

It is most probably this characteristic of the system which in the 90s led to the development of antagonistic molecules of the cannabinoid receptors, and more particularly to that of the CB1 receptor. The first antagonist to be developed was SR141716 (Rimonabant, Fig. **2**), and a great number of studies began with this molecule. Rimonabant is a selective antagonist of CB1 receptors, with little or no affinity for other receptors; CB2 included. However, there is a body of evidence that would lead one to think that Rimonabant should act more like an inverse agonist (i.e. displaying the opposite properties to those of an agonist), or that it would inhibit the constitutive activity of CB1 receptors [9, 18].

The effects of SR141716 on the regulation of food intake are highly conclusive. For example, the peripheral or central injection of anandamide in rodents leads to an increase in the quantity of ingested food, and this effect is blocked by SR141716 [13, 19, 20]. In parallel, SR141716 induces a reduction in the quantity of food ingested in treated mice and rats, as well as an increase in weight loss [21, 22]. This partly results in a strong and rapid reduction in food intake during the first days of treatment [22, 23], which can be explained by a hypothalamic co-localization of CB1 receptors with known neuropeptides, such as the “corticotropin releasing hormone” (CRH), the “cocaine amphetamine regulated transcript” (CART), the “melanin concentrating hormone” (MCH), and prepro-orexine, in order to modulate food intake [15]. However, we now know that the long-term effect of SR141716 on weight loss is most probably independent of food intake, but we will come back to this point later.

SR141716 CLINICAL STUDIES

Convincing results obtained with Rimonabant in rodents led the pharma industries to set up clinical studies in order to confirm these encouraging results in humans. The first of these studies was the Rimonabant study in Obesity (RIO) launched at the same time in Europe (RIO Europe) and the United States (Rio-North America), on more than 6600 overweight or obese patients [24, 25], treated for a period of 2 years (randomized control trial). The program also included the Rio-lipids study that was dedicated to overweight patients with dyslipidemia [26].

The majority of the results obtained from these various studies have allowed us to largely confirm the results obtained in animals, and in certain cases have even extended our knowledge much further. Indeed, initially, the postprandial plasma insulin levels, traditional markers of insulin-resistance, were significantly reduced among patients treated with Rimonabant versus the placebo [24-26]. This effect can no longer simply be explained by Rimonabant treatment and consecutive weight loss [27], which would seem to suggest that the molecule can have a more or less direct effect upon insulin sensitivity. It is possible that this effect can be related to the levels of adiponectin, the hormone produced by adipocytes and known to improve the action of insulin, since it has also been shown that SR141716 increases the plasma levels of adiponectin [26], with approximately 50 % of this effect not due to weight loss [26]. It is also possible that the reduction in postprandial insulin rates observed with Rimonabant could be due to the direct action of the molecule in the pancreas as it has been demonstrated that high glucose levels result in the secretion of endoCB by the β- pancreatic cells, and that endoCB stimulates the release of insulin [28]. It is thus possible that Rimonabant limits the stimulation of endoCB by insulin in βcells, leading to a reduction in postprandial insulin levels.

The compiled data from the Rio-Europe and Rio-Lipids studies have also shown that Rimonabant leads to a better reduction in plasma glucose levels than compared to the placebo, as well as a significant improvement in glucose tolerance. These findings would suggest a potential use of Rimonabant in the prevention of type II diabetes, as well as for the treatment of diabetic patients. These initial results were largely confirmed by the Rio-Diabetes, SERENADE and STRADIVARIUS studies [29-31], which demonstrated the real benefit of Rimonabant in the treatment of type II diabetes, even among patients treated with insulin [32].

The effects of Rimonabant are however not limited simply to the improvement of glucidic and insulinemic profiles of treated patients. Indeed, lipid parameters were also evaluated at the time of the various studies and, overall, the results were very positive. The data of the RIO program thus showed a reduction in the triglyceride levels and an increase in HDLs, which persisted beyond 2 years [24-26]. Some of these results can once again probably be attributed to the increase in plasma adiponectin levels, which are positively correlated with the levels of HDL and apoAI [26]. The recent Adagio-Lipids study was able to confirm these results, and in particular the reduction of CRP and the increase in adiponectin. The study also showed that Rimonabant is responsible for a reduction in the mass of visceral adipose tissue and hepatic fat [33].

PERIPHERAL ACTION OF SR141716

Although the molecule acts in an obvious way upon the regulation of appetite, with patients initially losing weight at the beginning of treatment, a great number of the effects of SR141716 seem however completely independent of weight loss. Thus, approximately 50% of the clinical effects observed on the levels of HDL-c, triglycerides, postprandial insulin, and on the resistance to insulin cannot be attributed to weight loss as a consequence of reduced food intake [27].

Rimonabant thus has an effect at the peripheral level, which in itself is not entirely surprising as a certain number of studies demonstrate clearly the hyper activation of the peripheral endoCB system (in particular at the adipocyte hepatic and pancreatic levels) as a result of a high-fat diet, or among obese patients [28, 34-36].

In the mouse, for example, a diet rich in fat increases the levels of anandamide, the number of CB1 receptors, as well as the synthesis of fatty-acids in the liver [36]. In obese women, the concentration of anandamide and 2-AG in the circulation are increased by 35% and 52% respectively, [35]. In addition, plasma 2-AG concentrations are clearly correlated with the visceral adipose tissue mass [34, 37] and the expression of CB1 within this tissue increases with BMI [38].

In fact, as far as the peripheral involvement of the endocannabinoid system is concerned, a number of arguments demonstrate that the disappearance or inhibition of the system would seem rather advantageous. Thus, in the liver, results obtained in mouse $CB1^{-/-}$ have already shown that the mice were protected from the development of fibrosis or hepatic steatosis induced by a high-fat diet [36] or via chemical means [39]. Treatment with Rimonabant led to the same protective effects in obese rats: improvement of hepatomegaly, steatosis, and damage to hepatic cells, associated with a reduction in the rates of hepatic and circulating TNF alpha levels, and with an increase in adiponectin levels [40]. These findings are similar in the mouse, where steatosis was chemically induced, with Rimonabant reducing the fibrotic activity of the hepatic myoblasts [39].

When one looks beyond the liver, Rimonabant could also have protective effects upon the pancreas, since the molecule seems to limit islets of Langerhans and beta cell death as was demonstrated in a diabetic rat model [41]. However, it is probably around adipose tissue that the most interest has developed, because this tissue is a major player in the development of metabolic disturbances associated with obesity [42, 43], and in addition, adipocytes secrete a large quantity of adiponectin. Moreover, CB1 receptor deficient mice are thin, and resistant to a high-fat diet [15, 17], and the treatment of obese mice with SR141716 reduces considerably the adipose mass as well as the size of adipocytes [44]. Lastly, human adipocytes express CB1 receptors and are able to produce and secrete endocannabinoids [45, 46]. All of these elements thus make adipose tissue, like pancreatic cells [28], a target of choice for the explanation of some of the effects of SR141716. Furthermore, Rimonabant seems able to increase the expression and the synthesis of adiponectin in the adipocytes of rodents [40, 47]. Moreover, the molecule inhibits the cellular proliferation of murine pre-adipocytes [40] as well as their differentiation [48]. However, these results have never been confirmed in human adipocytes and the work completed within our laboratory confirms only partially what has been demonstrated in murine models. We do, however, demonstrate that the treatment of mature human adipocytes with SR141716 does not have an influence on the expression and the production of adiponectin when the cells are in a non-inflammatory state, thus confirming the findings of a previous study [49]. On the contrary, the effects of treatment with bacterial LPS, leading to strong TNF alpha secretion and to a reduction in the secretion of adiponectin, are counterbalanced by co-treatment with SR141716 (unpublished data). As far as adipocyte differentiation is concerned, we have effectively demonstrated that SR141716 has an effect upon adiponectin expression, but this is not followed by an increase in adiponectin secretion (unpublished data). However, probably our most interesting result obtained with cultured adipocytes relates to inflammation, and TNF alpha. Indeed, we show that SR141716 strongly decreases the expression and the secretion of TNF alpha induced by LPS (unpublished data), as has already been described in macrophages [50, 51] or at the plasma level in the mouse [50, 52]. The strong anti-inflammatory effects of Rimonabant were certainly very largely neglected until recently and could probably help to explain the peripheral actions of the molecule. So, it is probable that this anti-inflammatory property is implicated in the increase of adiponectin serum levels, and in the improvement of the sensitivity to insulin found in patients treated with Rimonabant.

BAD END FOR A GOOD DRUG: HOW TO AVOID CNS ACTION?

With regards to the studies carried out with SR141716 *in vitro*, *in vivo*, and in clinical trials, it is clear that Rimonabant had a very good future as a drug blockbuster, whose indications could have been numerous. However, whereas the molecule was already authorized for use in Europe and in other countries (in particular Argentina), in June 2007 the FDA refused to allow Rimonabant onto the US market. More recently, in October 2008, the European Medicines Agency (EMEA) suspended the marketing authorization for Acomplia, the trade name of Rimonabant in Europe. As a consequence, on November 5th 2008, the manufacturer decided to halt all studies on the molecule, including those outside of the European Union. The reason for withdrawing these authorizations was due to the sometimes significant side-effects that the molecule can have on the central nervous system, and in particular on mood. Indeed, anxiety and depression were the two principal reasons for halting treatment in patients on the RIO program [53]. Generally, the risk from using the molecule was regarded as being too great compared to the benefits gained from treatment. Results obtained from the last study to be carried out show that the risk of psychiatric side-effects passes from 28.4% to 43.4% in patients treated with Rimonabant, which leaves little chance of a future for this molecule. It should be noted that all the laboratories that had developed a similar molecule; that is to say capable of acting upon the cannabinoid system (Fig. **2**), also decided to stop the clinical and commercial development of their molecules (Taranabant and Otenabant respectively from Merck and Pfizer).

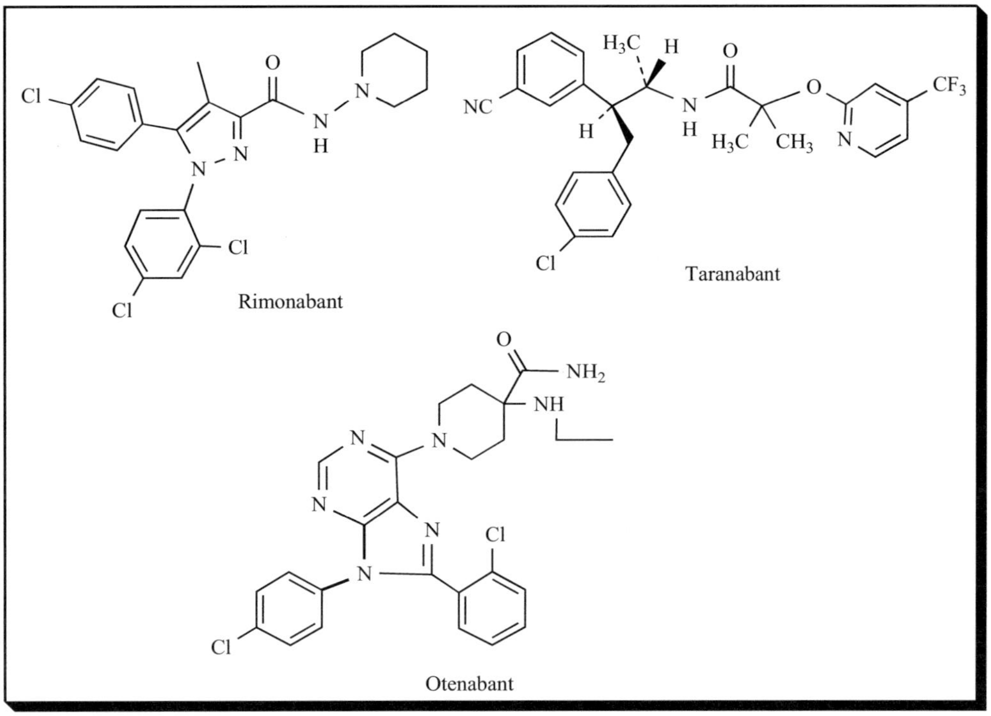

Fig. (2). Structures of the different CB1 receptor antagonists tested in clinical trials.

However, if one takes into account all of the mainly positive results obtained with Rimonabant, especially at the peripheral level, it seems rather a shame that the adventure should stop there. Indeed, it is clear that the problem with these molecules is related to their central effects, which in addition produce few advantages, except for a reduction in appetite. The development of new CB1 receptor antagonist molecules, unable to pass the hematoencephalic barrier would therefore be of enormous interest. A number of recent publications have in fact taken this direction. Initially, a very conclusive study using SR141716 established more clearly the differences in action between a central or peripheral antagonism of CB1 receptors. This work showed that the strictly peripheral effects are sufficient to decrease the production of glucose by the liver, to increase the mobilization of lipids by adipose tissue and to improve insulin sensitivity as well as glucose uptake; all this independently of a reduction in food intake [54].

In addition, another extremely interesting study showed that even the effects on appetite of the antagonists can be found, without the molecule binding to the central CB1 receptors. This is described by LoVerme *et al.*, with URB447 (Fig. **3**), a CB1 antagonist and CB2 agonist [55]. Indeed, following administration in the mouse, the molecule is not found in the brain, whereas it is largely detected in the blood, liver and adipose tissue. Furthermore, treatment of mice leads to a reduction in appetite as well as weight loss equivalent to that seen with Rimonabant [55]. Unfortunately, no data is available on the potential metabolic effects of this molecule.

Lastly, a study carried out with LH-21 (Fig. **3**), a neutral antagonist of CB1 receptors, showed rather surprisingly that this molecule reduces food intake and the weight of mice following treatment. However, these results were the same in control and $CB1^{-/-}$ mice [56], suggesting that the food intake mode of action of LH-21 is completely independent of CB1 receptors. This would seem to leave the question wide open concerning the global effects of the antagonists, with the possibility that the involvement of the endocannabinoid system is not absolutely necessary.

It is thus highly probable that this new class of molecule will become more and more common, and eventually lead to new clinical trials. However, before arriving at that point, it will of course be necessary to once again conduct most of the work that has already been carried out with SR141716, and in particular, to determine how adipose tissue is implicated in the observed peripheral effects, since it is clear that the role of the adipose tissue, if not major, is certainly far from being negligible.

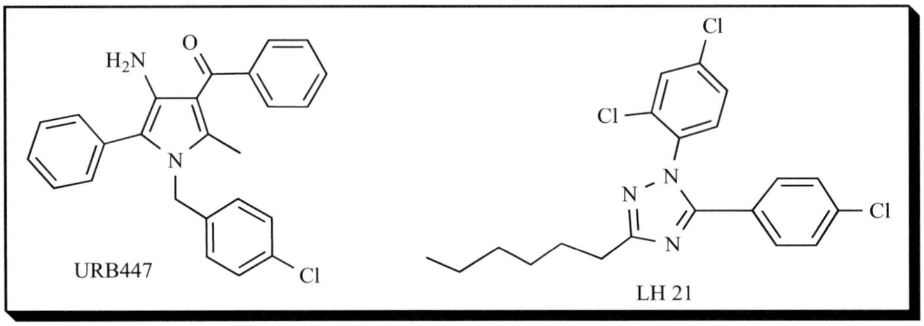

Fig. (3). Structures of new CB1 receptor antagonists.

FUTURE ADIPOSE TARGETS

In addition, even if the endocannabinoid system is of great interest, in the potential prevention of pathologies other than obesity (cardiovascular risks, insulin-resistance, dyslipidemia, etc), other types of targets are also very interesting from a tissue specificity point of view. Thus, as far as the regulation of the hypertriglyceridemias and cholesterol levels is concerned, it will undoubtedly be necessary to investigate in detail the cholesterol ester transfer protein (CETP), as well as the molecules capable of specifically inhibiting this transporter. In fact, approximately a third of the circulating CETP in humans is produced by adipose tissue. Moreover, the lipophilic nature of certain inhibitors could confer a relative tissue specificity upon them, in particular for adipose tissue, thus reducing the possibility of troublesome side effects. Currently, this type of molecule already gives good clinical results as far as lipid metabolism is concerned [57], and importantly, they do not possess a central action. Thus, in spite of the commercial failure of Torcetrapib, that was related to a strong increase in blood-pressure, independent of the inhibition of CETP [58], it is probable that in the coming years, we will see the development of several molecules with this therapeutic target with limited side-effects [59-61]. Nevertheless, it is certain that most of the molecules already developed, that are under development, or that will be developed in the future, for the treatment of pathologies more or less associated with obesity, will rely in some way or other upon adipose tissue.

REFERENCES

[1] Berry EM, Mechoulam R. Tetrahydrocannabinol and endocannabinoids in feeding and appetite. Pharmacol Ther 2002; 95(2): 185-90.

[2] Devane WA, Hanus L, Breuer A, *et al.* Isolation and structure of a brain constituent that binds to the cannabinoid receptor. Science 1992; 258(5090): 1946-49.

[3] Di Marzo V, Melck D, Bisogno T, De Petrocellis L. Endocannabinoids: endogenous cannabinoid receptor ligands with neuromodulatory action. Trends Neurosci 1998; 21(12): 521-8.

[4] Matsuda LA, Lolait SJ, Brownstein MJ, Young AC, Bonner TI. Structure of a cannabinoid receptor and functional expression of the cloned cDNA. Nature 1990; 346(6284): 561-4.

[5] Munro S, Thomas KL, Abu-Shaar M. Molecular characterization of a peripheral receptor for cannabinoids. Nature 1993; 365(6441): 61-5.

[6] Reggio PH. Endocannabinoid structure-activity relationships for interaction at the cannabinoid receptors. Prostaglandins Leukot Essent Fatty Acids 2002; 66(2-3): 143-60.

[7] Fride E. Endocannabinoids in the central nervous system--an overview. Prostaglandins Leukot Essent Fatty Acids 2002; 66(2-3): 221-33.

[8] Giuffrida A, Beltramo M, Piomelli D. Mechanisms of endocannabinoid inactivation: biochemistry and pharmacology. J Pharmacol Exp Ther 2001; 298(1): 7-14.

[9] Pertwee RG, Ross RA. Cannabinoid receptors and their ligands. Prostaglandins Leukot Essent Fatty Acids 2002; 66(2-3): 101-21.

[10] Van Sickle MD, Duncan M, Kingsley PJ, *et al.* Identification and functional characterization of brainstem cannabinoid CB2 receptors. Science 2005; 310(5746): 329-32.

[11] Abel EL. Cannabis: effects on hunger and thirst. Behav Biol 1975; 15(3): 255-81.

[12] Koch JE. Delta (9)-THC stimulates food intake in lewis rats: effects on chow, high-fat and sweet high-fat diets. Pharmacol Biochem Behav 2001; 68(3): 539-43.

[13] Williams CM, Rogers PJ, Kirkham TC. Hyperphagia in pre-fed rats following oral delta9-THC. Physiol Behav 1998; 65(2): 343-46.

[14] Howlett AC, Barth F, Bonner TI, *et al.* International union of pharmacology. XXVII. Classification of cannabinoid receptors. Pharmacol Rev 2002; 54(2): 161-202.

[15] Cota D, Marsicano G, Lutz B, *et al.* Endogenous cannabinoid system as a modulator of food intake. Int. J Obes Relat Metab Disord 2003; 27(3): 289-301.

[16] Mechoulam R, Fride E. Physiology. A hunger for cannabinoids. Nature 2001; 410(6830): 763-5.

[17] Ravinet Trillou C, Delgorge C, Menet C, Arnone M, Soubrié P. CB1 cannabinoid receptor knockout in mice leads to leanness, resistance to diet-induced obesity and enhanced leptin sensitivity. Int J Obes Relat Metab Disord 2004; 28(4): 640-8.

[18] Xie S, Furjanic MA, Ferrara JJ, *et al.* The endocannabinoid system and rimonabant: a new drug with a novel mechanism of action involving cannabinoid CB1 receptor antagonism--or inverse agonism--as potential obesity treatment and other therapeutic use. J Clin Pharm Ther 2007; 32(3): 209-31.

[19] Gomez R, Navarro M, Ferrer B, *et al.* A peripheral mechanism for CB1 cannabinoid receptor-dependent modulation of feeding. J Neurosci 2002; 22(21): 9612-7.

[20] Rinaldi-Carmona M, Barth F, Héaulme M, *et al.* SR141716A, a potent and selective antagonist of the brain cannabinoid receptor. FEBS Lett 1994; 350(2-3): 240-4.

[21] Chaperon F, Soubrié P, Puech AJ, Thiébot MH. Involvement of central cannabinoid (CB1) receptors in the establishment of place conditioning in rats. Psychopharmacology (Berl.) 1998; 135(4): 324-32.

[22] Colombo G, Agabio R, Diaz G, Lobina C, Reali R, Gessa GL. Appetite suppression and weight loss after the cannabinoid antagonist SR141716. Life Sci 1998; 63(8): PL113-7.

[23] Di Marzo V, Goparaju SK, Wang L, *et al.* Leptin-regulated endocannabinoids are involved in maintaining food intake. Nature 2001; 410(6830): 822-5.

[24] Pi-Sunyer FX, Aronne LJ, Heshmati HM, Devin J, Rosenstock J. Effect of rimonabant, a cannabinoid-1 receptor blocker, on weight and cardiometabolic risk factors in overweight or obese patients: RIO-North America: a randomized controlled trial. JAMA 2006; 295(7): 761-75.

[25] Van Gaal LF, Rissanen AM, Scheen AJ, Ziegler O, Rössner S. Effects of the cannabinoid-1 receptor blocker rimonabant on weight reduction and cardiovascular risk factors in overweight patients: 1-year experience from the RIO-Europe study. Lancet 2005; 365(9468): 1389-97.

[26] Després J, Golay A, Sjöström L. Effects of rimonabant on metabolic risk factors in overweight patients with dyslipidemia. N Engl J Med 2005; 353(20): 2121-34.

[27] Van Gaal L, Pi-Sunyer X, Després JP, McCarthy C, Scheen A. Efficacy and safety of rimonabant for improvement of multiple cardiometabolic risk factors in overweight/obese patients: pooled 1-year data from the rimonabant in obesity (RIO) program. Diabetes Care 2008; 31 (Suppl 2): S229-40.

[28] Matias I, Gonthier M, Orlando P, *et al.* Regulation, function, and dysregulation of endocannabinoids in models of adipose and beta-pancreatic cells and in obesity and hyperglycemia. J Clin Endocrinol Metab 2006; 91(8): 3171-80.

[29] Nissen SE, Nicholls SJ, Wolski K, *et al.* Effect of rimonabant on progression of atherosclerosis in patients with abdominal obesity and coronary artery disease: the STRADIVARIUS randomized controlled trial. JAMA 2008; 299(13): 1547-60.

[30] Rosenstock Rosenstock J, Hollander P, Chevalier S, Iranmanesh A. SERENADE: the study evaluating rimonabant efficacy in drug-naive diabetic patients: effects of monotherapy with rimonabant, the first selective CB1 receptor antagonist, on glycemic control, body weight, and lipid profile in drug-naive type 2 diabetes. Diabetes Care 2008; 31(11): 2169-76.

[31] Scheen AJ, Finer N, Hollander P, Jensen MD, Van Gaal LF. Efficacy and tolerability of rimonabant in overweight or obese patients with type 2 diabetes: a randomised controlled study. Lancet 2006; 368(9548): 1660-72.

[32] Hollander P. Endocannabinoid blockade for improving glycemic control and lipids in patients with type 2 diabetes mellitus. Am J Med 2007; 120(2 Suppl 1): S18-28; discussion S29-32.

[33] Després JP, Ross R, Boka G, Alméras N, Lemieux I. Effect of rimonabant on the high-triglyceride/ low-hdl-cholesterol dyslipidemia, intraabdominal adiposity, and liver fat: the adagio-lipids trial. Arterioscler Thromb Vasc Biol 2009; 29(3): 416-23.

[34] Blüher M, Engeli S, Klöting N, *et al.* Dysregulation of the peripheral and adipose tissue endocannabinoid system in human abdominal obesity. Diabetes 2006; 55(11): 3053-60.

[35] Engeli S, Böhnke J, Feldpausch M, *et al.* Activation of the peripheral endocannabinoid system in human obesity. Diabetes 2005; 54(10): 2838-43.

[36] Osei-Hyiaman D, DePetrillo M, Pacher P, *et al.* Endocannabinoid activation at hepatic cb1 receptors stimulates fatty acid synthesis and contributes to diet-induced obesity. J Clin Invest 2005; 115(5): 1298-305.

[37] Côté M, Matias I, Lemieux I, *et al.* Circulating endocannabinoid levels, abdominal adiposity and related cardiometabolic risk factors in obese men. Int J Obes (Lond) 2007; 31(4): 692-9.

[38] Sarzani R, Bordicchia M, Marcucci P, *et al.* Altered pattern of cannabinoid type 1 receptor expression in adipose tissue of dysmetabolic and overweight patients. Metab Clin Exp 2009; 58(3): 361-7.

[39] Teixeira-Clerc F, Julien B, Grenard P, *et al.* CB1 cannabinoid receptor antagonism: a new strategy for the treatment of liver fibrosis. Nat Med 2006; 12(6):671-6.

[40] Gary-Bobo M, Elachouri G, Gallas JF, *et al.* Rimonabant reduces obesity-associated hepatic steatosis and features of metabolic syndrome in obese zucker fa/fa rats. Hepatology 2007; 46(1): 122-9.

[41] Janiak P, Poirier B, Bidouard J, *et al.* Blockade of cannabinoid CB1 receptors improves renal function, metabolic profile, and increased survival of obese zucker rats. Kidney Int 2007; 72(11): 1345-57.

[42] Hotamisligil GS, Arner P, Caro JF, Atkinson RL, Spiegelman BM. Increased adipose tissue expression of tumor necrosis factor-alpha in human obesity and insulin resistance. J Clin Invest 199; 95(5): 2409-15.

[43] Trayhurn P, Wood IS. Adipokines: inflammation and the pleiotropic role of white adipose tissue. Br J Nutr 2004; 92(3): 347-55.

[44] Jbilo O, Ravinet-Trillou C, Arnone M, *et al.* The CB1 receptor antagonist rimonabant reverses the diet-induced obesity phenotype through the regulation of lipolysis and energy balance. FASEB J 2005; 19(11):1567-9.

[45] Gonthier M, Hoareau L, Festy F, *et al.* Identification of endocannabinoids and related compounds in human fat cells. Obesity (Silver Spring) 2007; 15(4): 837-45.

[46] Roche R, Hoareau L, Bes-Houtmann S, *et al.* Presence of the cannabinoid receptors, CB1 and cb2, in human omental and subcutaneous adipocytes. Histochem. Cell Biol 2006; 126(2): 177-87.

[47] Bensaid M, Gary-Bobo M, Esclangon A, *et al.* The cannabinoid CB1 receptor antagonist sr141716 increases acrp30 mrna expression in adipose tissue of obese fa/fa rats and in cultured adipocyte cells. Mol Pharmacol 2003; 63(4): 908-14.

[48] Yan ZC, Liu DY, Zhang LL, *et al.* Exercise reduces adipose tissue via cannabinoid receptor type 1 which is regulated by peroxisome proliferator-activated receptor-delta. Biochem Biophys Res Commun 2007; 354(2): 427-33.

[49] Pagano C, Pilon C, Calcagno A, *et al.* The endogenous cannabinoid system stimulates glucose uptake in human fat cells via phosphatidylinositol 3-kinase and calcium-dependent mechanisms. J Clin Endocrinol Metab 2007; 92(12): 4810-9.
[50] Dol-Gleizes F, Paumelle R, Visentin V, *et al.* Rimonabant, a selective cannabinoid CB1 receptor antagonist, inhibits atherosclerosis in LDL receptor-deficient mice. Arterioscler Thromb Vasc Biol 2009; 29(1): 12-8.
[51] Sugamura K, Sugiyama S, Nozaki T, *et al.* Activated endocannabinoid system in coronary artery disease and antiinflammatory effects of cannabinoid 1 receptor blockade on macrophages. Circulation 2009; 119(1): 28-36.
[52] Croci Croci T, Landi M, Galzin AM, Marini P. Role of cannabinoid cb1 receptors and tumor necrosis factor-alpha in the gut and systemic anti-inflammatory activity of SR141716 (rimonabant) in rodents. Br J Pharmacol 2003; 140(1): 115-22.
[53] Christensen R, Kristensen PK, Bartels EM, Bliddal H, Astrup A. Efficacy and safety of the weight-loss drug rimonabant: a meta-analysis of randomised trials. Lancet 2007; 370(9600): 1706-13.
[54] Nogueiras R, Veyrat-Durebex C, Suchanek PM, *et al.* Peripheral, but not central, CB1 antagonism provides food intake-independent metabolic benefits in diet-induced obese rats. Diabetes 2008; 57(11): 2977-91.
[55] LoVerme J, Duranti A, Tontini A, *et al.* Synthesis and characterization of a peripherally restricted cb1 cannabinoid antagonist, URB447, that reduces feeding and body-weight gain in mice. Bioorg Med Chem Lett 2009; 19(3): 639-43.
[56] Chen RZ, Frassetto A, Lao JZ, *et al.* Pharmacological evaluation of LH-21, a newly discovered molecule that binds to cannabinoid CB1 receptor. Eur J Pharmacol 2008; 584(2-3): 338-42.
[57] Bloomfield D, Carlson GL, Sapre A, *et al.* Efficacy and safety of the cholesteryl ester transfer protein inhibitor anacetrapib as monotherapy and coadministered with atorvastatin in dyslipidemic patients. Am Heart J 2009; 157(2): 352-60 E2.
[58] Hu X, Dietz JD, Xia C, *et al.* Torcetrapib induces aldosterone and cortisol production by an intracellular calcium-mediated mechanism independently of cholesteryl ester transfer protein inhibition. Endocrinology 2009; 150(5): 2211-9.
[59] Athyros VG, Kakafika A, Tziomalos K, Karagiannis A, Mikhailidis DP. Cholesteryl ester transfer protein inhibition and HDL increase: has the dream ended? Expert Opin Investig Drugs 2008; 17(4): 445-9.
[60] Krishna R, Anderson MS, Bergman AJ, *et al.* Effect of the cholesteryl ester transfer protein inhibitor, anacetrapib, on lipoproteins in patients with dyslipidaemia and on 24-h ambulatory blood pressure in healthy individuals: two double-blind, randomised placebo-controlled phase I studies. Lancet 2007; 370(9603): 1907-14.
[61] Rennings AJM, Stalenhoef AFH. JTT-705: is there still future for a CETP inhibitor after torcetrapib? Expert Opin Investig Drugs 2008; 17(10): 1589-97.

Gastric Endocrine Cell and Food Intake Regulation

Andreas Stengel, Miriam Goebel and Yvette Taché*

CURE: Digestive Diseases Research Center and Center for Neurovisceral Sciences and Women's Health, Digestive Diseases Division, David Geffen School of Medicine at UCLA and VA Greater Los Angeles Healthcare System, Los Angeles, California

Abstract: Specialized enteroendocrine cells are scattered within the gut mucosa and influenced by nutritional status. Released hormones are, besides other biological actions, involved in the regulation of food intake by mediating their information to brain centers involved in food intake regulation located in the brainstem as well as forebrain such as hypothalamic nuclei. Intestinal enteroendocrine cells produce a variety of gut peptides regulating food intake and were therefore the focus of many studies. However, recent evidence points towards a specific endocrine cell, the X/A-like cell, located within the stomach oxyntic mucosa as an important player in appetite control. Acylated ghrelin is the only known peripherally produced and centrally acting food intake-stimulatory (orexigenic) peptide so far. Its major source of production is gastric X/A-like cells. Desacyl ghrelin originates from the same cell and has been recently implicated in the regulation of food intake as well. Moreover, nesfatin-1, a novel food intake-inhibitory (anorexigenic) peptide, has been identified in ghrelin-positive cells of the stomach. This suggests an important role for gastric X/A-like cells to regulate food intake. Obestatin was initially described as a ghrelin gene product with anorexigenic properties. However, consecutive studies were not able to reproduce those findings and therefore its role as food intake regulating peptide remains equivocal. Ghrelin interacts with various other intestinal peptides to regulate food intake and body weight which has to be taken into account when targeting single peptides as a potential drug treatment for obesity.

Keywords: Desacyl ghrelin, food intake, ghrelin, nesfatin-1, NUCB2, obesity, obestatin.

INTRODUCTION

A variety of enteroendocrine cells located in the intestinal mucosa [1] release peptides in response to changing nutritional status and influence food intake in addition to other biological actions which are often exerted locally within the gut [2-4]. In the stomach four distinct endocrine cells were identified and mainly implicated in the physiological regulation of acid production and secretion. These cells encompass the gastrin-producing cells (G cells), somatostatin-releasing cells (D cells >20% of gastric oxyntic endocrine cells in humans whereas only 5-10% in rats), enterochromaffin-like cells releasing histamine (ECL, 30% in human and 65% in the rat,) and the less abundant serotonin-containing enterochromaffin (EC) cells [1, 5]. However, there is a 5th endocrine cell type that is located in the oxyntic glands of the stomach with (open-type) or without (close-type) connection to the lumen, which was previously classified as P/D_1 cell in men and X/A-like cell in rats and accounts for up to 20-30% of all oxyntic endocrine cells, thereby being the second most largest gastric endocrine cell population [1, 6]. The content of X cells in rats, which were also named A-like cells due to their similarity with pancreatic A-cells [6] and P/D_1 cells in humans remained unknown up to the discovery of ghrelin ten years ago by Kojima *et al.* [7]. The expression of ghrelin in rat X/A-like [7] and human P/D_1 cells [8] as the only peripherally produced and centrally acting peptide hormone known to increase food intake [7] has attracted much attention on this endocrine cell as regulator of appetite.

In addition to ghrelin, in the past few years, other peptides have been identified in rat X/A-like cells arising either from the ghrelin gene as a derived gene product (obestatin) [9], or differential posttranslational modification of proghrelin (des-octanoyl ghrelin, *n*-decanoyl ghrelin) [10, 11] or from the processing of a distinct gene (nucleobindin 2, NUCB2/nesfatin-1) (Table **1**) [12]. Evidence points towards a food intake-inhibitory action of nesfatin-1 [13] and desacyl ghrelin (Table **1**) [14]. However, the functions

*Corresponding author: Tel: 310-312-9275; Fax: 1-310-268-4963; E-mails: ytache@mednet.ucla.edu, astengel@mednet.ucla.edu

of obestatin have been largely unconfirmed in subsequent studies [15]. Taken together, these recent findings unraveled new functions for gastric endocrine cells with a prominent role of X/A-like cells which express peptides involved not only in the initiation but also suppression of food intake.

Table 1. Peptide Products from Rat X/A-Like Cells and Food Intake Response to Peripheral Administration in Mammals

Peptide	Effect on food intake	References
Acyl ghrelin	↑	[7, 10]
Desacyl ghrelin	↓/=/↑	[10, 14]
N-decanoyl ghrelin	↑	[11]
Obestatin	=/↓	[9, 15]
NUCB2/nesfatin-1	↓	[12, 16]

(↑) increase, (↓) decrease, (=) no effect.

Various other peptides that originate from intestinal endocrine cells and are implicated in the inhibition of food intake, namely cholecystokinin (CCK), peptide YY (PYY), oxyntomodulin (OXM), and glucagon-like peptide 1 (GLP-1) will not be discussed in this chapter since they are mainly produced outside the stomach (for detailed reviews see [3, 4]). These peptides are only taken into consideration in the context of their interactions with ghrelin's orexigenic action.

GENE PRODUCTS OF THE GASTRIC X/A-LIKE CELL

Ghrelin

Ghrelin is a 28-amino acid peptide which has a unique esterification of the serine-3 residue with n-octanoic acid resulting in increased lipophilicity Table (**2**) and was characterized by Kojima and colleagues in 1999 to be the endogenous ligand of the growth hormone secretagogue receptor 1a isoform (GHS-R1a) [7].

Table 2. Amino Acid Sequences of Rat Ghrelin, Obestatin and Nesfatin-1

Ghrelin	GSS(octanoyl)FL SPEHQ RVQQR KESKK PPAKL QPR
Obestatin	FNAPF DVGIK LSGAQ YQQHG RAL
Nesfatin-1	VPIDV DKTKV HNVEP VESAR IEPPD TGLYY DEYLK QVIEV LETDP HFREK LQKAD IEEIR SGRLS QELDL VSHKV RTRLD EL

Desacyl ghrelin is not posttranslationally modified, lacks the octanoyl group, and therefore does not bind to the GHS-R1a. The X/A-like endocrine cells of the stomach (Fig. **1**) are the major source of circulating ghrelin and desacyl ghrelin and initial studies indicated that the predominant circulating form is desacyl ghrelin as shown by an acyl/total ghrelin ratio of 1:55 [17]. However, data obtained using the recently developed RAPID method to process sampled blood using *R*educed temperatures, *A*cidification, *P*rotease inhibition, *I*sotopic exogenous controls and *D*ilution indicate a much higher yield of plasma acylated ghrelin with an acyl/total ghrelin ratio of 1:5 compared with 1:19 when detected using the standard method of blood processing (EDTA blood on ice) before simultaneous determination of acyl and total ghrelin levels by radioimmunoassay [18]. In addition to *n*-octanoyl ghrelin, another acyl-form of ghrelin has been recently identified in the same X/A-like cell, namely *n*-decanoyl ghrelin (D-ghrelin) in humans and rodents which accounts for 40-60% of circulating acylated ghrelin [11].

An important step forward was recently taken by two independent groups who identified the enzyme that acylates ghrelin in mice and humans [19, 20]. The enzyme is a member of the superfamily of membrane-bound *O*-acyltransferases (MBOATs) and was named *g*hrelin-*O*-*a*cyl*t*ransferase (GOAT). The enzyme octanoylates pro-ghrelin before it is transported to the Golgi apparatus where it is cleaved by prohormone convertase 1/3 (PC 1/3) to mature ghrelin [19]. Both medium chain fatty acids C8 and C10 are substrates for human GOAT resulting in octanoyl and decanoyl ghrelin [20]. *In situ* hybridization immunohistochemistry revealed that GOAT is highly co-expressed with ghrelin in cells of the mouse gastric oxyntic mucosa [21].

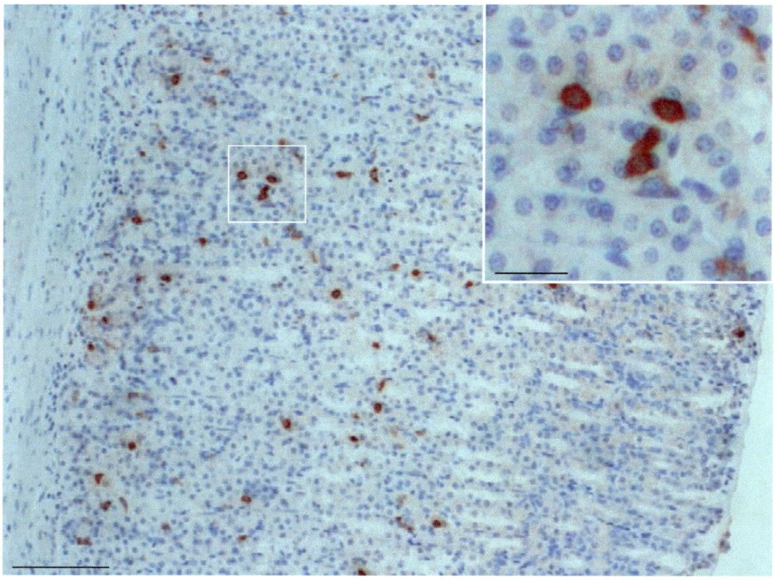

Fig. (1). Immunohistochemical illustration of ghrelin-containing cells in gastric oxyntic mucosa of a male freely fed Sprague-Dawley rat. Ghrelin-positive cells are brown cells distributed throughout the entire length of the glands. The insert shows the endocrine phenotype of the cells. Scale bars represent 100 μm in the overview and 25 μm in the insert.

Obestatin

Obestatin (or proghrelin$_{(53\text{-}75)}$) is a 23 amino acid amidated peptide (Table **2**) resulting from alternative splicing and posttranslational modification at a computer-based predicted cleavage site of the C-terminal pro-ghrelin [9, 22]. As expected for a peptide derived from the same gene as ghrelin, obestatin is expressed in the same cells as ghrelin in the human gastric mucosa and gastric endocrine tumors with subcellular distribution in secretory granules [23, 24]. Moreover, obestatin completely co-localizes with prepro-ghrelin in intracellular dense core granules in the rat gastric oxyntic mucosa, but only partly (60%) co-localizes with mature ghrelin indicating differential posttranslational expression [25].

Nesfatin-1

Nesfatin-1 is an 82 amino acid peptide (Table **2**) and was originally identified in the rat hypothalamus and shown to decrease food intake upon central administration and therefore named nesfatin for *N*UCB2 *e*ncoded *s*atiety and *fat*-*in*fluencing protei*n* [26]. We recently identified the expression of the nesfatin-1 precursor, NUCB2 in the gastric mucosa in significantly higher quantities compared to the brain (Fig. **2**)

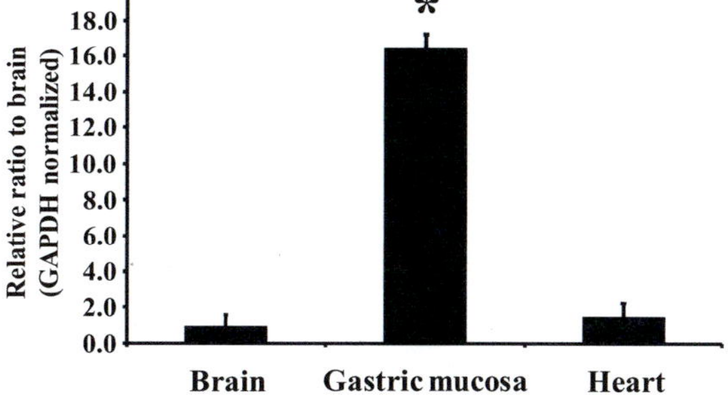

Fig. (2). NUCB2 mRNA expression in the stomach of *ad libitum* fed male Sprague-Dawley rats. The nesfatin-1 precursor, NUCB2 is highly expressed in the gastric oxyntic mucosa compared to brain or heart. Data are expressed as mean ± SD. * $p < 0.001$ *vs.* brain and heart. GAPDH: glyceraldehyde 3-phosphate dehydrogenase (housekeeping gene). (*Reproduced with permission from reference [12]; Copyright 2009, The Endocrine Society*).

[12]. Purification of small gastric endocrine cells revealed that NUCB2 mRNA is significantly expressed in those cells (Fig. **3**) [12].

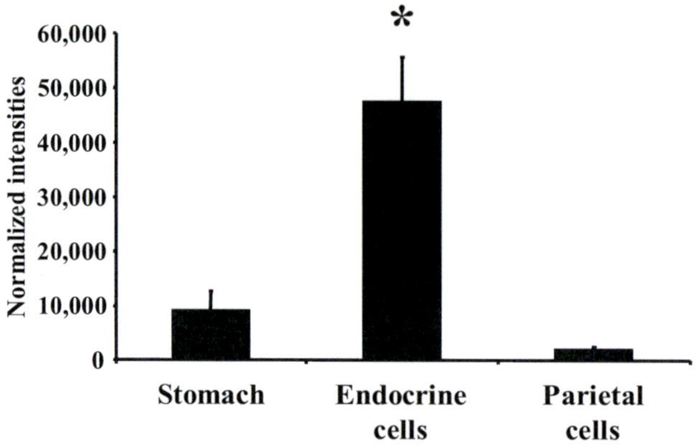

Fig. (3). Comparison of NUCB2 mRNA expression using whole-rat genome microarray expression analysis. NUCB2 expression is absent in purified gastric parietal cells but significantly increased in the purified small endocrine cell fraction compared to the whole stomach. Data are expressed as mean ± SD. * $p < 0.001$ *vs.* whole stomach and parietal cells respectively. (*Reproduced with permission from reference [12]; Copyright 2009, The Endocrine Society*).

Our recent studies in rats further established that nesfatin-1 and ghrelin are co-localized within the same cell although in different pools of vesicles (Fig. **4**) [12] providing novel evidence suggesting the production of nesfatin-1 in addition to ghrelin in gastric X/A-like cells. This contention is further supported by the presence of PC 1/3 in X/A-like cells [19] an enzyme involved in the processing of both ghrelin and nesfatin-1 consistent with NUCB2/nesfatin-1 and PC 1/3 being also co-localized in neuronal cells [27].

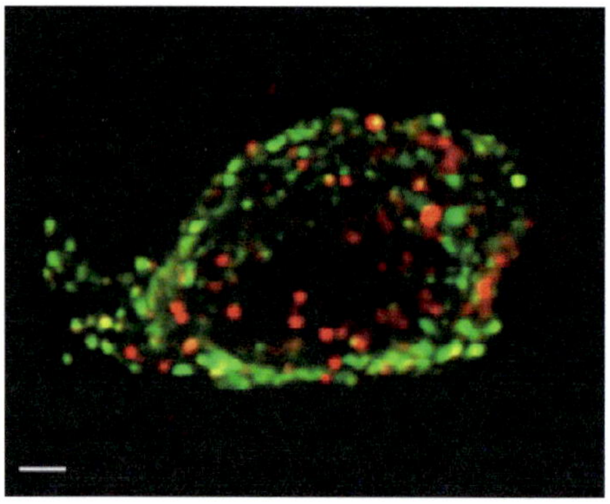

Fig. (4). High-resolution confocal microscopy of a single cell co-expressing ghrelin (green) and nesfatin-1 (red) located in cytoplasmic vesicles. Confocal microscopy was performed using a 100x objective and digital zoom, eight images in z-axis (stack size 24 x 24 x 7 µm) with dual laser excitation at 488 and 543 nm. Images were collected in two optical channels and photomultiplier tubes using FITC and TRITC filter sets, de-convoluted, and reconstructed into a three-dimensional image. The scale bar represents 1 µm. (*Reproduced with permission from reference [12]; Copyright 2009, The Endocrine Society*).

GHRELIN, DESACYL GHRELIN, OBESTATIN AND NESFATIN-1: REGULATION OF RELEASE AND INTERACTION WITH RECEPTORS

Ghrelin and Desacyl Ghrelin

As ghrelin is a circulating hormone a vast number of experimental and clinical studies have characterized circulating variations in response to various environmental conditions and stimuli. A well established finding is the inverse correlation between circulating ghrelin levels and the nutritional status and body mass index. Ghrelin plasma levels rise before a meal, during fasting and conditions of cachexia and anorexia and decline after food ingestion and under conditions of obesity in rodents and humans [28, 29]. Likewise, the concentration of the recently described n-decanoyl ghrelin increases in the mouse stomach and plasma during fasting [11]. Plasma ghrelin levels are also affected by a variety of peptides and immune cytokines. Somatostatin [30], cholecystokinin (CCK) [31], glucagon-like peptide 1 (GLP-1) [32], insulin [33], interleukin-1 [34] and prostacyclin [35] decrease circulating ghrelin upon peripheral administration in animals and humans, whereas adrenalin [36], secretin [36], central vagal stimulation [37] and stable analogs of the endogenous cannabinoid, anandamide [38] result in an increase. Whether these alterations of ghrelin levels reflect a direct action on ghrelin-synthesizing cells expressing cognate receptors for those peptides, lipids and cytokines still remains largely to be elucidated. However for some of the transmitters such as prostacyclin whose receptors have been detected on X/A-like cells by *in situ* hybridization, a direct action is most likely [35]. Further investigations with purified X/A-like cell preparations will be required to advance our understanding of the regulation of ghrelin release at the cellular level. Recently, Nakamura and colleagues showed preliminary results that ghrelin release is stimulated by adrenalin and noradrenalin in a cultured population of enriched X/A-like cells [39]. Another approach used genetic labeling of ghrelin cells with markers such as fluorescent proteins to obtain an enriched population of X/A cells [21].

Ghrelin is the endogenous ligand of the GHS-R1a which is highly expressed in the brain including the mesolimbic system, hypothalamus, medulla and vagal afferents corroborating ghrelin's role in the regulation of food intake and the hedonistic component of eating [40]. The octanoyl group on the serine is necessary for the activation of the receptor [7]. However, the active core of ghrelin consists of the first five N-terminal amino acids coupled to the hydrophobic residue which are also able to activate the receptor [41]. Ghrelin signaling is modulated by homo- or heterodimerization of the GHS-R1a as suggested by recent studies [40]. Homodimerization of GHS-R1a seems to contribute to the synergistic interaction between growth hormone-releasing hormone and ghrelin on growth hormone release [40]. In contrast, ghrelin responsiveness is reduced under conditions of heterodimerization of GHS-R1a and GHS-R1b whereas heterodimerization between GHSR-1a and cannabinoid 1 (CB_1) receptors could be involved in the stimulatory cross talk between the orexigenic interaction of ghrelin and cannabinoids [40]. Moreover, one has to take into consideration that the GHS-R1a is constitutively active in the absence of the endogenous ligand which results in basal signaling [42]. In contrast to ghrelin, desacyl ghrelin does not bind to the GHS-R1a and was therefore assumed to represent an inactive peptide [7]. However, ghrelin and desacyl ghrelin exert biological activities in a number of cells that do not express GHS-R1a pointing towards the existence of additional ghrelin receptor subtypes [22, 40].

Obestatin

Whereas circulating ghrelin levels as well as gastric content are altered by metabolic status, the density or intensity of obestatin immunoreactivity in the gastric mucosa does not change during food deprivation [25]. Moreover, circulating obestatin is below the detectable levels [43, 44] and neither affected by fasting nor feeding [9] except in one study [45]. Furthermore, obestatin immunoreactivity was not changed in gastric tumor endocrine cells [24]. Taken together, these data suggest differential mechanisms for ghrelin and obestatin regulating post-translational modification and cleavage in gastric X/A-like cells. Obestatin was initially reported to be the endogenous ligand of the seven transmembrane domain G protein-coupled receptor, GPR39 [9], which until then had been an orphan member of the ghrelin receptor family with high ligand-independent constitutive activity [46]. Later on, several independent groups [47-50] and even the original investigators themselves [51] failed to demonstrate binding of obestatin to tissue homogenates or cells transiently transfected with recombinant GPR39 or activation of GPR39 by obestatin. These findings convincingly refuted the initial claim that obestatin is the endogenous ligand of GPR39 and therefore it is still an orphan and the cognate receptor for obestatin remains to be characterized.

Nesfatin-1

We recently showed that fasting decreases NUCB2 mRNA expression in a pool of enriched gastric endocrine cells (Fig. **5**) using microarray analysis substantiated by RT-qPCR [12]. There is also a modest (20%) reduction of plasma levels of nesfatin-1 under conditions of overnight food deprivation in rats [52]. Mature nesfatin-1 was also detected in human plasma using Western blot analysis and possible changes of circulating nesfatin-1 concentrations under different metabolic conditions and the correlation with body mass index are under ongoing investigation [27]. Taken together these findings may support the hypothesis that NUCB2/nesfatin-1 expression and release are regulated by nutritional status corroborating the suggested role as physiological regulator of food intake. However, the cognate receptor for nesfatin-1 remains unknown so far and its identification will provide important insight to the action sites and the physiological role of nesfatin-1.

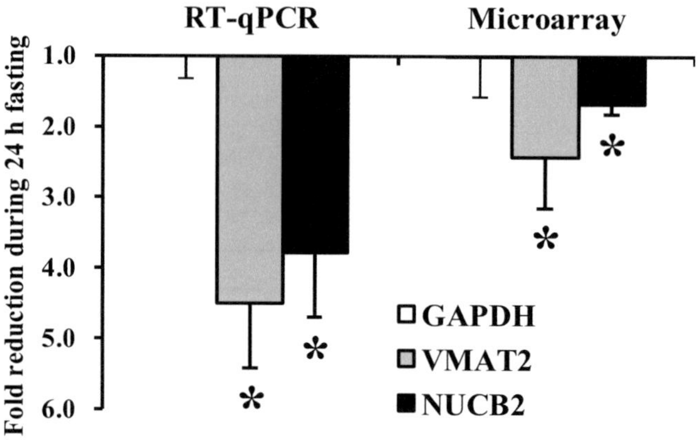

Fig. (5). Regulation of NUCB2 mRNA expression during fasting and *ad libitum* feeding conditions in rats. Fasting for 24 h results in a significant down-regulation of NUCB2 and VMAT2 in small gastric endocrine cells, whereas GAPDH expression does not change. Data are expressed as fold reduction of the mean of mRNA expression ratios ± SD. * $p < 0.05$ fasted vs. *ad libitum* fed. GAPDH: glyceraldehyde 3-phosphate dehydrogenase (housekeeping gene), VMAT2: vesicular monoamine transporter 2. (*Reproduced with permission from reference [12]; Copyright 2009, The Endocrine Society*).

EFFECTS OF X/A-LIKE CELL PEPTIDE PRODUCTS ON FOOD INTAKE

Ghrelin

Ghrelin is the only peripherally produced and centrally acting hormone known so far that stimulates food intake in freely fed rodents and in both lean and obese humans [53]. Acute peripheral as well as central injection of ghrelin promote food ingestion [54] and chronic application additionally increases body weight gain in rodents not only through increased appetite but rather promoting fat storage in white adipose tissue and reducing energy expenditure [28, 55]. N-decanoyl ghrelin has been less investigated than ghrelin but a recent report characterized its stimulatory effect on light phase food intake with similar potency as ghrelin in mice during the first 2 h post injection whereas the 24 h cumulative food intake was not altered [11]. Conversely, the use of GHS-R1a antagonists such as JMV 3002, 2959 and 2810 suppresses exogenous ghrelin-induced as well as fasting-induced food intake by modulating the activity of ghrelin-responsive cells in the hypothalamic arcuate nucleus [56].

Desacyl Ghrelin

In contrast to ghrelin, the role of desacyl ghrelin is much less well understood. However, the initial assumption of desacyl ghrelin being an inactive peptide is recently reconsidered based on reports that the peptide may serve as a possible anorexigenic hormone although some of the findings remain equivocal [14]. We could recently show that desacyl ghrelin blocks the stimulation of food intake induced by ghrelin upon simultaneous peripheral injection in rats [57]. However, the receptor for desacyl ghrelin action is yet to be identified to advance our understanding of desacyl ghrelin's function and sites of action.

Obestatin

The initial report on obestatin claimed an anorexigenic role for this peptide and the ability to counteract ghrelin's orexigenic action as well as decrease body weight gain upon chronic application [9]. However, only few subsequent studies [58-60] were able to partially reproduce those findings some of which have been recently retracted [61], whereas the vast majority conducted by several independent investigators failed to show that obestatin suppresses food intake, body weight gain or modulates ghrelin's effects (Table **3**) [44, 45, 48, 49, 62-73]. These negative findings were obtained under various experimental conditions: mimicking the conditions used in the initial experiment, including extensive dose ranges, different duration of monitoring, several sites of administration, circadian phase, metabolic state (fasted *vs. ad libitum* fed), state of acclimatization (habituated *vs.* non-habituated animals), different peptide diluents and different body weights of rodents (lean *vs.* diet-induced obese). For instance by using the originally described experimental setting no changes in food intake could be observed in rats either *ad libitum* fed or fasted after peripheral injection of obestatin (2520 – 12,600 μg/kg) during the light or dark phase [69]. Moreover, no change in Fos expression, a marker for neuronal activity and often used to investigate the effects of food intake regulatory peptides, was observed after intraperitoneal injection of obestatin whereas CCK increased Fos expression as expected in hypothalamic nuclei such as the paraventricular nucleus [69]. Therefore, evidence so far negates the biological action of obestatin as endogenous anorexigenic modulator of food intake as initially reported [9].

Table 3. Effect of Obestatin on Food Intake in Rodents

Site of Administration	Dose (µg/kg)	Feeding Condition	Circadian Phase	Species	Effect on Food Intake	Refs.
Icv	20	fas	light	mice	↓	[9]
Icv	17	ad lib, fas	light	rats	=	[62]
Icv	4 - 11	fas	light	rats	=,↓	[74]
Icv	1 - 8	ad lib, fas	light	rats	=	[65]
Icv	20 - 189	ad lib	n/a	rats	=	[68]
Icv	20	fas	light	mice	=	[67]
Icv	3 - 25	ad lib	dark, light	rats	↓	[59]
Icv	2 - 22	ad lib, fas	dark, light	mice, rats	=	[44]
Icv	20	fas	dark	mice	=	[71]
Ip	32 - 2520	fas	light	mice	↓	[9]
Ip	30 - 300	fas	light	mice, rats	=	[64]
Ip	320	fas	n/a	rats	↓	[58]
Ip	250-2500	ad lib, fas	n/a	mice	=	[49]
Ip	3 - 1260	ad lib, fas	dark, light	mice, rats	=	[68]
Ip	2520	ad lib, fas	dark	mice	=↓	[45]
Ip	2520	fas	light	mice	=	[48]
Ip	315	fas	light	mice	=	[75]
Ip	100-3000	ad lib, fas	dark, light	mice, rats	=	[76]
Ip	0.3 – 7.5	fas	light	mice	=	[66], retracted: [61]
Ip	25 or 250	ad lib, fas	dark, light	mice, rats	↓	[66], retracted: [61]
Ip	2500-7500	fas	light	mice	=	[66], retracted: [61]
Ip	109 - 202	ad lib	dark	mice	↓	[60]
Ip	2520-12,600	ad lib, fas	dark, light	mice, rats	=	[69]
Ip	315 -2520	ad lib	dark, light	mice	=	[44]
Ip	151 -1260	fas	light	mice	=	[70]
Ip	25 - 250	ad lib	n/a	rats	=,↓	[72]
Sc	378	ad lib	n/a	rats	=	[68]
Sc	252 -2520	ad lib	n/a	rats	=	[73]

icv: intracerebroventricular, ip: intraperitoneal, sc: subcutaneous, ad lib: ad libitum fed, fas: fasted, n/a: not applicable
(↑) increase, (↓) decrease, (=) no effect.

Nesfatin-1

The anorexigenic action of nesfatin-1 to reduce dark phase food intake in rats was reported by two independent groups of investigators [26, 52] and recently also observed in mice upon peripheral injection [16]. Furthermore, repeated intraperitoneal injections over a period of six days results in the inhibition of body weight gain [27]. The biological activity of nesfatin-1 seems to be exerted by the mid segment since peripheral injection of the 30-amino acid residue nesfatin-$1_{24\text{-}53}$ suppresses food intake in lean, *ob/ob* and high fat diet-induced obese mice, whereas the N-23 or C-29 amino acid terminal fragments have no effect [16]. Moreover, a recent report indicates that nesfatin-1 exerts a long-lasting inhibition of food intake following subcutaneous injection in mice or after intranasal administration in rats [27]. Therefore, evidence accumulated so far supports a suppressive action of peripheral nesfatin-1 on food intake in rodents. It remains to be investigated whether nesfatin-1 and ghrelin, both co-localized in the gastric X/A-like cells within different vesicles, are differentially released upon changes in metabolic conditions.

INTERACTION BETWEEN GHRELIN AND GUT PEPTIDES AS WELL AS BRAIN TRANSMITTERS REGULATING FOOD INTAKE

Interaction with Desacyl Ghrelin, CCK and Bombesin

The interaction of gut peptides has to be taken into account when investigating the regulation of food intake since peptides are not released separately but mostly simultaneously in response to changes in metabolic and nutritional status. Desacyl ghrelin was unable to influence food intake when injected alone [57], however, when injected simultaneously with ghrelin it completely abolished ghrelin's stimulatory action on food intake [57]. Also, CCK is able to completely eliminate the ghrelin-induced increase in food intake and Fos expression in hypothalamic nuclei regulating food intake [77]. Moreover, peripheral injection of bombesin abolishes ghrelin's orexigenic effect [78].

Interaction with Leptin

The anorexigenic protein hormone leptin is mainly derived from white adipose tissue [79] but also found in the gastric oxyntic mucosa [80]. Leptin-deficient *ob/ob* mice show increased ghrelin mRNA expression in the stomach [81] and exogenous application of leptin conversely decreases gastric ghrelin expression [81] indicative of a negative interaction between leptin and ghrelin. Moreover, central injection of ghrelin abolishes the central leptin-induced inhibition of food intake in rats [82] which may involve the suppression of the leptin-induced decrease in hypothalamic NPY mRNA levels [83]. Therefore, the interaction of leptin and ghrelin is also occurring centrally to modulate food intake-regulatory hypothalamic neuronal circuitries.

Interaction with Dopamine

Several studies suggest an involvement of ghrelin in reward mechanisms [84]. The mesocorticolimbic dopamine system is part of the circuitry involved in the reward for feeding [85] and investigated as potential target site of ghrelin action. Central as well as peripheral injection of ghrelin induces dopamine overflow in the nucleus accumbens of mice [86, 87]. Likewise, microinjection of ghrelin into the ventral tegmental area and latero-dorsal tegmental area increases the extracellular concentration of accumbal dopamine [88]. Ghrelin directly enhances the activity of dopaminergic cells in the nucleus accumbens of the ventral tegmental area by increasing dopamine turnover as shown by whole-cell patch clamp recordings in rodents [89]. Moreover, intra-tegmental microinfusion of ghrelin induces a significant increase in food intake [89]. Conversely, pharmacological blockade of the GHS-R1a in the ventral tegmental area reduces the re-feeding response following a fast as well as the food intake stimulatory action of exogenous ghrelin in mice [89]. Therefore, a direct action of ghrelin on dopamine-producing cells may contribute to ghrelin's effect on the reward system.

Interaction with Endocannabinoids

Ghrelin and the lipid transmitters endocannabinoids have similar effects on food intake and body weight which may indicate that they may act in series or recruit common pathways. The hypothalamic adenosine 5' monophosphate-activated protein kinase (AMPK) plays a major role in the regulation of food intake [90] and is involved in the mediation of the effects of several food intake regulatory hormones [91]. Both ghrelin and cannabinoids stimulate the hypothalamic AMPK [40]. The effect of exogenous ghrelin on activation of hypothalamic AMPK and consecutive stimulation of food intake is completely abolished in CB_1 knockout mice [92] indicating that the endocannabinoid signaling system is necessary for ghrelin's orexigenic effect. Moreover, peripheral application of the endocannabinoid anandamide stimulates ghrelin release and increases circulating ghrelin levels [38]. Conversely, treatment with rimonabant, a cannabinoid $(CB)_1$ receptor antagonist, reduces systemic ghrelin levels [93]. These data indicate a crosstalk between ghrelin and endocannabinoids which could take place on the receptor level based on the observation that the GHS-R1a and CB_1 are expressed in the hypothalamus and the assumption of the formation of heterodimers [40].

The complex interplay between the orexigenic ghrelin and other ligands modulating food intake are occurring both peripherally and centrally and understanding their mechanisms is important to take into account in the search for possible anti obesity targets where often single hormones are modulated.

GASTRIC X/A-LIKE CELL PEPTIDE PRODUCTS AS POTENTIAL TARGETS IN THE DRUG TREATMENT OF OBESITY

Overweight, obesity (body mass index, BMI > 30) and associated diseases are a major health problem both in the United States [94] and worldwide [95] mainly contributing to morbidity and mortality in Western countries [96]. Two thirds of the adult US American population are overweight or obese [97, 98] and the prevalence is rising [97] with an estimation of 704 million obese people in 2015 worldwide [95]. Therefore, the World Health Organization has declared obesity as the greatest threat to human health [99]. Public health initiatives have failed to reverse the rising incidence of obesity [100] and the drug treatment options so far are very limited [101] due to the lack of efficacy and/or adverse side effects [102]. Bariatric surgery is the most effective treatment for long-term weight loss in morbidly obese patients so far with Roux-en-Y gastric bypass (RYGB) being the most commonly performed (Table **4**) [103]. Emerging evidence indicates that gut hormone alterations may play a role in the mediation of the weight-reducing effects of bariatric surgery [104]. Therefore, gut peptides regulating food intake are perceived as potential, efficient and safe novel targets to curtail obesity and associated diseases.

Table 4. Clinical Studies Investigating the Effects of Roux-en-Y Gastric Bypass on Body Weight Loss in Obese Patients Observed Over a Period of Longer than One Year

Body Weight Loss (%)	Follow Up Period	Participants (n)	Reference
28	10	1025	[105]
25	10	34	[106]
31	5	251	[107]
35	4	39	[108]
30	3	157	[109]

Ghrelin has been the focus of several studies as a promising target in the stimulation as well as inhibition of food intake. For instance, randomized placebo-controlled trials show that ghrelin is able to stimulate food intake in patients with impaired appetite as seen under conditions of cancer or end-stage kidney disease [110]. With regards to curtail appetite in order to reduce food intake and fat deposition, several investigations have been directed to block ghrelin signaling using various techniques. Administration of an antibody specifically recognizing the acylated form of ghrelin was able to acutely reduce food intake but failed to decrease body weight in diet-induced obese mice (Table **5**) [111]. Also, the vaccination against ghrelin gave very encouraging results in pre-clinical studies [112] but failed to induce body weight loss in obese human subjects (Table **5**) [113]. This is likely due to compensatory mechanisms [40] which may become apparent during the longer observation period in the clinical study (24 weeks) [113] compared to preclinical studies (e.g. 13 weeks in [112]). Another experimental approach is the use of synthetic L-isomer oligonucleotides, called Spiegelmers (Spiegel = German for mirror), specifically recognizing ghrelin but because of their L-RNA structure, these oligonucleotides are not recognized by endogenous nucleases resulting in a long half life (Fig. **6**) [114].

The anti-ghrelin Spiegelmer, NOX-B11 administered peripherally completely abolished the ghrelin-induced food intake as well as neuronal activation in the arcuate nucleus in the hypothalamus in rats (Table **5**) [114]. Likewise, GHS-R1a antagonists that cross the blood-brain barrier are able to reduce food intake in lean and obese mice (Table **5**) [115]. Moreover, repeated application of the Spiegelmer or the GHS-R1a antagonist reduces body weight gain in mice (Table **5**) [115, 116]. However, until now no anti-obesity drugs targeting ghrelin or its receptor are currently on the market which is mainly due to lack of sustained body weight loss which is most likely caused by associated compensatory and redundant mechanisms [40].

Also additional ghrelin receptor subtypes which remain to be identified [40] may contribute to compensatory mechanisms and therefore the lack of sustained drug-induced weight loss.

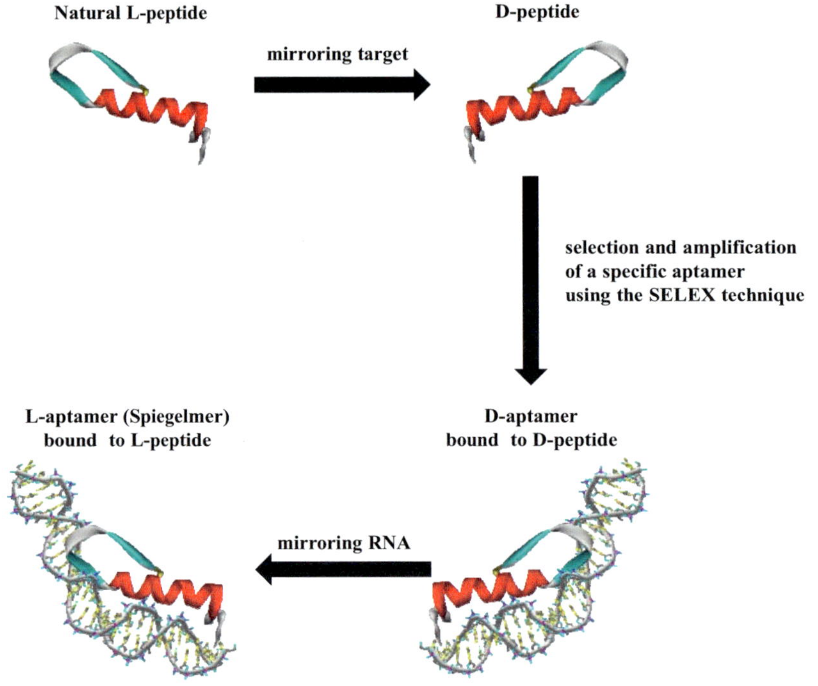

Fig. (6). Development of Spiegelmers. The selective RNA is identified and synthesized using the SELEX (*S*ystematic *E*volution of *L*igands by *Ex*ponential enrichment) technique. This scheme is oriented on a chart of NOXXON Pharma AG.

Table 5. Pre-Clinical and Clinical Studies to Decrease Food Intake and Body Weight by Targeting Ghrelin

	Pre-clinical studies		
	GHS-R1a antagonist	**Anti-ghrelin oligonucleotide**	**Anti-ghrelin vaccination/ Anti-ghrelin antibody**
Species	mice	rats, mice	mice, rats, pigs
Route	ip	ip, sc	ip, sc
Conditions	lean and diet-induced obese	normal body weight or diet-induced obese	normal body weight or diet-induced obese
Duration	5 days	acute (1 day) and 13 days	4 – 22 weeks
Effect	food intake ↓, body weight ↓	food intake ↓, neuronal activation ↓, body weight ↓	food intake ↓/=, body weight ↓/=
Reference	[115]	[114, 116]	[111, 112, 117, 118]
	Clinical study		
	Anti-ghrelin vaccination		
Route	not mentioned		
Conditions	obese patients		
Duration	24 weeks		
Effect	body weight =		
Reference	[113]		

(↑) increase, (↓) decrease, (=) no effect, ip: intraperitoneal, sc: subcutaneous.

Although bariatric surgery, most commonly Roux-en-Y gastric bypass, results in a pronounced decrease of blood ghrelin levels which are only partially recovered, it is questionable whether such a change contributes to the long-lasting body weight loss observed in those obese patients [29] based on lack of efficacy reported in other blocking studies. In addition, circulating ghrelin levels increase in obese patients after diet-induced weight loss. This phenomenon can be interpreted as a response to a state of starvation to restore the previous obese state, which was perceived as "normal" due to the long existence of this situation and re-setting of the homeostatic balance [119].

Another pharmacological approach in development is based on the recent characterization of the ghrelin-acylating enzyme GOAT and the possibility to interfere with the activity of this enzyme [120] to decrease acylated ghrelin levels and concomitantly induce a relative increase of desacyl ghrelin. Acylated pentapeptides were able to inhibit GOAT activity but follow-up studies [120] are needed to develop GOAT inhibitors without GHS-R1a activating properties. Another study investigating GOAT knockout or GOAT and human ghrelin over-expressing mice hypothesized that the ghrelin-GOAT system is a lipid sensor not only in the absence of food but rather when high caloric food is available based on the observations that GOAT is regulated by ingested nutrients especially lipids [121]. This finding will have to be confirmed in subsequent studies.

With regard to nesfatin-1 a recent study indicates that the anorexigenic effect of peripheral administration of nesfatin-1 is leptin-independent [16] as indicated by unchanged food intake-reducing activity after peripheral injection of nesfatin-1 in leptin receptor-deficient *db/db* mice. Since leptin resistance or decreased leptin sensitivity is a common phenomenon in obese subjects [27] nesfatin-1 may be a promising target in the drug treatment of obesity [27].

CONCLUSION

After the discovery of the potent orexigenic effect of ghrelin, gastric X/A-like cells were considered to uniquely express and selectively release this orexigenic hormone. However, new findings including the description of nesfatin-1 in X/A-like cells and the possible anorexigenic or ghrelin-modulating effect of desacyl ghrelin expand the function of this cell type to a stimulatory as well as inhibitory action on food intake as well as modulation of ghrelin's effect. In addition, the ghrelin action can be modulated by a variety of food intake-regulatory gut peptides, proteins and lipids forming a complex intertwined food intake-regulatory network. The identification of the yet unknown receptors for desacyl ghrelin and nesfatin-1 as well as possible additional ghrelin receptor subtypes will markedly deepen our understanding of the peptides' as well as X/A-like cells' physiology. Since incidence and prevalence of overweight, obesity and associated diseases such as diabetes mellitus type 2, hypertension, osteoarthrosis, and certain forms of cancer are rising along with medical costs for treating these conditions and in the absence of sufficient drug therapy options new therapeutic strategies are needed. Therefore, products of the X/A-like cell may be promising drug candidates although so far no anti-ghrelin drugs seem to show efficacy. However, mechanistic studies at the cellular and subcelluar level will be required to understand the regulation/secretion of the different peptide products derived from the gastric X/A-like endocrine cell.

ACKNOWLEDGEMENTS

Y.T. is in receipt of VA Research Career Scientist Award and NIH R01grants DK 33061 and DK 57238. A.S. and M.G. are supported by the German Research Foundation grants STE 1765/1-1 and GO 1718/1-1. We thank Ms. Eugenia Hu for careful review of the manuscript.

REFERENCES

[1] Rindi G, Leiter AB, Kopin AS, Bordi C, Solcia E. The "normal" endocrine cell of the gut: changing concepts and new evidences. Ann N Y Acad Sci 2004; 1014: 1-12.

[2] Hameed S, Dhillo WS, Bloom SR. Gut hormones and appetite control. Oral Dis 2009; 15: 18-26.

[3] Moran TH, Dailey MJ. Minireview: Gut peptides: targets for anti obesity drug development? Endocrinology 2009; 150: 2526-30.

[4] Karra E, Batterham RL. The role of gut hormones in the regulation of body weight and energy homeostasis. Mol Cell Endocrinol 2010; 316: 120-8.

[5] Prinz C, Kajimura M, Scott DR, Mercier F, Helander HF, Sachs G. Histamine secretion from rat enterochromaffinlike cells. Gastroenterology 1993; 105: 449-61.

[6] Bordi C, D'Adda T, Azzoni C, Ferraro G. Classification of gastric endocrine cells at the light and electron microscopical levels. Microsc Res Tech 2000; 48: 258-71.

[7] Kojima M, Hosoda H, Date Y, Nakazato M, Matsuo H, Kangawa K. Ghrelin is a growth-hormone-releasing acylated peptide from stomach. Nature 1999; 402: 656-60.

[8] Rindi G, Necchi V, Savio A, *et al.* Characterisation of gastric ghrelin cells in man and other mammals: studies in adult and fetal tissues. Histochem Cell Biol 2002; 117: 511-9.

[9] Zhang JV, Ren PG, Avsian-Kretchmer O, *et al.* Obestatin, a peptide encoded by the ghrelin gene, opposes ghrelin's effects on food intake. Science 2005; 310: 996-9.

[10] Date Y, Kojima M, Hosoda H, Sawaguchi A, *et al.* Ghrelin, a novel growth hormone-releasing acylated peptide, is synthesized in a distinct endocrine cell type in the gastrointestinal tracts of rats and humans. Endocrinology 2000; 141: 4255-61.

[11] Hiejima H, Nishi Y, Hosoda H, *et al.* Regional distribution and the dynamics of n-decanoyl ghrelin, another acyl-form of ghrelin, upon fasting in rodents. Regul Pept 2009; 156: 47-56.

[12] Stengel A, Goebel M, Yakubov I, *et al.* Identification and characterization of nesfatin-1 immunoreactivity in endocrine cell types of the rat gastric oxyntic mucosa. Endocrinology 2009; 150: 232-8.

[13] Shimizu H, Ohsaki A, Oh IS, Okada S, Mori M. A new anorexigenic protein, nesfatin-1. Peptides 2009; 30: 995-8.

[14] Inhoff T, Wiedenmann B, Klapp BF, Mönnikes H, Kobelt P. Is desacyl ghrelin a modulator of food intake? Peptides 2009; 30: 991-4.

[15] Goebel M, Stengel A, Taché Y. Continued controversy on obestatin as a gut hormone influencing food intake and gastrointestinal motility. Obes Metab 2008; 4: 143-8.

[16] Shimizu H, Oh-I S, Hashimoto K, *et al.* Peripheral Administration of Nesfatin-1 Reduces Food Intake in Mice: The leptin-independent mechanism. Endocrinology 2009; 150: 662-71.

[17] Hosoda H, Kojima M, Matsuo H, Kangawa K. Ghrelin and des-acyl ghrelin: two major forms of rat ghrelin peptide in gastrointestinal tissue. Biochem Biophys Res Commun 2000; 279: 909-13.

[18] Stengel A, Keire D, Goebel M, *et al.* The RAPID method for blood processing yields new insight in plasma concentrations and molecular forms of circulating gut peptides. Endocrinology 2009; 150: 5113-8.

[19] Yang J, Brown MS, Liang G, Grishin NV, Goldstein JL. Identification of the acyltransferase that octanoylates ghrelin, an appetite-stimulating peptide hormone. Cell 2008; 132: 387-96.

[20] Gutierrez JA, Solenberg PJ, Perkins DR, *et al.* Ghrelin octanoylation mediated by an orphan lipid transferase. Proc Natl Acad Sci USA 2008; 105: 6320-5.

[21] Sakata I, Yang J, Lee CE, *et al.* Colocalization of ghrelin O-acyltransferase and ghrelin in gastric mucosal cells. Am J Physiol Endocrinol Metab 2009; 297: E134-141.

[22] Soares JB, Leite-Moreira AF. Ghrelin, des-acyl ghrelin and obestatin: Three pieces of the same puzzle. Peptides 2008; 29: 1255-70.

[23] Gronberg M, Tsolakis AV, Magnusson L, Janson ET, Saras J. Distribution of Obestatin and Ghrelin in Human Tissues: Immunoreactive Cells in the Gastrointestinal Tract, Pancreas, and Mammary Glands. J Histochem Cytochem 2008; 56: 793-801.

[24] Tsolakis AV, Grimelius L, Stridsberg M, *et al.* Obestatin/ghrelin cells in normal mucosa and endocrine tumours of the stomach. Eur J Endocrinol 2009; 160: 941-9.

[25] Zhao CM, Furnes MW, Stenstrom B, Kulseng B, Chen D. Characterization of obestatin- and ghrelin-producing cells in the gastrointestinal tract and pancreas of rats: an immunohistochemical and electron-microscopic study. Cell Tissue Res 2008; 331: 575-87.

[26] Oh-I S, Shimizu H, Satoh T, Okada S, *et al.* Identification of nesfatin-1 as a satiety molecule in the hypothalamus. Nature 2006; 443: 709-12.

[27] Shimizu H, Oh-I S, Okada S, Mori M. Nesfatin-1: An overview and future clinical application. Endocr J 2009; 56: 537-43.

[28] Tschöp M, Smiley DL, Heiman ML. Ghrelin induces adiposity in rodents. Nature 2000; 407: 908-13.

[29] Cummings DE, Weigle DS, Frayo RS, *et al.* Plasma ghrelin levels after diet-induced weight loss or gastric bypass surgery. N Engl J Med 2002; 346: 1623-30.

[30] Shimada M, Date Y, Mondal MS, *et al.* Somatostatin suppresses ghrelin secretion from the rat stomach. Biochem Biophys Res Commun 2003; 302: 520-5.

[31] Brennan IM, Otto B, Feltrin KL, Meyer JH, Horowitz M, Feinle-Bisset C. Intravenous CCK-8, but not GLP-1, suppresses ghrelin and stimulates PYY release in healthy men. Peptides 2007; 28: 607-11.

[32] Hagemann D, Holst JJ, Gethmann A, Banasch M, Schmidt WE, Meier JJ. Glucagon-like peptide 1 (GLP-1) suppresses ghrelin levels in humans via increased insulin secretion. Regul Pept 2007; 143: 64-8.

[33] Saad MF, Bernaba B, Hwu CM, *et al.* Insulin regulates plasma ghrelin concentration. J Clin Endocrinol Metab 2002; 87: 3997-4000.

[34] Wang L, Basa NR, Shaikh A, *et al.* LPS inhibits fasted plasma ghrelin levels in rats: role of IL-1 and PGs and functional implications. Am J Physiol Gastrointest Liver Physiol 2006; 291: G611-20.

[35] Madison LD, Scarlett JM, Levasseur P, *et al.* Prostacyclin signaling regulates circulating ghrelin during acute inflammation. J Endocrinol 2008; 196: 263-73.

[36] de la Cour CD, Norlen P, Hakanson R. Secretion of ghrelin from rat stomach ghrelin cells in response to local microinfusion of candidate messenger compounds: a microdialysis study. Regul Pept 2007; 143: 118-26.

[37] Ao Y, Go VL, Toy N, *et al.* Brainstem thyrotropin-releasing hormone regulates food intake through vagal-dependent cholinergic stimulation of ghrelin secretion. Endocrinology 2006; 147: 6004-10.

[38] Zbucki RL, Sawicki B, Hryniewicz A, Winnicka MM. Cannabinoids enhance gastric X/A-like cells activity. Folia Histochem Cytobiol 2008; 46: 219-24.

[39] Nakamura E, Hasumura M, Gabriel AS, Uneyama H, Torii K. Functional Characterization of Cultured a-Like Cells Isolated from Rat Gastric Mucosa. Gastroenterology 2009; 136 (S1): S1617.

[40] Schellekens H, Dinan TG, Cryan JF. Lean Mean Fat Reducing "Ghrelin" Machine: Hypothalamic Ghrelin and Ghrelin Receptors as Therapeutic Targets in Obesity. Neuropharmacology 2010; 58: 2-16.

[41] Bednarek MA, Feighner SD, Pong SS, *et al.* Structure-function studies on the new growth hormone-releasing peptide, ghrelin: minimal sequence of ghrelin necessary for activation of growth hormone secretagogue receptor 1a. J Med Chem 2000; 43: 4370-6.

[42] Holst B, Schwartz TW. Constitutive ghrelin receptor activity as a signaling set-point in appetite regulation. Trends Pharmacol Sci 2004; 25: 113-7.

[43] Bang AS, Soule SG, Yandle TG, Richards AM, Pemberton CJ. Characterisation of proghrelin peptides in mammalian tissue and plasma. J Endocrinol 2007; 192: 313-3.

[44] Mondal M, Toshinai K, Ueno H, Koshinaka K, Nakazato M. Characterization of obestatin in rat and human stomach and plasma, and its lack of acute effect on feeding behavior in rodents. J Endocrinol 2008; 198: 339-46.

[45] Zizzari P, Longchamps R, Epelbaum J, Bluet-Pajot MT. Obestatin partially affects ghrelin stimulation of food intake and growth hormone secretion in rodents. Endocrinology 2007; 148: 1648-53.
[46] Holst B, Holliday ND, Bach A, Elling CE, Cox HM, Schwartz TW. Common structural basis for constitutive activity of the ghrelin receptor family. J Biol Chem 2004; 279: 53806-17.
[47] Lauwers E, Landuyt B, Arckens L, Schoofs L, Luyten W. Obestatin does not activate orphan G protein-coupled receptor GPR39. Biochem Biophys Res Commun 2006; 351: 21-5.
[48] Tremblay F, Perreault M, Klaman LD, Tobin JF, Smith E, Gimeno RE. Normal food intake and body weight in mice lacking the G protein-coupled receptor GPR39. Endocrinology 2007; 148: 501-6.
[49] Holst B, Egerod KL, Schild E, *et al.* GPR39 signaling is stimulated by zinc ions but not by obestatin. Endocrinology 2007; 148: 13-20.
[50] Chartrel N, Alvear-Perez R, Leprince J, *et al.* Comment on "Obestatin, a peptide encoded by the ghrelin gene, opposes ghrelin's effects on food intake". Science 2007; 315: 766; author reply 766.
[51] Zhang JV, Klein C, Ren P-G, *et al.* Response to Comment on "Obestatin, a Peptide Encoded by the Ghrelin Gene, Opposes Ghrelin's Effects on Food Intake". Science 2007; 315: 766d.
[52] Stengel A, Goebel M, Wang L, *et al.* Central Nesfatin-1 Reduces Dark Phase Food Intake and Gastric Emptying in Rats: Differential Role of Corticotropin-Releasing Factor2 Receptor. Endocrinology 2009; 150: 4911-9.
[53] Druce MR, Wren AM, Park AJ, *et al.* Ghrelin increases food intake in obese as well as lean subjects. Int J Obes (Lond) 2005; 29: 1130-6.
[54] Wren AM, Small CJ, Ward HL, *et al.* The novel hypothalamic peptide ghrelin stimulates food intake and growth hormone secretion. Endocrinology 2000; 141: 4325-8.
[55] Davies JS, Kotokorpi P, Eccles SR, *et al.* Ghrelin induces abdominal obesity via GHS-R-dependent lipid retention. Mol Endocrinol 2009; 23: 914-24.
[56] Salome N, Haage D, Perrissoud D, *et al.* Anorexigenic and electrophysiological actions of novel ghrelin receptor (GHS-R1A) antagonists in rats. Eur J Pharmacol 2009; 612: 167-73.
[57] Inhoff T, Mönnikes H, Noetzel S, *et al.* Desacyl ghrelin inhibits the orexigenic effect of peripherally injected ghrelin in rats. Peptides 2008; 29: 2159-68.
[58] Bresciani E, Rapetti D, Dona F, *et al.* Obestatin inhibits feeding but does not modulate GH and corticosterone secretion in the rat. J Endocrinol Invest 2006; 29: RC16-8.
[59] Carlini VP, Schioth HB, Debarioglio SR. Obestatin improves memory performance and causes anxiolytic effects in rats. Biochem Biophys Res Commun 2007; 352: 907-12.
[60] Nagaraj S, Peddha MS, Manjappara UV. Fragments of obestatin as modulators of feed intake, circulating lipids, and stored fat. Biochem Biophys Res Commun 2008; 366: 731-7.
[61] Lagaud GJ, Young A, Acena A, Morton MF, Barrett TD, Shankley NP. Retracted notice to: ''Obestatin reduces food intake and suppresses body 4 weight gain in rodents" Biochem Biophys Res Commun 2009; 388: 619.
[62] Seoane LM, Al-Massadi O, Pazos Y, Pagotto U, Casanueva FF. Central obestatin administration does not modify either spontaneous or ghrelin-induced food intake in rats. J Endocrinol Invest 2006; 29: RC13-15.
[63] Moechars D, Depoortere I, Moreaux B, *et al.* Altered gastrointestinal and metabolic function in the GPR39-obestatin receptor-knockout mouse. Gastroenterology 2006; 131: 1131-41.
[64] Gourcerol G, Million M, Adelson DW, *et al.* Lack of interaction between peripheral injection of CCK and obestatin in the regulation of gastric satiety signaling in rodents. Peptides 2006; 27: 2811-9.
[65] Samson WK, White MM, Price C, Ferguson AV. Obestatin acts in brain to inhibit thirst. Am J Physiol Regul Integr Comp Physiol 2007; 292: R637-43.
[66] Lagaud GJ, Young A, Acena A, Morton MF, Barrett TD, Shankley NP. Obestatin reduces food intake and suppresses body weight gain in rodents. Biochem Biophys Res Commun 2007; 357: 264-9.
[67] Yamamoto D, Ikeshita N, Daito R, *et al.* Neither intravenous nor intracerebroventricular administration of obestatin affects the secretion of GH, PRL, TSH and ACTH in rats. Regul Pept 2007; 138: 141-4.
[68] Nogueiras R, Pfluger P, Tovar S, *et al.* Effects of obestatin on energy balance and growth hormone secretion in rodents. Endocrinology 2007; 148: 21-6.
[69] Kobelt P, Wisser AS, Stengel A, *et al.* Peripheral obestatin has no effect on feeding behavior and brain Fos expression in rodents. Peptides 2008; 29: 1018-27.
[70] Depoortere I, Thijs T, Moechars D, De Smet B, Ver Donck L, Peeters TL. Effect of peripheral obestatin on food intake and gastric emptying in ghrelin-knockout mice. Br J Pharmacol 2008; 153: 1550-7.
[71] Annemie VD, Debby VD, Valentijn V, *et al.* Central administration of obestatin fails to show inhibitory effects on food and water intake in mice. Regul Pept 2009; 156: 77-82.
[72] Brunetti L, Leone S, Orlando G, *et al.* Effects of obestatin on feeding and body weight after standard or cafeteria diet in the rat. Peptides 2009; 30: 1323-7.
[73] Unniappan S, Speck M, Kieffer TJ. Metabolic effects of chronic obestatin infusion in rats. Peptides 2008; 29: 1354-61.
[74] Sibilia V, Bresciani E, Lattuada N, *et al.* Intracerebroventricular acute and chronic administration of obestatin minimally affect food intake but not weight gain in the rat. J Endocrinol Invest 2006; 29: RC31-4.
[75] De Smet B, Thijs T, Peeters TL, Depoortere I. Effect of peripheral obestatin on gastric emptying and intestinal contractility in rodents. Neurogastroenterol Motil 2007; 19: 211-7.
[76] Gourcerol G, Coskun T, Craft LS, *et al.* Preproghrelin-derived peptide, obestatin, fails to influence food intake in lean or obese rodents. Obesity (Silver Spring) 2007; 15: 2643-52.
[77] Kobelt P, Tebbe JJ, Tjandra I, *et al.* CCK inhibits the orexigenic effect of peripheral ghrelin. Am J Physiol Regul Integr Comp Physiol 2005; 288: R751-8.
[78] Kobelt P, Goebel M, Stengel A, *et al.* Bombesin, but not amylin, blocks the orexigenic effect of peripheral ghrelin. Am J Physiol Regul Integr Comp Physiol 2006; 291: R903-13.
[79] Friedman JM, Halaas JL. Leptin and the regulation of body weight in mammals. Nature 1998; 395: 763-70.
[80] Bado A, Levasseur S, Attoub S, *et al.* The stomach is a source of leptin. Nature 1998; 394: 790-793.
[81] Asakawa A, Inui A, Kaga T, *et al.* Ghrelin is an appetite-stimulatory signal from stomach with structural resemblance to motilin. Gastroenterology 2001; 120: 337-45.
[82] Nakazato M, Murakami N, Date Y, *et al.* A role for ghrelin in the central regulation of feeding. Nature 2001; 409: 194-8.

[83] Shintani M, Ogawa Y, Ebihara K, *et al.* Ghrelin, an endogenous growth hormone secretagogue, is a novel orexigenic peptide that antagonizes leptin action through the activation of hypothalamic neuropeptide Y/Y1 receptor pathway. Diabetes 2001; 50: 227-32.
[84] Jerlhag E, Egecioglu E, Landgren S, *et al.* Requirement of central ghrelin signaling for alcohol reward. Proc Natl Acad Sci USA 2009; 106: 11318-23.
[85] Saper CB, Chou TC, Elmquist JK. The need to feed: homeostatic and hedonic control of eating. Neuron 2002; 36: 199-211.
[86] Jerlhag E, Egecioglu E, Dickson SL, Andersson M, Svensson L, Engel JA. Ghrelin stimulates locomotor activity and accumbal dopamine-overflow via central cholinergic systems in mice: implications for its involvement in brain reward. Addict Biol 2006; 11: 45-54.
[87] Jerlhag E. Systemic administration of ghrelin induces conditioned place preference and stimulates accumbal dopamine. Addict Biol 2008; 13: 358-363.
[88] Jerlhag E, Egecioglu E, Dickson SL, Douhan A, Svensson L, Engel JA. Ghrelin administration into tegmental areas stimulates locomotor activity and increases extracellular concentration of dopamine in the nucleus accumbens. Addict Biol 2007; 12: 6-16.
[89] Abizaid A, Liu ZW, Andrews ZB, *et al.* Ghrelin modulates the activity and synaptic input organization of midbrain dopamine neurons while promoting appetite. J Clin Invest 2006; 116: 3229-39.
[90] Minokoshi Y, Alquier T, Furukawa N, *et al.* AMP-kinase regulates food intake by responding to hormonal and nutrient signals in the hypothalamus. Nature 2004; 428: 569-74.
[91] Kola B, Korbonits M. Shedding light on the intricate puzzle of ghrelin's effects on appetite regulation. J Endocrinol 2009; 202: 191-8.
[92] Kola B, Farkas I, Christ-Crain M, *et al.* The orexigenic effect of ghrelin is mediated through central activation of the endogenous cannabinoid system. PLoS One 2008; 3: e1797.
[93] Cani PD, Montoya ML, Neyrinck AM, Delzenne NM, Lambert DM. Potential modulation of plasma ghrelin and glucagon-like peptide-1 by anorexigenic cannabinoid compounds, SR141716A (rimonabant) and oleoylethanolamide. Br J Nutr 2004; 92: 757-761.
[94] Ogden CL, Carroll MD, Curtin LR, McDowell MA, Tabak CJ, Flegal KM. Prevalence of overweight and obesity in the US, 1999-2004. JAMA 2006; 295: 1549-1555.
[95] James WP. The epidemiology of obesity: the size of the problem. J Intern Med 2008; 263: 336-52.
[96] Flegal KM, Graubard BI, Williamson DF, Gail MH. Cause-specific excess deaths associated with underweight, overweight, and obesity. JAMA 2007; 298: 2028-37.
[97] Flegal KM, Carroll MD, Kuczmarski RJ, Johnson CL. Overweight and obesity in the United States: prevalence and trends, 1960-1994. Int J Obes Relat Metab Disord 1998; 22: 39-47.
[98] Marx J. Cellular warriors at the battle of the bulge. Science 2003; 299: 846-9.
[99] Wynne K, Stanley S, Bloom S. The gut and regulation of body weight. J Clin Endocrinol Metab 2004; 89: 2576-82.
[100] Wren AM, Bloom SR. Gut hormones and appetite control. Gastroenterology 2007; 132: 2116-30.
[101] Gura T. Obesity drug pipeline not so fat. Science 2003; 299: 849-52.
[102] Isidro ML, Cordido F. Drug treatment of obesity: established and emerging therapies. Mini Rev Med Chem 2009; 9: 664-73.
[103] Tanner BD, Allen JW. Complications of bariatric surgery: implications for the covering physician. Am Surg 2009; 75: 103-12.
[104] Pournaras DJ, le Roux CW. Obesity, Gut Hormones, and Bariatric Surgery. World J Surg 2009; 33: 1983-8.
[105] Sugerman HJ, Wolfe LG, Sica DA, Clore JN. Diabetes and hypertension in severe obesity and effects of gastric bypass-induced weight loss. Ann Surg 2003; 237: 751-6; discussion 757-8.
[106] Sjostrom L, Lindroos AK, Peltonen M, *et al.* Lifestyle, diabetes, and cardiovascular risk factors 10 years after bariatric surgery. N Engl J Med 2004; 351: 2683-93.
[107] Yale CE. Gastric surgery for morbid obesity. Complications and long-term weight control. Arch Surg 1989; 124: 941-6.
[108] Balsiger BM, Kennedy FP, Abu-Lebdeh HS. Prospective evaluation of Roux-en-Y gastric bypass as primary operation for medically complicated obesity. Mayo Clin Proc 2000; 75: 673-80.
[109] Waters GS, Pories WJ, Swanson MS, Meelheim HD, Flickinger EG, May HJ. Long-term studies of mental health after the Greenville gastric bypass operation for morbid obesity. Am J Surg 1991; 161: 154-7; discussion 157-8.
[110] Cheung WW, Mak RH. Ghrelin and its analogues as therapeutic agents for anorexia and cachexia in end-stage renal disease. Kidney Int 2009; 76: 135-7.
[111] Lu SC, Xu J, Chinookoswong N, *et al.* An acyl-ghrelin-specific neutralizing antibody inhibits the acute ghrelin-mediated orexigenic effects in mice. Mol Pharmacol 2009; 75: 901-7.
[112] Zorrilla EP, Iwasaki S, Moss JA, *et al.* Vaccination against weight gain. Proc Natl Acad Sci USA 2006; 103: 13226-31.
[113] Biotechnology C. Phase I/IIa clinical trial with obese individuals shows no effect of CYT009-GhrQb on weight loss. Cytos Biotechnology: Press Release November 7, 2006.
[114] Kobelt P, Helmling S, Stengel A, *et al.* Anti-ghrelin Spiegelmer NOX-B11 inhibits neurostimulatory and orexigenic effects of peripheral ghrelin in rats. Gut 2006; 55: 788-92.
[115] Asakawa A, Inui A, Kaga T, *et al.* Antagonism of ghrelin receptor reduces food intake and body weight gain in mice. Gut 2003; 52: 947-52.
[116] Shearman LP, Wang SP, Helmling S, *et al.* Ghrelin neutralization by a ribonucleic acid-SPM ameliorates obesity in diet-induced obese mice. Endocrinology 2006; 147: 1517-26.
[117] Kellokoski E, Kummu O, Serpi R, *et al.* Ghrelin vaccination decreases plasma MCP-1 level in LDLR(-/-) -mice. Peptides 2009; 30: 2292-300.
[118] Vizcarra JA, Kirby JD, Kim SK, Galyean ML. Active immunization against ghrelin decreases weight gain and alters plasma concentrations of growth hormone in growing pigs. Domest Anim Endocrinol 2007; 33: 176-89.
[119] Wells T. Ghrelin - Defender of fat. Prog Lipid Res 2009; 48: 257-74.
[120] Yang J, Zhao TJ, Goldstein JL, Brown MS. Inhibition of ghrelin O-acyltransferase (GOAT) by octanoylated pentapeptides. Proc Natl Acad Sci USA 2008; 105: 10750-5.
[121] Kirchner H, Gutierrez JA, Solenberg PJ, *et al.* GOAT links dietary lipids with the endocrine control of energy balance. Nat Med 2009; 15: 741-5.

Mitigation Strategies of Obesity-Induced Inflammation and Metabolic Syndrome

Andreas D. Flouris[*,1], Andres E. Carrillo[1] and Giorgos S. Metsios[2]

[1]*FAME Laboratory, Institute of Human Performance and Rehabilitation, Centre for Research and Technology Thessaly, Karies, Trikala, 42100 Greece*

[2]*School of Sports, Performing Arts and Leisure, University of Wolverhampton, Walsall Campus, Gorway Road, Walsall, WS1 3BD UK*

Abstract: Obesity is a major global epidemic involving children and adults. According to the World Health Organization, obesity incidence will continue to rise with global estimations reaching 700 million by 2015. Thus, it is essential to investigate the nature of the obesity epidemic and potential mitigating mechanisms. In this chapter, we explore the association between obesity and inflammation and the efficacy of biochemical mimetics such a ghrelin and leptin for exercise and diet in the control of obesity-induced inflammation. We also review non-pharmaceutical obesity interventions and non-invasive means for predicting metabolic syndrome development as well as methods of obesity assessment.

Keywords: Ghrelin, leptin, exercise, diet, vitamin D, body fat.

INTRODUCTION

Obesity is a major global epidemic involving both children and adults. In adults, ample epidemiological evidence demonstrates a positive association between obesity and a greater risk of all-cause mortality, particularly from coronary heart disease (CHD) [1]. Similarly, overweight or obese children are more likely to display aberrant CHD risk factor profiles [2-6], develop a distorted self-image that appears to persist into adulthood [7], and are at increased risk for becoming overweight and/or obese adults [8]. On a global scale, over 1 billion adults are overweight, and at least 300 million are obese. According to the World Health Organization, obesity incidence will continue to rise with global estimations reaching 700 million by 2015 [9]. The financial burden associated with obesity is overwhelming; for example, ~8% of the total EU health care budget is allocated for obesity-related treatment [9]. This financial burden is further inflated with the consideration of obesity as a contributing factor to the development of several chronic conditions, such as type 2 diabetes, atherosclerosis, and hypertension. In this light, it is necessary to investigate the nature of the obesity epidemic and to explore potential mitigating mechanisms. In this chapter, we investigate the association between obesity and inflammation and the efficacy of biochemical mimetics such a ghrelin and leptin for exercise and diet in the control of obesity-induced inflammation. We also review non-pharmaceutical obesity interventions and non-invasive means for predicting metabolic syndrome development as well as methods of obesity assessment.

OBESITY AND INFLAMMATION: A DISEASE-DRIVEN COLLABORATION

Obesity disturbs the human biological system and thus creates an environment that succumbs to disease infiltration. According to recent evidence increased adipose tissue and its invisible accomplice—inflammation—fuel obesity-related disease development [10]. It is not accurate, however, to simply imply that a positive relationship exists between adipose tissue and inflammation. Instead, it has recently been suggested that adipose tissue acts as motor for the inflammation associated with obesity [11]. Indeed, increased adipose tissue 1) produces and secretes pro-inflammatory cytokines [2, 12] secretes adipokines that interact with immune cells to release inflammatory proteins [3, 13] recruits immune cells, such as macrophage precursors (monocytes), into adipose tissue that subsequently produces and releases pro-inflammatory mediators [13]. Pharmaceutical interventions that target the aforementioned adipose tissue-induced progression of inflammatory stress *via* adipose-immune interactions may be valuable in alleviating obesity-associated disease development.

* Corresponding author: Tel: +302431047055; Fax: +302431047056; E-mail: aflouris@cereteth.gr

Atta-ur-Rahman / M. Iqbal Choudhary (Eds.)

Activation of transcription factors, such as nuclear factor-κB (NFκB) that bind to relevant DNA binding sites in immune cells, promote the production of pro-inflammatory cytokines that are frequently observed with increased body fat [14]. Furthermore, humans contain at least two monocyte sub-populations with differing phenotypes—that is, classical and inflammatory monocytes. Inflammatory monocytes account for only 10% of all circulating monocytes in healthy humans [15]. Increased NFκB activation and a disturbed distribution of monocyte sub-populations, has recently been observed in obese individuals [16]; favoring a shift toward the inflammatory monocyte phenotype that may be caused by a disruption in adipokine secretion. Further, inflammatory monocytes have a functional role in the pathogenesis of chronic disease [17, 18], and are major producers of pro-inflammatory proteins [19]. Increased concentrations of circulating tumor necrosis factor alpha (TNF-α), interleukin-6 (IL-6) and C-reactive protein (CRP) characterize inflammatory stress associated with obesity [20, 21].

The importance of targeting obesity-associated inflammation in anti-obesity drug development is highlighted in a recent review article describing inflammation (IL-6 and CRP) as a predictor for the development of type 2 diabetes [22]. Given that over 90% of type 2 diabetics are overweight or obese [9], it reasonable to suggest that obesity-associated inflammation contributes substantially to the development of this disease. Furthermore, other chronic conditions that develop or worsen with obesity, such as cardiovascular disease (CVD), also contain a strong inflammatory component. Indeed, systemic inflammatory stress has been linked to the increased risk of development of CVD [23]. Research investigating the aforementioned mechanistic properties of potential anti-inflammatory strategies that target obesity-induced inflammation is particularly important to anti-obesity pharmacological development—to control the obesity-induced inflammation that leads to disease progression. The following sections will focus on certain biological attributes frequently impaired with obesity that may have valuable implications for developing anti-obesity agents that target inflammation and lessen disease risk—that is, ghrelin and vitamin D status.

GHRELIN EXERTS ANTI-INFLAMMATORY PROPERTIES

Ghrelin is the appetite-stimulating hormone predominantly synthesized and secreted from the stomach and small intestine [24, 25]; and is typically reduced in obese individuals [26]. Ghrelin is the endogenous ligand for the growth hormone secretagogue receptor (GHS-R), which is expressed on the surface of human monocytes; this suggests a multi-functional role for ghrelin that includes immune regulation [27]. Indeed, data from a recent *in vitro* experiment indicates a dose-dependant inhibition of IL-1β and IL-6 production from human monocytes, following incubation with varied ghrelin concentrations [27]. This ghrelin-induced inhibition of pro-inflammatory cytokine expression appears to occur *via* the interaction with the GHS-R and a shared antagonistic relationship with the hormone leptin [27]. Leptin is synthesized by adipocytes, and is elevated in obese individuals due to increased amounts of leptin-secreting adipose tissue. Contrary to ghrelin, elevated leptin concentrations stimulate pro-inflammatory cytokine production occurring *via* interaction with leptin receptor (Ob-R)—expressed on ~25% of monocytes [27]. Interestingly, ghrelin inhibits leptin-induced pro-inflammatory cytokine expression [27]. It is, therefore, suggested that reduced ghrelin combined with increased leptin may lead to an increase in inflammation, potentially among obese individuals [28]. Understanding the mechanisms responsible for a variety of ghrelin-governing functions, including inflammation, will provide valuable insight on its use as a potential therapeutic target in obesity and inflammation.

GHRELIN: EXERCISE TRAINING MIMETIC FOR CONTROLLING OBESITY-INDUCED INFLAMMATION?

As mentioned above, evidence suggests a strong link between inflammation and chronic disease [12, 13, 23]. Exercise training, however, has recently been shown to have potent anti-inflammatory actions [28-30]. Indeed, McFarlin *et al.* [31] observed elevated levels of lipopolysaccharide (LPS)-stimulated IL-6, IL-1β, and TNF-α production in sedentary younger (18 – 30 years) and older (60 – 80 years) participants versus age-matched physically active controls (LPS is found in the outer membrane of Gram-negative bacteria that stimulates an inflammatory cascade following interaction with its receptor on monocytes). Similarly, Stewart *et al.* reported a significant reduction in CRP after a 12-week exercise intervention program in both younger (18 – 35 years) and older (65 – 85 years) sedentary subjects [32]. Interestingly, the intensity and type of exercise training appears to reflect the observed exercise-induced metabolic and adipokine response [33]. Specifically, greater changes in body composition—such as increased muscle mass and resting energy expenditure (REE)—observed with resistance training may induce a greater anti-inflammatory response. A change in body composition alters secretion of ghrelin [34]; which has been suggested as a possible mechanism responsible for the anti-inflammatory effects of exercise.

The multi-functional nature of the orexigenic hormone, ghrelin, identifies its potential as a target for anti-obesity (and its associated inflammation) drug development. The majority of research examining exercise-induced changes in circulating ghrelin, without a reduction in body weight, have shown only minor effects. For example, Leidy, *et al.* [34] reported a significant increase in circulating ghrelin in women following a combined treatment of weight loss (diet) and aerobic exercise; there was, however, no change in ghrelin among the exercise-only women who remained weight stable. Furthermore, Foster-Schubert *et al.* [35] examined changes in ghrelin following participation in a 1 year exercise training program and reported higher levels of ghrelin among all participants, with greater increases among subjects who lost more weight. A more recent study documented a significant increase in circulating ghrelin among older adults participating in a higher intensity 12-week resistance training program. Interestingly, the significant increase in ghrelin was reported without any significant alterations in body weight or body fat %, and was negatively correlated with the change in the percentage of monocytes exhibiting the inflammatory phenotype [36]. Using a protocol similar the one mentioned previously, 12-weeks of resistance training in older adults increased muscle protein synthesis rate [37]; it is, therefore, logical to speculate that the potential gain in fat free mass (FFM) following 12-weeks of training influences metabolic activity and overall energy balance. Similar to weight loss, the metabolic alterations and potential lean mass gains that occur with resistance training may alter ghrelin secretion in response to negative energy balance.

Higher intensity exercise training appears to elevate circulating ghrelin concentrations [35, 36], that, in turn, may be partially responsible for the anti-inflammatory effects of exercise [28]. Given the biological abnormalities (i.e. increased leptin, inflammatory monocytes, low metabolic rate, etc.) observed in obese individuals, the development of pharmaceutical interventions aimed at normalizing ghrelin concentrations mimics the relevant hormonal changes observed after exercise training and weight loss; thus, alleviating leptin-mediated pro-inflammatory cytokine secretion, and obesity-associated inflammation that will subsequently reduce disease risk. This highlights the importance of ghrelin as an anti-inflammatory player, important in coordinating metabolic-immune interactions; highly relevant for anti-obesity drug development.

GHRELIN: CALORIC RESTRICTION MIMETIC FOR CONTROLLING OBESITY-INDUCED INFLAMMATION?

Reduced ghrelin observed with obesity is correlated with obesity-associated inflammation [38]. Moreover, increased ghrelin observed with caloric restriction (CR) is associated with reduced inflammation [39, 40]. Individuals living in a state of chronic negative energy balance elicited by CR experience an improved immune response; that is only a small portion of the pleiotropic effects induced by CR [41-43]. In fact, CR is the only genetic-independent approach to extend lifespan; tested using various experimental models [44]. Several CR reports reveal its effects on mononuclear cells (including monocytes) to reduce inflammatory cytokine secretion; including TNF-α and IL-6 [45]. Other related work shows positive CR-induced changes that occur within the immune system—including the enhancement of the T cell response, and natural killer cell activity [46, 47]. It has been suggested that the neuroendocrine factors regulating energy balance, influence immune function during CR [48]. Given that CR is a state of chronic negative energy balance, hunger stimulating hormones—ghrelin—are released following central nervous system activation. Indeed, ghrelin and leptin are metabolic regulators that are altered during CR [48]. Dixit *et al.* has eloquently examined the potent anti-inflammatory effects of ghrelin in T cells, monocytes and endothelial cells *via* ghrelin interaction with GHS-R [27, 48]. Given the aforementioned ghrelin-induced anti-inflammatory effects, and its alterations in response to changes in energy balance, this orexigenic hormone is important in coupling the metabolic and immune systems. In turn, ghrelin may be a valuable target to pursue as a potential compound that mimics the biological changes evident during CR. Further, it has been suggested that ghrelin analogues or receptor agonists may be effective as a class of CR mimetic that may alleviate inflammation associated with obesity [48].

OBESITY AND VITAMIN D DEFICIENCY

Overall, obese individuals have the ability to synthesize and metabolize vitamin D, just as effectively as lean individuals. Despite this, deficiency in vitamin D—as measured by serum 25-hydroxyvitamin D [25(OH)D]—is commonly observed with obesity [49, 50]. Controlled research investigating ultraviolet

(UV) radiation treatment to obese individuals reveals obesity-associated vitamin D deficiency is caused as a result of decreased bioavailability. Specifically, vitamin D [25(OH)D] stores become difficult to access and are essentially sequestered in adipocytes among individuals with high body fat [51]. Given this, in addition to the concern that vitamin D is not commonly found in most foods, and specific combinations of environmental factors (i.e. latitude and season) are essential for vitamin D synthesis *via* UV radiation—vitamin D deficiency is considered to be a global concern [52, 53]. This is particularly important among obese individuals that are living in most of Europe, Canada, and northern USA; because vitamin D synthesis is impaired at the aforementioned latitudes during winter. In fact, an article published in March of this year proposes that the reduction in vitamin D status is the stimulus for the accumulation of body fat during winter [54]. Without intervention, this will eventually turn into a downward spiral of accumulating body fat and vitamin D deficiency. Current supplementation recommendations do not elevate vitamin D status [25(OH)D] to sufficient levels [55]; which is even less in obese individuals [51]. Current research shows that vitamin D deficiency is related to the development of certain chronic conditions; such as type 2 diabetes and hypertension [56]. Interestingly, chronic conditions associated with vitamin D deficiency are at least in part, characterized by inflammation [57]. This reflects the importance of vitamin D-induced anti-inflammatory actions. Monitoring vitamin D status and supplementing with a specific dosage to elevate 25(OH) D to sufficient levels, rather than suggesting a specific dose for everyone may alleviate inflammation associated with obesity; and thus, improve disease risk.

VITAMIN D EXERTS ANTI-INFLAMMATORY EFFECTS

Vitamin D exerts its effects on several cells of the immune system, and thus, appears to have anti-inflammatory actions [58]. Recent reports indicate associations existing between vitamin D deficiency and lower circulating CRP and other pro-inflammatory cytokines [59, 60]. Furthermore, cell culture studies suggest a vitamin D-induced reduction in pro-inflammatory markers such as TNF-α [61]. Specifically, Cohen *et al.* [61] incubated human macrophages with various concentrations of the active vitamin D metabolite [$1,25(OH_2)D_3$] followed by an lipopolysaccharide (LPS) incubation period, and showed a significant inhibitory effect of $1,25(OH_2)D_3$ on LPS-stimulated production of TNF-α. Similarly, Riancho *et al.* [62] showed a significant reduction in TNF-α secretion from peripheral blood mononuclear cells (PBMC) acquired from 7 hemodialysis patients after 1-month of oral vitamin D supplementation (0.5 μg/day). The vitamin D-induced reductions in TNF-α and CRP have significant practical implications, as these biomarkers of systemic inflammation are often elevated with obesity and are associated with elevated disease risk [63, 64].

Considering the increasing number of targets for $1,25(OH_2)D_3$ among immune cells, it is difficult to elucidate the precise mechanism responsible for the anti-inflammatory actions of $1,25(OH_2)D_3$ [58]. There is emerging evidence that the transcription factor NFκB is a potential target for vitamin D-induced reductions in inflammatory biomarkers [65, 66]. Cohen-Lahav *et al.*, [65] showed an increase in mRNA and protein levels of the NFκB inhibitor IκB in murine macrophage cells following a $1,25(OH_2)D_3$ and subsequent LPS incubation period. Using mouse embryonic fibroblasts from vitamin D receptor knockout mice, Sun *et al.*, [66] showed a significant increase in NFκB activity and elevated circulating TNF-α and IL-6, likely due to a reduction in the NFκB inhibitor (IκB). Vitamin D may illicit its anti-inflammatory effects by binding to vitamin D receptors on monocytes and/or stimulating gene expression of proteins, such as cathelicidin, that interfere with inflammatory pathways. Cathelicidin is an anti-microbial peptide that binds to, and thus inhibits LPS-stimulated pro-inflammatory cytokine secretion [67]. Vitamin D up-regulates cathelicidin gene expression [68], which may partly explain the mechanism behind vitamin D's anti-inflammatory actions. Vitamin D deficiency is analogous with obesity [49, 50], and vitamin D status is associated with circulating cathelicidin levels in humans [69], it is, therefore, reasonable to suggest that obese individuals have low cathelicidin—and that it may be linked to obesity-associated inflammation. Normalizing vitamin D status *via* appropriate supplementation strategies, specific to the given population, may be effective in alleviating inflammation associated with obesity. In addition, knowledge of specific mechanisms responsible for the anti-inflammatory actions of vitamin D may serve as potential targets important for pharmaceutical development aiming to lessen the inflammatory stress associated with obesity.

NON PHARMACEUTICAL OBESITY INTERVENTIONS

Exercise

Exercise has well been recognized as an important non-pharmaceutical intervention to ameliorate symptoms in the most common chronic diseases such as rheumatoid arthritis, cardiovascular disease and cancer [70-72]. This is due to the beneficial adaptations that occur as a result of the physical stress imposed on the human biological system during increased physical effort. More specifically, exercise has been implicated in the improvement of vascular function, muscular strength and balance, cardiac and respiratory structure and function as well as significant changes in body composition. The latter represents perhaps the most commonly stated rational for embarking in exercise regimes, as these programs have obvious short term effects on body fatness. Alongside this, evidence from large studies supports that increased involvement in physical activity may prevent the development of undesirable body composition changes leading to overweight and obesity [73].

The adipose tissue is the body's most plentiful source of energy. Fat-derived energy can be produced from the following major sources: triglycerides that are stored within the muscle close to mitochondria and also circulating triglycerides and/or free fatty acids. *Via* these sources, fat is broken down to generate energy, a physiological process known as lipolysis. This process is significantly enhanced during and post exercise, which is the main reason that in the long-term the size of adipose tissue significantly reduces.

During Exercise

Adipocytes synthesize and store triglycerides. Hormone sensitive lipase is a hormone that catalyses the breakdown of triglycerides and enables them to diffuse into the circulation. With the help of albumin they are transferred to the active exercising muscle fibres as free fatty acids. Although the free fatty acids may again form triglycerides when located in close proximity to mitochondria, during physical effort they enter the mithochondria and provide energy. The most commonly prescribed exercise regime in overweight and obese individuals, demands progressive increases in physical effort which mainly utilizes the contribution of slow-twitch muscle fiber mobilization within the muscle. The large numbers of mitochondria and blood supply in these fibers makes them the predominant units responsible for fat breakdown. The adipose-derived triglycerides are broken down in glycerol and fatty acids. Glycerol can be converted to glucose by the liver and provide energy for cellular metabolism. *Via* beta oxidization, the fatty acid compounds converts to acetyl-coA within the mitochondrion and then transferred into the citric acid cycle for energy generation. These biochemical pathways mainly materialize in the presence of the aerobic metabolism since in anaerobic conditions; fat catabolism is not used as the primer pathway for energy generation. Apart from these processes, lipoprotein lipase, an enzyme that is found in endothelial cells lining the capillaries, catalyses triglycerides and enables them to be transferred into cells in order to provide energy (or triglyceride resynthesis).

Post Exercise

It has been well documented that both aerobic as well as resistance training may promote significant changes in the body that favors a healthy body composition and lead to reduced body fat accumulation. Both long term structured aerobic (at 60-75% of the maximum aerobic capacity) and resistance (at 60-75% of one maximum repetition) exercise training programs significantly decrease adipose tissue and increase muscle mass [74]. These beneficial adaptations occur irrespective of the presence of a chronic disease, such as cardiovascular disease of arthritis, in both males and females. The exercise-induced fat depletion leads to a decrease in fat mass size in the long term and the subsequent reduction in weight. This decrease in adipose tissue is accompanied by a significantly favorable health profile, as the adipose tissue is a major source of pro-inflammatory cytokines. Increase expression of specific cytokines (proteins) may be deleterious for health as it may unbalance major biological processes related to homeostasis and thus, well-being.

Resistance training has a significant impact of muscle metabolism, function and size. Initial gains in strength are attributed to neural muscle adaptations that may occur in the absence of muscle size [75]. These are the enhanced recruitment of neurons, better central nervous system activation and increased synchronization of the motor units. In contrast, long term resistance exercise increases the size of the muscles by hypertrophying the muscle fibers. This is a physiological adaptation that occurs irrespective of age and gender as human physiological pathways respond to specific stimuli in the same manner at all ages and in both genders (e.g. aerobic exercise will always stimulate increased lipolysis); regarding the latter, the differences in specific hormones (e.g. testosterone) between genders favor the increased strength levels found in males. Resistance training works as a mechanical stress stimulus, which enhances protein signaling towards increased synthesis. The muscle cell myofibril enlarges and also increases in number forming additional sarcomeres, the basic unit of the muscle's myofibril. As these adaptations result in increased muscle size, resting energy expenditure increases concomitantly [76]. Therefore, increased expenditure at rest may further compensate for the changes in body composition in response to exercise.

Diet

Diet is also recognized as the other most important non-pharmaceutical intervention to combat obesity. The cause of obesity is the disruption of the equilibrium between energy intake and expenditure. Diet significantly affects the former particularly nowadays where the frequently adopted westernized lifestyle is characterized by less involvement in physical exercise (i.e. decreased expenditure) and increased calorie intake due to the insufficient quality of fast food. Moreover, everyday tasks that required physical involvement (such as washing) have been replaced by equipment (e.g. washing machine), that although made our lives easier they have contributed to a generalized attitude towards avoiding physical tasks and subsequent less energy expenditure.

The advances of science in energy intake and dieting have become increasingly effective and therefore weight loss can be mathematically and theoretically achieved when solely based on the calculation between intake and expenditure. However, the highly variable human behavior when dieting makes diet interventions very challenging. This is perhaps the reason that after an effective weight reduction intervention, in many occasions the individuals regain their weight within 3-5 years [77].

To date, there are many variations regarding the effectiveness of different energy input interventions ranging from low-carbohydrate/high protein diets to extreme high protein diets. Scientists have long been investigating the sufficient formula that will achieve and maintain desirable body composition results. Excellent systematic reviews and meta-analyzed reveal that the simple approach of reducing calorie intake with any means (e.g. low fat or low-glycemic load diets) is as effective as the more complex diets and, although it may be sufficient in the short term in combating obesity, weight gain will almost definitely increase after the end of the intervention if weight reduction is not accompanied by a behavioral change towards dieting [78]. The most commonly adopted strategies that achieve beneficial results when applied with an effective diet regime are:

- ∞ General change in lifestyle to incorporate increases in physical activity and,
- ∞ Developing skills to replace existing routines with new ones such as eating before shopping grocery are also effective.

Caution should be exercised when prescribing diets, as existing extreme approaches may result in loss of weight in the short-term but may have concomitant detrimental health effects. An example of such an extreme approach is the ketonic diets with low carbohydrate intake: the concept behind this is that fat storage depletes more easily in the absence of carbohydrate intake. However, the significant intake of fat as well as protein may result in other harmful health effects such as a high increase in cholesterol, which is a major factor leading to cardiovascular disease. In general, extreme diet intervention serves the willingness of the dieters to lose weight using a "quick fix" without taking into consideration the adverse effects that these may have on human health. Besides, a balanced low-calorie diet coupled with a behavioral change is a much more effective way of combating obesity and may have better and permanent effects [79].

NON-INVASIVE MEANS FOR PREDICTING METABOLIC SYNDROME DEVELOPMENT

The metabolic syndrome has been described as a link amongst insulin resistance, hypertension, dyslipidemia, type 2 diabetes, and other metabolic abnormalities associated with an increased risk of atherosclerotic cardiovascular disease in adults. The metabolic syndrome is prevalent in approximately 15%, 35% and 13.5% of adults in Europe, the US and China, respectively and has been recognized [80] as a secondary target of risk-reduction therapy by the World Health Organization and the US National Cholesterol Education Program Adult Treatment Panel III [80], because it places individuals at risk for type 2 diabetes [81] and cardiovascular disease [82].

Obesity, the most common cause of insulin resistance in children, is, similarly to the metabolic syndrome, associated with dyslipidemia, type 2 diabetes, and long-term vascular complications. Obesity, is prevalent in approximately 18%, 30% and 20% of adults in Europe, the US and China, respectively and is unanimously acknowledged as a major global epidemic involving both children and adults. In adults, ample epidemiological evidence demonstrates a positive association between obesity and a greater risk of all-cause mortality, particularly from cardiovascular disease [1]. Similarly, overweight or obese children are more likely to display aberrant cardiovascular disease risk factor profiles [2], develop a distorted self-image that appears to persist into adulthood [7], and are at increased risk for becoming overweight and/or obese adults [8].

The pathogeneses of metabolic syndrome and obesity are exceedingly complex and, to date, not entirely understood; yet the interaction of sedentary lifestyle, dietary elements and obesity in childhood and adolescence together with genetic factors have been suggested to contribute to its development [83-85]. As the number of overweight and obese children is increasing [84-86] and it has become clearly evident that the pathology of the metabolic syndrome begins early in life [87, 88], it is vital to study the etiology of metabolic syndrome and obesity in childhood in order to understand their implications later in life and to limit them by introducing strong prevention strategies and comprehensive screening in childhood and adolescence.

SCREENING CUTOFFS FOR METABOLIC SYNDROME

In order to aid in the development of pediatric guidelines that will allow comprehensive screening for metabolic syndrome, we recently generated longitudinal preventive-screening cutoffs for this syndrome in adolescents by detecting demarcation points in key and easy-to-monitor parameters that enable – as early as five years in advance – the successful detection of metabolic syndrome that develops at the age of 17 years [MS_{17} [5]]. The gathered data covered metabolic syndrome risk factors as well as fitness, habitual physical activity, and dietary elements. The study adopted a 6-year design incorporating 4 data collection time points. The volunteers were assessed prospectively at the ages of 12, 13, 14 and 17 years with 210, 204, 198 and 187 adolescents volunteering at each data collection time point, respectively.

Our results showed that 12% of the participants, most of them boys, were diagnosed with MS_{17} and that the prevalence of MS_{17} increased from 5.3% to 31% and to 62.5% in normal, overweight, and obese participants, respectively [5]. More importantly, through receiver operating characteristics curve analyses it was possible to correctly diagnose MS_{17} in 12-, 13-, and 14-year old boys and girls using either BMI, or adiposity, or aerobic fitness levels. The BMI cutoffs for boys were set at 20.9, 22.5, 22.5 and 23.5 in ages 12, 13, 14 and 17 years, respectively (cutoffs henceforth are reported in an identical age-related sequence). The BMI cutoffs for girls were set at 21.2, 22.2, 22.7 and 23.0. The adiposity cutoffs for boys were set at 21.6%, 20.8%, 19.4% and 18.6%. The equivalent cutoffs for girls were set at 25.7%, 26.4%, 26.4% and 26.4%. The aerobic fitness cutoffs for boys were set at 31.8, 37.5, 37.8 and 38.5 $ml \cdot kg^{-1} \cdot min^{-1}$. The equivalent cutoffs for girls were set at 26.8, 28.3, 28.3 and 27.6 $ml \cdot kg^{-1} \cdot min^{-1}$.

The discovered longitudinal preventive-screening cut-offs for MS_{17} were found statistically valid and can be adopted as practical pediatric guidelines for mitigating future increases in the prevalence of metabolic syndrome because they allow for mass MS_{17} screening with minimal equipment and cost. For instance, the sensitivity and specificity for the BMI cutoffs indicated that should the proposed cutoffs be used to screen for MS_{17} in a population with 1000 boys and 1000 girls 12 years of age, 141 of 160 boys and 47 of 70 girls with MS_{17} would be identified. On the other hand, 235 boys and 279 girls would be misdiagnosed if the BMI cutoff was used alone. Therefore, further confirmatory testing with appropriate criteria such as the National Cholesterol Education Program - Adult Treatment Panel III definition would be required for a total of 702 (35.1%) of the 2000 children being tested. This would reduce the cost of diagnosis from the present situation, which requires screening of all children using criteria such as those of the National Cholesterol Education Program - Adult Treatment Panel III and, as such, is prohibitively expensive. This is noteworthy, considering that this five-years-in-advance diagnosis is achieved through simple height and weight measurements.

INVOLVEMENT OF ADIPOSITY

The early identification of children at high risk for developing metabolic syndrome in the years to come may help to develop strategies by focusing on the syndrome's underlying pathophysiology, particularly because the metabolic syndrome phenotype persists over time and tends to progress clinically with type 2 diabetes being imminent [89]. This is especially true for overweight and obese adolescents who are at higher risk for developing the metabolic syndrome and who, generally, become obese adults. Indeed, previous research has confirmed that the key elements of the metabolic syndrome are excess bodyweight, physical inactivity and a genetic predisposition to develop insulin resistance [88]. Furthermore, it has become apparent that excess bodyweight is a root cause in the development of this syndrome, due to its known link with insulin resistance [90]. Adipose tissue is also an important endocrinological component expressing adipocytokines, including adiponectin, interleukin-6, angiotensinogen/angiotensin II, plasminogen activator inhibitor type 1 and tumor necrosis factor-alpha, all of which contribute to the development of coronary heart disease [88]. Previous work from our group has shown that development of adiposity is longitudinally associated inversely with physical activity and aerobic fitness, but it shows no link with total energy intake [85]. These findings are in line with longitudinal data from other European [91] and North-American [92] groups showing adiposity to be inversely related to physical activity and aerobic fitness levels.

Physical activity, which has a marked seasonal pattern in children [84], is hypothesized to protect from the development of obesity through two main channels. First, through increased energy expenditure, mainly due to the high cost of activity itself, which normally appears with concomitant increases in resting metabolic rate [93]. This limits the likelihood of positive energy balance. Second, physical activity has beneficial effects on substrate metabolism, with an increased reliance on fat, relative to carbohydrate, for muscular fuel utilization [94]. In general, the effect of physical activity on caloric expenditure is accumulative, and with time, small amounts of activity can add up to significant weight loss. In children, however, aspects related to growth and development affect fat and weight regulation in different ways in boys and girls [95]. Unlike males, adequate body fat in young females is necessary for menarche to occur and this can be partly achieved through reduced physical activity levels. Indeed, a 50% reduction in physical activity has been observed prior to female puberty [96] indicating the existence of a biologically-regulated energy-conserving mechanism in favor of fat accumulation.

METHODS OF OBESITY ASSESSMENT

The prevalence of human obesity has dramatically increased over the last decades justifying its given characterization of an "epidemic" [97]. The rapid increase in obesity prevalence is a fact that intensifies the necessity to systematically monitor the phenomenon using reliable and valid measures of adiposity. To date, there are many available methods for estimating changes in weight and body composition whereas the advantages and limitations of each method vary.

BODY MASS INDEX (BMI)

Despite being controversial, BMI is the most frequently utilized method in epidemiological and clinical research to record body mass. It is calculated after the assessment of weight and height *via* the equation:

$$\text{BMI} = \text{weight (kg)} / \text{height (cm)}^2$$

Based solely on the assessment of weight and height therefore, BMI does not take into account adiposity and/or fat-free mass contents of human body, the two components of body composition; this represents apparently the major limitation of this method. For example, in large cohort studies, BMI may misclassify both muscular individuals of normal and/or short stature as obese [98]. This may also be the case as well in diseased populations in which body composition has been altered due to disease-related manifestations [99]. In contrast, the major advantage of BMI is that is a very quick method of assessing body mass, it can be performed by anyone without specific skills, does not require expensive equipment for its calculation and finally, it provides values that can be then compared amongst research studies. Moreover, in large cohort and epidemiological studies of non-specific athletic populations (e.g. weight lifters) it may detect trends towards the risk of cardiovascular disease risk factors [100], suggesting that it may be used as a prognostic proxy.

SKINFOLD MEASUREMENT

This is perhaps the most commonly used method of assessing body fat percentage in athletic populations. Its rationale is based on the interrelation that subcutaneous fat has with adipose and internal fat. It assesses the skinfold thickness (i.e. subcutaneous fat) in mm using specific calipers that have developed for this particular assessment. There are a lot of variations in the selection of the skinfold sites which may range from four to nine skinfolds as suggested by the American College of Sports Medicine guidelines [74]. Subsequently, different equations are available to calculate percentage body fat depending on the number of the skinfolds used. More recently, improved prediction equations have been developed for the assessment of skinfold thickness that may improve the prediction power of this method considerably [101]. The right side of the body is the one utilized at all times for these assessments whereas the anatomic location of the skinfolds is the following:

∞ *Triceps*: Vertical fold of the posterior midline of the upper part of the arm while it rests free on the side of the body. The calipers record the subcutaneous fat in the halfway from the top of the shoulder and the lower end of the elbow.

∞ *Biceps*: Vertical fold at the front midline of the arm, approximately one cm above the triceps skinfold.

∞ *Chest*: Right diagonal fold directed toward the nipple on the anterior axillary line as high as possible.

∞ *Midaxillary*: Vertical fold on the midaxillary line of the xiphoid process of the sternum.

∞ *Subscapular*: Diagonal fold below the tip of the scapula.

∞ *Iliac*: Diagonal fold above the bone of the hip following the natural line of the iliac creast.

∞ *Abdomen*: Vertical fold at the right side (approximately 2 cm) of the umbilicus.

∞ *Thigh*: Vertical fold at the middle of the thigh between the proximal border of patella and the inguinal crease.

∞ *Calf*: Vertical fold taken at the maximum circumference of the calf.

The main limitations of the skinfold method when utilized in normal non-athletic populations are the inability of the calliper jaws to fit the large folds of overweight and obese individuals resulting in reduced precision in predicting body fat and also the increased difficulty to find the appropriate landmarks. As such, its validity and reproducibility varies and therefore, its use for the assessment of overall adiposity is not recommended.

WAIST CIRCUMFERENCE

Abdominal obesity is recognized as amongst the important health factors that predispose to cardiovascular diseases, such as hypertension and diabetes. Therefore, the waist to hip ratio has been frequently used to detect body fat in epidemiological research which has been progressively been replaced by researchers with waist circumference alone. A waist circumference above 102 cm for men and 88 cm for women indicates a significantly increased risk for cardiovascular disease [102]. Similarly to BMI, although this method does not distinguish between muscle and fat tissues, it is a good predictor of adiposity and heart disease in epidemiological studies

UNDERWATER HYDROSTATIC WEIGHING

This methods of assessment is based on one of the Archimedes principles suggesting that when a mass is submerged into water, it displaces an amount of water volume that is equal to this mass. Underwater weighing assumes that fat and fat-free mass densities are constant: fat-free mass such as bone and muscle are denser than water whereas fat tissue is less dense than water. Hence, an individual with more body fat will weigh less underwater and be more buoyant compared to a muscular individual who will weigh more under the water. The assessment requires the individual to first be correctly weighted in air before submerged using standard weighing procedures. Sitting in a specific area and wearing appropriate minimal clothing, the individual then produces a forced maximal expiration and slowly is fully submerged underwater. The temperature of the water should be similar to the skin temperature. In order to take an accurate estimate the individual has to stay motionless for five to eight seconds. This procedure is repeated several times (from three to 12) and the average recording is filled in as the individual's underwater weight. Thereafter, body density is calculated using the following formula:

$$\text{Body Density} = \text{mass} / \text{volume} = W_a / [(W_a - W_w) / T_w] - LV$$

where W_a = normal weight measured in air, W_w = weight measured underwater, T_w = water temperature correction and LV = lung volume. After the calculation of body density, body fat percentage can then be estimated using the popular Siri equation.

This technique was considered to be and still is amongst the gold standard techniques for assessing body composition. However, it needs long testing hours, specific laboratory equipment specialized personnel whereas the individuals assessed have to undergo all these complicated procedures which may be inconvenient especially for diseased and/or large population studies. Thus, this method is not used often particularly given the availability of new accurate means of body composition assessment.

MAGNETIC RESONANCE IMAGING

This is one of the most commonly used imaging methods of body composition assessments that provide valuable information for body tissue compartments. Despite the need for specialized equipment and personnel and the long time for assessment, this methods is frequently used in both research and the clinical setting (e.g. for the diagnosis of muscle atrophy) as it is a non-invasive method and does not use radiation (such as the computed tomography method). Magnetic resonance imaging is based on the principle that when the body is subjected to a strong magnetic field, a certain amount of the body's nuclei will align with or against the magnetic field, and in particular its hydrogen atoms. The amount of nuclei that do align project a detectable signal that can be rearranged to represent bodily structures, such as adipose, muscle and bone tissues. To obtain a full body assessment, this technique requires a series of time consuming multiple scans along the length of the body (approximately 30 min). One of the major advantages of the magnetic resonance imaging scans is its ability to differentiate between visceral and subcutaneous adipose tissue, which make it an assessment that provides very valuable information. This information can be also obtained from the computed tomography, but the latter uses radiation to collect the required data, which has many adverse health effects.

COMPUTED TOMOGRAPHY

This is one of the most advanced and recent means available for assessing body composition and fatness. It generates dimensional images of body segments from a large series of two dimensional x-ray images captured around a single axis of rotation, covering a full 360° arc. The tomography technique utilizes x-rays that are collimated to provide a beam, which passes through the body, while the detectors positioned on the opposite side of the body of the participant are used to detect the transmitted radiation. Based on the on the fact that different tissues will have a different ability to block the he X-ray/Röntgen beam, computed tomography may generate information about the body's total tissue area, overall fat and muscle mass content as well as the volume and thickness of the tissue within a specific organ [103]. Hence, the images can separate the adipose tissue in subcutaneous and visceral mass, or the lean tissues into skeletal muscle and visceral mass.

To produce actual data obtained from a body scan, reconstruction algorithms have been developed and are available. The advantage of computed tomography over magnetic resonance imaging is that it also provides additional data for the tissue's true density at each pixel. When this information is coupled with the pixel's anatomical location, then this image can be used to identify adipose tissue, as well other tissues (e.g. viscera, muscle and bone). Using 10 cm intervals based on scan taken along the body have been show to be both valid and reliable [104]. The disadvantage of computed tomography however, is mainly the use of radiation to obtain the required data for the calculation of relevant bodily masses. Hence, this technique is not the preferable method used in research as the harmful effects of radiation can be severe and therefore unethical to subject individuals to it, particularly given that other techniques do exist with similar validity and reliability.

DUAL ENERGY X-RAY ABSORPTIOMETRY

Dual Energy X-Ray Absorptiometry (DEXA) is perhaps the most commonly used imaging technique for the determination of body composition. The wide use of DEXA for the determination of body composition components is interesting, given that its clinic use mainly concentrates on the lumbar spine, proximal femur, forearm and total body [105]. However, this is because DEXA is valid and reliable and is able to detect changes in body composition as well as bone mineral density after an intervention or over a period of time.

Despite the use of different types of DEXA, they all operate on the same principles. During the assessment, a radiation source is aimed at a radiation detector which is placed directly opposite of the body part that is measured. The person assessed is placed on a specific table in a supine position while the detector assembly scans across the body or specific body region. DEXA technology can virtually assess any skeletal site whereas the apparatus that are available are full table systems or peripheral systems. Given that the latter are limited to measuring the peripheral sites of the body, full table DEXA is the current clinical and research choice for body composition assessment. Moreover, new technology full table scanners, despite being more expensive, they utilise multiple detectors which are swept across the measurement region of the body and provide better accuracy. Fan beam provides the advantage of decreased scan times compared with the old DEXA machines which used single-beam systems. Fan-beam systems use either a single-view or multiple views to image the body.

DEXA scanning uses two low energy x-ray beams that penetrate the human body at a depth of ~30 cm. After the assessment which lasts approximately 30 minutes, including participant preparation and assessment (15 minutes), a computer software generates an image based on the projected x-ray beams, and can differentiate amongst bone mineral density, fat and fat-free mass for which it gives exact information. Although highly valid and reproducible, the major disadvantage of DEXA is the radiation, which however, is significantly reduced compared to computerised tomography. This is perhaps the reason why it explains its wide use over computed tomography.

OTHER METHODS

Less common methods for the determination of body fatness are the near-infrared interactance, the use of the ultrasound, and air displacement plethysmography.

NEAR-INFRARED INTERACTANCE

This technique uses near-infrared light (low energy beam) that is emitted by a probe in the anterior midline surface of the dominant bicep of the tested individual. Using specific technologies to measure light absorption and reflection as well as specific algorithms, this method can then estimate percentage body fat and fat-free mass. The high variability of near-infrared interactance as well as its lack to demonstrate validity against established methods, makes it a non popular method which is not frequently used, particularly given that less invasive but quicker methods (e.g. skinfold assessment) may provide better results.

ULTRASOUND

Via the use of a probe, ultrasound converts energy into high frequency sound waves that reach the underline tissues of the body. Using specific apparatus and software the sound waves that reflect on the body tissues can be used to produce real time images. *Via* the use of ultrasound method and technology, researchers and/or clinicians can now evaluate the thickness of muscle and fat tissues as well as the muscles cross sectional area. Other uses of the ultrasound include the assessment of vascular endothelial function using the flow mediated vasodilation technique as well as the evaluation of the fetus well-being during pregnancy.

AIR DISPLACEMENT PLETHYSMOGRAPHY

This is a new, practical and promising technique for the assessment of body composition. The BOD POD is the first commercially available apparatus to measure body composition using this technique, and only lasts approximately five minutes. The BOD POD apparatus is a small chamber with enough space for an individual to sit. The machine first measures the volume of the chamber when empty and then the volume when the tested individual sits inside. By comparing the two volumes and also subtracting the individual's lung volume, the BOD POD can then estimate body volume which can be then converted to body fat percentage using the popular Siri equation.

REFERENCES

[1] Wilson P, D' Agostino R, Sullivan L, Parise H, Kannel W. Overweight and obesity as determinants of cardiovascular risk: the Framingham experience. Arch Intern Med 2002; 162: 1867-72.

[2] Ball G, Marshall J, McCargar L. Fatness and fitness in obese children at low and high health risk. Ped Exerc Sci 2003; 15: 392-405.

[3] Flouris AD, Bouziotas C, Faught BE, Koutedakis Y, Dobbin S. Risk factor profiles of coronary heart disease in peri-adolescent youth in Canada and Greece. Br J Sports Med 2003; 37(5): 468.

[4] Flouris AD, Canham CH, Faught BE, Klentrou P. Prevalence of cardiovascular disease risk in Ontario adolescents. Arch Dis Child 2007; 92(6): 521-3.

[5] Flouris AD, Bouziotas C, Christodoulos AD, Koutedakis Y. Longitudinal preventive-screening cutoffs for metabolic syndrome in adolescents. Int J Obes (Lond) 2008; 32(10): 1506-12.

[6] Flouris AD, Faught BE, Klentrou P. Cardiovascular disease risk in adolescent smokers: evidence of a 'smoker lifestyle'. J Child Health Care 2008; 12(3): 217-27.

[7] Wabitsch M. Overweight and obesity in European children: definition and diagnostic procedures, risk factors and consequences for later health outcome. Eur J Pediatr 2000; 159 (Suppl 1): S8-S13.

[8] Togashi K, Masuda H, Rankinen T, Tanaka S, Bouchard C, Kamiya H. A 12-year follow-up study of treated obese children in Japan. Int J Obes Relat Metab Disord 2002; 26(6): 770-7.

[9] WHO. Obesity and overweight. World Health Organization: Global Strategy on Diet, Physical Activity and Health 2006.

[10] Meshkani R, Adeli K. Hepatic insulin resistance, metabolic syndrome and cardiovascular disease. Clin Biochem 2009; 42(13-14): 1331-46.

[11] Vachharajani V, Granger DN. Adipose tissue: a motor for the inflammation associated with obesity. IUBMB Life 2009; 61(4): 424-30.

[12] Shah A, Mehta N, Reilly MP. Adipose inflammation, insulin resistance, and cardiovascular disease. JPEN J Parenter Enteral Nutr 2008; 32(6): 638-44.

[13] Gutierrez DA, Puglisi MJ, Hasty AH. Impact of increased adipose tissue mass on inflammation, insulin resistance, and dyslipidemia. Curr Diab Rep 2009; 9(1): 26-32.

[14] Triantafilou M, Triantafilou K. Lipopolysaccharide recognition: CD14, TLRs and the LPS-activation cluster. Trends Immunol 2002; 23(6): 301-4.

[15] Passlick B, Flieger D, Ziegler-Heitbrock HW. Identification and characterization of a novel monocyte subpopulation in human peripheral blood. Blood 1989; 74(7): 2527-34.

[16] Markofski MM, Flynn MG, Sedlock DA, Campbell WW, Carrillo AE, Eds. Inflammatory monocyte (CD14+CD16+) percentage is high among physically inactive adults and highest in obese, inactive adults. Int Soc Exerc Immunol Ann Meet 2009; Tubingen, Germany.

[17] Kawanaka N, Yamamura M, Aita T, *et al.* CD14+, CD16+ blood monocytes and joint inflammation in rheumatoid arthritis. Arthritis Rheum 2002; 46(10): 2578-86.

[18] Schlitt A, Heine GH, Blankenberg S, *et al.* CD14+CD16+ monocytes in coronary artery disease and their relationship to serum TNF-alpha levels. Thromb Haemost 2004; 92(2): 419-24.

[19] Belge KU, Dayyani F, Horelt A, *et al.* The proinflammatory CD14+CD16+DR++ monocytes are a major source of TNF. J Immunol 2002; 168(7): 3536-42.

[20] Festa A, D'Agostino R, Jr., Williams K, *et al.* The relation of body fat mass and distribution to markers of chronic inflammation. Int J Obes Relat Metab Disord 2001 Oct; 25(10): 1407-15.

[21] Kao TW, Lu IS, Liao KC, Lai HY, Loh CH, Kuo HK. Associations between body mass index and serum levels of C-reactive protein. S Afr Med J 2009; 99(5): 326-30.

[22] Sattar N, Wannamethee SG, Forouhi NG. Novel biochemical risk factors for type 2 diabetes: pathogenic insights or prediction possibilities? Diabetologia 2008; 51(6): 926-40.

[23] Li JJ, Fang CH. C-reactive protein is not only an inflammatory marker but also a direct cause of cardiovascular diseases. Med Hypotheses 2004; 62(4): 499-506.

[24] Date Y, Kojima M, Hosoda H, *et al.* Ghrelin, a novel growth hormone-releasing acylated peptide, is synthesized in a distinct endocrine cell type in the gastrointestinal tracts of rats and humans. Endocrinology 2000; 141(11): 4255-61.

[25] Kojima M, Hosoda H, Date Y, Nakazato M, Matsuo H, Kangawa K. Ghrelin is a growth-hormone-releasing acylated peptide from stomach. Nature 1999; 402(6762): 656-60.

[26] Tschop M, Weyer C, Tataranni PA, Devanarayan V, Ravussin E, Heiman ML. Circulating ghrelin levels are decreased in human obesity. Diabetes 2001; 50(4): 707-9.

[27] Dixit VD, Schaffer EM, Pyle RS, *et al.* Ghrelin inhibits leptin- and activation-induced proinflammatory cytokine expression by human monocytes and T cells. J Clin Invest 2004; 114(1): 57-66.

[28] Flynn MG, McFarlin BK, Markofski MM. The Anti-Inflammatory Actions of Exercise Training. Am J Lifestyle Med 2007; 1(10): 1-16.

[29] McFarlin BK, Flynn MG, Campbell WW, Stewart LK, Timmerman KL. TLR4 is lower in resistance-trained older women and related to inflammatory cytokines. Med Sci Sports Exerc 2004; 36(11): 1876-83.

[30] Stewart LK, Flynn MG, Campbell WW, *et al.* Influence of exercise training and age on CD14+ cell-surface expression of toll-like receptor 2 and 4. Brain Behav Immun 2005; 19(5): 389-97.

[31] McFarlin BK, Flynn MG, Campbell WW, *et al.* Physical activity status, but not age, influences inflammatory biomarkers and toll-like receptor 4. J Gerontol A Biol Sci Med Sci 2006; 61(4): 388-93.

[32] Stewart LK, Flynn MG, Campbell WW, *et al.* The influence of exercise training on inflammatory cytokines and C-reactive protein. Med Sci Sports Exerc 2007; 39(10): 1714-9.

[33] Fatouros IG, Tournis S, Leontsini DJ, *et al.* Leptin and adiponectin responses in overweight inactive elderly following resistance training and detraining are intensity related. J Clin Endocrinol Metab 2005; 90(11): 5970-7.

[34] Leidy HJ, Gardner JK, Frye BR, *et al.* Circulating ghrelin is sensitive to changes in body weight during a diet and exercise program in normal-weight young women. J Clin Endocrinol Metab 2004; 89(6): 2659-64.

[35] Foster-Schubert KE, McTiernan A, Frayo RS, *et al.* Human plasma ghrelin levels increase during a one-year exercise program. J Clin Endocrinol Metab 2005; 90(2): 820-5.

[36] Carrillo AE, Flynn MG, Timmerman KL, Coen PM, Markofski MM, Pence BD. Changes in plasma ghrelin are associated with human monocyte phenotype following exercise training. Med Sci in Sports Exerc 2008; 40(5): S433.
[37] Greiwe JS, Cheng B, Rubin DC, Yarasheski KE, Semenkovich CF. Resistance exercise decreases skeletal muscle tumor necrosis factor alpha in frail elderly humans. FASEB J 2001; 15(2): 475-82.
[38] Wiedmer P, Nogueiras R, Broglio F, D'Alessio D, Tschop MH. Ghrelin, obesity and diabetes. Nat Clin Pract Endocrinol Metab 2007; 3(10): 705-12.
[39] Dixit VD, Taub DD. Ghrelin and immunity: a young player in an old field. Exp Gerontol 2005; 40(11): 900-10.
[40] Yang H, Youm YH, Nakata C, Dixit VD. Chronic caloric restriction induces forestomach hypertrophy with enhanced ghrelin levels during aging. Peptides 2007; 28(10): 1931-6.
[41] Nikolich-Zugich J, Messaoudi I. Mice and flies and monkeys too: caloric restriction rejuvenates the aging immune system of non-human primates. Exp Gerontol 2005; 40(11): 884-93.
[42] Spaulding CC, Walford RL, Effros RB. Calorie restriction inhibits the age-related dysregulation of the cytokines TNF-alpha and IL-6 in C3B10RF1 mice. Mech Ageing Dev 1997; 93(1-3): 87-94.
[43] Spaulding CC, Walford RL, Effros RB. The accumulation of non-replicative, non-functional, senescent T cells with age is avoided in calorically restricted mice by an enhancement of T cell apoptosis. Mech Ageing Dev 1997; 93(1-3): 25-33.
[44] Bishop NA, Guarente L. Genetic links between diet and lifespan: shared mechanisms from yeast to humans. Nat Rev Genet 2007; 8(11): 835-44.
[45] Messaoudi I, Warner J, Fischer M, *et al.* Delay of T cell senescence by caloric restriction in aged long-lived nonhuman primates. Proc Natl Acad Sci USA 2006; 103(51): 19448-53.
[46] Jolly CA. Dietary restriction and immune function. J Nutr 2004 Aug; 134(8): 1853-6.
[47] Weindruch R. Effect of caloric restriction on age-associated cancers. Exp Gerontol 1992; 27(5-6): 575-81.
[48] Dixit VD. Adipose-immune interactions during obesity and caloric restriction: reciprocal mechanisms regulating immunity and health span. J Leukoc Biol 2008; 84(4): 882-92.
[49] Blum M, Dolnikowski G, Seyoum E, *et al.* Vitamin D(3) in fat tissue. Endocrine 2008; 33(1): 90-4.
[50] Goldner WS, Stoner JA, Thompson J, *et al.* Prevalence of vitamin D insufficiency and deficiency in morbidly obese patients: a comparison with non-obese controls. Obes Surg 2008; 18(2): 145-50.
[51] Wortsman J, Matsuoka LY, Chen TC, Lu Z, Holick MF. Decreased bioavailability of vitamin D in obesity. Am J Clin Nutr 2000; 72(3): 690-3.
[52] Moreno-Reyes R, Carpentier YA, Boelaert M, *et al.* Vitamin D deficiency and hyperparathyroidism in relation to ethnicity: a cross-sectional survey in healthy adults. Eur J Nutr 2009; 48(1): 31-7.
[53] Passeri G, Vescovini R, Sansoni P, Galli C, Franceschi C, Passeri M. Calcium metabolism and vitamin D in the extreme longevity. Exp Gerontol 2008; 43(2): 79-87.
[54] Foss YJ. Vitamin D deficiency is the cause of common obesity. Med Hypotheses 2009; 72(3): 314-21.
[55] Heaney RP. Vitamin D: criteria for safety and efficacy. Nutr Rev 2008; 66 (10 Suppl 2): S178-81.
[56] Holick MF. Vitamin D: important for prevention of osteoporosis, cardiovascular heart disease, type 1 diabetes, autoimmune diseases, and some cancers. South Med J 2005; 98(10): 1024-7.
[57] Dandona P, Aljada A, Bandyopadhyay A. Inflammation: the link between insulin resistance, obesity and diabetes. Trends Immunol 2004; 25(1): 4-7.
[58] May E, Asadullah K, Zugel U. Immunoregulation through 1, 25-dihydroxyvitamin D3 and its analogs. Curr Drug Targets Inflamm Allergy 2004; 3(4): 377-93.
[59] Cigolini M, Iagulli MP, Miconi V, Galiotto M, Lombardi S, Targher G. Serum 25-hydroxyvitamin D3 concentrations and prevalence of cardiovascular disease among type 2 diabetic patients. Diabetes Care 2006; 29(3): 722-4.
[60] Timms PM, Mannan N, Hitman GA, *et al.* Circulating MMP9, vitamin D and variation in the TIMP-1 response with VDR genotype: mechanisms for inflammatory damage in chronic disorders? Qjm 2002; 95(12): 787-96.
[61] Cohen ML, Douvdevani A, Chaimovitz C, Shany S. Regulation of TNF-alpha by 1alpha,25-dihydroxyvitamin D3 in human macrophages from CAPD patients. Kidney Int 2001; 59(1): 69-75.
[62] Riancho JA, Zarrabeitia MT, de Francisco AL, *et al.* Vitamin D therapy modulates cytokine secretion in patients with renal failure. Nephron 1993; 65(3): 364-8.
[63] Romero-Corral A, Sierra-Johnson J, Lopez-Jimenez F, *et al.* Relationships between leptin and C-reactive protein with cardiovascular disease in the adult general population. Nat Clin Pract Cardiovasc Med 2008 Apr 22.
[64] Lechleitner M, Herold M, Dzien-Bischinger C, Hoppichler F, Dzien A. Tumour necrosis factor-alpha plasma levels in elderly patients with Type 2 diabetes mellitus-observations over 2 years. Diabet Med 2002; 19(11): 949-53.
[65] Cohen-Lahav M, Shany S, Tobvin D, Chaimovitz C, Douvdevani A. Vitamin D decreases NFkappaB activity by increasing IkappaBalpha levels. Nephrol Dial Transplant 2006; 21(4): 889-97.
[66] Sun J, Kong J, Duan Y, *et al.* Increased NF-kappaB activity in fibroblasts lacking the vitamin D receptor. Am J Physiol Endocrinol Metab 2006; 291(2): E315-22.
[67] Pinheiro da Silva F, Gallo RL, Nizet V. Differing effects of exogenous or endogenous cathelicidin on macrophage toll-like receptor signaling. Immunol Cell Biol 2009 Apr 7
[68] Cannell JJ, Hollis BW. Use of vitamin D in clinical practice. Altern Med Rev 2008; 13(1): 6-20.
[69] Jeng L, Yamshchikov AV, Judd SE, *et al.* Alterations in vitamin D status and anti-microbial peptide levels in patients in the intensive care unit with sepsis. J Transl Med 2009; 7: 28.
[70] Metsios GS, Stavropoulos-Kalinoglou A, Veldhuijzen van Zanten JJ, *et al.* Rheumatoid arthritis, cardiovascular disease and physical exercise: a systematic review. Rheumatology (Oxford). 2008; 47(3): 239-48.
[71] Kodama S, Saito K, Tanaka S, *et al.* Cardiorespiratory fitness as a quantitative predictor of all-cause mortality and cardiovascular events in healthy men and women: a meta-analysis. JAMA 2009; 301(19): 2024-35.
[72] Markes M, Brockow T, Resch KL. Exercise for women receiving adjuvant therapy for breast cancer. Cochrane Database Syst Rev 2006(4): CD005001.
[73] Shaw K, Gennat H, O'Rourke P, Del Mar C. Exercise for overweight or obesity. Cochrane Database Syst Rev 2006(4): CD003817.
[74] ACSM. Guidelines for exercise testing and prescription. 7 ed. Philadelphia, PA: Lippincott Wiliams & Wilkins; 2005.
[75] Staron RS, Karapondo DL, Kraemer WJ, *et al.* Skeletal muscle adaptations during early phase of heavy-resistance training in men and women. J Appl Physiol 1994; 76(3): 1247-55.

[76] Hunter GR, McCarthy JP, Bamman MM. Effects of resistance training on older adults. Sports Med 2004; 34(5): 329-48.

[77] Miller WC. How effective are traditional dietary and exercise interventions for weight loss? Med Sci Sports Exerc 1999; 31(8): 1129-34.

[78] Summerbell CD, Cameron C, Glasziou PP. WITHDRAWN: Advice on low-fat diets for obesity. Cochrane Database Syst Rev 2008(3): CD003640.

[79] McArdle WD, Katch FI, Katch VL. Exercise Physiology. Energy, Nutrition, and Human Performance. Fifth ed. USA: Lippincott Williams & Wilkins; 2001.

[80] Adult Treatment Panel III. Executive summary of the third report of the national cholesterol education program (NCEP) expert panel on detection, evaluation, and treatment of high blood cholesterol in adults. JAMA 2001; 285(19): 2486-97.

[81] Laaksonen DE, Lakka HM, Niskanen LK, Kaplan GA, Salonen JT, Lakka TA. Metabolic syndrome and development of diabetes mellitus: application and validation of recently suggested definitions of the metabolic syndrome in a prospective cohort study. Am J Epidemiol 2002; 156(11): 1070-7.

[82] Lakka HM, Laaksonen DE, Lakka TA, *et al.* The metabolic syndrome and total and cardiovascular disease mortality in middle-aged men. JAMA 2002; 288(21): 2709-16.

[83] Hu G, Qiao Q, Tuomilehto J, Balkau B, Borch-Johnsen K, Pyorala K. Prevalence of the metabolic syndrome and its relation to all-cause and cardiovascular mortality in nondiabetic European men and women. Arch Intern Med 2004; 164(10): 1066-76.

[84] Christodoulos AD, Flouris AD, Tokmakidis SP. Obesity and physical fitness of pre-adolescent children during the academic year and the summer period: effects of organized physical activity. J Child Health Care 2006; 10(3): 199-212.

[85] Koutedakis Y, Bouziotas C, Flouris AD, Nelson PN. Longitudinal modeling of adiposity in periadolescent Greek schoolchildren. Med Sci Sports Exerc 2005; 37(12): 2070-4.

[86] Bouziotas C, Koutedakis Y, Shiner R, Pananakakis Y, Fotopoulou V, Gara S. The prevalence of selected modifiable coronary heart disease risk factors in 12-year-old Greek boys and girls. Pediatr Exerc Sci 2001; 13: 173-84.

[87] Cruz ML, Goran MI. The metabolic syndrome in children and adolescents. Curr Diab Rep 2004; 4(1): 53-62.

[88] Shirai K. Obesity as the core of the metabolic syndrome and the management of coronary heart disease. Curr Med Res Opin 2004; 20(3): 295-304.

[89] Weiss R, Dziura J, Burgert TS, *et al.* Obesity and the metabolic syndrome in children and adolescents. N Engl J Med 2004; 350(23): 2362-74.

[90] Kahn BB, Flier JS. Obesity and insulin resistance. J Clin Invest 2000; 106(4): 473-81.

[91] Raitakari O, Porkka K, Taimela S, Telama R, Rasanen L, Viikari J. Effects of persistent physical activity and inactivity on coronary risk factors in children and young adults. The Cardiovascular Risk in Young Finns Study. Am J Epidemiol 1994; 140(3): 195-205.

[92] Johnson M, Figueroa-Colon R, Herd S, *et al.* Aerobic fitness, not energy expenditure, influences subsequent increase in adiposity in black and white children. Pediatrics 2000; 106(4): E50.

[93] Poehlman ET. A review: exercise and its influence on resting energy metabolism in man. Med Sci Sports Exerc 1989; 21(5): 515-25.

[94] Almeras N, Lavallee N, Despres JP, Bouchard C, Tremblay A. Exercise and energy intake: effect of substrate oxidation. Physiol Behav 1995; 57(5): 995-1000.

[95] Kanbur N, Derman O, Kinik E. Prevalence of obesity in adolescents and the impact of sexual maturation stage on body mass index in obese adolescents. Int J Adolesc Med Health 2002; 14: 61-5.

[96] Goran MI, Reynolds KD, Lindquist CH. Role of physical activity in the prevention of obesity in children. Int J Obes Relat Metab Disord 1999; 23 (Suppl 3): S18-33.

[97] Davey RC. The obesity epidemic: too much food for thought? Br J Sports Med 2004; 38(3): 360-3; discussion 3.

[98] Nevill AM, Stewart AD, Olds T, Holder RL. The relationship between adiposity and body size reveals the limitations of BMI. Am J Phys Anthropol 2006; 129: 151-6.

[99] Stavropoulos-Kalinoglou A, Metsios GS, Koutedakis Y, *et al.* Redefining overweight and obesity in rheumatoid arthritis patients. Ann Rheum Dis 2007; 66(10): 1316-21.

[100] Stavropoulos-Kalinoglou A, Metsios GS, Panoulas VF, *et al.* Associations of obesity with modifiable risk factors for the development of cardiovascular disease in patients with rheumatoid arthritis. Ann Rheum Dis 2009; 68(2): 242-5.

[101] Nevill AM, Metsios GS, Jackson AS, Wang J, Thornton J, Gallagher D. Can we use the Jackson and Pollock equations to predict body density/fat of obese individuals in the 21st century? Internation J Body Compos Res 2008; 6(3): 114-21.

[102] Clinical guidelines on the identification, evaluation, and treatment of overweight and obesity in adults: executive summary. Expert Panel on the Identification, Evaluation, and Treatment of Overweight in Adults. Am J Clin Nutr 1998; 68(4): 899-917.

[103] Goodpaster BH, Thaete FL, Kelley DE. Composition of skeletal muscle evaluated with computed tomography. Ann N Y Acad Sci 2000; 904: 18-24.

[104] Sjostrom L. A computer-tomography based multicompartment body composition technique and anthropometric predictions of lean body mass, total and subcutaneous adipose tissue. Int J Obes 1991; 15 (Suppl 2): 19-30.

[105] Hans D, Downs RW, Jr., Duboeuf F, *et al.* Skeletal sites for osteoporosis diagnosis: the 2005 ISCD Official Positions. J Clin Densitom 2006; 9(1): 15-21.

Medication Absorption Post-Bariatric Surgery with Emphasis on Management of Vitamin Deficiencies

Susan Jacob*, Nhu Nguyen, Christian S. Jackson and Stewart Rendon

Department of Veterans Affairs Loma Linda, Western University of Health Sciences, Pomona, CA, USA

Abstract: The increased prevalence of obesity worldwide has led to a rise in bariatric surgeries performed each year. Bariatric surgery is currently one of the most effective interventions for weight loss. The most common procedures include gastric bypass, adjustable gastric band, jejuno-ileal bypass, vertical banded gastroplasty, and biliopancreatic diversion with duodenal switch. Bariatric surgery can improve various medical conditions including but not limited to diabetes, hypertension, dyslipidemia, reflux, and obstructive sleep apnea. Patients with type 2 diabetes develop increased insulin sensitivity and improvements in glucose metabolism within days after surgery. As weight loss occurs, blood pressure and cholesterol levels may improve post operatively, allowing discontinuation of medications. Due to the possible achlorhydric nature of the gastrointestinal tract, post surgery patients often do not require acid suppressing agents for reflux. Medication absorption is highly affected by post gastric bypass surgery, specifically drug solubility and surface area for absorption. These changes warrant manipulation in drug route or dose to ensure adequate delivery. As weight loss occurs, medication adjustments are essential to provide optimal bioavailability for various health related conditions. Consideration should be made for certain medications that depend on absorption site and pH of the gastrointestinal tract for solubility and proper absorption. Non-steroidal anti-inflammatory drugs, aspirin, and bisphosphonates, should be discontinued as these can cause an increased risk of stomach ulcerations if continued post surgery. Long acting and enteric coated formulations will not be absorbed as they require an extended period of time in the intestines for drug dissolution and metabolism. Patients undergoing bariatric surgery have alterations in the digestive anatomy resulting in micronutrient and mineral deficiencies requiring immediate postoperative vitamin supplementations. Nutrient deficiencies include calcium, fat soluble vitamins (A, D, E, K), thiamine, iron, folic acid, and cyanocobalamin. Calcium and vitamin D deficiencies may cause secondary hyperparathyroidism and bone softening diseases. Cyanocobalamin deficiency may lead to irreversible peripheral neuropathy. Wernicke's encephalopathy is common in patients with thiamine deficiency. Anemia may develop in patients with iron deficiency. Due to rapid weight loss and physiological changes, patient monitoring for therapeutic effects is crucial. Recent developments in anti-obesity therapies such as bariatric surgery have revealed improvements or complete remission of multiple chronic diseases. Manipulation of the gastrointestinal tract post bariatric surgery requires medication adjustments and vitamin supplementation for optimal patient care.

Keywords: Bariatric surgery, vitamin deficiency, medication adjustments.

INTRODUCTION

Obesity results from the excessive accumulation of fat that exceeds the body's skeletal and physical standards. According to the National Institutes of Health (NIH), an increase of 20 percent or more above one's "ideal body weight" is the point at which excess weight becomes a health risk. Today, over 200 million Americans, approximately two-thirds of the adult population, are overweight or obese. An estimated nine million of those are considered morbidly obese. Obesity is a major cause of premature death and its prevalence is ubiquitous among all ages, genders, and education levels, racial, ethnic, and even smoking levels [1, 2].

Obesity becomes "morbid" or "clinically severe obesity" when it reaches the point of significantly increasing the risk of one or more obesity-related health conditions or serious diseases that result either in significant physical disability or death. Thus obesity is defined as a BMI of at least 30 [3]. Morbid obesity

*Corresponding author: Tel: (909) 469-5696; Fax: (909) 469-5539; E-mails: jacobss@westernu.edu, Susan.Jacob2@va.gov

Atta-ur-Rahman / M. Iqbal Choudhary (Eds.)

is typically defined as being 100 pounds or more over ideal body weight or having a Body Mass Index (BMI) of 40 or greater (see Table **1**). BMI is calculated as weight in kilograms divided by the square of the height in meters [4]. According to the American Society of Metabolic and Bariatric Surgeons, morbid obesity is defined as a chronic disease with symptoms that develop slowly over an extended period of time [5].

Table 1. Summary of Classifications of Obesity Based on BMI and their Recommended Therapeutic Modalities

BMI (kg/m^2)	Weight Category	Recommended Weight Loss Treatment Modality
<18.5	Underweight	N/A
18.5-24.9	Normal Weight	N/A
25.0-29.9	Overweight	Dietary changes, exercise, behavioral therapy, counseling; consider pharmacotherapy in the presence of co-morbidities
30.0-34.9	Class I Obesity	Similar to above, plus pharmacotherapy
35.0-39.9	Class II Obesity	Similar to above; bariatric surgery to be considered in the presence of co-morbidities
≥ 40.0	Class III Obesity	Bariatric Surgery

BMI = body mass index; N/A = not applicable
Adapted from Chan LN, Downing J. Management of Patients Receiving Bariatric Surgery. Pharmacotherapy Self-Assessment Program, 6th ed. 63-75.

Morbid obesity is a complex, multi-factorial chronic disease. The increased prevalence of obesity worldwide has lead to a rise in bariatric surgeries performed each year. Diet therapy with and without support organizations is not a durable means of treating morbid obesity. Pharmacologic agents (see Table **2**) have not been shown to be effective in treating morbid obesity [6, 7]. Weight loss surgery, when compared to other interventions, has provided the longest period of sustained weight loss in patients for whom all other therapies have failed [8]. Patients who have had bariatric procedures and are benefiting from the results report improvements in their quality of life, social interactions, psychological well-being, employment opportunities, and economic condition.

Table 2. Drugs for Weight Loss

Drug	Dose (mg)
FDA Approved	
Phentermine	15-37.5 mg daily
Orlistat	60-120 mg three times daily
Sibutramine	1-15 mg daily
Off Label Use	***Dose Studied***
Buproprion	300-400 mg daily
Fluoxetine	60 mg daily
Metformin	850 mg twice daily
Setraline	150-200 mg daily
Topiramate	96-192 mg daily
Zonisamide	100 mg daily, titrate up to 600 mg daily

Adapted from Chan LN, Downing J. Management of Patients Receiving Bariatric Surgery. Pharmacotherapy Self-Assessment Program, 6th ed. 63-75.

CURRENT TREATMENTS OPTIONS FOR OBESITY

Routine health screening should incorporate measurement of BMI and waist circumference. The goal for screening patients is to prevent excessive weight gain and delay co-morbid factors which include but are not restricted to: cardiovascular disease, diabetes, hypertension, dyslipidemia, sleep apnea, cerebral vascular accidents, asthma, back and lower extremity weight bearing degenerative problems, and several forms of cancer [8, 9]. Patient intervention is indicated based on obesity related co-morbid conditions, laboratory abnormalities, and dietary pattern. Factors which can contribute to significant weight gain must be evaluated which may include clinical depression, mood disorders, and eating disorders. Careful examination of barriers to weight loss should be taken into consideration prior to surgical therapy.

In a recent study of morbidly obese patients, bariatric surgery has shown an 83% resolution of type 2 diabetes, 85% resolution of obstructive sleep apnea, 75% resolution of hypertension, and 93% decrease of hyperlipidemia and hypercholesterolemia [10]. There is evidence to show that patients with type 2 diabetes develop increased insulin sensitivity with improvements in glucose metabolism within days after surgery. As weight loss occurs, blood pressure and cholesterol levels may improve post operatively, allowing the discontinuation of medications [11].

BARIATRIC SURGICAL OPTIONS

The American Society for Metabolic and Bariatric Surgeons describes two basic approaches, and a combination of procedures weight loss surgery must achieve (see Table **3**):

∞ Restrictive procedures

∞ Malabsorptive procedures

∞ Combination restrictive/malabsorptive procedures

There are several procedures that combine the restrictive and malabsorptive mechanisms of weight loss surgery. The risks of complications and side effects generally increase with the alteration of the digestive process.

RESTRICTIVE PROCEDURES

Restrictive weight loss surgery works by reducing the amount of food consumed at one time. It does not, however, interfere with the normal absorption and digestion of food or medication. In a restrictive procedure, the surgeon creates a smaller upper-stomach pouch. The pouch, with a capacity of approximately one-half to one ounce (15 to 30 ml), connects to the rest of the stomach through an outlet known as a "stoma." In a cooperative and compliant patient, the reduced stomach capacity, along with behavioral changes, can result in consistently lower caloric intake resulting in a significant weight loss.

MALABSORPTIVE PROCEDURES

Malabsorptive procedures alter digestion, causing food to be poorly digested and incompletely absorbed so that it is eliminated in the stool. In addition to restriction, these techniques involve a bypass of the small intestine, limiting the absorption of calories. Malabsorptive or malabsorptive/restrictive procedures result in an overall increase in the loss of excess weight compared to purely restrictive procedures. The risk of complications generally increases with the lengthening of the small intestine bypass [12].

COMBINATION RESTRICTIVE AND MALABSORPTIVE PROCEDURES

A combination approach to weight loss surgery is one in which the procedure utilizes both restrictive and malabsorptive approaches. The Roux-en-Y Gastric Bypass (RYGB) procedure is the most utilized technique, comprising greater than 75 % of bariatric surgical procedures. An average of 77 % of excess body weight loss had been noted one year after surgery. Studies have shown that after 10 to 14 years, patients have maintained 60 % of excess body weight loss [10].

Table 3. Classifications of Bariatric Procedures

Type	Mechanism	Procedure
Restrictive	Weight loss is accomplished by decreased food intake due to the reduced food reservoir in the gastrointestinal tract, especially the stomach	Vertical-banded gastroplasty Adjustable gastric banding (including laparoscopic adjustable gastric banding) Sleeve gastrectomy (lesser curve pouch)
Malabsorptive	Weight loss is accomplished by significant nutrient malabsorption	Jejuno-ileal bypass Biliopancreatic diversion (malabsorption is the primary mechanism as the flow of food from the remaining stomach into the small intestine is not regulated due to the absence of the pyloric sphincter)
Combined Restrictive and Malabsorptive		Rou-en-Y gastric bypass (restriction is the primary mechanism because it is the rate-limiting step for food intake; the malabsorption component is only mild with proximal Roux-en-Y) Biliopancreatic diversion with duodenal switch (pylorus is preserved and thus increases the significance of the restrictive component) Sleeve gastrectomy

Adapted from Chan LN, Downing J. Management of Patients Receiving Bariatric Surgery. Pharmacotherapy Self-Assessment Program, 6th ed. 63-75.

AN OVERVIEW OF WEIGHT LOSS SURGERY OPTIONS

The following is an overview of the bariatric surgical procedures, although an in depth discussion is far beyond the scope of this text. Surgical options will include the advantages and disadvantages. Over the last few decades, these procedures have been continually refined in order to improve results and to minimize risks. Laparoscopy has made these procedures more accessible and has decreased complications rates.

VERTICAL BANDED GASTROPLASTY

Vertical Banded Gastroplasty (VBG) is purely a restrictive procedure (see Fig. **1**). In this procedure, the upper stomach near the esophagus at the Angle of His is stapled vertically about 2.5 inches to create a small

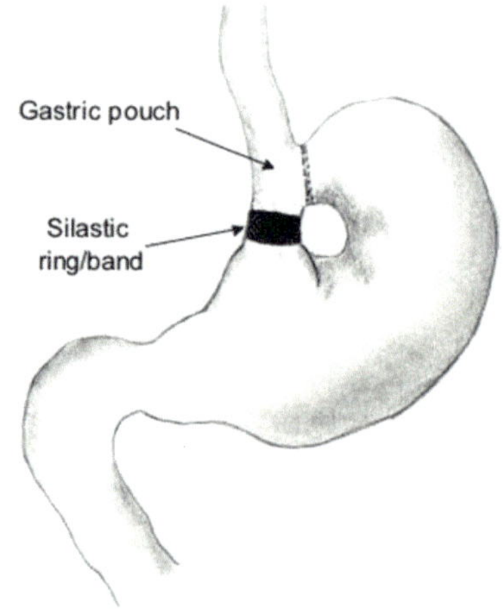

Fig. (1). Vertical banded gastroplasty (VBG). A vertical pouch is created by stapling the front of the stomach to the back wall, below the esophagogastric junction. The end of the newly created gastric pouch is constricted with either a 1-cm diameter polypropylene band (VBG) or a 1-cm silastic ring (vertical ring-banded gastroplasty). *Reprinted with permission from Medscape General Medicine 2004; 6(2): 15.*

stomach pouch. The outlet from the pouch is restricted by a marlex band or a silastic ring that slows the emptying of the food, helping to create the feeling of fullness. The primary advantage of this restrictive procedure is that a reduced amount of food enters and passes through the digestive tract. Nutrients and vitamins are fully absorbed into the body in the normal fashion. After five years, studies show that patients can maintain 50 % of targeted excess weight loss [10].

Postoperatively, stapling of the stomach carries with it the risk of staple-line disruption that can result in leakage and/or serious infection. This may require prolonged hospitalization with antibiotic treatment and/or additional operations. Staple-line disruption may also lead to weight regain. For this reason, some surgeons divide the staple-line wall of the pouch from the rest of the stomach to reduce the risk of long-term staple-line disruption. The band or ring applied may lead to obstruction or perforation requiring surgical intervention. Characteristically, these procedures, while creating an earlier sense of fullness, do not provide the necessary feeling of satiety. Because restrictive procedures rely solely on a small stomach pouch to reduce food intake, there is the risk of the pouch stretching or of the restricting band or ring at the pouch outlet breaking or dislodging. About 40 percent of patients undergoing these procedures have lost about a half of their excess body weight.

LAPAROSCOPIC ADJUSTABLE GASTRIC BAND

Laparoscopic adjustable gastric banding (LABG) or adjustable gastric banding (see Fig. **2**) is similar to VBG. It is a purely restrictive surgical procedure in which an inflatable silicon band is placed around the proximal aspect of the stomach to create a small gastric pouch. Tubing connects the band to an access port which is placed in the abdominal wall, subcutaneous fat tissue. Access to this port can be performed with or without radiologic guidance by a non-coring needle, which allows adjustment of the band. The instillation of saline tightens the stoma, decreasing the area between the proximal gastric pouch and rest of the stomach. This gives the patient the impression of early satiety [11]. Food digestion occurs through the normal digestive and absorption process, but the band restricts the amount of food that can be consumed at any meal. Food consumed passes through the digestive tract in the usual manner, allowing it to be fully absorbed into the body. The band can be adjusted to increase or decrease the restriction according to what the patient is reporting. The uniqueness of this procedure is that it can be reversed with minimal to no complications. Complications such as port displacement, infection, explanation, gastric slippage, and erosion may require reoperation around 10-13% of the time [13]. Other complications may include nausea, vomiting, outlet obstruction, pouch dilation, band migration.

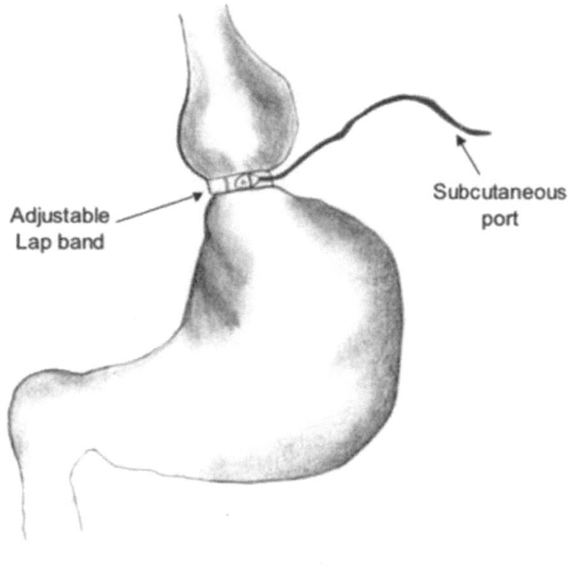

Fig. (2). Adjustable laparoscopic banding. A band is laparoscopically placed around the upper stomach to create a restrictive pouch. The balloon in the band is connected to a port that is placed subcutaneously and can be accessed to inflate or deflate the balloon, consequently changing the size of the band circumference. *Reprinted with permission from Medscape General Medicine 2004; 6(2): 15.*

Patients who should be considered for LABG are those who have multiple co-morbidities which would not make them candidates for other types of bariatric surgeries, but who still would see benefit from weight loss. The low mortality, morbidity, and relative ease of placement laparoscopically, short operating rooms times, and short hospital stays make this restrictive procedure an attractive option for patients and surgeons. The aforementioned factors have led LABG to replace VBG as a purely restrictive procedure of choice [11].

In recent years, a better clinical understanding of procedures combining restrictive and malabsorptive approaches has increased the choices of effective weight loss surgery for thousands of patients. By adding malabsorption, food is delayed in mixing with bile and pancreatic juices that aid in the absorption of nutrients. The result can be an early sense of fullness, combined with a sense of satisfaction, which reduces the desire to eat.

ROUX-EN-Y GASTRIC BYPASS (RYGB)

The Roux-en-Y Gastric Bypass is the most commonly performed weight loss surgery in the United States. The RYGB (see Fig. **3**) is both a malabsorptive and restrictive operation. Three components constitute a successful RYGB: the gastric pouch should be less than $30cm^3$, a Roux limb which ranges from 60 to 250cm to alter malabsorption, and a small gastrojejunostomy of approximately 12mm in diameter. Malabsorption may be added to the RYBG to potentiate further weight loss. This can occur by varying the length of the Roux limb and the biliopancreatic limb. There is evidence to suggest that for a BMI > 50, a 150cm Roux limb may impart greater weight loss than a 75cm limb without increasing metabolic consequences [14]. Because the antrum, duodenum, and part of the jejunum are bypassed, this may provide additional benefits in the treatment of diabetes by alternating gut signaling mechanisms which enhance the treatment of insulin resistance when compared to other restrictive operations [15].

There are short and long term complications related to the procedure, such as leakage at the gastrojejunal anastomosis, remnant stomach, jejujunostomy, and pouch. Other complications may include marginal ulcerations or strictures and internal hernias. The development of metabolic abnormalities, such as deficiencies in calcium, iron, folic acid, copper, zinc, thiamine, and vitamin B_{12} may occur. There is also difficulty in accessing the excluded stomach and duodenum, making the diagnosis of pathology in this region difficult. Patients will need to be compliant secondary to the need for dietary supplementation necessary after this type of operation. There is some evidence to show that preoperative BMI, race, and marriage status may have an effect on mean excess body weight loss [16].

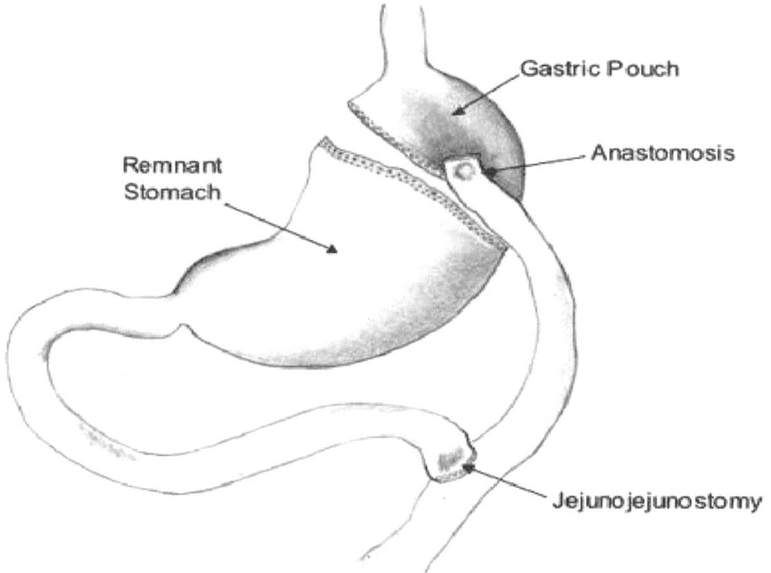

Fig. (3). Roux-en-Y gastric bypass (RYGBP) surgery. A small pouch is created by either stapling or transecting the stomach. The pouch is then connected to and empties into the Roux limb of the jejunum, which is approximately 50-100 cm in length. *Reprinted with permission from Medscape General Medicine 2004; 6(2): 15.*

http://www.medscape.com/viewarticle/471952 © 2004, Medscape

BILIOPANCREATIC DIVERSION/DUODENAL SWITCH

Biliopancreatic Diversion (BPD) is a malabsorptive procedure, a partial gastrectomy which leaves a small gastric pouch which empties into the Roux limb with an approximately 50cm common channel for absorption (see Fig **4a**).

The Biliopancreatic Diversion with "Duodenal Switch" (BPD/DS) is a variation of the BPD (see Fig **4b**) which is designed to decrease marginal ulceration, metabolic derangements such as vitamin deficiencies, iron deficiency, and protein calorie malnutrition. This is achieved by creating a gastric sleeve, preserving the pylorus, and lengthening the common channel in which stomach removal is restricted to the outer margin, leaving a sleeve of stomach with the pylorus and the beginning of the duodenum intact.

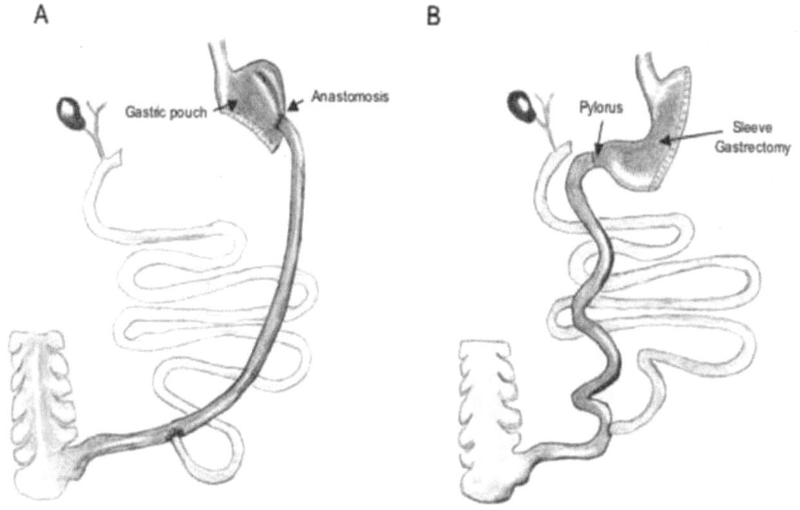

Fig. (4). (A) Biliopancreatic diversion (BPD). A limited gastrectomy is created, and the transected ileum is anastomosed to the gastric pouch. **(B)** BPD with duodenal switch. A sleeve gastrectomy is created to maintain the pylorus and avoid anastomotic complications. Similar to classic BPD, the transected, distal small bowel is connected to the stomach via a small part of the first potion of the duodenum. *Reprinted with permission from Medscape General Medicine 2004; 6(2): 15.*

This particular malabsorptive procedure has the advantage of providing excellent results, especially in those patients with a BMI < 50. In patients with a BMI > 50, 92% of patients achieve a BMI < 35, and 83% of patients with a BMI > 50 achieve a BMI < 35 after BPD/DS. In addition, medications can be discontinued in 92% of diabetics, cardiac risk index can be reduced, and continuous positive airway pressure can be discontinued in 90% if those with obstructive sleep apnea. Though decreased absorption occurs, there is a potential for the patient to consume larger amounts of food secondary to the larger gastric reservoir. Most complications are related to the short common channel and malabsorption, which has the potential for fat soluble vitamin deficiency and protein malnutrition [17].

MEDICATION MANAGEMENT

After surgery, obesity-related medical co-morbidities may improve dramatically. Many chronic medical conditions require monitoring, as well as adjustments in the medications prescribed for those conditions.

Diabetes Management

Well maintained glucose management during the perioperative period is important to improve the outcome of bariatric surgery. The ideal glycemic range for this patient population is unknown; however, an upper limit of serum glucose less than 150mg/dl is a reasonable goal.

After surgery, patients with type 2 diabetes develop increased insulin sensitivity and improvements in glucose metabolism within days. A patient's dietary intake is dramatically limited after surgery, and weight loss can be significant during the first month which can lead to an increase in insulin sensitivity. After RYGB, exposure of the distal jejunum to undigested nutrients elevates peptide YY glucagon-like peptide-1 and glucose-dependent insulinotropic polypeptide, resulting in insulin modifications leading to improvements in glucose metabolism [18].

Oral antidiabetic agents such as sulfonylureas or thiazolidinediones place patients at a high risk of hypoglycemia. Metformin is not associated with hypoglycemia, but absorption is compromised as it is not completely absorbed in the duodenum. After surgery patients are additionally at high risk of dehydration, leading to acute renal failure especially if dumping syndrome occurs. Careful consideration should be given before reinitiating metformin as the patient may be at higher risk of lactic acidosis. Therefore, it is recommended that all oral antidiabetic agents should be discontinued prior to surgery. Insulin is the preferred medication for post-operative diabetes management.

Postoperatively, patients have a significant reduction of glucose and caloric intake and are at a high risk of hypoglycemia. Frequent monitoring of blood glucose is imperative in the early postoperative period and should be managed with both basal and pre-prandial insulin. Patients already on an insulin regimen should have their basal insulin decreased by 50% starting the night before surgery, and may need a further decrease before discharge home to prevent hypoglycemia. Patient's pre-prandial insulin regimen should not be initiated until blood glucose normalizes and after the patient is eating. Pre-prandial insulin should then be adjusted to half or less than half of the standard regime with a correction dose of ~2 units for every 50mg/dl above 120mg/dl for rise in blood glucose [19]. Due to vast differences in insulin resistance, carbohydrate intake, and patient weight, insulin doses can vary and should be individualized for each patient. Providers must be extremely careful that a patient's diabetes regimen does not place the patient at risk for hypoglycemia as the patients' ability to correct hypoglycemia is restricted because of food intake restrictions. Upon discharge, patients should be educated on medication changes, blood sugar management, and provided with a glucagon kit to prevent severe hypoglycemia.

Many patients will have remission of type 2 diabetes within one year after surgery. For those that do not experience diminution of diabetes, medication requirements will be substantially reduced. Due to the rapid weight loss during the first year and improved insulin sensitivity, patients require close follow up and medication adjustments.

Hypertension Management

Blood pressure often decreases post operatively, allowing discontinuation of antihypertensive medications. Hypotension is common in the early postoperative period, especially if fluid intake is poor or the patient experiences persistent vomiting. Diuretics should be discontinued for at least one month after surgery because of the high risk of significant dehydration. Blood pressure should be monitored monthly until blood pressure stabilizes. Improvement of hypertension may occur as early as one month postoperative and is more common in patients with a shorter preoperative duration of disease. Patients with preexisting hypertension of less than four years are more likely to have resolution of hypertension following surgery. Hypertension is not always related to obesity and dietary changes do not ensure normalization of blood pressure. Patients who have suffered from hypertension for a longer period have more functional and structural changes accompany the disease and it is more difficult for the disease to resolve [20]. Some patients may need to resume antihypertensive medications, but usually at adjusted doses.

Reflux

Due to the possible achlorhydric nature of the gastrointestinal tract after the Roux-en-Y bypass and banding, patients often do not require acid suppressing agents for reflux. Over time, patients have decreased acid reflux due to decreased intra-abdominal pressure secondary to weight loss [9]. It would be appropriate to discontinue acid suppressing agents after surgery. They can be reinitiated if symptoms reoccur.

Contraception

For female patients undergoing malabsorptive bariatric surgery, the absorption of oral contraceptives will be compromised and patients should be educated that oral contraceptives will be less effective after the procedure [21]. The estrogen component of hormonal contraceptives additionally place patient at increased risk of thromboembolic complications. Ideally oral contraceptives should be discontinued one week before surgery. After surgery, patients should use barrier methods to prevent contraception. The American College of Obstetrics and Gynecology recommends that an alternative to oral hormonal contraceptives should be considered in women who have undergone malabsorptive bariatric surgery who desire hormonal contraception [22]. Patient should be encouraged to use condoms and spermicides for contraception prevention. For patients desiring hormonal contraception methods, they may be offered (patch, injection, or intra-uterine device). It is critical to obtain screen folate levels and pregnancy testing in sexually active women of child bearing age.

Weight loss after surgery may also lead to greater fertility. Women should be advised of the increased possibility of pregnancy. Women should be advised to delay pregnancy for at least 12-18 months after surgery, which is the rapid weight loss period. For female patients who still plan to become pregnant, the lap band may be a preferred procedure, as the band can be adjusted to accommodate the patient's needs during pregnancy. Women who become pregnant should be referred to a high risk obstetric clinic for management and be evaluated for nutritional deficiencies and the need for additional vitamin supplementation.

Psychiatric Disorders

Dramatic weight loss after surgery can be associated with emotional stress. Patients on psychiatric medications should continue on their current regimen during the postoperative period. Medications should be adjusted to ensure adequate absorption after surgery to formulations that will provide optimal availability. Careful psychiatric monitoring of the patient is imperative to ensure optimal medication efficacy and to address the patient's changing emotional needs.

Thromboembolic Complications

Venous thromboembolism (VTE) is one of the leading causes of complication within 30 days after bariatric surgery. Obesity itself increases patient risk of VTE. Surgery also causes an increase of clotting factors related to hypercoagulability and venous stasis. Patients with a previous history of thromboembolic events, BMI over 60 kg/m^2, BMI over 50 kg/m_2 with chronic venous stasis, obstructive sleep apnea, a hospital stay longer than five days, or patients who have received RYGB are at greater risk of developing VTE after surgery. A national guideline on postoperative VTE prophylaxis after initial discharge has not been established and dosing in the severely obese is controversial. Based on available research conducted in patients receiving RYGB, enoxaparin 40mg subcutaneously twice daily appears to be the most efficacious without causing excessive bleeding. In the male population with BMI over 60 kg/m^2 enoxaparin 60mg subcutaneously twice daily may be offered as they are at a higher risk of DVT/PE. Many institutions extend the postoperative VTE prophylaxis regimen for up to four weeks [23]. Alternatively an IVC filter maybe placed to prevent VTE.

Medication Absorption after Bariatric Surgery

To prevent stress and tearing of the anastomoses site after surgery, patients should be transitioned to liquid or crushable forms of all their medication. It may take up to two months before the patient is able to swallow whole pills again [24]. Even then, pill size should be considered as large pills may get trapped in the stomach pouch and cause ulceration. Patients should be advised to not take any pills larger than a pencil tip eraser. If the pill is large, it will require splitting, crushing, or grinding to increase absorption of the medication. Large capsules should be opened and can be mixed with food such as applesauce. Gel capsules (e.g. docusate) are difficult to open, and therefore should be changed to alternative formulations. All medications should be taken with water or a calorie free, sugar free, or caffeine free beverage.

Medication absorption is highly affected post gastric bypass surgery; specifically drug solubility and surface area for absorption depending upon type of surgery performed (see Table **4**). Blood perfusion to the gastrointestinal tract highly influences drug bioavailability and oral absorption. These changes warrant manipulation in drug route or dose to ensure adequate delivery. Drug preparations in aqueous solutions are more rapidly absorbed than those in other formulations (oily solutions, suspensions, or solid forms) [25]. When medications are given in solid form, the times to disintegration and dissolution are highly affected [21]. Drug disintegration is the rate-limiting step in most solid dosage forms [26].

Alternative medications formulations include sublingual, buccal, chewable, spray, inhaled, intranasal, subcutaneous, and intramuscular topical, shampoo, and medication contained in lollipops are available to patients. Liquid formulations also a good alternative, but the provider should ensure that the medications do not contain sorbitol, as this can cause diarrhea which places patient at increased risk of dehydration. Transdermal medications provide a way to avoid first-pass hepatic metabolism through the liver. Suppositories should be avoided in case the patient develops diarrhea or dumping syndrome which will affect absorption of medication.

Table 4. Effects on Drug Absorption

Factor Influencing Absorption	**Surgery**					
Drug Disintegration and Dissolution	**GB**	**VBG**	**SG**	**RYGB**	**BPD**	**JIB**
Gastric Mixing	x	x	x	x	x	
Gastric pH		x	x	x	x	
Gastric Emptying				x	x	
Bile Salt Solubilization and Enterohepatic Recirculation				x	x	x
Drug Disintegration and Dissolution						
Length of Bypassed Segment and Transit Time				x	x	x
Intestinal Adaptation				x	x	x
Absorption Across Intestine						
Metabolism				x	x	x
Efflux				x	x	x

GB = Gastric Bypass, VBG = Vertical Banded Gastroplasty, SG = Sleeve Gastrectomy,
RYGB = Rou-en-Y Gastric Bypass, BPD = Bioliopancreatic Diversion, JIB = Jejuno-ileal bypass
Adapted from: Padwal R, Brocks D, Sharma AM. A Systematic Review of Drug Absorption Following Bariatric Surgery and its Theoretical Implications. Obesity Reviews 2009; 1-10.

Drug Solubility

Consideration should be given to certain medications that depend on absorption site and pH of the gastrointestinal tract for solubility and proper absorption. In patients who have undergone gastric bypass surgery, the small pouch located at the top of the stomach produces less hydrochloric acid than before, leading to decreased absorption of medications dependent on an acidic environment for solubility or absorption. Drugs that are more soluble at an acidic pH are absorbed in the stomach, and those soluble in alkaline environments are absorbed in the small intestine [21]. Enteric coated and film coated products may exhibit incomplete dissolution, and therefore should be changed to alternative formulations.

Drug Absorption

Roux-ex-Y bypass procedures circumvent the major portion of the small intestine, reducing the surface area available for drug absorption. The small intestine has a much greater surface area due to villi and microvilli in comparison to the large intestine [27]. Therefore a large loss of surface area results from bypassing the duodenum and jejunum. These changes warrant manipulation of drug route or dose to ensure adequate delivery. Long acting formulations that require extended periods of time in the intestines for absorption are likely to exhibit decreased bioavailability and erratic absorption after surgery. It is generally recommended that extended release or delayed release medications should be converted to the equivalent immediate release products (Table **5**).

Gastrointestinal Injury

Many medications have the potential to cause gastrointestinal injury after bariatric surgery. Nonsteroidal anti-inflammatory drugs (NSAIDs) may cause injury to the pouch due to the acidic property of the drug and to the systemic effect of inhibition of prostaglandin synthesis. A reduction in prostaglandin synthesis causes decreased mucous production which exposes the stomach to damage leading to ulceration

Table 5. Medications that may Present Decreased Absorption in Patients who have Undergone Bariatric Surgery

Drug	Possible Absorption Site	Recommendation
	Cardiolovascular/Endocrine Medications	
Enalapril	Hydrolyzed to active form (enalaprilat) in stomach and absorbed in small intestine[a]	May consider an alternative Angiotensin Converting Enzyme Inhibitor (ACEI).
Ramipril	Unknown absorption but decreased absorption documented in patients with steatorrhea and malabsorption[b]	Monitor blood pressure postoperatively; may consider alternative agents. Need for antihypertensive may decrease post surgery.
Metoprolol	Rapid and complete absorption at stomach and duodenum[c]	Monitor blood pressure; medication requirements may decrease as weight loss occurs.
Simvastatin	Hydrolyzed to the active form in stomach[d]	Consider other HMG-cOA reductase inhibitors.
Niacin	Primarily absorbed in duodenum[e]	Consider other agents; Administer with low-fat snack may improve absorption. Avoid use of aspirin to prevent flushing due to increased risk of gastrointestinal ulcers.
Metformin	Slowly and incompletely absorbed in duodenum[f]	Increase monitoring for blood glucose; drug requirements can decrease as weight loss occurs. For poorly controlled diabetics, consider the use of insulin.
Thyroxine	Acidic gastric environment appears important for maximal absorption[g]	Monitor TSH and T_4 levels more frequently.
	Psychiatry/Neurology Medications	
Lamotrigine	Rapid and complete absorption likely at stomach and proximal small intestine[h]	Monitor for decreased efficacy.
Olanzapine	Absorption is primarily in the stomach[i]	Monitor for decreased efficacy. Orally disintegrating tablet will not increase absorption
Quetiapine fumarate	Exact location unknown, but likely stomach and duodenum due to rapid absorption[j]	Monitor for decreased efficacy.
Phenytoin	Absorption slow and erratic. Absorption greatest at the duodenum and continues at a slower rate in the jejunum and ileum[k]	Monitor for efficacy and serum level monitoring warranted.
	Psychiatry/Neurology Medications	
Zolpidem	Absorbed rapidly and completely[l]	Absorption time may be increase, resulting in delay to effect. Recommend to take on an empty stomach.
Certain Antidepressants	*In Vitro* studies showed that possibly Amitriptyline, Fluoxetine, Paroxetine, Sertraline, and Bupropion could be affected post surgery[m]	May consider switching to Citalopram, Venlafaxine[m].
Clonazepam	*In Vitro* studies showed that absorption may be affected[m]	May consider switching to: Buspirone, Diazepam, Lorazepam, Trazodone, or Zolpidem[m].
Certain Antipyschotic	Clozapine, Olanzapine, Quetiapine, Risperidone, Ziprasidone, Lithium carbonate	May consider switching to: Haloperidol, Methylpheniate, or Oxcarbazepine[m].

(Table 5) Contd......

Drug	Possible Absorption Site	Recommendation
	Infectious Disease/Transplant	
Amoxicillin	Well absorbed in the duodenum and jejunum[n]	Consider alternative antibiotic.
Nitrofurantoin (Macrodantin)	Macrocrystalline form has a slower rate of dissolution and absorption[g]	Consider use of Nitrofurantion Monohydrate (Macrobid).
Rifampin	Absorption may be decreased (solubility depends on acidic environment)[g]	Monitor chest x-ray more often.
Ketoconazole	Acidic environment required for absorption (stomach)[o]	Consider alternative agents.
Cyclosporine	Enterohepatic recirculation prolongs elimination time[g]	Monitor Cyclosporine levels.
Tacrolimus	Low bioavailability (20-30%) with incomplete and variable absorption. Primary site of absorption at the jejunum[g]	Monitor Tacrolimus levels.
	Women's health	
Oral contraceptives	May undergo extensive first pass metabolism and enterohepatic recirculation	Consider use of alternative routes of administration (patch, injections, intrauterine device, etc.)

[a]Vasotec (Enalapril) package insert. Morrisville, NC: Biovail Pharmaceuticals; 2—2 Aug.; [b]Data on file. King Pharmaceuticals, Bristol, TN; 2004 Feb.; [c]Lopressor (metoprolol tartrate) package insert. Suffern, NY: Novartis; 2004 Nov.; [d]Vickers S, Duncan CA, Chen IW *et al.* Metabolic disposition studies on simvastatin, a cholesterol lowering prodrug. Drug Metab Dispos 1900; 18:138-45. [e]Data on file. Kos Pharmaceuticals, Cranbury, NJ; 2005 Aug.; [f]Vidon N, Chaussade S, Noel M *et al.* Metformin in the digestive tract. Diabetes Res Chlin Pract 1988; 4: 223-9.; [g]R. Padwal, D. Brocks and A. M. Sharma. "A systematic review of drug absorption following bariatric surgery and its theoretical implications." International Assocation for the Study of Obesity. Obesity reviews. doi:10.111/j:1467-789x.2009.00614.x.; [h]Lamical (lamotrigine) package insert. Research Triangle Park, NC; GlaxoSmithKline; 2005 Aug.; [i]Data on file. Eli Lilly Pharmaceuticals, Indianapolis; 2005 Oct.; [j]Seroquel (quetiapine fumarate) package insert. New York: Sanofi-Synthelabo; 2003 Mar.; [k]Garnett WR. Gastrointestinal and hepatic disease. Ettinger AB and Devinsky O, Eds. Managing epilepsy and co-existing disorders. Boston: Butterworth- Heinemann; 2002; 63-74. Last access: 09/04/2009. http://professionals.epilepsy.com/page/gieffects_phenytoin.html.; [l]Ambien (zolpidem) package insert. New York: Sanofi-Synthelabo; 2004 Mar.; [m]Jeff S Seaman, Steven P Bowers, Patricia Dixon, Libby Schindler. "Dissolution of common Psychiatric Medications in a Roux-en-Y Gastric Bypass Model." Psychosomatics 46: 3. May-June 2005.; [n]William H Barr PhD, Elizabeth M Zola PharmD, Edrick L Candler PhD, Shie-Ming Hwang PhD, Amol V Tendolkar PhD, Robert Shamburek MD, Bertram Parker MD and Milo D Hilty MD. "Differential absorption of amoxicillin from the human small and large intestine." Clinical Pharmacology and Therapeutics (1994).; [o]Data on file. Janssen Pharmaceuticals, Titusville, NJ. *Adapted from: Miller AD, Smith KM. Medication and nutrient administration considerations after bariatric surgery." Am J health- Syst Pharm. Vol 63. Oct 1, 2006.*

[12]. A retrospective study of 1001 RYGB recipients showed that recent NSAID use was associated with an 11-fold higher risk for developing marginal ulcers as diagnosed by endoscopy. Based on these findings, the short-term use of NSAIDs should be discouraged, and their chronic use should be avoided in RYGB recipients [24]. It is also not recommended for patients taking daily doses of aspirin, aspirin-containing products, or anticoagulants unless deemed absolutely necessary. The oral bisphosphonates may present problems due to the reduced pouch size increasing the risk of gastrointestinal ulceration [28]. The risks versus benefit of using non-steroidal anti-inflammatory drugs (NSAIDs), aspirin, antiplatelet agents, corticosteroids, and bisphosphonates should be carefully assessed. Patients currently taking the above medications should discontinue them one week before surgery. Medications should not be started until the pouch has completely healed. The need for postoperative ulcer prophylactic therapy remains a current controversial topic, and further studies are warranted.

Warfarin

Patients currently taking warfarin for long term anticoagulation may pose a clinical challenge when considering surgery. Laparoscopic bariatric surgery can be performed relatively safely in morbidly obese patients requiring chronic oral anticoagulation. Warfarin should be stopped five days before surgery and patients should be placed on bridging therapy with a low molecular weight heparin injection if clinically indicated. There have been reports of hemorrhagic complications in patients receiving chronic anticoagulation after surgery. Therefore, a careful evaluation of a patient's bleeding risk versus the risk of thromboembolic complication is critical to determine the optimal postoperative bridging protocol [29, 30]. Patient should not start warfarin until complete healing has occurred. Patients who undergo malabsorptive procedures may demonstrate resistance to warfarin therapy and require much higher doses than before surgery. Absorption of warfarin is variable and the patient should be referred to an anticoagulation specialist for close monitoring and dosage adjustments to maintain therapeutic effects in these patients [30].

Nutrient Absorption

After bariatric surgery micronutrient and mineral deficiencies may occur, particularly after gastric bypass, because of inadequate intake of nutrients and changes in the digestive anatomy from the surgery [31] (Table **6**).

Table 6. Vitamin Deficiency Supplementation Recommendations*

Vitamin/Nutrient	Clinical Presentation	Recommended Dose
Calcium	Asymptomatic unless severe deficiency has occurred. Altered mental status, tetanus, and generalized weakness may occur	500mg calcium citrate orally 4 times daily
Copper	Fatigue, cardiomegaly, anemia, growth retardation, defective keratinization and pigmentation of hair, hypothermia	2.4mg intravenously for 6 days, then 8mg daily orally for 30 days[1]
Folic acid	Megaloblastic anemia glossitis, pharyngeal ulcers, and impaired immunity	1600 mcg orally daily for 12 months
Iron	Anemia, tiredness, shortness of breath, malaise	150-300 mg elemental iron orally daily (taken with 500mg of vitamin C for optimal absorption)
Thiamine	Wernicke-Korsakoff encephalopathy, peripheral neuropathy, beriberi	100 mg intravenously every 6 hours for 2 days, then 200mg orally twice daily for 30 days, then 100mg daily Wernicke encephalopathy: 100 mg intravenously, then 50-100 intramuscularly or intravenously daily until consuming a regular balanced diet Beriberi: 5-30 mg intramuscularly or intravenously 3 times daily (if critically ill); then 5-30 mg orally daily for 1 month
Vitamin A	Night vision	100,000 units orally daily for 3 days, then 50,000 units orally daily for 14 days
Vitamin B_{12}	Anemia, Neuropathy	30 mcg intramuscular daily for 5-10 days, then 100-200 mcg once monthly
Vitamin D	Osteomalacia	10,000 units orally daily for 6 weeks
Vitamin E	Rash, Neurologic (ataxia)	400 units orally daily
Vitamin K	Coagulopathy	1 mg orally daily
Zinc	Dwarfism, hypogonadism, dermatitis, and T-cell immunodeficiency	25-50 mg elemental zinc orally divided 3 times daily

*The recommended duration of therapy post surgery is 12 months or longer in certain cases.

1. Based on case reports, no current studies with appropriate regiment for copper supplementation. Griffith DP, Lift DA, Ziegler TR, Esper GJ, Winton EF. Acquired Copper Deficiency: A Potentially Serious and Preventable complication Following Gastric Bypass Surgery. Obesity. 2009; 17:827-831.

Adapted from Chan LN, Downing J. Management of Patients Receiving Bariatric Surgery. Pharmacotherapy Self-Assessment Program, 6th Ed. 63-75. Schweitzer DH, Posthuma EF. Prevention of Vitamin and Mineral Deficiencies after Bariatric Surgery: Evidence and Algorithms. Obes Surg. 2008; 18:1485-1488.

Multivitamin

Patients should take a daily multivitamin indefinitely. Vitamin supplements should be reviewed to ensure they meet recommended daily values for adults (see Table **7**). Some patients may tolerate a liquid vitamin preparation better as pills are sometimes not tolerated by the stomach pouch. For patients with anemia, additional iron, vitamin B_{12}, and folic acid supplementation may be necessary. Prenatal vitamin formulations may be beneficial for patients who are at risk of iron or folic acid deficiency.

Iron and Cyanocobalamin (Vitamin B_{12})

The duodenum is the primary site for iron absorption, which is bypassed in the RYGB procedure, creating the potential for iron deficiency. Iron is consumed in the ferric form (Fe^{3+}) and reduced to the ferrous state (Fe^{2+}) in the acidic environment of the stomach to be absorbed in the duodenum. In patients who have had gastric bypass surgery, iron salts should be combined with Vitamin C (ascorbic acid) to acidify the stomach environment and facilitate absorption [32]. Patients at risk of iron deficiency, such as menstruating women, should take iron supplementation of 40-65 mg of elemental iron (Ferrous sulfate

325mg contains 65 mg of elemental iron). Those who develop iron deficiency anemia should receive 150-300 mg of elemental iron daily.

Table 7. Supplementation after Roux-en-y Bypass*

Lifelong Maintenance of Vitamin Supplementation	Recommendations
Multivitamins containing minerals	1-2 tablets a day, should minimally contain: ◦ Vitamin B_1 (Thiamine): 1.2 mg ◦ Vitamin K: 120 mcg for men; 90 mcg for women ◦ Biotin: 30 mcg ◦ Zinc 11 mg for men; 8 mg for women ◦ Folic Acid: 400 mcg ◦ Iron: 18 mg
Calcium Citrate	1200-2000 mg daily
Vitamin D	400-800 international units daily (2000 international units daily for long limb RYGB)
Iron	Elemental iron: ◦ 40-65 mg/day for premenopausal women ◦ 18-27 mg/day for others (may be included in the multivitamin) recommend to take with vitamin C to aid the absorption
Vitamin B_{12}	◦ Oral or Sublingual: 1000 mcg daily ◦ Intramuscular: 1000 mcg/week or 3000 mcg every 6 months ◦ Intranasal: 500 mcg/week
Protein	60 grams daily ◦ Protein-rich foods include: lean meat, low-fat milk, dairy products, beans, peas, lentils, and eggs

* Patients with deficiency states will need treatment beyond these recommendations.
Adapted from: Mechanick, JI, Kushner, RF, Sugerman, HJ, et al. American Association of Clinical Endocrinologists, the Obesity Society, and American Society for Metabolic & Bariatric Surgery Medical guidelines for clinical practice for the perioperative nutritional, metabolic, and Nonsurgical support of the bariatric surgery patient. Endocr Pract 2008; 14 Suppl 1:1.

Cyanocobalamin (Vitamin B_{12}) absorption depends on the presence of intrinsic factors produced in the parietal cells of the stomach and hydrochloric acid necessary to break down cyanocobalamin. Patients do not produce intrinsic factors further decreasing the absorption of cyanocobalamin from the terminal ileum. Cyanocobalamin has a higher transcellular uptake while bound to an intrinsic factor. Exclusion of the gastric parietal cells, such as in the case of sleeve gastrectomy or RYGB, affects the absorption of cyanocobalamin, especially in those with a pH-sensitive absorption pattern. After surgery, patients have an achlorhydric environment, which affects absorption of food and protein-bound cyanocobalamin. This can lead to cyanocobalamin deficiency in patients after gastric bypass surgery. Patient should be provided with oral Cyanocobalamin 1000 μg daily or once-monthly injections [33].

Calcium and Vitamin D

After gastric bypass procedures, patients are prone to deficiencies in fat soluble vitamins (A, D, E, and K) and calcium. Long-term deficiencies of calcium and vitamin D can lead to complications such as osteoporosis and metabolic bone disease.

Calcium deficiency is one of the most common problems after bariatric surgery and early bone density monitoring would be prudent. Calcium is absorbed in the body through the duodenum which is bypassed after RYGB surgery. It is important to address calcium intake as soon as possible after surgery. After bariatric surgery there is a dramatic decrease in the production of hydrochloric acid affecting the absorption of calcium carbonate. Calcium citrate is the preferred formulation after bariatric surgery. One study comparing the bioavailability of both products in achlorhydric patients found the bioavailability of calcium carbonate and calcium citrate to be 4% and 45% respectively [34]. Patients should be educated to take their calcium with food but not with iron supplementation because calcium may impair iron absorption. The recommended daily dose for most patients is calcium citrate 500mg three times daily.

There is a high incidence of low vitamin D in obese patients. Patients should receive 400-800 international units of Vitamin D through a multivitamin or additional vitamin D supplementation if necessary. Baseline serum 25-hydroxyvitamin D concentration should be measured before bariatric surgery for a goal of 30 micrograms/milliliter (mcg/mL) or higher and corrected if necessary. If the 25-hydroxyvitmian D serum is low, the parathyroid hormone should also be checked. If patients have a 25-hydroxyvitamin serum level 20-30 nanogram/milliliter (ng/ml) they should be given oral Vitamin D 1000 International Units (IU) daily for 12 weeks. Patients with a serum level of 9-19ng/ml should take oral Vitamin D 50,000 IU once weekly for eight weeks. Patients with a severe deficiency of less than 8ng/ml should be provided with oral Vitamin D 50,000 IU twice weekly for eight weeks. A repeat serum 25-hydroxyvitamin concentration should be checked after 8-12 weeks to evaluate adequacy of replacement. Patients should be maintained with Vitamin D 1000 IU daily. For patients receiving a long-limb Roux-en-Y bypass, at least 2,000 IU of vitamin D should be taken daily. Doses should be adjusted based on 25-hydroxyvitamin D concentrations, which should be monitored no less than annually [35].

Thiamine (B_1)

Thiamine deficiency has been increasingly reported in bariatric surgery patients and presents as progressive joint and muscle pain, peripheral neuropathy, beriberi, acute psychosis, and in some serious cases as Wernicke's encephalopathy. Thiamine deficiency is a chronic disorder that develops over weeks or months of insufficient intake. Patients should take a multivitamin with the daily recommended amount of thiamine. Patients with persistent vomiting or other causes of inadequate nutrient intake should receive an additional 50mg of thiamine daily [24]. Intestinal thiamine absorption is saturable at 25mg, therefore higher oral doses are needed for optimal absorption.

Nutrient Deficiency Management

Patients undergoing bariatric surgery have alterations in the digestive anatomy resulting in inadequate intake of nutrient which creates micronutrient and mineral deficiencies. Patients who undergo adjustable laparoscopic banding do not present with micronutrient deficiencies with the exception of folate and fat soluble vitamins (A, D, E, and K). Macronutrient deficiencies are very rare unless the patient is nonadherent to dietary recommendations, experiences severe surgical complications (i.e anastomotic leaks), or has an eating disorder. Patients who undergo jejuno-ileal bypass, biliopancreatic diversion, or procedures involving the resection of the small bowel have a higher incidence of nutrient deficiencies. Patients who have undergone distal RYGB are also at higher risk of nutrient deficiencies than those compared to proximal RYGB [17].

Nutrient deficiencies include but are not limited to: calcium, fat-soluble vitamins (A, D, E, and K), thiamine, iron, folic acid, copper, and cyanocobalamin (Vitamin B_{12}). A retrospective study with 232 preoperative patients and 149 postoperative patients showed anemia in 17% of patients, low ferritin levels in 15%, low vitamin B_{12} in 11%, and low red blood cell folate in 12% of patients [36]. Close monitoring of pertinent labs should be routinely done at baseline, three months, six months, and annually thereafter in order to prevent such deficiencies (see Table **8**). Patients with a history of malnutrition and dumping associated with malabsorptive surgery are especially at risk of deficiency in Vitamin A, Vitamin C, carnitine, and essential fatty acids [24]. The deficiencies mentioned above can be managed through proper diet and vitamin supplements. Supplementation varies with the degree of deficiency and surgical anatomic changes to the gut. Due to the loss of surface area and possible saturation of the transport mechanisms, there may be a reduction of overall nutrient absorptive capacity. Optimal absorption can be achieved by increasing the frequency, dosage, and duration of the daily recommended vitamin supplementation. At this time, there is limited data for nutrient deficiency management after bariatric surgery.

Calcium and Vitamin D

Calcium and Vitamin D deficiencies may cause secondary hyperparathyroidism and bone softening diseases. Women should be aware of the potential for heightened bone calcium loss. Bypassing the duodenum has caused metabolic bone disease in some patients, resulting in bone pain, loss of height, humped back, and fractures of the ribs and hip bones. The oral bisphosphonates should not be given to patients after surgery as they can increase the risk of gastrointestinal ulceration [37]. Patients who are at risk for osteoporosis due to decreased calcium absorption should be provided with calcium citrate 500mg four times daily in addition to alternative treatment options such as calcitonin salmon nasal spray, zoledronic acid, teriparatide, or raloxifene for women.

Table 8. Summary of Recommended Tests to Assess for Nutritional Deficiency

Recommended Tests	
24 hour urine calcium	Folate
25-hydroxyvitamin D	Glucose
Albumin	Glycosylated hemoglobin A1c
Alkaline phosphatase	Helicobacter Pylori
Aminotransferase	Iron studies (Serum Iron, Total iron binding capacity, ferritin)
Bilirubin	Lipid profile
Body Mass Index (BMI)	Liver profile
Complete blood count	Parathyroid hormone (PTH), intact
Copper	Thiamine
Cyanocobalamin (Vitamin B_{12})	Thyroid Stimulating Hormone (TSH)
DEXA Scan	Uric Acid
Electrolytes	Weight
Fat Soluble Vitamins	

Adapted from: MechanickJI, Kushner RF, Sugerman HJ, Gonzales-Campoy JM, Collazo-Clavell ML, Guven S, Spitz AF, Apovian CM, Livingston EH, Brolin R, Sarwer, DB, Anderson WA, Dixon J. American Association of Clinical Endocrinologist, The Obesity Society, and American Society for Metabolic & Bariatric Surgery Medical Guidelines for Clinical Practice for the Perioperative Nutritional, Metabolic, and Nonsurgical Support of the Bariatric Surgery Patient. Endocr Prac 2008; 14:1-83.

Vitamin D deficiency may be secondary to insufficient dietary intake, decreased sun exposure, and reduced bioavailability of Vitamin D from sequestration in fat [38-40]. Patients with low Vitamin D levels after surgery may benefit from supplementation with Vitamin D aqueous solution 10,000 units daily for six weeks. Patients should have close lab monitoring of pertinent labs to ensure that Vitamin D levels are corrected.

Cyanocobalamin (Vitamin B_{12}) and Folic Acid

The incidence of cyanocobalamin (Vitamin B_{12}) deficiency is reportedly between 26% and 70% in patients post Roux-en-Y gastric bypass. Cyanocobalamin deficiency may lead to several hematological, neurological, and psychiatric complications. Cyanocobalamin deficiency can be associated with irreversible peripheral neuropathy and paresthesias. Patients may suffer from megaloblastic anemia. Pancytopenia, leucopenia, and thrombocytopenia have been reported with advanced disease. Symptoms of irritability, personality changes, mild memory impairment or dementia-like behavior, depression, and psychosis have also been noted. Cyanocobalamin deficiency is best managed in this patient population by subcutaneous injections. Patients may benefit from Cyanocobalamin intramuscular injections at 30 micrograms daily for 5-10 days, and 100-200 micrograms monthly for correcting the deficiency for one-year post surgery [41].

Thiamine (B_1)

Thiamine deficiency has been increasingly identified following bariatric surgery. Patients may experience progressive joint and muscle pain, peripheral neuropathy, beriberi, Wernicke's encephalopathy, and acute psychosis. Development of thiamine deficiency may take weeks to months. For patients with low thiamine levels, supplementation with oral thiamine 200mg twice daily for 30 days and then 100mg daily thereafter may correct the deficiency. Patients with intolerance to oral administration of thiamine secondary to persistent nausea and vomiting may be provided with intravenous thiamine. Thiamine should be given 100mg intravenously every six hours for two days, then 100mg orally twice daily for 30 days until levels normalize. Thiamine can then be continued at 100mg once daily for one-year post surgery [37, 42].

CONCLUSION

Weight loss surgery is a major surgery. Although most patients enjoy an improvement in obesity-related conditions (mobility, self-image, and self-esteem) after the successful results of weight loss surgery, these results should not be the overriding motivation for having the procedure. Recent developments in anti-obesity therapies such as bariatric surgery have revealed improvements or complete remission of multiple chronic diseases. Manipulation of the gastrointestinal tract post bariatric surgery requires medication adjustments and vitamin supplementation for optimal patient care. The decision to have weight loss surgery should only be made after careful consideration and consultation with an experienced bariatric surgeon and a multidisciplinary health care team [24]. With recent advancements and emerging therapies in anti-obesity research, it is imperative that health care providers and patients have a clear understanding that any bariatric procedure carries the risk of nutritional deficiencies. Patients should be closely monitored indefinitely to detect complications and therapy should be administered to prevent irreversible clinical outcomes.

REFERENCES

[1] American Society for Bariatric Surgery. Surgery for morbid obesity: what patients should know? Toronto: FD-Communications Inc. 2000.

[2] Mokdad AH, Ford ES, Bowman BA, *et al.* Prevalence of obesity, diabetes, and obesity related health risk factors, 2001. JAMA 2003; 289: 76-9.

[3] Clinical Guidance on the Identification, Evaluation and Treatment of Overweight and Obesity in Adults: The Evidence Report. National Institutes of Health. Obes Res 1988; 6: 51S-209S.

[4] Deitel M. Overweight and obesity worldwide now estimated to involve 1.7 billion people. Obes Surg 2003; 13(3): 329-30.

[5] National Institutes of Health (NIH). Gastrointestinal surgery for severe obesity. National Institute of Health Consensus Development Program. March 25-27, 1991. [Accessed 01 September 2009].

[6] North American Association for the Study of Obesity and the National Heart, Lung, and Blood Institute. The practical guide: identification, evaluation, and treatment of overweight and obesity in adults. Bethesda, MD: National Institutes of Health; 2000. NIH publication 00-4084.

[7] North American Association for the Study of Obesity (NAASO) and the National Heart. Clinical guidelines on the identification, evaluation, and treatment of overweight and obesity in adults: The Evidence Report. Bethesda, MD: National Institutes of Health; 1998. NIH publication 98-4083.

[8] Sjöström L, Narbro K, Sjöström CD, *et al.* Effects of bariatric surgery on mortality in Swedish obese subjects. N Engl J Med 2007; 357: 741-52.

[9] Must A, Spadano J, Coakley EH, Field AE, Colditz G, Dietz WH. The disease burden associated with overweight and obesity. JAMA 1999; 282: 1523-9.

[10] Pories WJ, Swanson MS, MacDonald KG, *et al.* Who would have thought it? An operation proves to be the most effective therapy for adult onset diabetes mellitus. Ann Surg 1995; 222: 339-53.

[11] MechanickJI, Kushner RF, Sugerman HJ, *et al.* American association of clinical endocrinologist, the obesity society, and american society for metabolic & bariatric surgery medical guidelines for clinical practice for the perioperative nutritional, metabolic, and nonsurgical support of the bariatric surgery patient. Endocr Pract 2008; 14: 1-83.

[12] American Society for Metabolic and Bariatric Surgery, 2009. www.asbs.org Accessed September 9, 2009.

[13] Ren C, Horgan S, Ponce J. US Experience with the Lap-Band System. Am J Surg 2002; 184: 46S-50S.

[14] Brolin RE, Kenler HA, Gorman JH. Long limb gastric bypass: a five-year prospective randomized study. Ann Surg 1992; 215: 123-43.

[15] Rubino F, Gagner M. Potential of surgery curing type 2 diabetes mellitus. Ann Surg 2002; 236: 554-59.

[16] Lutfi R, Torquati A, Sekhar N, Richards WO. Predictors of success after laparoscopic gastric bypass: a multivariate analysis of socioeconomic factors. Surg Endosc 2006; 20: 864-7.

[17] Poitou BC, Ciangura C, Coupaye M, Czernichow S, Bouillot JL, Basdevant A. nutritional deficiency after gastric bypass: diagnosis prevention and treatment. Diabetes Metab 2007; 33: 13-24.

[18] Thompson GB, Service FJ, Andrews JC, Collazo-Clavell ML, Lloyd RV. Hyperinsulinemic hypoglycemia with nesidioblastosis after gastric-bypass surgery. N Engl J Med 2005; 353: 249-54.

[19] Dunn JP, Jagasia SM. Management of Type 2 diabetes after bariatric surgery. Clin Diab 2007; 25: 112-4.

[20] Hinojosa MW, Varela JE, Smith BR, Che F, Nguyen NT. Resolution of systemic hypertension after laparoscopic gastric bypass. J Gastrointest Surg 2009; 13: 793-7.

[21] Miller AD, Smith KM. Medication and nutrient administration considerations after bariatric surgery. Am J Health-Syst Pharm 2006; 63: 1852-7.

[22] ACOG Committee opinion number 315: Obesity in pregnancy. Obstet Gynecol 2005; 106: 671-5.

[23] Ojo P, Asiyanbola B, Valin E, Reinhold R. Post discharge prophylactic anticoagulation in gastric bypass patient – how safe? Obes Surg 2008; 18: 197-796.

[24] Chan LN, Downing J. Management of patients receiving bariatric surgery. Pharmacotherpay self-assessment program, 6th ed. pp. 63-75.

[25] Benet LZ, Kroetz DL, Sheiner LB. Pharmacokinetics: The dynamics of drug absorption, distribution, and elimination. In: Hardman JG, Limbird LE, Eds. Goodman and Gilman's the pharmacological basis of therapeutics. 10th ed. New York: McGraw-Hill 2001; pp. 3-29.

[26] Gubbins PO, Bertch KE. Drug absorption in gastrointestinal disease and surgery. Clin Pharmacokinet 1991; 21: 431-47.

[27] (a) Fosamax (alendronate sodium) package insert. Whitehouse Station, NJ: Merck & Co. Inc.; Jul 2005. (b) Rowland M, Tozer TN. Absorption. In: Clinical pharmacokinetics: concepts and applications. 3rd ed. Philadelphia: Lippincott: Williams, and Wilkins 1995; pp. 119-36.

[28] Mourelo R, Kaidar-Person O, Fajnwaks P, *et al.* Hemorrhagic and thromboembolic complications after bariatric surgery in patients receiving chronic anticoagulation therapy. Obes Surg 2008; 18: 167-70.

[29] Coumadin (warfarin sodium) package insert. Bristol-Myers Squibb Company.

[30] Bloomberg RD, Fleishman A, Nalle JE, Herron DM, Kini S. Nutritional deficiencies following bariatric surgery: what have we learned? Obes Surg 2005; 15: 145-54.

[31] Rhode BM, Shustik C, Christou NV, MacLead LD. Iron absorption and therapy after gastric bypass. Obes Surg 1999; 9: 17-21.

[32] Behrns KE, Smith CD, Sarr MG. Prospective evaluation of gastric acid secretion and cobalamin absorption following gastric bypass for clinically severe obesity. Dig Dis Sci 1994; 39: 315-20.

[33] Recker RR. Calcium absorption and achlorhydria. N Eng J Med 1985; 313: 70-3.

[34] Compher CW, Badellino KO, Boullata JL. Vitamin D and the bariatric surgical patient: a review. Obes Surg 2008; 18: 220-4.

[35] Toh SY, Zarshenas N, Jorgensen J. Prevalence of nutrient deficiencies in bariatric patients. Nutrition 2009; 25(11-12): 1150-6.

[36] Schweitzer DH, Posthuma EF. Prevention of vitamin and mineral deficiencies after bariatric surgery: evidence and algorithms. Obes Surg 2008; 18: 1485-8.

[37] Hamoui N, Anthone G, Crookes PF. Calcium metabolism in the morbidly obese. Obes Surg 2004; 14: 9-12.

[38] Sánchez-Hernández J, Ybarra J, Gich I, *et al.* Effects of bariatric surgery on vitamin d status and secondary hyperparathyroidism: a prospective study. Obes Surg 2005; 15: 1389-95.

[39] Hamoui N, Kim K, Anthone G, Crookes PF. The significance of elevated levels of parathyroid hormone in patients with morbid obesity before and after bariatric surgery. Arch Surg 2003; 138: 891-7.

[40] Oh R, Brown DL. Vitamin B_{12} deficiency. Am Fam Phys 2003; 67: 979-86.

[41] Carrodeguas L, Kaidar-Person O, Szomstein S, Antozzi P, Rosenthal R. Preoperative Thiamine deficiency in obese population undergoing laparoscopic bariatric surgery. Surg Obes Rel Dis 2005; 8: 517-22.

[42] Wittgrove AC, Clark GW. Laparoscopic gastric bypass roux-en-y 500 patients: technique and results with 3-60 month follow-up. Obes Surg 2000; 10: 233-9.

Author Index

Made in the USA
Las Vegas, NV
10 November 2026

57858718R00176